ANNUAL PROGRESS
IN CHILD PSYCHIATRY AND
CHILD DEVELOPMENT
1973

ANNUAL PROGRESS IN CHILD PSYCHIATRY AND CHILD DEVELOPMENT 1973

Edited by

STELLA CHESS, M.D.

Professor of Child Psychiatry
New York University Medical Center

and

ALEXANDER THOMAS, M.D.

Professor of Psychiatry
New York University Medical Center
Director, Psychiatric Division, Bellevue Hospital

BRUNNER/MAZEL *Publishers* • New York

published by
BRUNNER/MAZEL, INC.
64 University Place
New York, N. Y. 10003

Library of Congress Catalog Card No. 68-23452
SBN 87630-062-x

MANUFACTURED IN THE UNITED STATES OF AMERICA

PREFACE

This is the sixth volume in our annual series devoted to outstanding articles on child psychiatry and child development. The continued favorable response to these annual volumes affirms our own judgment that their publication is useful to a wide range of professional workers.

We have continued the brief introductions to each section, started in last year's volume. We have attempted in these introductions to highlight the most notable trends represented by the articles selected.

As in previous volumes, all the articles are presented in their entirety as first published in English-speaking professional journals, in this case during 1972. The articles selected either report original work, offer systematic reviews in an important area, or discuss significant professional and social issues affecting the approach to work with children.

We are grateful to the authors and the journal publishers for their cooperation.

The preparation of this volume was a painful task for us because of the untimely tragic deaths early in the year and within a day of each other of our dear friends and colleagues, Dr. Herbert Birch and Dr. Samuel Sillen. Dr. Birch was an outstanding figure in the international research community who was at the height of his enormously productive and creative career at the time of his sudden death. His passing is indeed a great loss, not only to our own friends, but to society at large because of his central concern to link his research and that of others with broad social questions. Those of us who worked with him and knew him personally can never forget the stimulation, imaginativeness and profound intelligence he brought to any discussion. The task of selecting one of Dr. Birch's final articles for inclusion in this volume was a painful reminder of what we will miss in future years.

Dr. Sillen was our close editorial associate and co-author for many years on a number of projects. We could not have begun this annual series without his work in organizing the search of the literature and establishing with us criteria for the selection of appropriate articles. His own previous professional background in the field of literature proved uniquely useful when combined with his extraordinary ability to master the central questions in psychology and psychiatry. Looking at these issues analytically from the outside, so to speak, he was always able not only to broaden and deepen our formulations but frequently to add significant insights of his own. For the two of us he is irreplaceable, both as a friend and as a collaborator.

STELLA CHESS, M.D.
ALEXANDER THOMAS, M.D.

CONTENTS

Part I

INFANCY STUDIES

This year has seen the publication of an unusually large number of fruitful studies on infancy (as well as on developmental questions, which are considered in the next section). The infancy studies are focused on several broad issues. Three articles take up the nature of infants' responses to stimulation. Yarrow and his colleagues add a further dimension to the identification and differentiation of essential elements in effective stimulation of early infant development. Human and inanimate stimulation are separated, and their relative independence of each other is emphasized. Brackbill demonstrates anew that infants can distinguish temporal patterns as early as the second month of life. Korner and Thoman explore certain infant responses which are usually attributed to contact and identify them as actually due to proprioceptive stimulation.

Two separate reports challenge conventional formulations regarding infant intelligence. Lewis and McGurk's data challenge the concept that scores on infant intelligence tests can properly be generalized to issues beyond the specific ability being measured by a particular test item. The authors are highly critical, therefore, of the attempts to use global infant intelligence scales to assess the effect of specific intervention procedures. McCall and his coauthors emphasize the need to consider intelligence developmentally and not as a fixed, unchangeable quality.

Werner's paper reviews 50 contemporary cross-cultural studies of infant psychomotor development in five continents. Her data pose a number of questions, including one relating to the significance for later development of early acceleration.

1

1

DIMENSIONS OF EARLY STIMULATION AND THEIR DIFFERENTIAL EFFECTS ON INFANT DEVELOPMENT

Leon J. Yarrow, Judith L. Rubenstein,

Frank A. Pedersen, and Joseph J. Jankowski

National Institute of Child Health and Human Development
Social and Behavioral Sciences Branch

To some extent experimental studies have confirmed the general premise that marked trauma and extreme deprivation can have significant effects. The impact of less extreme variations in experiences, experiences within the "normal" range, is much less clear. This is due in part to a lack of differentiation of environments, and to our difficulties in describing and measuring with any degree of precision the dimensions of natural environments. In this study we have looked at a range of variation in experiences of five- to six-month-old infants on a concrete behavioral level, and have conceptualized these discrete behaviors.

Our major objectives in this study were (a) to differentiate the natural environment in conceptually meaningful terms through detailed analysis of caretaker's behavior and properties of the proximal inanimate stimuli

Reprinted from MERRILL-PALMER QUARTERLY OF BEHAVIOR AND DEVELOPMENT, Volume 18, No. 3, 1972, pp. 205-218.

This paper is a condensation of four papers presented at a symposium at the biennial meeting of the Society for Research in Child Development, April 4, 1971, Minneapolis, Minnesota. We are indebted to Mrs. Myrna Fivel and Miss Joan Durfee for their assistance in the development of the observation scale and their dedicated work in the collection of data; and to Mr. Richard Cain for his arduous labor on the data analyses.

in the infant's environment; (b) to determine whether inanimate stimulation on the one hand, and social stimulation on the other, are related to different facets of the infant's development; and (c) to determine the extent to which separate dimensions or components of these variables (e.g., variety, complexity, and responsiveness of inanimate stimuli; level and variety of social stimulation; and the expression of positive affect) have different orders of relationships to the development of early infant functions.

This study represents a convergence of applied and theoretical interests. We are especially interested in assessing the impact on development of so-called "disadvantaged" environments in early infancy. Limited observational data are available on mother-infant interaction in disadvantaged groups. Moreover, we thought environmental effects might be highlighted in these settings. Our sample, however, represents a wide continuum on environmental variables. Therefore, the implications of this research go beyond disadvantaged or depriving environments; the findings have relevance for understanding a broad range of environmental influences on development.

METHOD

The sample consisted of 41 black infants, 21 boys and 20 girls, who had been cared for by a stable "primary caretaker." The mother was the primary caretaker in 30 cases, a relative (usually the maternal grandmother) in 6 cases, and an unrelated babysitter in 5 cases. Of this group, 34 were recruited through two public well-baby clinics. Their fathers had completed 6 to 12 years of schools, with a mean of 10.9 years. They were engaged in primarily semi-skilled and unskilled occupations. To extend the range of environmental variables, 7 black infants were obtained through a private group medical program. These families were all intact, and the fathers' education ranged from one year of college through graduate school; the mean education level was 14.6 years. All infants were of normal birth weight, were free from gross complications in pregnancy or delivery, and were screened by a pediatrician to eliminate cases in which there were any indications of neurological damage.

The basic data were obtained through time-sampling observations in the home when the infants were five months of age.* The mother or baby's caretaker was encouraged to go about her usual activities. Two home observations about a week apart were conducted; each involved three hours of time-sampling while the baby was awake. The time-

---

* The manual describing the observation categories is available from the authors.

sampling cycle consisted of a 30 second observation period and a 60 second recording period repeated through 120 cycles each day. There are a total of 240 time-sample units, or six hours, for each child and caretaker.

Approximately 60 categories of events were monitored in each interval. Selected infant behaviors observed included positive vocalizations, fussing or irritable vocalizations, and whether the infant was engaging in focused manipulation of play objects or directing his visual attention to the mother. Approximately 45 categories of caretaker behavior were recorded describing aspects of social stimulation. There were in addition several time-sample measures of the proximal inanimate environment. The categories of social stimulation can be classified in the following areas: (a) *Sensory modality* of social stimulation (e.g., visual, auditory, tactile, and kinesthetic stimulation, as exemplified by looking at, talking to, and holding the baby; (b) The *intensity* or rate of stimulus change (for example, passive holding is distinguished from active touching or moving the baby); (c) Whether stimulation is *contingent* on certain infant behaviors (for example, social soothing in response to distress states, contingent vocal response to the infant's positive vocalizations); and (d) The *type* or class of behavior the caretaker is attempting to evoke (for example, the attainment of motor skills such as postural control or locomotion, or fostering interest in play materials by highlighting the properties of toys or positioning them for the baby). In addition, ratings were made of the caretaker's expression of positive affect toward the infant, and contingency of response to distress.

To measure perceptual-sensory stimulation from the proximal inanimate environment, the observers recorded all play materials and household objects within reach of the infant during each time-sampling interval. At a later time similar objects were obtained and rated in terms of their complexity and responsiveness.

Three young women served as observers; one with a doctorate in developmental psychology; one with an M.A. degree; and one with a B.A. degree. Observer reliability was established on 20 cases before data collection was initiated. The correlations ranged from .96 to .99 on the time-sampling variables, and from .72 to .91 on the ratings.

Environmental Variables

Our basic strategy in choosing variables for differential analysis of the natural environment was to order the infant's experiences in terms of a conceptual framework. The selection of the parameters of the environment was guided by concepts from several theoretical orientations, such as, information theory, adaptation level theory, operant learning theory, and Piagetian developmental theory.

The inanimate environment was analyzed in terms of three major dimensions: variety, responsiveness, and complexity. Although the deprivation literature has particularly emphasized quantity of sensory or social stimulation, theoretical thinking and some experimental studies in recent years have pointed to the crudeness of sheer amount of stimulation. Several theoretical positions, especially information theory, have emphasized the importance of variety. Variety in this study was measured in terms of the number of different objects within reach of the infant during the six hours of observation. The interobserver reliability was .99.

Our second dimension, responsiveness, an index of the feedback potential inherent in objects, derives from several theoretical sources. In a loose sense it is related to the contingency concept in operant learning theory; it is also related to Hunt's (1965) thinking about intrinsic motivation. The basic hypothesis is that an object that changes in response to some action on the part of the infant may affect the infant's rudimentary sense of mastery, the conviction that he can have an effective impact on the environment. This variable was measured in terms of the extent to which objects change in visual, auditory, and tactile properties as a result of the infant's behavior. There are four subscales: moving parts, change in shape and contour, reflected image, and noise production. The subscale scores for each toy were added; a subject's score was the average for all his toys. Interrater reliability on this measure was .90.

The third dimension of the inanimate environment, complexity, derives its meaning from information theory, particularly Berlyne's (1960) theoretical formulations. Theories regarding complexity emphasize a golden mean, that is, an optimal degree of complexity based on the organism's capacity to assimilate the information provided. Complexity represents the extent to which objects provide information through various modalities. Criteria of complexity include number of colors, number of different shapes and variation in contour, the amount of visual and tactile pattern, and the degree of responsiveness of the object. A subject's score is the average for his toys (interrater reliability .83).

Theories regarding the influence of social stimulation are more diverse, more wide-ranging, and less explicit than theories about the inanimate environment. In this study, the social environment was observed at the level of discrete behaviors of the mother, for example, talking to the infant, smiling, touching him, moving him, etc. These behaviors formed the basis for higher order categories similar to some of the dimensions of the inanimate environment, such as, level of social stimulation and variety of social stimulation. Other dimensions like contingency of maternal response and expression of positive affect were more distinctive to the human environment.

Level of social stimulation was a composite of the amount and intensity of stimulation by the caretaker. We obtained through time-sampling the frequency with which the mother was within view or within reach of the infant; and the frequency with which she talked to the infant, touched or held him, or engaged him in vigorous play. These discrete behaviors were weighted on a five-point scale so that vigorous play involving intense stimulation and several modalities received a higher score than stimulation of low intensity in one modality, such as touching the baby (composite reliability .99).

Variety of social stimulation is an unweighted sum of different types of social stimulation. Examples of these are play, encouraging motor responses, presentation of play objects, the range of affect which the caretaker exhibited, and the number of different physical settings in which social stimulation occurred (composite reliability .95).

Two indices of contingency were used: (a) frequency of contingent responses to positive vocalizations by the infant obtained through time-sampling (interobserver reliability .96); and (b) contingency of response to distress, a five-point rating scale based on latency of response to the infant's distress signals (interrater reliability .91). These variables are derived from operant learning theory (Gewirtz, 1969), and other formulations (Ainsworth, 1967; Lewis & Goldberg, 1968) emphasizing the importance of early intervention in distress states.

The variable, expression of positive affect, was based on ratings by the observers following the time-sampling observations. It is a measure of the characteristic level of demonstrativeness of the mother or caretaker (interrater reliability .72).

THE INFANT VARIABLES

The dependent variables were derived from two procedures, a research from the Bayley Scales of Infant Development (administered in the fifth month) and a structured situational test measuring exploratory behavior and preference for novel stimuli (administered in the sixth month). In addition to the Mental Developmental Index and Psychomotor Developmental Index which the Bayley yields, eight more differentiated clusters were developed. Items were grouped on the basis of their apparent conceptual coherence. Split-half and part-whole analyses provided a statistical basis for further refinement. The final split-half reliabilities ranged from .74 to .92. The clusters include: *Social Responsiveness, Language, Fine Motor, Gross Motor,* and four measures that we considered indices of cognitive-motivational functions—*Goal Orientation, Reaching and Grasping, Secondary Circular Reaction,* and *Object Permanence.* Another cluster, *Problem Solving*—a measure of rudimentary means-ends relationships—was developed from four supplementary items administered after the Bayley Test.

The procedure to measure exploratory behavior and preference for novel stimuli, functions that we also labelled cognitive-motivational, has been described in detail by Rubenstein (1967). Essentially it involves presenting the baby with an attractive, novel toy—a bell—for ten minutes. The amount of exploratory interest shown by looking and manipulating was recorded; then a series of ten new toys were presented one at a time for one-minute intervals paired with the bell, which had become more familiar. Preference for novel stimuli was expressed by measures of differential looking or manipulation, that is, the difference between time directed to the novel toy vs. the more familiar bell.

RESULTS

Differentiation of the Environment

Table 1 indicates the interrelationships among the social and inanimate variables. Among the social variables, level, variety, and positive affect are all rather strongly interrelated. In fact, level has considerable generality with all other social stimulation variables. In regard to the two contingency measures, there is a relatively low relationship between the frequency measure, contingent response to positive vocalization, and the latency measure, contingent response to distress ($r = .31$). This suggests that maternal responsiveness is itself not a highly general trait.

Within the dimensions of inanimate stimulation, variety of play objects is independent of responsiveness and complexity. On the other hand, the correlation between responsiveness and complexity is .70, in part because responsiveness is one of the components of the complexity scale.

Perhaps the most important generalization to be made from Table 1 is that the dimensions of the social environment are largely independent of dimensions of the inanimate environment. This differentiation sug-

TABLE 1

Interrelationships Among the Social and Inanimate Variables

	Social				Inanimate		
	Variety	Posi-tive Affect	Cont. R. to Pos. Voc.	Cont. R. to Distress	Respon-siveness	Com-plexity	Variety
Social							
Level	.76	.62	.64	.53	—	—	—
Variety		.64	.45	.48	.33	—	.29
Positive Affect			.51	.23	.23	—	.20
Contingent Response to Positive Vocalization				.31	—	—	—
Contingent Response to Distress					—	—	.31
Inanimate							
Responsiveness						.70	—
Complexity							—
Variety							

For $p = .05$, one-tailed test, $r = .26$.
— indicates r less than .20

gests that global characterizations of environments as "depriving" or "stimulating" are oversimplified.

Relations Between the Social Environment and Infant Functioning

Both Level and Variety of social stimulation are thought of as having an arousal function, serving to activate the infant and increase his responsiveness to the environment. The general pattern of relationships seen in Table 2 is quite similar for these two variables, although a greater number of significant correlations are found with variety.

The variables were defined quite differently. Level is defined in terms of characteristics of the stimuli themselves, amount weighted by different degrees of intensity. Variety was defined in terms of the types of behavior elicited by the caretaker and the different physical settings where interaction occurred. It is the frequency of interactive play, motor training, presentation and highlighting of play objects, and the number of changes in the location of interaction with the baby, such as an infant seat, the

TABLE 2

Correlations Between Social Stimulation Variables and Infant Functioning

Infant Functioning	Social Stimulation Variables				
	Level	Variety	Positive Affect	Cont. R. Pos. Voc.	Cont. R. Distress
General Status					
Mental Dev. Index	.32*	.34*	.23	—	.32*
Psychomotor Dev. Index	—	.23	—	—	.37*
Social Responsiveness	.35*	.34*	.26*	.22	—
Language					
Vocal. to Bell	—	.31*	.24	.30*	—
Language Quality	—	—	—	—	—
Motor Development					
Gross	—	—	—	—	.28*
Fine	—	.26*	—	—	.33*
Goal-Directed Behaviors					
Goal Orientation	.45**	.48**	.30*	—	.38**
Reaching & Grasping	.25	.28	—	—	.29*
Secondary Circular Reaction	.32*	.35*	.30*	—	.30*
Cognitive Functions					
Problem Solving	.21	.20	—	—	—
Object Permanence	.31*	.47**	—	—	—
Exploratory Behavior					
Looking at Bell	—	—	—	−.37	—
Manipulating Bell	—	.32*	—	—	.21
Looking at Novel	—	—	—	—	—
Manipulating Novel	—	—	.28*	.31*	.24

* $p < .05$; one-tailed test.
** $p < .01$; one-tailed test.
— indicates r less than .20.

caretaker's lap, or the floor. The essence of variety is the encouragement of more differentiated responses on the part of the infant, whereas level is defined in terms of the stimulus characteristics.

As with level and variety, contingent response to distress is also significantly related to the Mental Development Index and to the measures of goal-directed behavior. These results seem to support the Ainsworth

(1967) or the Lewis and Goldberg (1968) interpretation of what happens when one responds to the infant's cry; relatively early intervention in distress states may have a general facilitating effect, either by freeing the infant to respond to external stimuli or by making him aware of a contingent relationship with the caretaker.

There are two language measures. Vocalize to Bell is a measure of *amount* of vocalization obtained during the test of exploratory behavior, the ten minute period when the infant had the interesting toy. Its significant relationship with the mother's contingent response to infant vocalization has special conceptual interest. This relationship found in the natural environment adds to the generalizability to life settings of the operant laboratory studies of the social reinforcement of vocalization rates (Rheingold, Gewirtz, & Ross, 1959; Weisberg, 1963; Todd & Palmer, 1968). Another measure, the mother's spontaneous vocalizations (that is, total vocalization minus contingent vocalization), was not related to the infant's vocal output. This finding, as well as the lack of relationship to the other measure of contingency, underscores the specificity of this effect and buttresses the operant learning interpretation.

The second language measure is a cluster of eight Bayley items dealing with the qualitative aspects of language. The measure was not related to any environmental variables. Although language quality at five to six months may be more important conceptually than amount of vocalization, it is probably too unstable developmentally or too complex to measure adequately with a few test items.

More evidence of differential effects is seen in relation to social responsiveness. This cluster of eight Bayley items includes vocalizing to a social stimulus, anticipatory adjustment to lifting, enjoying frolic play, and approaching and smiling to a mirror image. Instigating stimuli, that is, level, variety, and expression of positive affect, are all significantly correlated with social responsiveness; whereas the soothing stimuli, contingent response to distress, are unrelated to social responsiveness.

The strongest grouping of significant relationships is in the cognitive-motivational set called goal-directed behaviors. *Goal orientation* is a cluster of six Bayley items, primarily motivational in nature, including such behaviors as persistent and purposeful attempts to secure objects just out of reach. This measure has very high generality with many other dependent variables; it correlates .86 with the total Bayley Mental Developmental Index, higher than any other cluster. The results suggest that motivational differences in infants are particularly sensitive to the social environment.

The cluster *Reaching and Grasping* consists of nine Bayley items and emphasizes especially visual-motor coordination and fine motor skills in transactions with play objects. It probably has more of a skill emphasis than other variables in this group, and that may account for the weaker relationships.

Secondary Circular Reaction, as defined by Piaget, is the repetition of behavior which produces interesting results. It reflects an intentionality to maintain interesting activities, and it is thought of as a precursor of instrumental behavior requiring an appreciation of means-ends relationships. The cluster consisted of only two items, banging in play and enjoying sound production. Despite the sharp restriction in range of the dependent variable, there are four correlations significant at the .05 level. A supplementary test item with high face validity was also devised for measuring secondary circular reactions; the results were essentially the same as for the Bayley cluster.

Relations Between the Inanimate Environment and Infant Functioning

Table 3 presents the results. A striking specificity of effect is seen for properties of the inanimate environment. Variety, responsiveness, and complexity show no significant relationships with language or social responsiveness. In contrast, there are many significant relationships with the cognitive-motivational and the fine motor variables, all measures which involve responses to inanimate objects.

Responsiveness, which is defined in terms of the feedback potential of objects, is most highly related to the variable that specifically tests the infant's repeated efforts to evoke feedback from objects, namely secondary circular reactions. Responsiveness is also related to goal orientation and reaching and grasping; to fine motor development; and to a measure of exploratory behavior, preference for looking at novel stimuli. Our findings suggest that the responsiveness of objects in the infant's natural environment may facilitate both motivational and skill components of development.

Consistent with expectations, complexity is related to infant measures that reflect receptivity to stimulation: preference for novel stimuli; reaching and grasping objects; and repeating actions which produce changes in stimulation, that is, secondary circular reactions. Contrary to expectation, complexity is not significantly related to the Bayley Mental Developmental Index, goal orientation, or problem solving ability.

Of the three dimensions of the inanimate environment, variety of inanimate objects is the strongest antecedent, in terms of both the

TABLE 3

Relations Between Dimensions of Inanimate Stimulation and Infant Functioning

Infant Functioning	Inanimate Stimulation		
	Responsiveness	Complexity	Variety
General Status			
Mental Developmental Index	.27*	—	.36*
Psychomotor Developmental Index	.28*	—	.51**
Social Responsiveness	.21	—	—
Language			
Voc. to Bell	—	—	—
Language Quality	—	—	—
Motor Development			
Gross	.27*	.22	.42**
Fine	.33*	—	.37*
Goal-Directed Behaviors			
Goal Orientation	.30*	—	.41**
Reaching and Grasping	.46**	.32*	.38*
Secondary Circular Reaction	.51**	.46**	.33*
Cognitive Functions			
Problem Solving	—	—	.50**
Object Permanence	—	—	.30*
Exploratory Behavior			
Looking at Bell	—	—	—
Manipulating Bell	.21	—	.40**
Looking at Novel	.28*	.30*	.35*
Manipulating Novel	—	.35*	.48**

* $p < .05$.
** $p < .01$.
— indicates r less than .20.

number of significant relationships with developmental outcomes and the magnitude of these correlations. Variety is related to nearly all the infant measures dealing with inanimate objects, and it correlates more highly than does complexity or responsiveness with most of them.

Variety is the one parameter of inanimate objects that is significantly related to object permanence and problem solving. Both these measures involve the infant's reaction to inanimate objects that are not immediately available or easily accessible. At this developmental level object permanence measures primarily the baby's tendency to look for an object that is out of reach and going out of view; problem solving measures his efforts and ability to use one object as a means to another that is in view but out of reach. The results suggest that it is the variety of objects with which the baby comes in contact, rather than complexity or feedback potential, that relates to the ability to secure and follow visually objects not immediately accessible.

Variety of inanimate objects also shows strong relationships with exploratory behavior. The high relationship between variety and manipulating novel objects ($r = .48$) is consistent with several theoretical views. Piaget emphasizes that assimilating and accommodating to varying properties of objects is instrumental in differentiating basic schemata. Variety may also affect the arousal level of the infant, keeping him alert and ready to "tune in" to the environment (Schaffer & Emerson, 1968); and it may lead to an adaptation level (Helson, 1964) for more novel input, strengthening the infant's motivation to maintain high degrees of variation in stimulation.

Sex Differences

Although results have been reported for the group as a whole, the data have also been analyzed separately for males and females. Generally, the direction of the relationships tends to be similar for boys and girls. However, the magnitude of relationships between environmental and infant variables is higher for females. Among the girls there are 23 correlations that are .50 or higher. In contrast, no correlation as high as .50 is found for the boys.

DISCUSSION

Several issues important for developmental theory and research are highlighted by these findings. We have shown that the natural environment of the young infant can be differentiated into many discrete behaviors of the caretaker, and the properties of objects available to the infant can be subjected to very detailed analyses.

We have shown that events in the natural environment can be coordinated with theoretical concepts. We have isolated specific variables in the natural environment and we have explored their relationships to specific aspects of infant development, for example, the relationship between responsiveness of objects in the home and the emergence of secondary circular reactions; the relationship between the mother's contingent responsiveness to the infant's vocalizations and rate of vocalization in the exploratory behavior situation. These findings suggest that some relationships found in the laboratory can be generalized to life settings.

Another issue highlighted by the findings of this study concerns the level at which one characterizes environments. The findings underscore the inadequacy of global characterizations of environments, and emphasize the value of differentiating the dimensions and characteristics of stimulation. The relatively low relationships between variables of the inanimate environment and variables of the social environment suggest that, for this particular sample at least, it may not be very meaningful to label environments grossly as depriving.

A third issue, a very complex and controversial one, concerns the relative importance of human and inanimate stimulation. There has been a tendency in recent years in theory and in experimental research to focus on cognitive stimulation variables, and to deemphasize the affective components of the mother-infant relationship. Our findings of a relative independence of the inanimate and the social environments, in conjunction with the specific relationships between social stimulation and social responsiveness and language, on the one hand, and between properties of inanimate stimulation and exploratory behavior, on the other hand, emphasize the importance of both the human and the inanimate environment.

A fourth issue has to do with the simple correlational model we have used. We recognize that looking at relationships between single variables is a very simple model that ignores the realities of environment-child interaction. Although there are many significant correlations between environmental variables and infant characteristics, the magnitude of many of the correlations is not very high. These associations exceed chance expectations and, in general, are consistent with theoretical assumptions, but they do not permit predictions with any high degree of accuracy. It is likely that these environmental variables interact in many complex ways. We cannot conclude that any single variable alone is decisive for any particular infant function. It is meaningful, however, to ask to what extent a given environmental variable makes a special contribution to some aspect of infant functioning.

We also need to ask more complex questions, such as, whether certain environmental variables may be interchangeable; whether certain combinations of variables are additive in their effects; and to what extent certain variables interact to strengthen or diminish each other's impact. We must also recognize that the relationship between environmental variables and infant behavior is not a simple unidirectional one. There is a reciprocal interaction between infant characteristics and environmental events. It is likely that an active and responsive infant elicits more social response from others as well as greater inanimate stimulation than a lethargic withdrawn infant.

We have been particularly interested in the group of infant behaviors that we have called cognitive-motivational functions. One striking finding of this study is the extent to which these functions seem to be amenable to environmental influences in early infancy. These results support Provence and Lipton's (1961) impressions that motivational functions may be more vulnerable to depriving institutional environments than are specific emerging skills.

Motivation, as we have used it, is not an abstract intervening variable. It refers to clearly specified behaviors, such as reaching persistently for objects, attempting to have an effect on and elicit responses from objects, showing preferential attention to and manipulation of novel objects. These behaviors might be considered expressions of the infant's motivation to assimilate, to learn about, and to master the environment. They may be viewed as an early expression of a competence or an effectance motive (White, 1959). The importance of these relationships lies in their convergence with a number of theoretical formulations based primarily on laboratory studies. Lewis and Goldberg (1969) have formulated a "generalized expectancy model," emphasizing the role of contingent mother-infant interaction in the development of the child's belief that he can affect his environment, that he can bring about reinforcement by his actions. Watson (1966) speaks of "contingency awareness" as a precondition for later learning. The common thread in these formulations is the active, information processing organism, initiating transactions with the environment and in turn being influenced by these transactions.

One last point in regard to the significance of motivational functions. It is likely that the infant's orientation to objects and to people very early becomes part of a feedback system with the environment. His smiling, vocalizing, and reaching out to people; his visually attending to and manipulating objects tend to be self-reinforcing and thus, to some extent, self-perpetuating. These behaviors become part of a system of reciprocal interactions which may characterize a given infant's transactions with the environment over a long period of time. This orientation to the world may be a more consistent and more significant characteristic of the young infant than any specific cognitive ability. We might speculate that the infant's orientation to his environment adds to the continuity of his experiences. If this is so, then the fact that these aspects of functioning seem to be related to identifiable aspects of the environment during the first six months may have great significance not only for developmental theory, but for intervention programs as well.

REFERENCES

AINSWORTH, M.: *Infancy in Uganda: Infant Care and the Growth of Love.* Baltimore: Johns Hopkins, 1967.

BERLYNE, D.: *Conflict, Arousal and Curiosity.* New York: McGraw-Hill, 1960.

GEWIRTZ, J.: Mechanisms of social learning: Some roles of stimulation and behavior in early human development. In D. Goslin (Ed.): *Handbook of Socialization Theory and Research.* Chicago: Rand McNally, 1969.

HELSON, H.: *Adaptation Level Theory.* New York: Harper & Row, 1964.

HUNT, J. McV.: Intrinsic motivation and its role in psychological development. In D. Levine (Ed.): *Nebraska Symposium on Motivation.* Lincoln: University of Nebraska Press, 1965. Pp. 189-282.

LEWIS, M. & GOLDBERG, S.: Perceptual-cognitive development in infancy: A generalized expectancy model as a function of the mother-infant relationship. *Merrill-Palmer Quarterly,* 1969, Vol. 15, 81-100.

PROVENCE, S. & LIPTON, R.: *Infants in Institutions.* New York: International University Press, 1961.

RHEINGOLD, H., GEWIRTZ, J., & ROSS, H.: Social conditioning of vocalizations in the infant. *Journal of Comparative and Physiological Psychology,* 1959. Vol. 52, 68-73.

RUBENSTEIN, J.: Maternal attentiveness and subsequent exploratory behavior. *Child Development,* 1967, Vol. 38, 1089-1100.

SCHAFFER, H. & EMERSON, P.: The effects of experimentally administered stimulation on developmental quotients of infants. *British Journal of Social and Clinical Psychology,* 1968, Vol. 7, 61-67.

TODD, G. & PALMER, B.: Social reinforcement of infant babbling. *Child Development,* 1968, Vol. 39, 591-596.

WATSON, J.: The development and generalization of contingency awareness in early infancy: Some hypotheses. *Merrill-Palmer Quarterly,* 1966, Vol. 12, 123-135.

WEISBERG, P.: Social and nonsocial conditioning of infant vocalizations. *Child Development,* 1963, Vol. 34, 377-388.

WHITE, R.: Motivation reconsidered: The concept of competence. *Psychological Review,* 1959, Vol. 66, 297-323.

2

STEREOTYPE TEMPORAL CONDI-
TIONING IN INFANTS

Yvonne Brackbill, Ph.D.

Professor of Obstetrics and Gynecology
Georgetown University Medical School

and

Hiram E. Fitzgerald, Ph.D.

Michigan State University

ABSTRACT: This study investigated stereotype temporal conditioning of pupillary dilation and constriction in infants. Stereotype conditioning of dilation was obtained, though it was less uniform over subjects than simple temporal conditioning of the same responses. Relevant speculative concepts concerning the physiological basis of discriminating time and ordinal position are presented.

DESCRIPTORS: Temporal conditioning, Time discrimination, Conditioned stereotype, Pupillary reflex, Infancy.

Increasing attention is being devoted to the importance of temporal and rhythmical phenomena in human behavior and development. The focus of much of this research has been on the ontogeny of temporal regularity. For example, Hellbrügge (1960) has investigated the early

Reprinted from PSYCHOPHYSIOLOGY, Vol. 9, No. 6, pp. 569-577. Copyright © 1972 by The Society for Psychophysiological Research.

This research was supported in part by Research Career Award MH 5925 from NIMH and Research Grant GB 15155 from NSF to the first author.

development of such endogenous biological rhythms as body temperature, skin resistance, heart rate, and sleepwaking activity; Wolff (1967) has studied the rhythmical qualities of the infant's sucking and crying behavior; other investigators have rescribed REM-NREM cycles (e.g., Stern, Parmelee, Akiyama, Schultz, & Wenner, 1969). Yet, biological rhythms comprise only one aspect of temporal regularity. An equally important aspect is the organism's ability to discriminate one temporal interval from another and to respond on the basis of such discrimination.

For several years we have been investigating, through the Pavlovian method of temporal conditioning, the human infant's ability to accurately perceive the passage of time. For example, Brackbill, Fitzgerald, and Lintz (1967) and Brackbill and Fitzgerald (1969) demonstrated simple temporal conditioning of pupillary dilation and constriction in one- to three-month-old infants. Acquisition of both conditioned responses proceeded rapidly and uniformly for all infants. The human infant has proved to be an excellent subject for these investigations because he is yet uncluttered by cognitive or attitudinal factors that methodologically contaminate studies of time discrimination in adult subjects (see Brackbill et al., 1967; Fitzgerald & Brackbill, 1968). Successful demonstration of simple temporal conditioning in infants permits one to investigate the next step in the ontogeny of time discrimination, i.e., the organism's ability to discriminate temporal *patterns.*

The general purpose of the present experiment was to investigate the applicability of the Pavlovian procedure of stereotype conditioning for the study of the infant's ability to discriminate temporal patterns. *Stereotype conditioning* refers to a classical conditioning procedure whereby a conditioned sequence of responses is formed by repeatedly presenting a series of conditional stimuli in the same order. (Note that the term "stereotype" is not equivalent to the clinical term "stereotype" which refers to abnormal mannerisms or auto-erotic activities.) Stereotype paradigms have been used to investigate various parameters of patterned responding in a variety of animals (Asratyan & associates, 1968; Burdina, 1960; Dumenko, 1961; Gantt, 1940; Gorbatsevich, 1959; Maizelis, 1959; Norkina, 1958; Vedent'yeva, 1961), in adult human beings (Maizelis, 1961; Naidel, 1959; Samsonova, 1959), in children (Degtyar, 1961; Koltsova, 1961), and in pilot work with infants (Brackbill et al., 1967).

The basic design for stereotype conditioning is illustrated in Fig. 1A. The major dimensions of the stereotype are the number and pattern of conditional stimuli involved. Operationally, when the focus of interest is on the conditional stimuli themselves, and when real, external events serve as CSs, the length of the interstimulus interval (ISI) is variable and

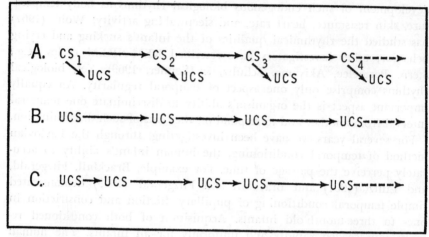

Fig. 1. Classical conditioning designs. A. Basic stereotype conditioning. B. Simple temporal conditioning. C. Stereotype temporal conditioning.

random. On the other hand, when the focus of interest is on the temporal relationship between stimuli, external CSs are eliminated and the constant ISI becomes in effect the CS. This is the paradigm for temporal conditioning, the simplest case of which is presented in Fig. 1B. Here there are no external CSs. The unconditioned stimulus (UCS) is applied at regular, constant-length intervals during conditioning and is withheld on test trials. If the subject responds on a test trial at that point in time when the UCS should have been applied, it is inferred that he has accurately perceived the passage of time during the ISI. The CS in this case—if it is appropriate to speak of one at all—is equivalent to an internalized version of the ISI ('interiorization" in Pavlovian terminology).

Simple temporal condition does not necessarily involve patterned responding. *Stereotype temporal conditioning* does, however. Fig. 1C illustrates the paradigm used for stereotype temporal conditioning, the design used in the present study. Here there are two ISIs—both of constant though differing lengths—applied in an alternating sequence. A test trial consists in the withholding of as many reinforcements as there are ISIs of differing lengths (e.g., two in the illustration) and noting whether a response occurs despite the absence of the UCS.

The studies previously cited have demonstrated two basic differences between simple conditioning and stereotype conditioning. The first difference is that acquisition of a stereotype proceeds more slowly than simple conditioning, because stereotype conditioning demands more complex behavioral change than does simple conditioning. The second difference is that stereotype conditioning shows greater individual differences in acquisition than does the simple conditioning, presumably because it is more dependent than simple conditioning on variables such as "temperament" or personality characteristics (Pavlov, 1941; Teplov, 1964).

Thus, the specific purposes of the present experiment were first to test the possibility of conditioning a temporal stereotype in infants, and second, to see if simple and stereotype temporal conditioning show the same acquisition differences in terms of speed and uniformity that have been documented for simple and stereotype nontemporal conditioning.

METHOD

Subjects

Thirty-nine full-term infants from a residential nursery served as subjects (Ss). All infants were judged clinically normal by the attending obstetrician. Results for an additional 9 Ss were discarded because these infants were unable to tolerate the long experimental procedure and yielded insufficient data for analysis. (The minimum number of conditioning trials had been set at 32, to allow comparison with data of previous studies.)

There were two experimental groups with 15 Ss per group. Ss in the first experimental group, conditioned pupillary dilation, had a median age of 44.5 days at the beginning of experimentation; 12 were white and 3, black; 8 were female and 7, male; 11 were blue eyed and 4, brown-eyed. Ss in the second experimental group, conditioned pupillary constriction, had a median age of 38.5 days at the beginning of experimentation; 12 were white and 3, black; 9 were male and 6, female; 10 were blue-eyed and 5, brown-eyed. There were no significant differences in conditionability for either group as a function of S's age, race, sex, or eye color—a finding that accords with previously published pupillary conditioning results obtained with infants (Brackbill et al., 1967; Fitzgerald, Lintz, Brackbill, & Adams, 1967) and with adults (Fitzgerald & Brackbill, 1968).

Design and Procedure

The basic design used in this experiment for temporal stereotype conditioning is outlined in Fig. 1C. Operationally, 1 stereotype conditioning trial lasted 58 sec and contained two interstimulus intervals: ISI_{20}, a 20-sec period of elapsed time followed by a 4-sec UCS, and ISI_{30}, a 30-second period of elapsed time followed by a 4-sec UCS. The same UCS, a change in illumination, followed each ISI. For 15 Ss the UCS was light offset and the UCR, pupillary dilation; for the remaining 15 Ss the UCS was light onset and the UCR, pupillary constriction. The UCS was provided by turning on or off a 100-watt blue bulb. (Further details are presented below.) Test trials were randomly distributed among conditioning trials at a ratio of 1:3.5.

Testing took place inside a small sound-attenuated booth. A hole in one side of the booth allowed a camera to photograph the infant's pupillary responses. Inside the booth were the S, propped in an infant seat, and one experimenter (E) who held the S's head in position at all times so that camera focus could be maintained. If the infant became drowsy during the session, E also held his eyelid open. A second E outside the booth operated the camera as well as a switch that eliminated the UCS on designated test trials. The experimental session began approximately one-half hour after infants had been fed to satiety.

Apparatus

The UCS for pupillary conditioning was a change in illumination level; for conditioning pupillary constriction, a 100-watt blue bulb mounted in a reflector housing 15 in. from S was turned on, and for conditioning pupillary dilation the same bulb was turned off. The duration and timing of the stimuli was determined by electronic recycling sequence timers.

Pupil responses were photographed and subsequently measured from photographic frames. The photographs were taken on Eastman HIR-430 infrared film with a Bolex H16 reflex camera, Kodak Cine Ektar 102 mm f:2.7 lens with extension tubes, and a Wratten A 25 red gelatin filter. The film speed was one frame per sec with a 1/35 sec exposure. The distance from camera to S was 26 inches. Light for photography came from two 25-watt red bulbs located 12 inches from S's eyes. A small red pilot bulb, within the camera field but shielded from S's view, was connected in parallel with the UCS lamp and provided a photographic record of events. The camera focused on an image of S's left eye reflected through an opening in the wall of the soundproofed booth by a front-surfaced mirror.

The films, developed by a commercial firm, were projected on a Kodak Model 10 Recordak viewer which provided a linear enlargement

23 times the original. Pupil diameter was measured to the nearest .01 mm by data reduction equipment built by an engineering specialist in the behavioral sciences. This equipment included a Philbrick operational amplifier, Electro Instruments digital voltmeter, and Clary digital printer connected in sequence. For analog-to-digital conversion of pupil diameters from projected film records, the sensing element was a vernier caliper mechanically coupled to a ten-turn Helipot. Both the zero point and the scale of the digital printout were selected by varying parameters of the operational amplifier, so that the printed data represented actual pupil diameters in mm.

After adjusting the caliper to match the projected diameter of the pupil, the scorer depressed a "record" button which triggered the data reduction apparatus. This method of mechanically recording the pupil diameter has the practical advantage of minimizing scoring bias in that the scorer is never aware of the numerical value of his measurements. Both naive and sophisticated scorers were used to determine interscorer reliability for measures to the nearest .01 mm. As previously reported (Fitzgerald et al., 1967) reliability ranged from .90 to .96 (median, .94) for all scorers.

RESULTS

Stereotype Temporal Conditioning

It was intended that each conditioning session would last 80 minutes and consist of 18 test trials randomly distributed among 64 conditioning trials in a 1:3.5 ratio. In practice, however, an 80-minute session turned out to be too demanding on infants of this age, so that only 1 of the 30 Ss completed all 18 test trials. For the 15 Ss exposed to pupillary dilation condition, the mean number of test trials was 13.43 (range, 9-16), and the mean number of reinforced trials was 46.87 (range 32-59). For Ss exposed to pupillary constriction conditioning, mean number of test trials was 14.83 (range, 9-18), and mean number of reinforced trials was 49.53 (range, 32-64).

The data on pupil size for all difference-score comparisons to be presented are from the 4 photographic frames collected during the 4 sec immediately preceding a test trial and the 4 sec of the test trial itself. For dilation, difference-scores were obtained by subtracting the single largest pupil diameter during a test trial from the single largest pupil diameter during the preceding 4 sec of the ISI. For constriction, difference scores were obtained by subtracting the single smallest pupil diameter during a test trial from the single smallest pupil diameter during

TABLE 1

Stereotype pupillary conditioning

| Measures | Mean Diameters and Differences in mm | | | |
| | Dilation | | Constriction | |
	ISI_{20}	ISI_{30}	ISI_{20}	ISI_{30}
No. Ss	15		15	
Mean No. Cond. Trials	46.86		49.50	
Pretest Mean	2.299	2.285	2.601	2.609
Test Mean	2.393	2.378	2.578	2.571
M_D	+.094	+.093	−.023	−.038
S_{MD}	.038	.034	.028	.042
t ($df = 14$)	2.47*	2.74**	.82	.90

* $p < .05$.
** $p < .02$.

the 4 pretest sec. A mean difference score for each S was calculated. Differences between these difference scores were then analyzed via a t-test for correlated means.

These mean differences and t-test results are shown in Table 1. There is statistically significant evidence of conditioning for both interstimulus intervals among Ss in the dilation group, but no evidence of conditioning among Ss in the constriction group. These results are similar to those obtained from pilot Ss in the previous study of stereotype temporal conditioning (Brackbill et al., 1967, p. 44, Table 11). Those results indicated less successful stereotype conditioning for constriction than for dilation, a finding difficult to explain insofar as constriction is the stronger UCR (Adler, 1965).

Differential conditionability as a function of this type of response did not, however, characterize the results obtained from the study of simple temporal conditioning carried out by Brackbill et al. (1967). (See also Fitzgerald et al., 1967.) In that study, both dilation and constriction were successfully conditioned. Furthermore, a smaller number of reinforcements (32) was needed to effect conditioning in that study than in the present study, in which the mean number of UCS presentations was 48.2 for both groups combined. This suggestion of lessened dependence of stereotype conditionability on external, task-related variables is supported by the fact that when dilation results from the present study were examined on an individual basis, mean number of reinforcements was negatively related to the likelihood of conditioning. For the 5 Ss who showed clear evidence of conditioning, the median number of reinforcements was 44, whereas for those Ss who showed little or no evidence of conditioning the median number of reinforcements was 54. A diminution in the influence of number of reinforced trials on stereotype conditioning outcome has already been noted in Soviet research (Teplov, 1964) —as well as in second-order operant conditioning schedules (Kelleher, 1966)—and is one of the reasons for inferring that stereotype conditioning reflects organismic variables to a greater extent than does simple conditioning.

In summary, the differences in results between present and previous studies suggest at the very least that stereotype temporal conditioning is indeed slower and subject to greater individual difference variability than is simple temporal conditioning. The most probable explanation for these differences lies in the different levels of complexity or difficulty of the tasks involved. However, the previous and present studies did make use of different subject samples (although they were drawn from the same population). Therefore, in order to be more sure that the difference between studies was not attributable to some kind of systematic difference between the two subject samples, it was decided to follow up the present experiment by exposing the same Ss to simple temporal conditioning.

Simple Temporal Conditioning Follow-Up

The design for simple temporal conditioning is shown in Fig. 1B. Operationally, 1 conditioning trial lasted 24 seconds and consisted of a 20-second ISI followed by a 4-second UCS. The procedure, apparatus, etc., were otherwise identical to those described for stereotype conditioning and to those employed in the previous studies of temporal pupillary conditioning (Brackbill et al., 1967; Fitzgerald et al., 1967).

Sixteen of the 30 Ss were still available for the follow-up procedure. The remaining infants had been adopted before a second experimental session could be scheduled for them. Time between the original conditioning and follow-up ranged from 1 week to 10 days. (Recall that, at least for infants, pupillary conditioning is not age-dependent [Brackbill et al., 1967; Fitzgerald et al., 1967]).

Despite the reduction in sample size there is clear evidence of success in simple temporal conditioning for both dilation and constriction responses (Table 2).

TABLE 2
Simple conditioning follow-up

Measures	Mean Diameters and Differences in mm	
	Dilation	Constriction
No. Ss	6	10
No. Cond. Trials	32 .	32
Pretest Mean	2.507	2.637
Test Mean	2.603	2.497
M_D	+.096	−.140
S_{MD}	.013	.042
t	7.38**	3.33*

* $p < .01$ $(df = 9)$.
** $p < .001$ $(df = 5)$.

DISCUSSION

This study was designed to investigate infants' ability to discriminate temporal patterns. To measure this ability we used the Pavlovian procedure of stereotype conditioning. Results suggest that such conditioned responding is possible, although the success in conditionability as well as the rate of acquisition of the conditioned stereotype is more variable than is the case for simple temporal conditioning. Apparently, perception of temporal *patterns* is a more difficult task for young infants than is the perception of simple temporal intervals.

There is considerable behavioral evidence attesting to the ability of many organisms to perceive time, i.e., to respond correctly on the basis of temporal intervals. Migrating and hibernating animals match their peripatetic and torporous behaviors with remarkable accuracy to long temporal intervals (weeks and months). Furthermore, although these behaviors can be modified by such nontemporal factors as light and temperature, they are not completely controlled by them. (See, for example, Pengelley & Asmundson, 1971.) Many organisms, including man, are also able to respond correctly to short intervals of time (seconds, minutes) under controlled laboratory conditions such as those used in this experiment. For example, such responses as brain wave activity (Holubár, 1969) and electrodermal activity (Holubár, 1969; Lockhart, 1966) have been temporally conditioned in human adults to time intervals less than 1 minute. Even human infants manifest this ability, as we have demonstrated in the present and previous studies.

How does the organism accomplish this? What physiological mechanisms mediate this ability? Through what anatomical sites? Surprisingly enough, the abundant behavioral evidence on time discrimination has no counterpart in physiological or anatomical research—either in terms of quantity of output or in terms of successful outcome. Concerning discrimination of longer time intervals, current speculation in biology now suggests that the accumulation of metabolites during hibernation may be responsible for the onset of arousal either during or at the end of hibernation, but there are no viable hypotheses concerning the physiological mediators of the onset of hibernation itself (Strumwasser, Schlechte, & Streeter, 1967). Research has been equally unproductive in identifying the physiological basis for discrimination of short time intervals. Physiological measures for short-interval time discrimination have variously been referred to the nervous system as a whole (Cloudsley-Thompson, 1966; Pavlov, 1927), all cortical cells (Dmitriev & Kochigina, 1959), the septal area (Ellen, Wilson, & Powell, 1964), the prefrontal cortex and thalamus (Dimond, 1964), the hypothalamus (Richter, 1965), and the cortex, as a separate modality or sensory analyzer.

A possible explanatory mechanism of a quite different nature is suggested by the recent discovery of Thompson, Mayers, Robertson, and Patterson (1970) of individual "counting" cells in the associational areas of the cat's cortex. These cells are single neurons that fire in response to a particular *ordinal* stimulus within a sequence of stimuli, e.g., to the 6th stimulus in a sequence of 10. The authors call this effect "number coding" and conclude that it is independent of stimulus modality, intensity, and interstimulus interval. However, and most important for our purposes here, although their procedure has employed ISIs of differing absolute lengths between experiments, the ISIs have been of constant unvarying lengths within experiments. Thus, what the authors have apparently found is evidence of single cell component contributions to temporal-ordinal pattern perception.

Although the conclusion drawn by Thompson et al. may be accurate and sufficient for cats, cortical programming of ordinal events in higher organisms must represent a more complex stage of physiological affairs. In human beings, the probability of occurrence of any sequential response is *not* solely dependent on the ordinal position of the stimulus for that response. For example, "switching" the significance of the *n*th stimulus in a series so that it indicates the arrival of an appetitive UCS rather than an aversive UCS does cause some disruption of a conditioned stereotype (Degtyar, 1961). Nevertheless, much greater response disruption is caused by changing the ordinal positions of the component stimuli in the stereotype pattern (Asratyan, 1968; Degtyar, 1961; Kolt-sova, 1961). This suggests that maintaining the unaltered ordinal position of component stimuli within a series of stimuli is not the only determinant of stereotype performance, but it is probably the most important determinant. Thus, the Thompson et al. formulation of neuronal specificity with respect to ordinal position may be the most promising lead to understanding the physiological basis of stereotype temporal conditioning and, perhaps, patterned or sequential responding in general.

REFERENCES

ADLER, F. H.: Physiology of the Eye. St. Louis: C. V. Mosby, 1965.
ASRATYAN, E. A.: Some peculiarities of formation, functioning and inhibition of con-ditioned reflexes with two-way connections. In E. A. Asratyan (Ed.): Progress in Brain Research. Vol. 22. Brain Reflexes. Amsterdam: Elsevier, 1968. Pp. 8-20.
BRACKBILL, Y. & FITZGERALD, H. E.: Development of the sensory analyzers during in-fancy. In L. P. Lipsitt & H. W. Reese (Eds.): Advances in Child Development and Behavior. Vol. 4. New York: Academic Press, 1969. Pp. 174-208.
BRACKBILL, Y., FITZGERALD, H. E., & LINTZ, L. M.: A developmental study of classical conditioning. Monographs of the Society for Research in Child Development, 1967, 32, No. 8.
BURDINA, V. N.: The use of stereotype of two stimuli for the nervous system typing of dogs. Pavlov Journal of Higher Nervous Activity, 1960, 10, 238-245.
CLOUDSLEY-THOMPSON, J. L.: Time sense in animals. In J. T. Fraser (Ed.), The Voices of Time. New York: Braziller, 1966. Pp. 296-311.
DEGTYAR, E. N.: Interaction between temporary connections of different types in the elaboration of a stereotype in children. Pavlov Journal of Higher Nervous Ac-tivity, 1961, 11, 663-668.
DIMOND, S. J.: The structural basis of timing. Psychological Bulletin, 1964, 62, 348-350.
DMITRIEV, A. S., & KOCHIGINA, A. M.: The importance of time as stimulus of condi-tioned reflex activity. Psychological Bulletin, 1959, 56, 106-132.
DUMENNO, V. N.: Changes in the electrical activity of the cerebral cortex of dogs during the formation of a stereotype of motor-conditioned reflexes. Pavlov Jour-nal of Higher Nervous Activity, 1961, 11, 292-298.
ELLEN, P., WILSON, A. S., & POWELL, E. W.: Septal inhibition and timing behavior in the rat. Experimental Neurology, 1964, 10, 120-132.
FITZGERALD, H. E. & BRACKBILL, Y.: Interstimulus interval in classical pupillary con-ditioning. Psychological Reports, 1968, 23, 369-370.
FITZGERALD, H. E., LINTZ, L. M., BRACKBILL, Y., & ADAMS, G.: Time perception and conditioning an autonomic response in young infants. Perceptual & Motor Skills, 1967, 24, 479-486.
GANTT, W. H.: The role of the isolated conditioned stimulus in the integrated re-sponse pattern, and the relation of pattern changes to psychopathology. Journal of General Psychology, 1940, 23, 3-16.
GORBATSEVICH, L. I.: The development of the fever reaction in certain disorders of higher nervous activity in dogs. Pavlov Journal of Higher Nervous Activity, 1959, 9, 166-176.
HELLBRÜGGE, T.: The development of circadian rhythms in infants. In Cold Spring Harbor Symposium on Quantitative Biology. Vol. 25. Biological Clocks. Cold Spring Harbor, New York: Biological Laboratory, 1960. Pp. 311-323.

HOLUBAR, J.: *The Sense of Time*. (Trans. J. S. Barlow) Cambridge, Mass.: The Massachusetts Institute of Technology Press, 1969.

KELLEHER, R. T.: Chaining and conditioned reinforcement. In W. K. Honig (Ed.), *Operant Behavior: Areas of Research and Application*. New York: Appleton-Century-Crofts, 1966. Pp. 160-212.

KOLSOVA, M. M.: The role of temporary connections of associative type in the development of systematized activity. *Pavlov Journal of Higher Nervous Activity*, 1961, 11, 56-60.

LOCKHART, R. A.: Importance of a stereotype of eating, muscular activity, and sleeping in the regulation of physiological functions. *Pavlov Journal of Nervous Activity*, 1959, 6, 845-850.

MAIZELIS, M. R.: Importance of a stereotype of eating, muscular activity, and sleeping in the regulation of physiological functions. *Pavlov Journal of Higher Nervous Activity*, 1959, 6, 845-850.

NAIDEL, A. V.: Interaction of two conditioned reflex processes in a dynamic stereotype. *Pavlov Journal of Higher Nervous Activity*, 1959, 9, 591-596.

NORKINA, K. N.: The production of experimental neurotic states in the lower apes. *Pavlov Journal of Nervous Activity*, 1958, 8, 52-58.

PAVLOV, I. P.: *Conditioned Reflexes*. London: Oxford University Press, 1927.

PAVLOV, I. P.: *Lectures on Conditioned Reflexes: Conditioned Reflexes and Psychiatry*. Vol. 2. (Trans. & Ed., W. Gantt) New York: International, 1941.

PENGELLEY, E. T., & ASMUNDSON, S. J.: Annual biological clocks. *Scientific American*, 1971, 224, 72-79.

RICHTER, C. P.: *Biological Clocks in Medicine and Psychiatry*. Springfield, Ill.: Charles C Thomas, 1965.

SAMSONOVA, V. G.: The effect of establishing a complex motor stereotype, and replacing one of its components by a new one, on visual discrimination. *Pavlov Journal of Higher Nervous Activity*, 1959, 9, 166-176.

STERN, E., PARMELEE, A. H., AKIYAMA, Y., SCHULTZ, M. A., & WENNER, W. H.: Sleep cycle characteristics in infants. *Pediatrics*, 1969, 43, 65-70.

STRUMWASSER, F., SCHLECHTE, F. R., & STREETER, J.: The internal rhythms of hibernators. In K. C. Fisher, A. R. Dawe, C. P. Lyman, E. Schönbaum, & F. E. South, Jr. (Eds.): *Mammalian Hibernation*. III. New York: American Elsevier, 1967. Pp. 110-139.

TEPLOV, B. M.: Problems in the study of general types of higher nervous activity in man and animals. In J. A. Gray (Ed.): *Pavlov's Typology*. New York: Macmillan, 1964. Pp. 3-153.

THOMPSON, R. F., MAYERS, K. S., ROBERTSON, R. T., & PATTERSON, C. J.: Number coding in association cortex of the cat. *Science*, 1970, 168, 271-273.

VEDENT'YEVA, R. A.: Features of the inhibition of vascular reactions on disturbance of an experimental stereotype in dogs. *Pavlov Journal of Higher Nervous Activity*, 1961, 11, 974-978.

WOLFF, P. H.: The role of biological rhythms in early psychological development. *Bulletin of the Menninger Clinic*, 1967, 31, 197-218.

3

THE RELATIVE EFFICACY OF CONTACT AND VESTIBULAR-PROPRIOCEPTIVE STIMULATION IN SOOTHING NEONATES

Anneliese F. Korner, Ph.D.

Senior Scientist, Department of Psychiatry,
Stanford University Medical Center

and

Evelyn B. Thoman, Ph.D.

Associate Professor, Department of Biobehavioral Sciences
University of Connecticut

Forty 2- to 4-day old healthy full-term newborns, equally divided between males and females and breast- and bottle-fed infants, were given, in random order, 6 interventions which replicated common maternal soothing techniques. The interventions entailed, singly or in combination, con-

Reprinted from CHILD DEVELOPMENT, 1972, 43, No. 2, June 443-453. © 1972 by the Society for Research in Child Development, Inc. All rights reserved.

This study was supported by Public Health Service grant HD-03591 from the National Institute of Child Health and Human Development and by Public Health Service Training grants MH-8304 and 5 TO 1 HD-00049 and also a grant (RR-81) from the General Clinical Research Center's Program of the Division of Research Resources, National Institutes of Health. We thank Dr. Helena Kraemer for assisting in the statistical analyses of the data and Lynn Beason for acting as mother substitute to the infants. The cooperation of the nursing staff of Stanford Hospital and the Department of Pediatrics made this study possible.

tact and vestibular-proprioceptive stimulation with and without the upright position. Crying time was recorded for 30 seconds during and after each intervention. Vestibular stimulation had a highly potent soothing effect both during and after the interventions. Contact had a lesser effect during, and none following, the interventions. The results suggest that the soothing effects usually attributed to contact comfort may be largely a function of vestibular-proprioceptive stimulation which attends most contacts between mother and child. Significant individual differences in soothability were found among the infants. While mode of feeding was not related to how much the infants cried while being soothed, breast-fed infants cried significantly more after the interventions, possibly because they were hungrier.

Mothers the world over have been concerned since time immemorial with soothing their infants. Yet it has been only in the last decade that researchers have become interested in investigating systematically the effects of various soothing methods on newborns. Judging from the literature, many different stimuli are capable of soothing newborns. For example, continuous, monotonous, or rhythmical forms of stimulation are rocking (J. A. Ambrose, personal communication, August 28, 1968; Pederson, Champagne, & Pederson 1969), swaddling (Lipton, Steinschneider, & Richmond 1965), continuous sound, particularly white noise (Wolff 1966), the human heartbeat (Brackbill, Adams, Crowell, & Gray 1966; Salk 1965), other sustained sounds (Birns, Blank, Bridger, & Escalona 1965; Brackbill et al. 1966), bright overhead lights (Wolff 1966), and sucking on a pacifier. Various brief, discontinuous types of stimulation have also been found to be soothing to young infants (Birns, Blank, & Bridger 1966; Bridger & Birns 1963; Kopp 1971; Sternglanz 1969). Sternglanz (1969) found significant differences in the effectiveness of various soothing devices for neonates, and Kopp (1971) did so for somewhat older children. By contrast, Bridger and Birns (1963) and Birns et al. (1966) found no significant differences among the soothing techniques they used.

Contact comfort has been described in the literature as a most important soother during infancy (e.g., Bowlby 1958; Harlow 1958; Ribble 1944). Several different forms of stimulation are involved in contact comfort, including tactile, cutaneous, olfactory, thermal, and usually kinesthetic and vestibular-proprioceptive stimulation as well. We had noted that these different forms of stimulation had a highly differential effect on another type of neonatal behavior, namely, visual alerting

(Korner & Thoman 1970). In the present study, we addressed ourselves to the question of whether common types of maternal interventions which entailed, singly or in combination, contact and vestibular-proprioceptive stimulation all had an equal effect in calming infants (as had the interventions of Bridger & Birns [1963] and Birns et al. [1966]); or whether, in fact, some of the component stimulations inherent in common maternal interventions are more effective than others in soothing infants. We also assessed whether some infants are more easily comforted than others and whether males differed from females in this respect. Furthermore, we examined whether breast-fed infants cry less than bottle-fed infants, as was suggested by Simmons, Ottinger, and Haugk's study (1967), or whether they actually cry more as Bell's (1966) data indicate.

METHOD

Subjects.—The Ss were 40 infants equally divided between males and females and breast- and bottle-fed infants. To control for the possible effects of parity on the neonates' behavior (Thoman, Turner, Leiderman, & Barnett 1970; Weller & Bell 1965), only infants born to multiparae were included. All infants were Caucasian. The infants were 2 days old or older to allow for recovery from birth (range, 47-116 hours; mean, 59 hours). Since the infant's proneness to cry can be influenced by pre- and postnatal complications, stringent criteria were used to select for inclusion in the study only healthy, full-term babies. Their weights ranged from 6 lb 5 oz to 9 lb 14 oz (mean, 7 lb 9 oz). Apgar ratings were 8 or above at 1 minute. Infants suspected of any fetal or postnatal anoxia were excluded. Analgesic used during labor was below 200 mg 1-6 hours prior to delivery, and maternal labor neither exceeded 13 hours nor was less than 1 hour. All infants were judged to be normal newborns on physical examination. A lapse of a minimum of 24 hours since circumcision was required for boys to be included.

Procedure.—The infants were brought individually from the newborn nursery into an adjacent treatment room by a nurse. This treatment room was dimly lit, quiet, and physically separated from the activities of the nurses' station and from the crying of other newborns in the nursery. To provide uniform treatment for all Ss, the assistant first diapered each infant, regardless of need. The infant was then lifted from his bassinet and placed in the supine position on the examining table.

Six interventions were made with each infant, each of which replicated common experiences attending child care in the earliest weeks of life. The interventions entailed, singly and in combination, contact, along with the forms of stimulation which attend contact, and the experience of being moved. The latter invariably provides vestibular stimulation as well as the concomitant activation of the proprioceptive receptors. These receptors, particularly those which are located in the neck muscles, inevitably become activated whenever the head is moved. The following is a description of these interventions, with the types of stimulation provided in each given in parentheses:

1. The infant was lifted from the examining table and put to the shoulder with the head supported and with the face just above shoulder level (upright, vestibular-proprioceptive, and contact).

2. The infant was lifted horizontally and was cradled in the arms in the nursing position (vestibular-proprioceptive and contact).

3. The assistant, bending over the supine infant on the examining table and leaning on one elbow, held the infant close, simulating the nursing position commonly assumed in the maternal bed. In so doing, the infant was not moved in any way (contact only).

4. The infant, who had been previously placed in a "Baby Line" infant seat, was raised to the upright position with the back of the infant seat at a 55° angle to the table (upright and vestibular-proprioceptive).

5. The infant, having been previously placed in the infant seat, was moved to and fro horizontally as if in a perambulator. With an 18-inch total displacement, the infant was given 14 excursions during the time treatment was provided (vestibular-proprioceptive only).

6. The infant, lying supine on the examining table, was talked to at a standard distance in a high-pitched female voice, simulating "mother talk." The voice was used as a marker to avoid arbitrariness or bias in picking a time during which to observe crying in the absence of any intervention. This was decided after a preliminary study established that the voice diminished crying more than would have occurred spontaneously without any intervention.

Each intervention lasted 30 seconds and provided stimulation for that period. Each intervention involving contact provided contact identical in form, in that each included containment, olfactory stimuli, and ventral body contact. The quality and quantity of vestibular-proprioceptive stimulation was directly comparable only in interventions 1 and 4. In each of these interventions, the infant was lifted and put in the vertical position, which provided both angular acceleration and the sustained vestibular-proprioceptive stimulation entailed in maintaining the upright position. The type of vestibular-proprioceptive stimulation given during interventions 2 and 5 differed in that during intervention 5 the infant was given continuous linear acceleration over the 30-second period and during intervention 2 only momentary linear acceleration was provided.

To avoid an order effect of presentation, the six interventions were made in a computer-programmed, random order. For comparability of handling, the same person did all the interventions with all babies. To avoid the cumulative effects of soothing interventions given in rapid succession, a minimum of 2 minutes was required between interventions and the point in time when the infant was last touched. Thus, when an infant was placed in the infant seat, at least 2 minutes had to elapse before the next intervention was given. To ensure reasonable comparability of prestimulus arousal, interventions were made only after the infant fussed for at least a minute and cried vigorously for 10 seconds. Nothing was done before or during the experiment to induce crying in the infant, partly to avoid differential reactions to such manipulations, partly to keep constant the amount of stimulation given each S. This often made it difficult to complete the observations. Six Ss had to be eliminated from the study for this reason. Crying time was measured both during the interventions (Crying A) and immediately following the interventions (Crying B). A stopwatch was activated whenever any crying was heard during the 30-second intervals. Two observers independently recorded the crying time of 24 infants. In order to assess observer reliability, the trials in which no crying occurred during the interventions or after the interventions were excluded from the calculations. The average time discrepancy between two observers for Crying A was 0.07 seconds (SD=1.35) and for Crying B 0.16 seconds (SD=1.07).

RESULTS

An analysis of variance was used to assess simultaneously the differential effects of the interventions and differences between the sexes, individual infants, and breast- and bottle-fed infants. The data analyses also included comparisons of relevant interventions to assess the effectiveness of specific types of stimulation for soothing the infants. The data were analyzed separately for crying observed during the 30-second intervention (Crying A) and that observed during the 30-second period immediately following the intervention (Crying B).

Differential effects of types of stimulation in soothing infants.—Table 1 shows the means and standard errors of crying time during and after each intervention. The analysis of variance showed that the interventions differed significantly in their effectiveness in reducing or stopping crying and in their aftereffects, Crying A: $F(5,180)=19.53$, $p<.001$; Crying B: $F(5,180)=11.76$, $p<.001$.

We next assessed the efficacy of contact and of vestibular-proprioceptive stimulation in soothing the infants. To assess the contribution of each, four interventions were chosen for an analysis of variance which were balanced as to the type of stimulation provided. Thus, to assess the effect of vestibular-proprioceptive stimulation, crying time during two interventions providing 30 seconds of comparable types of vestibular-proprioceptive stimulation (being lifted and kept in the upright) was compared with crying time during two interventions which did not entail any vestibular-proprioceptive stimulation (interventions 1 and 4 vs. 3 and 6). Similarly, to assess the effect of contact, crying time during two interventions providing 30 seconds of contact was compared with crying time during two interventions which provided no contact (interventions 1 and 3 vs. 4 and 6). The analysis for these comparisons showed that contact had a significant effect, Crying A: $F(1,180)=7.1$, $p<.01$. This analysis also showed that the vestibular-proprioceptive stimulation entailed in being lifted and maintained in the upright had a powerful soothing effect, Crying A: $F(1,180)=86.0$, $p<.001$.

The differences in F values for these two forms of stimulation clearly show a difference in the magnitude of the effect. This difference was also highlighted in a direct comparison of the means of the four interventions. The mean difference between the interventions which entailed contact and those that did not was 3.3 seconds, whereas the difference for the relevant comparisons involving vestibular-proprioceptive stimulation was 11.5 seconds.

The effects of the two forms of stimulation on crying time during the 30 seconds immediately following the intervention (Crying B) were assessed by means of the same comparisons. During this period, contact did not have a significant effect, whereas vestibular-proprioceptive stimulation had a marked impact, $F(1,180)=25.5$, $p<.001$. The mean differences between intervention with and without contact was 0.07 seconds. The mean difference between interventions with and without vestibular-proprioceptive stimulation was 7.5 seconds.

Differences among infants.—There were no significant sex differences in crying time either during or after the interventions. By contrast, there were highly significant individual differences in the extent to which different infants were soothed both during and immediately following the interventions, Crying A: $F(36,180)=2.09$, $p<.001$; Crying B:

TABLE 1

MEAN CRYING TIME DURING AND AFTER INTERVENTIONS

Intervention	Stimulation[a]	Mean Crying Seconds during Intervention	SEM	Mean Crying Seconds after Intervention	SEM
1. To shoulder	CVU	11.23	1.34	15.32	1.67
2. To breast	CV	21.25	1.37	19.45	1.77
3. Held close	C	23.00	1.28	19.28	1.91
4. Infant seat up	VU	14.80	1.63	11.85	1.83
5. Infant seat to side	V	17.65	1.38	9.48	1.81
6. Female voice	...	26.00	1.02	22.90	1.69

a Stimulation: C = contact; V = vestibular-proprioceptive; U = upright.

$F(36,180)=2.59$, $p<.001$. Further evidence of differences in individual responsiveness to soothing was shown by a correlation of $r=.50$, $p<.01$, between the infants' crying time during and after the interventions.

Differences due to mode of feeding.—There were no significant differences between breast- and bottle-fed infants in the degree to which they were soothed during the interventions. By contrast, highly significant differences were found between these two groups in crying time after the interventions, Crying B: $F(1,36)=9.59$, $p<.001$. The breast-fed infants cried significantly more after the interventions than the bottle-fed infants.

DISCUSSION

In this paper, we have explored the differential soothing effects of various types of common maternal interventions on the crying of neonates. These interventions entailed, singly or in combination, contact and vestibular-proprioceptive stimulation with or without the upright position. Our data indicate that the interventions provided differed in their effectiveness in calming newborns to a highly significant degree. This finding is at variance with the results of Bridger and Birns (1963) and Birns et al. (1966), which indicate that no one of their interventions was more effective in soothing infants than any other.

When one reviews the literature on the types of interventions which have been found to be soothing to neonates, it becomes apparent that two general conditions predictably bring about this effect: (1) Continuous monotonous or rhythmical stimulation will lead to a lowering of arousal and to a peripheral and possibly also a central inhibition (e.g., rocking, swaddling, continuous sound—be it white noise, the human heartbeat, or a continuous loud tone—bright overhead light, or sucking on a pacifier). (2) Briefer forms of stimulation, which, in terms of the organism's stage of neurophysiological development, must be adequate in duration and intensity to diminish or disrupt an ongoing activity, in this case crying. This disruption in crying, in some instances at least, may be the consequence of an orienting response. In our study, we found brief vestibular-proprioceptive stimulation to be a most potent stimulus of the second variety.

The discrepancy between our findings, that stimuli differ with respect to their effectiveness for soothing, and the findings by Bridger and Birns (1963) and by Birns et al. (1966), which indicate a lack of differential effectiveness, can be explained on several grounds. In one of their studies, Birns et al. (1966) used stimulation that persisted for 60 seconds, which is a more continuous form of stimulation than the 30 seconds we used. Also, the types of stimulation they used were, for the most part, highly adequate soothers of infants (i.e., sucking on a sweetened pacifier, gentle rocking, continuous loud tone, and the immersion of the infant's foot, with body position unspecified, in warm water). In the earlier study (Bridger & Birns 1963), brief stimulations were used. One involved sucking on a sweetened pacifier; the other entailed gentle rocking of the infant's head in an elevated body position, an intervention which, in effect, provided vestibular-proprioceptive stimulation. Considering our findings regarding the soothing efficacy of this form of stimulation, it is not too surprising that these two interventions proved equally effective.

It is of interest that, while continuous vestibular-proprioceptive stimulation (as provided during rocking) has long been known to calm infants, the soothing effect of brief vestibular-proprioceptive stimulation provided by changes in body position has not been sufficiently stressed in the literature. Perhaps the reason why vestibular-proprioceptive stimulation is such an adequate soother for the newborn lies in the fact that the vestibular component of this stimulation, at least, is transmitted by a highly mature system which functions well long before birth. According to Humphrey (1965), the vestibular nuclei are "unquestionably functional at 21 weeks of gestation." Also, Langworthy (1933) demonstrated that myelinization of the vestibular system begins at 4 months of gestational age, is well underway in the fetus of 6 months, and is quite heavy at term.

Some forms of vestibular-proprioceptive stimulation, whether continuous or brief, seem to be more potent than others in soothing newborns. For example, in continuous vestibular-proprioceptive stimulation, Pederson et al. (1969) found that up-and-down motion was a much more effective soother than side-to-side motion. Ambrose (personal communication) found that 60-70 rocking oscillations per minute were more effective in stopping crying than slower rates. It seems likely that the most effective soothers involve rhythms and types of motions experienced in utero. In our study, in which brief vestibular-proprioceptive stimulation was used, we found that, within the limits of our interventions, those which entailed the most rapid and the most drastic positional change were the most effective in reducing crying (interventions 1, 4, and 5).

Our study showed that contact, too, had a significant effect in calming the infants; however, this effect was not nearly as potent as that of vestibular-proprioceptive stimulation. When, during intervention 3, the effect of contact alone was compared with that of the voice, which a preliminary study revealed to have no more than a chance effect, the infants cried on the average only 3 seconds less when they were given contact. It seems probable that the reason why contact has been viewed as such an excellent soother for young infants for so long lies in the fact that there is hardly any contact between mother and child which does not also involve vestibular-proprioceptive stimulation. In almost any caretaking act, the infant is not only touched but also moved in space.

We observed an interesting parallel in an animal study in which we investigated the effects of vestibular-proprioceptive stimulation on the behavior and development of infant rats (Thoman & Korner 1971). In this study, we provided contact for one group of newborn rats by swaddling them. Another group was given vestibular-proprioceptive stimulation in addition to contact by being rotated on a drum while swaddled in an identical manner. Like newborn humans, the infant rats responded from day 1 to vestibular-proprioceptive stimulation by an almost complete cessation of distress calls. As soon as the rotation stopped, the pups resumed vocalizing to the level of the group which was swaddled only, a level which was markedly higher than that of the experimental group during rotation.

Like Bridger and Birns (1963) and Birns et al. (1966), we found highly significant individual differences among the infants in how soothable they were. They differed significantly from each other not only during the interventions but also in the poststimulation soothing effects. In addition, the infants' response was reasonably self-consistent during and after the interventions, $r=.50$, $p<.01$. This differential soothability, combined with the differences which exist in the infants' capacity for self-comforting (see Korner & Kraemer 1972), must have important implications both for early experience and the beginning mother-infant relationship.

When responsiveness of breast- and bottle-fed infants was compared, we found that they were equally soothable during the interventions, but that after the interventions, the breast-fed infants cried significantly more than the bottle-fed infants. Simmons et al. (1967) found that breast-fed neonates (age unspecified) cried significantly less than bottle-fed infants, and they raised the question of whether the tactile stimulation and the sucking at the breast did not make for more satisfied and optimally stimulated babies. By contrast, Bell (1966) found that 3- to 4-day-old breast-fed infants cried more and showed higher levels of arousal than bottle-fed infants. He invoked as one possible explanation that breast-fed infants were hungrier because of the delayed onset of the mother's milk flow. Our data on 2- to 4-day-old babies are consistent with Bell's (1966) findings. While during the interventions the soothing effects seemed to override the group differences, breast- and bottle-fed infants did differ in response after the interventions. This probably was true because the breast-fed infants were hungrier. Our results underscore Bell's warning that, because mode of feeding can affect the infant's behavior, this factor needs to be controlled in sampling for neonatal studies.

REFERENCES

BELL, R. Q.: Level of arousal in breast-fed and bottle-fed human newborns. *Psychosomatic Medicine,* 1966, 28, 177-180.

BIRNS, B., BLANK, M., & BRIDGER, W. H.: The effectiveness of various soothing techniques on human neonates. *Psychosomatic Medicine,* 1966, 28, 316-322.

BIRNS, B., BLANK, M., BRIDGER, W. H., & ESCALONA, S. K.: Behavioral inhibition in neonates produced by auditory stimuli. *Child Development,* 1965, 36, 639-645.

BOWLBY, J.: The child's tie to his mother. *International Journal of Psychoanalysis,* 1958, 39, 350-373.

BRACKBILL, Y., ADAMS, G., CROWELL, D. H., & GRAY, L.: Arousal level in neonates and preschool children under continuous auditory stimulation. *Journal of Experimental Child Psychology,* 1966, 4, 178-188.

BRIDGER, W. H. & BIRNS, B.: Neonates' behavioral and autonomic responses to stress during soothing. *Recent Advances in Biological Psychiatry,* 1963, 5, 1-6.

HARLOW, H.: The nature of love. *American Psychologist,* 1958, 13, 673-685.

HUMPHREY, T.: The embryologic differentiation of the vestibular nuclei in man correlated with functional development. In *International Symposium on Vestibular and Oculomotor Problems.* Tokyo: Nippoon-Hoechst, 1965. Pp. 51-56.

KOPP, C.: Inhibition of infant crying: A comparison of stimuli. Paper presented at the meeting of the Society for Research in Child Development, Minneapolis, April 1971.

KORNER, A. F. & KRAEMER, H. C.: Individual differences in spontaneous oral behavior in neonates. In J. F. Bosma (Ed.): *Third Symposium on Oral Sensation and Perception: The Mouth of the Infant.* Springfield, Ill.: Thomas, 1972, in press.

KORNER, A. F. & THOMAN, E. B.: Visual alertness in neonates as evoked by maternal care. *Journal of Experimental Child Psychology,* 1970, 10, 67-78.

LANGWORTHY, O. R.: Development of behavior patterns and myelinization of the nervous system in the human fetus and infant. *Carnegie Institution of Washington Contributions to Embryology,* 1933, 24, 1-57.

LIPTON, E. L., STEINSCHNEIDER, A., & RICHMOND, J. B.: Swaddling, a child care practice: Historical, cultural and experimental observations. *Pediatrics,* 1965, 35 (Suppl.), 521-567.

PEDERSON, D. R., CHAMPAGNE, L., & PEDERSON, L.: Relative soothing effects of vertical and horizontal rocking. Paper presented at the meeting of the Society for Research in Child Development, Santa Monica, California, March 1969.

RIBBLE, M. A.: Infantile experience in relation to personality development. In J. McV. Hunt (Ed.): *Personality and the Behavior Disorders.* Vol. 2. New York: Ronald, 1944. Pp. 621-651.

SALK, L.: The heart beat rhythm as a prenatal stimulus: Experiments, observations and thoughts. Paper presented at the meeting of the American Orthopsychiatric Association, New York, March 1965.

SIMMONS, J. E., OTTINGER, D., & HAUGK, E.: Maternal variables and neonate behavior. *Journal of the American Academy of Child Psychiatry*, 1967, 6, 174-183.

STERNGLANZ, S. H.: Neonatal quieters. Paper presented at the meeting of the Society for Research in Child Development, Santa Monica, California, March 1969.

THOMAN, E. B. & KORNER, A. F.: Effects of vestibular stimulation on the behavior and development of infant rats. *Developmental Psychology*, 1971, 5, 92-98.

THOMAN, E. B., TURNER, A., LEIDERMAN, P. H., & BARNETT, C. R.: Neonate-mother interaction: Effects of parity on feeding behavior. *Child Development*, 1970, 41, 1103-1111.

WELLER, C. M. & BELL, R. Q.: Basal skin conductance and neonatal state. *Child Development*, 1965, 36, 647-657.

WOLFF, P. H.: The causes, controls and organization of behavior in the neonate. *Psychological Issues*, 1966, 5 (1, Whole No. 17).

4

EVALUATION OF INFANT INTELLIGENCE

Infant Intelligence Scores — True or False?

Michael Lewis, Ph.D.

Director, Infant Laboratory, Educational Testing Service (Princeton)
Clinical Professor of Pediatric Psychology, Columbia University

and

Harry McGurk, Ph.D.

University of Surrey (England)

The late Sir Cyril Burt once remarked of intelligence, "Of all our mental qualities, it is the most far-reaching; fortunately it can be measured with accuracy and ease" (1, p. 28). Although much progress has been made in the field of psychometrics since Burt's statement, his early confidence has hardly been justified with respect to the measurement of intelligence during the early stages of human development. In common with many others, Burt espoused the view that intelligence is a finite potential with which the individual is endowed at conception; the manifestations of this intelligence increase at a stable rate during the growth process, but intelligence is subject neither to qualitative change nor to environmental influence. "It is inherited, or at least innate, not due to teaching or training; it is intellectual, not emotional or moral, and remains uninfluenced by industry or "zeal" (1, p. 29).

Reprinted from Science, Vol. 178, December 15, 1972, pp. 1174-1177. Copyright 1972 by the American Association for the Advancement of Science.

It is a *sine qua non* of this view that measures of intelligence have high predictive validity from one age to another. Such validity is singularly lacking in every scale used to assess intelligence during early infancy. For example, Bayley (2), employing an early version of her infant development scales, reported correlations between scores at 1, 2, and 3 months and scores at 18 to 36 months which ranged between —.04 and .09. Recently, Bayley (3, p. 1174) has concluded, "The findings of these early studies of mental growth of infants have been repeated sufficiently often so that it is now well established that test scores earned in the first year or two have relatively little predictive validity." Stott and Ball (4) and Thomas (5), after extensive reviews of a wide variety of infant intelligence scales, arrived at essentially similar conclusions.

Despite these acknowledged limitations, infant intelligence scales are widely used in clinical situations, in the belief that, although lacking in predictive validity, these scales are valuable in assessing the overall health and developmental status of babies at the particular time of testing, relative to other babies of the same age. This use of infant intelligence scales is justified only if, in interpreting the resultant scores, the scores are regarded solely as measures of present performance and not as indices of future potential. What this performance may mean is questionable, since it is possible that "superior" performance may be indicative of poor performance later. For example, Bayley shows a correlation of —.30 between males' earlier test behavior and their IQ (intelligence quotient) at ages 16 to 18 (6). Infant intelligence scales are invalid as measures of future potential; the necessity for caution in this respect cannot be overstressed.

Intelligence test scores are frequently used as a criterion in evaluating the efficiency of infant intervention, or enrichment, programs. Typically, a sample of subjects from some specified population is exposed to a program of stimulation and interaction beyond the normal experience of that population. At various points in the program, intelligence test scores are obtained and compared with the scores of a control sample. If the scores of the former are higher than those of the latter, the program is evaluated positively; if not, it is evaluated negatively. Two assumptions underlie such procedures—one explicit, the other implicit. Explicitly, it is assumed that, while the limits of intellectual achievement may be genetically determined, mental development is strongly influenced by environmental factors. This view enjoys considerable support, but it is not the focus of our interest here. Implicitly, it is assumed that infant intelligence is a general, unitary capacity and that mental development can be enhanced by enriching the infant's experience in a few specific

TABLE 1

MEAN AND STANDARD DEVIATION (S.D.) OF MENTAL
DEVELOPMENT INDEX SCORES

Age (months)	Mean	S.D.
3	101.64	14.9
6	110.05	20.6
9	109.45	13.3
12	113.40	11.6
18	113.63	17.8
24	126.42	18.9

areas. Similarly, it is assumed that infant intelligence scales can reflect any improvement in competence that results from a specific enrichment experience. Data collected in the course of our longitudinal study of infant affective and cognitive development during the first 24 months of life allow us to consider whether there is any justification for the implicit assumptions.

Our study involved a sample of approximately 20 infants who were tested at regular intervals during their first 24 months (7). There were approximately equal numbers of males and females, and the sample was heterogeneous with respect to social class, although it was slightly skewed toward the upper-middle classes. The mental scale of the Bayley Scale of Infant Development was administered at 3, 6, 9, 12, 18, and 24 months, as was the object permanence scale from Escalona and Corman's (8) Scales of Sensori-motor Development. In addition, at 24 months, infants were given language comprehension and production tasks. These tasks were based on items selected from the Peabody Picture Vocabulary Test. For the comprehension task, standard Peabody instructions were followed, although a restricted number of items were employed. For the production task, subjects were shown individual pictures adopted from the Peabody test and asked, "What is this called?" or "Can you tell me what this is?" Seventeen comprehension and 17 production items were administered to each subject.

Table 1 presents the mean (X) Bayley Mental Development Index (MDI) for each age, together with standard deviations (S.D.). It will be noted that at all ages the mean scores for the MDI are consistently higher than the mean scores for Bayley's standardization sample ($X = 100$; S.D. $= 16$). We believe these differences to be a reflection of the relatively high socioeconomic composition of our sample.

TABLE 2

Mean and Standard Deviation (S.D.) for Object Permanence Scale of Escalona and Corman Scales of Sensori-Motor Development

Age (months)	Mean	S.D.
3	1.10	0.77
6	5.10	1.65
9	8.45	1.90
12	11.80	2.31
18	14.90	1.77
24	15.95	1.39

Table 2 presents mean scores and standard deviations for the object permanence scale of Sensori-motor Development. The scale is constructed to reflect the infant's acquisition of the concept of objects (9); such acquisition is evidenced in our sample by the regular increase in mean score from one age to the next. Mean scores and standard deviations for the language production and comprehension tasks at the age of 24 months are $X = 11.53$, S.D. $= 4.66$ and $X = 11.79$, S.D. $= 4.43$, respectively.

Intercorrelations among the MDI scores at different ages and among the scores on the object permanence scale at different ages are presented in Table 3. As can be seen, of the 30 correlations shown, only four are significant beyond the $P < .05$ level. For the MDI scores, correlations between 3- and 9-month-olds and between 6- and 24-month-olds reached significance, although in each case the correlation (.45 and .54, respec-

TABLE 3

Interage Correlations for the Mental Development Index (Upper Right) and the Permanence Scale (Lower Left)

Age (months)	3	6	Age (months) 9	12	18	24
6		.20	.45*	.06	—.01	—.25
6	—.10		.08	.34	.37	.54*
9	—.10	.00		.40	.13	.00
12	.48*	.16	.31		.29	.26
18	46*	.07	—.13	.32		.36
24	.05	.39	—.07	.08	.05	

* $P < .05$

TABLE 4

CORRELATIONS OF THE THREE MEASURES OF INTELLECTUAL SKILLS
(MDI IS THE MENTAL DEVELOPMENT INDEX)

	Age (months)					
	3	6	9	12	18	24
Correlations of MDI with object permanence	.24	.60*	.16	.09	.23	.02
Correlations of MDI with language at 24 months						
Comprehension	—.19	.40	.10	.22	.42	.49†
Production	—.24	.14	.04	.21	.57*	.48†
Correlation of object permanence with language at 24 months						
Comprehension	.13	.39	—.28	.17	.38	.21
Production	.21	.26	—.34	—.23	—.15	.31

* $P < .01$
† $P < .01$

tively) is relatively low and accounts for less than 30 percent of the variance—relatively useless for predictive purposes. All other MDI correlations are low. Moreover, the data fail to reveal either simplex or other patterns of correlation; for example, MDI scores of 3-month-olds predict neither their scores at 6 months nor their scores at 24 months (indeed, in the latter instance, the correlation is negative). These findings apply across all ages tested (10).

Correlations among scores on the object permanence scale are correspondingly low. Again, only two of them, between 3- and 12-month-olds and between 3- and 18-month-olds, reach significance. Each of these correlations accounts for less than 25 percent of the variance. As with the MDI scores, there is no clear pattern of interrelation in the infant's performance on a sensorimotor function. To further stress the lack of interrelation, we would point out that other work (11) has indicated little or no interrelation over a variety of sensorimotor scales at any particular age. Thus, although for our sample there is an increase in the mean score from one age to another, there is no indication that successful performance at the simpler level is predictive of an infant's ability to succeed in the more complex items when he is older.

Correlations between MDI and object performance at each age and between language development at 24 months and MDI and object permanence at each age are presented in Table 4. The results reveal an interesting pattern of development among the intercorrelations. First, the MDI scales are most closely related to the object permanence scales in the first 6 months of infancy, while the MDI scales are most closely related to language at 18 and 24 months. This result makes good sense, since the early items from the MDI are closely related to sensorimotor functions, while the later MDI items are more closely related to language. Finally, there was no significant relation between the object permanence scale and language ability at the age of 24 months. In fact, there are some rather high negative correlations at 9 months.

A number of general conclusions are justified on the basis of these data. Concerning the lack of predictive validity in infant intelligence scales, there is little to add; as is the case with so many other longitudinal studies, our results indicate that there is no reliable relation between successive measures of infant intelligence during the first 24 months of life. A similar picture emerges with respect to the measure of sensorimotor development—the object permanence scale—employed in our study. Although there was a regular increase in mean scores on this scale from one age to the next, and although the majority of subjects showed a steady rise in scores over the 24-month period (8), high scores at an early age were not predictive of high scores later.

Only at the earlier ages was there any significant association between object permanence and MDI scores, and we attribute this to the fact that, for these ages, both scales measure sensorimotor abilities. After the age of 9 months, none of the correlations between the two scales was significant. There was no association between the early MDI scores and the scores on the language tests at 24 months; however, there were significant correlations between the MDI scores at 18 and 24 months and the language scores at 24 months. There was no association whatever between scores on the object permanence scale and scores on the language tests. For 24-month-olds, of course, the Bayley test has a considerable verbal loading, whereas the object permanence scale has none.

All in all, these findings cast serious doubt on the notion that the concept of general intelligence is applicable to the period of infancy. We have found no evidence to support the view that intelligence is a capacity which unfolds at a steady rate throughout the process of development and which increases only quantitatively from one age to the next. Rather, our data tend to support the view, advanced by Bayley (3), that at each stage of infant development intelligence comprises a set of relatively discrete abilities, or factors. During the early period of development, according to Bayley, these clusters of abilities are relatively age- or stage-specific; therefore there is no necessary continuity between intelligence as defined at one stage of development and as defined at another. Our data, as well as other information (11), indicate that, even with respect to sensorimotor functions, there is a lack of continuity.

Our data also cast doubt on the notion that scores on infant intelligence scales can be generalized beyond the particular set of abilities, or factors, sampled by the items administered at the time of testing. Thus, an infant who showed dramatic gains in tasks involving sensorimotor function would not necessarily manifest such gains on tasks involving verbal skills.

The implications of these conclusions for evaluation of infant intervention programs seem clear. Simply stated, infant intelligence scales are unsuitable instruments for assessing the effects of specific intervention procedures. This is true primarily because infant intelligence is not a general, unitary trait, but is, rather, a composite of skills and abilities that are not necessarily covariant. Such a view of intelligence is by no means new (12), but it is one that appears to require constant restating in order to counteract a tendency to reify simple, single measures of infant intelligence.

Frequently, evaluations of infant intervention programs have been confused because of a failure both to specify clearly the particular set of skills which the program seeks to emphasize and to develop specific criteria for tests of those skills. Consider an intervention procedure that is primarily intended to influence sensorimotor intelligence—for example, the development of object permanence. An appropriate curriculum might involve training subjects in a variety of peek-a-boo and hide-and-seek tasks. It is clear from our data and from the arguments presented above that a standard infant intelligence scale would be the *wrong* instrument to use in assessing the efficiency of such a program and, further, that the use of such an instrument is likely to lead to erroneous conclusions about the program's efficiency. Even more serious is the possibility that, by using the wrong instrument of evaluation in a large number of programs, one would erroneously conclude that intervention in general is ineffective in improving intellectual ability, thereby supporting the view that environment is ineffective in modifying intellgence. There are few who would suggest that schoolchildren should be administered a standard intelligence test after, say, a course in geography. Yet, such a procedure would be analogous to using an intelligence test to measure the success of attempts to teach the object concept to infants. Clearly, the success of a geography course is best assessed by tests of geographical knowledge and understanding; by the same token, the success of a program stressing sensorimotor skill is best assessed by specific tests of sensorimotor ability. In both cases, there may be some instances of improvement in intelligence test scores, but such improvement has to be regarded as fortuitous.

It cannot be emphasized too strongly that the success of specific intervention programs must be assessed according to specific criteria related to the content of the program. By focusing attention upon the criteria for evaluating programs, the necessity for careful specification of the program's goals will be emphasized. As argued above, the failure to specify goals has been a contributing factor in the confusion over means of evaluating intervention programs.

The nature and structure of infant intelligence is a complex and, as yet, unsolved problem. In our search for social relevance, we must not be misled into thinking that the worth of our efforts can be determined solely by the magnitude of infants' scores on intelligence tests of demonstrably limited generality.

REFERENCES

1. BURT, C., JONES, E., MILLER, E., & MOODIE, W.: *How the Mind Works*. New York: Appleton-Century-Crofts, 1934.
2. BAYLEY, N.: *Genet. Psychol. Monogr.*, 14, 1, 1933.
3. BAYLEY, N.: in P. H. Mussen (Ed.), *Carmichael's Manual of Child Psychology*. New York: Wiley, 1970, pp. 1163-1209.
4. STOTT, L. H. & BALL, R. S.: *Infant and Preschool Mental Tests: Review and Evaluation* (Monographs of the Society for Research in Child Development No. 30, serial No. 3, Chicago: Univ. of Chicago Press, 1965).
5. THOMAS, H.: *Merrill-Palmer Quart. Behav. Develop.*, 16 (No. 2), 179, 1970.
6. BAYLEY, N.: *Amer. Psychol.*, 10, 805, 1955.
7. Not all infants were able to complete all tests. The smallest N for which data are reported here is 19. Data from an additional 120 infants, seen cross-sectionally at 3, 6, 9, 12, 18, and 24 months (20 infants at each age), were essentially similar to those reported here.
8. ESCALONA, S. K., & CORMAN, H. H.: "The validation of Piaget's hypotheses concerning the development of sensori-motor intelligence: methodological issues," paper presented at the meeting of the Society for Research in Child Development, New York, 1967.
9. PIAGET, J.: *The Origins of Intelligence in Children*. M. Cook (Transl.). New York: International Universities Press, 1952.
10. These results cannot be attributed to low instrument reliability. Bayley has reported split-half reliabilities ranging from .81 to .92, although she too fails to obtain any stability across these early ages (*Manual of Bayley Scales of Infant Development*. New York: Psychological Corporation, 1969).
11. KING, W. & SEEGMILLER, B.: "Cognitive development from 14-22 months of age in black, male, first-born infants by the Bayley and Hunt-Uzgiris scales." Paper presented at a meeting of the Society for Research in Child Development, Minneapolis, 1971.
12. GUILFORD, J. P.: *Amer. Psychol.*, 14, 469, 1959.
13. This research was supported by National Science Foundation grant 28105 and a grant from the Spencer Foundation.

5

TRANSITIONS IN INFANT SENSORI-MOTOR DEVELOPMENT AND THE PREDICTION OF CHILDHOOD IQ

Robert B. McCall, Pamela Savoy Hogarty, and

Nancy Hurlburt

Fels Research Institute, Yellow Springs, Ohio

Over the last 50 years, there have been numerous attempts to relate developmental test scores, obtained during infancy, to standardized intelligence tests, given later in adolescence and adulthood. Reviews of this literature (Bayley, 1970; Rutter, 1970; Stott & Ball, 1965; Thomas, 1970) tend to concur with Bayley's summarization:

> The findings of these early studies of mental growth of infants have been repeated sufficiently often so that it is now well-established that test scores earned in the first year or two have relatively little predictive validity (in contrast to tests at school age or later), although they may have high validity as measures of the children's cognitive ability at the time [p. 1174].

Reprinted from AMERICAN PSYCHOLOGIST, Vol. 27, No. 8, August 1972, pp. 728-748. Copyright 1972 by the American Psychological Association and reproduced by permission.

This research was supported by Grant HD-04160 to the senior author; by United States Public Health Service Grants FR-05537, HD-00686, and FR-00222 to the Fels Research Institute; and by the Fels Fund of Philadelphia. Portions of this report would not be possible without the 42 years of effort by the staff of the Fels Research Institute and its Director Emeritus, L. W. Sontag, and by the continuing support of the Fels Fund of Philadelphia. The authors thank John Bench, Virginia Crandall, Jerome Kagan, and A. F. Roche for their insightful comments on early forms of this manuscript.

This conclusion is disappointing and perhaps perplexing to some. It is disappointing because if one could predict later mental performance, one might be able to select certain infants for specialized early educational experiences, detect incipient mental abnormalities, evaluate obstetric and pediatric practices, etc. The conclusion may be perplexing, because one might wonder how it is possible for a test to have concurrent but not predictive validity as an index of mental ability.

The apparent paradox may dissolve for one of at least two classes of reasons. First, perhaps correlations are low for some psychometric circumstance (Rutter, 1970). For example, correlations with later IQ could be depressed if the infant test has poor reliability or if sex differences exist but combined-sex samples are used. Moreover, predictions might increase if the infant test score were used in combination with other information (e.g., parental socioeconomic status) or if specific item subsets rather than the total score were examined. However, a second explanation for the apparent failure to predict later IQ may lie implicitly in the basic concept of "intelligence." One may need to discard the reified notion of intelligence as an unchanging characteristic that governs nearly all of an individual's mental performance at every age. Despite the incredibly pervasive and restrictive character of this assumption, psychologists have apparently been willing to make it, explicitly or implicitly, throughout most of modern psychological history. There are many alternatives to this conception, for example: (a) The nature of general intelligence changes with development, and thus correlations are minimal between tests of mental ability assessed at developmentally distant ages; (b) there is no such thing as "general intelligence" or "g" at any age, but there are skills which have functional utility at a given developmental level that may emerge, change, and/or disappear as development progresses; or (c) there is neither general intelligence nor much continuity from one age to another in the performance of so-called mental tasks, at least during infancy and early childhood.

The purpose of this article is twofold. First, the empirical literature concerning the prediction of childhood and adult IQ scores from infancy is reviewed, with a special focus on the possibility of psychometric factors clouding long-term prediction. Second, since most of that research was inspired by and executed under the assumption of an immutable, pervasive, general intellectual trait, the other goal of this article is to consider an alternative conception of intelligence, to describe its theoretical nature, and to illustrate empirically its possible character.

TABLE 1

MEDIAN CORRELATIONS BETWEEN INFANT TESTS AND
CHILDHOOD IQ FOR NORMAL CHILDREN

Childhood age (years)	Age in infancy (months)			
	1–6	7–12	13–18	19–30
8–18	.01 (12/4)	.20 (8/2)	.21 (6/2)	.49 (9/2)
5–7	.01 (7/5)	.06 (5/4)	.30 (5/4)	.41 (16/4)
3–4	.23 (7/4)	.33 (5/3)	.47 (6/4)	.54 (16/3)

Note.—The number of correlations entering into the median and the number of different studies included are found in parentheses.

EARLY RESEARCH

Prediction from Infancy

Normal children. It is something of an overstatement to say that there is "no prediction" from the infancy period to childhood IQ. There are correlations that attain statistical significance between certain ages for some tests, but the size of the relationships is not particularly impressive and certainly not adequate for clinical application (e.g., see Table 1). Table 1 displays the median level of prediction from several ages during the first 30 months of life to childhood IQ measured between 3 and 18 years. This table was compiled by taking the data from L. D. Anderson (1939), Bayley (1949), Cavanaugh, Cohen, Dunphy, Ringwell and Goldberg (1957), Escalona and Moriarty (1961), Honzik (1938), Moore (1967), Nelson and Richards (1938, 1939), and Werner, Honzik, and Smith (1968). All correlations from these studies were used, and the table presents the median correlation for the different age combinations. The number of correlations entering into the median and the number of different studies included are found in parentheses. These data ignore the fact that different tests were used, that correlations in different cells are not always independent of one another, and that these results are weighted heavily with Bayley's (1949) and Honzik's (1938) data. Nevertheless, these data do give a descriptive impression of the level of prediction for normal children.

There are two obvious trends in the table. The first is that when predicting to any age in childhood, the later the test is given during the infancy period, the higher the relationship. Second, correlations to IQ at 3-4 years are higher than with IQ scores assessed thereafter.

Nonnormal samples. One purpose of developing infant tests was to detect children who might have severe pathologies. Attempts have been made to detect mental retardation (Hunt & Bayley, 1971; Illingworth, 1961), prematurity (Drillien, 1961), schizophrenia (Fish, 1957, 1960; Fish, Shapiro, Halpern, & Wile, 1965), and neonatal apnea (Stechler, 1964). Several studies have correlated total score on infant tests with later IQ for samples involving subjects having extremely low infant test scores or subjects having known or suspected abnormalities. For example, Werner et al. (1968) correlated the score on the Cattell Infant Scale given at 20 months with 10-year Primary Mental Ability scores. While the correlation for a normal group of children was .49, those subjects scoring below 80 on the infant test had a correlation of .71 with 10-year Primary Mental Ability scores. In a series of reports, Knobloch and Pasamanick (1960, 1963, 1967) have shown that the prediction from the Gesell given within the first year of life to childhood IQ is much better for a clinical population than for a normal group. For example, the correlation between 40-week Gesell and 3-year Gesell was .74 for a group of 48 infants considered abnormal, but only .43 for normal children.[*] They also indicate that prediction between infancy and childhood IQ for those infants scoring below 80 is higher than for subjects scoring above 80 ($r = .66$ versus .46, respectively). Greater predictability for low scores on the Bayley has also been reported by Ireton, Thwing, and Gravem (1970). These several authors concluded that the Gesell test may have predictive value for clinic populations.

This view is supported further by the data of Honzik, Hutchings, and Burnip (1965). Pediatricians examined the birth records of a large sample of infants and categorized them on the basis of birth records into groups ranging between "definitely suspect" and "normal." The Bayley Infant Scale was administered to these infants at 8 months without knowledge of this categorization. Infants ranked "definitely suspect" on the basis of birth information had lower scores on the Bayley at 8 months. Given the probable basis of the pediatricians' rankings and the nature of the 8-month Bayley, this result likely indicates at least short-term continuity in neuromotor abnormalities. Further, Werner et al. (1968) reported impressive information that either a low score on the Cattell *or* a bad prognosis by a pediatrician at 20 months has fairly

---

[*] Unfortunately, Knobloch and Pasamanick's (1960) concurrent correlations have been erroneously reported as predictive relationships in some secondary sources. The correlation between 3-year Gesell (*not* 40-week Gesell) and 3-year Binet was .87.

accurate prognostic value in indicating low levels of Primary Mental Ability performance at 10 years. Briefly, infant tests may have contemporary as well as predictive utility in identifying pathological and "suspect" conditions in infancy, and a very low score on an infant test, even though a pediatrician does not classify the child as abnormal (and vice versa), may have diagnostic value.

While the correlations for suspect and clinical populations are high, they must be applied with caution. Often, correlations in the range of .70-.80 for special clinical populations are cited as justification for use of the assessment instrument to screen more randomly selected populations. This is not always practical because of the difference in base rate of abnormality in the clinical versus the random sample. Consider the following hypothetical illustration. Suppose a test correctly diagnoses 90% of the infants known to have mental deficiency while incorrectly classifying only 15% of normal infants as being deficient when two groups of 100 definitely abnormals and 100 normals are studied. This would be regarded as an excellent testimony to the validity of the test. However, when a random sample of 1,000 infants is selected, only 50 of whom are truly deficient, while the test correctly identifies 90% or 45 of the 50 abnormals, it also labels 15% or 142 normals as being deficient. The false-positive *rate* is tolerable, but the *absolute number* of false positives in a randomly selected population would make the test impractical as a screening device.

Caution should also be invoked on theoretical grounds. The correlations reported for clinical samples may merely reflect the presence of some subjects whose deficiencies are so marked that there is practically no behavior to assess at either age. Such low scores by "default" can produce sizable correlations in an otherwise variable sample, but they are neither theoretically nor practically interesting. Consequently, infant tests in concert with other assessment techniques may have value in detecting neuromotor abnormalities, but sole reliance on the test in applied clinical situations must be tempered by the size and source of the correlations as well as by considerations of base rate.

Reliability of Infant Scales

Whenever one fails to get a relationship between two test scores, one of the first concerns is the reliability of the instruments. Few people question the reliability of childhood IQ scores since test-retest correlations with as long as three years between testings rarely fall below .85. In contrast, many people suspect that the infant tests are unreliable, but this does not seem to be the case.

The most exhaustively researched infant test is the Bayley Infant Scale. In general, the split-half and test-retest reliabilities of these scales are quite good after 3 months of age, though there is some suggestion that the mental scale is slightly more reliable than the motor. For the original version of the test, Bayley (1931) reported split-half coefficients corrected by the Spearman-Brown formula of approximately .63 during the first 3 months and .93 from 3 to 12 months for the total mental score. Test-retest correlations with a 1-month interval between testings were approximately .58 for the first 4 months, but in the high .80s thereafter. The motor scale was found to have less reliability and relatively little cross-age consistency compared to the mental scale, though the motor test has considerably fewer items (Bayley, 1935).

The reliability of the revised Bayley (1965) scales is equally impressive. The internal consistency (Kuder-Richardson correction) for the mental scales is .79 during the first month and .84-.94 between 2 and 15 months. The internal consistency of the motor scale increases from .57 at 1 month to .89 at 6 months, the coefficients being relatively stable thereafter. Finally, in a study using two observers as well as a test-retest paradigm (1-week interval), test-retest agreement was achieved on 76% of the items for both the mental and motor scales, but the inter-observer agreement was 89% for the mental and 93% for the motor scale (Werner & Bayley, 1966).

The picture is similar for other infant scales (see review by Werner & Bayley, 1966). The corrected split-half coefficients for the Gesell test at 6, 12, and 18 months were .89, .84, and .79, respectively (Richards & Nelson, 1939), figures comparable to those obtained with the Linfert-Hierholzer test (Furfey & Muehlenbein, 1932). For the Cattell scale, test-retest reliabilities (interval of 1½-7 days) at 16-29 months were .80-.96, and the comparable figures for the Kuhlmann test were .79-.85 (Harms & Spiker, 1959).

Consequently, while the reliabilities are not particularly high during the first 3 months (though there are reliable neonatal examinations), the internal consistency and the test-retest comparability of infant scales after 3 months of age (particularly for the mental scales) are substantial (high .80s and low .90s). Since the infant tests are approximately as reliable as the childhood IQ assessments, reliability does not appear to be a major factor in the failure to obtain prediction from infancy to later intelligence.

Sex Differences

Almost all of the reports of infant-childhood test correlations described above used mixed samples with respect to sex. While sex differences are not usually found for the general scores from the Bayley (1933, 1935, 1965) or the Gesell tests (Nelson & Richards, 1938, 1939; but see Dales, 1969; Goffeney, Henderson, & Butler, 1971; Willerman, Broman, & Fielder, 1970), this fact does not obviate differences in cross-age correlations for the sexes. If the sexes differ in the nature of the relationship between infant performance and later IQ, combining the sexes into a single sample might prevent these relationships from appearing.

Working with the London longitudinal data, Moore (1967) correlated scores on the Griffiths Baby Scale at 6 and 18 months with Binet IQs at 3, 5, and 8 years, separately for each sex. While the correlations from infancy to the 3-year Binet are not different for the sexes, the relations with the 5-year and 8-year Binet are higher for females than for males, though not significantly so. Werner et al. (1968) found no sex differences in the prediction from 20-month Cattell scores to 10-year Primary Mental Abilities performance; but Goffeney et al. (1971) correlated Bayley mental and motor scores (gross and fine) assessed at 8 months with the Wechsler Intelligence Scale for Children (WISC) at 7 years and found somewhat more significant correlations for girls than for boys. This was especially true for black subjects (none of the 12 correlations was significant for black males). Hunt and Bayley (1971) reported unpublished work by Bruehl indicating that there were more positive predictors for girls but more negative predictors for boys between the "age at first passage" of Bayley test items and Wechsler subtest scores between 16 and 36 years for the Berkeley Growth Study sample.

While Nelson and Richards (1938, 1939) reported correlations between infant scores and early childhood IQ for the data from the Fels Research Institute's longitudinal study, they did not separate the sexes. This sample* is now considerably larger, and Table 2 presents the correlations between the Gesell test given at 6, 12, 18, and 24 months and Stanford-Binet at 3½, 6, and 10 years. Tests for sex differences at each age are given also. Note first that these correlations are generally higher than for other studies (see Table 1). Second, a rather consistent pattern

---

* All subjects in the Fels study with at least one pair of infant-childhood mental assessments were included in this analysis. This sample is described in detail elsewhere (e.g., Kagan & Moss, 1962; Sontag, Baker, & Nelon, 1958), and is composed of middle- and upper-middle-class children born after April 1930, and living in rural and small-town Ohio. Omitted or ambiguous items on the Gesell were counted as missed.

TABLE 2

Correlations of Total Gesell Scores in Infancy with Childhood Stanford–Binet IQ (Fels Data)

Gesell test given at:		Girls			Boys			Sex difference test	
			Age of childhood IQ test (years)						
	3½	6	10	3½	6	10	3½	6	10
6 months									
r	.26**	.22*	.05	−.01	−.06	.07	z 1.99	1.70	.12
N	102	79	68	112	71	72	p .02	.045	.45
12 months									
r	.57***	.51***	.37**	.16	.22*	.12	z 3.53	2.03	1.55
N	105	80	67	112	70	75	p .0002	.02	.06
18 months									
r	.50***	.43***	.42**	.35***	.28*	.27*	z 1.26	.90	.90
N	94	70	57	99	61	62	p .10	.18	.18
24 months									
r	.74***	.65***	.53***	.58***	.39***	.59***	z 1.95	1.04	−.24
N	88	69	58	100	63	59	p .025	.15	.41

* $p < .05$, one-tailed.
** $p < .01$, one-tailed.
*** $p < .001$, one-tailed.

of sex differences emerges, though the correlations are not independent of one another because of substantial (but not total) overlap in the samples at different age periods. Except for the fact that there is no significant prediction from 6 months to 10 years for either sex, the correlations from 6 and 12 months to other childhood ages are all significantly higher for girls than for boys. Predicting from 2 years of age, girls show greater short-term consistency, but the two sexes are equal in forecasting 10-year Binet IQ.

While Werner et al. (1968) found no sex differences in the prediction from 20-month Cattell to 10-year Primary Mental Abilities scores and Moore (1967) reported only minor sex differences in the relationship between the Griffiths Infant Scale and a modified Binet, the Fels data using the Gesell test are particularly emphatic in illustrating greater predictability for females than for males, especially for assessments made in the first year of life.

Unfortunately, these conflicting results are difficult to interpret. The studies differ in sample characteristics, national origin, infant and childhood tests, etc. One of several hypotheses is that the Gesell infant test might be a better predictor of childhood Binet IQ, especially for girls, than other infant mental assessment techniques. Regrettably, there are very few comparisons of infant tests. The only data that can be cited indicate that scores on the Gesell test may not be as comparable to other infant tests. For example, Caldwell and Drachman (1964) examined the Cattell, Griffiths, and a "composite test" that the authors constructed mostly from Gesell items. They tested infants between 6 weeks and 2 years of age (both whites and blacks in the sample). The Cattell and Griffiths scales correlated .84-.94 at various ages in the infancy period. The "composite test" (i.e., modified Gesell) correlated only .46-.77 with the Cattell and Griffiths during the first year of life but .89-.97 thereafter. There were also mean differences in scores between the tests. Therefore, despite considerable item overlap among infant tests, there may be nontrivial differences between them, particularly during the first year.

Moreover, there are additional suggestions that the Gesell may predict later IQ measures better than other infant tests. Some of the highest correlations in the literature between infant behavior and childhood IQ have been based on Gesell scores (Knobloch & Pasamanick, 1960; Nelson & Richards, 1938, 1939), although a firm conclusion cannot be drawn because of the many differences between studies using different tests. Nevertheless, the data are consistent with the suspicion that Gesell predictions to childhood IQ may be higher than for other infant tests and that girls may be more predictable from the first year of life than boys, but long-term predictability from later in the infancy period appears to be comparable for the two sexes.

Socioeconomic Status

The infant test might predict later mental performance better if its score were used in combination with some other variable, such as the socioeconomic (occupational and/or educational) status of the parents.

In considering this hypothesis, one observes that parental socioeconomic status does not relate to infant test performance until the second or third year of life* (Bayley, 1933, 1935, 1954, 1965; Golden & Birns, 1968; Golden, Birns, Bridger, & Moss, 1971; Honzik, 1963; Kagan & Moss, 1959; MacRae, 1955; Willerman et al., 1970). Bayley's (1954) data relating midparent education and child IQ indicate a rather sharp rise in the correlation from zero to an asymptote of .60 between 1½ and 4 years (peak rise at 2 years). Other studies find similar results, but the age at which the relationship begins (2-5 years) and the nature of sex differences (girls earlier than boys) vary somewhat from study to study (e.g., Honzik, 1963; Kagan & Moss, 1959). Honzik's (1957) demonstration that these identical relationships hold for adopted children and their biological mother's education but not for their rearing mother's education suggests that these data reflect the changing nature of the mental ability required by these tests rather than the potential of the environment to mold IQ test performance (though other data suggest that socioeconomic status is a factor). Furthermore, these results imply that parental education may be a better predictor of childhood IQ than an assessment on the child during the first 2 years of life.

Several researchers have attempted to increase the level of prediction by combining some measure of socioeconomic status with the infant test score in a multiple-regression formula. One of the first was by L. D. Anderson (1939), who in a post hoc manner tried to increase the level of prediction by picking only those items on his infant test that seemed to discriminate between children having exceptionally low Binet scores at 5 years. He then attempted to add mother's and father's educational level into a multiple regression and found correlations increased by approximately .10 over item predictions alone. More recently, Knobloch and Pasamanick (1967) gave 123 children the Gesell at 4-12 months and the Binet at 6-10 years. A multiple regression including the Gesell score,

---

* Parental socioeconomic status does relate to certain specific behavior (e.g., some Piaget tests) during early infancy. (Décarie, 1965; Wachs, Uzgiris, & Hunt, 1971).

socioeconomic status, and the persistence of convulsive seizures produced an R of .84 versus an R of .70 for the Gesell alone. For subjects scoring lower than .80 on the Gesell, the multiple R was .90 versus .71. It is difficult to evaluate these figures for the present purpose because of the mixed nature of the sample (clinic and normal subjects) and the impossibility of separating the contribution of seizures from socioeconomic status to the multiple R.

Hindley and Munro (1970) factor analyzed the Griffiths Infant Scale given at 18 months and then attempted to predict later IQ with the factor scores and social class. These analyses produced several interesting results. First, parental social class correlated with child 11-year Binet at a much higher level for both males and females (.50, .56) than did the infant test (.10, .39). Social class did not produce significant correlations with the infant test, though they were opposite in sign for males and females. The multiple correlations between socioeconomic status-infant test and 11-year Binet were relatively equivalent for both sexes (.55, .62) but not a great deal higher than the bivariate correlations between socioeconomic status alone and childhood Binet. Moreover, statistical control of the general infant factor did not greatly alter the relationship between socioeconomic status and 11-year Binet (partial $rs = .55, .50$). Thus, the infant test did not appear related to the socioeconomic status-childhood IQ association. The overriding impression is that the social class of the parents is a moderately good predictor of the child's 11-year IQ and that the infant test is of little additional value.

Similar conclusions were reached by Ireton et al. (1970), who examined the relationship between 8-month Bayley scores, socioeconomic status, and 4-year Binet performance. Their data indicated that while both measures related to later IQ, socioeconomic status is a better predictor than the infant test, predictive correlations derive mostly from low scores for the infant test but from the entire range of socioeconomic status, and low mental score in infancy is a better predictor of low childhood IQ than low socioeconomic status. The infant test apparently has value in picking out relatively permanent deficits in neuromotor functioning, but socioeconomic status is a better predictor than the infant test for the average and above average infant.

These results prompted examination of the Fels data regarding the correlation between Gesell tests administered during the first 2 years and childhood IQ. The education score from the Hollingshead two-factor index of social position was obtained for the parents of the children providing the data in Table 2. Gesell total scores at 6, 12, 18, and 24 months were entered separately into a multiple regression with

TABLE 3

BIVARIATE AND MULTIPLE CORRELATIONS OF INFANT GESELL SCORE AND PARENTAL EDUCATION WITH CHILDHOOD STANFORD–BINET IQ FOR DIFFERENT AGE COMBINATIONS (FELS DATA)

Age at testing		Males			Females		
Infant (months)	Child (years)	Gesell-IQ	Parental education-IQ	Multiple R	Gesell-IQ	Parental education-IQ	Multiple R
6	3½	−.01	.36***	.36*	.26**	.40***	.49***
6	6	−.06	.33**	.33*	.22*	.50***	.56***
6	10	.07	.47***	.49***	.05	.42***	.43**
12	3½	.16	.36***	.39*	.57***	.40***	.68***
12	6	.22*	.33**	.39*	.51***	.50***	.69***
12	10	.12	.47***	.48***	.37**	.42***	.54***
18	3½	.35***	.36***	.53***	.50***	.40***	.67***
18	6	.28*	.33**	.46***	.43***	.50***	.69***
18	10	.27*	.47***	.57***	.42**	.42***	.63***
24	3½	.58***	.36***	.68***	.74***	.40***	.80***
24	6	.39***	.33**	.51***	.65***	.50***	.77***
24	10	.59***	.47***	.75***	.53***	.42***	.63***

Note.—Gesell and parental education: $r = −.17, .04, .10, .01$ at 6, 12, 18, 24 months, respectively, for males; $−.07, .06, −.10, .15$ for females. Ns between 57 and 112 (see Table 2).

* $p < .05$.
** $p < .01$.
*** $p < .001$, all one-tailed.

parental education level to predict childhood Binet score at 3½, 6, and 10 years. These data are presented in Table 3, which displays the Infant × Childhood age combination in the lefthand column, the bivariate correlation between the Gesell and the childhood Binet at the ages indicated on that row (data the same as in Table 2), the bivariate correlation between parental education and childhood IQ, and the multiple correlation between Gesell test and parental education with childhood IQ.

There are several things to observe in this table. First, as expected, the relationship between Gesell score and parental education (indicated at the bottom of Table 3) was quite minimal. Second, when predicting from the 6-month Gesell, the multiple correlation involving both the Gesell and parental education is not much better at predicting later IQ than parental education alone. In short, at 6 months, one might as well disregard the infant test and use parental education alone as a predictor of childhood IQ. At 12 months, there is still almost no advantage in using the infant test in addition to parental education for boys, but there is some for girls: the combination of Gesell and parental education raises the level of prediction .10-.20 over the bivariate relationships. By 18 months, there is some degree of advantage in using both the infant test and parental education for both sexes.

In summary, there appears to be some justification for considering other variables in concert with the infant test when attempting to predict later IQ. Specifically, for normal infants parental education or socioeconomic status is probably a better single predictor than the infant test during the first 12-18 months of life. Thereafter, the level of prediction may be elevated slightly by adding the infant test score into a multiple regression with socioeconomic status, and the multivariate advantage may occur at an earlier age for girls than for boys.

Specific Items and Abilities

Another approach to the problem of prediction from infancy is based on the proposition that specific subgroups of items within the test might have greater predictive saliency than the total score. If many of the items on an infant test are irrelevant to the future course of cognitive growth, they would contribute "noise" to the total score which would mask the effect of items that actually are predictors of later mental performance. For example, Filmore (1936) found that while the total score of a test given at 12 months correlated only .19 with IQ at 2-3 years, some individual items had biserial correlations as high as .47 (e.g., "piling some blocks"). Similarly, Hunt and Bayley (1971) have isolated subsets of items that are relatively "hard" or "easy" for mental retardates. Further, Nelson and Richards (1938, 1939) observed that relatively few of the items on the 6-month and 12-month Gesell that correlated with IQ at age 3 were also among the leading item correlates of the Gesell total score. This implies that the total score did not reflect faithfully the infant's performance on items that showed the greatest correlation with later intelligence.

Following Nelson and Richards, infants were selected from the Fels study who had at least one Gesell test at either 6, 12, 18, and/or 24 months and who also had at least one of the following general IQ scores: the Binet at 3½, 6, and 10 years; the WISC at 7 or 11 years; and/or the Wechsler-Bellevue at 13 years. The 15 items on each of the four Gesell tests which had the highest correlation with the total score at that age were defined arbitrarily as the set most representative of the test (i.e., the total score). Then all items on the four Gesell tests which had significant ($p < .05$) relationships with any one of the childhood IQ tests were selected, and it was asked if the childhood correlates and the infant total score correlates were the same items. Several patterns of results emerged. First, the percentage of items that predicted later IQ and also correlated in the top 15 with the Gesell total score was smaller at the younger than at the older infant ages (25%, 38%, 43%, 46%, respectively, at 6, 12, 18, and 24 months). This seems to imply that the Gesell total score may be somewhat less representative of the predictive power of the item pool in the first than in the second year of life. Second, across all four Gesell tests there were more items that predicted later IQ for girls than for boys (96 versus 68), and more of these predicting items were among the 15 most highly correlated with the total Gesell score for girls than for boys (39 versus 27). However, the *percentage* of predicting items that were also correlated with the total score was essentially the same for the two sexes (41% versus 40%). These observations suggest that while girls show more Gesell item predictions to later IQ, the total score on the Gesell is equally reflective of the potential of the test for predicting IQ for each sex. It seems that specific items and abilities might be more predictive of later IQ than the total score of an infant test and that there may be sex differences with respect to which items and skills are most predictive. Of course, one would expect that some individual items would correlate with later intelligence more than others in normal children (L. D. Anderson, 1939) and in retardates or children having suspected neurological impairments (Honzik, Hutchings, & Burnit, 1965; Hunt & Bayley, 1971). The issue is whether there is any consistency in the general nature of items that predict later mental ability versus items that do not.

The most replicable item subset which predicts from infancy to later IQ involves early vocalization behavior, and the predictions are found more frequently for girls than for boys. Kagan (1969, 1971), who conducted a longitudinal study of the first 3 years of life, reported that the amount of vocalization an infant female made to the presentation of facial stimuli was relatively stable over three assessments during the first year and that these responses predicted spontaneous verbal behavior at 2½ years (but not general IQ). The stability and predictive power occurred for girls but not for boys. In England, Moore (1967) found that the "speech quotient" on the 1954 Griffiths Infant Scale was fairly stable between 6 and 18 months of life for girls ($r = .51$) but not for boys (.15), and that the 18-month speech quotient predicted vocabulary (.55), comprehension (.53), and general IQ (.50), at 8 years of age for girls but not for boys (—.06, .12, and .20, respectively). Moreover, Cameron, Livson, and Bayley (1967) clustered the age-of-first-passage of the items on the Bayley Infant Scale for the Berkeley Growth Study sample. Since the Bayley test had been given monthly for the first 15 months, for any particular item the child received a number corresponding to his age when he first passed that item. When these scores were clustered, one grouping that was weighted heavily with vocalization items (e.g., vocalizes eagerness, displeasure, interjections; says "da-da," two words, etc.) showed a correlation with verbal IQ that rose throughout life to an impressive peak of approximately .74 at 26 years. Again, this was true only for girls.

In summary, three studies indicate that vocalization in infancy may have a special salience for females that it does not connote for males with respect to predicting later mental performance. It is unlikely that this sex difference is merely a simple reflection of precocious verbal behavior on the part of females relative to males. If this were true, then the age-of-first-passing scores (Cameron et al., 1967) would merely be a few months younger for girls than for boys, and such a difference in the means of these distributions should not influence the correlation. Thus, there may be some qualitative sense in which early vocalization behavior has special meaning for girls.

What might be the predictor for males that is analogous to vocalization? One hint comes from Bayley's (1970) report in which she subjected the age-of-first-passing scores for the items from the California First Year Mental Scale (Bayley Scale) and the California Preschool Scale to a cluster analysis. Two of the 12 clusters showed some prediction to later

IQ. The first-year cluster was the vocalization grouping described above and reported by Cameron et al. (1967). While it did predict later verbal intelligence for the girls through 26 years, it did so for boys only through 3 years of age (Bayley, 1966; Cameron et al., 1967). A preschool factor called "verbal knowledge" ("What runs? What cries? Place a block in, on, under, behind, etc.") correlated with IQ for both sexes ($rs = .40$-$.75$) until age 18, after which the correlations continued through age 36 for males but declined for females. It is difficult to interpret this sex difference, since the mental test used in the Berkeley Growth Study was the Binet up to age 18 when the Wechsler tests were introduced and used thereafter. It may be that sex differences in the prediction of later intelligence are not only linked with particular items and certain infant tests but also with the particular test used to assess later IQ (see following discussion).

SOME REDIRECTION

Basic Concept of Development

The search for correlational stability across vastly different ages implies a faith in a developmentally constant, general conception of intelligence that presumably governs an enormous variety of mental activities. Under that assumption, the nature of the behavioral manifestations of "g" would change from age to age, but g itself is presumed constant, and thus mental precocity at one age should predict mental precocity at another. Confronted with the evidence reviewed above, this g model of mental development must be questioned. Voices dissonant with the general intelligence conception were heard early, but they were in the minority. J. E. Anderson (1939) suggested that there is actually no prediction of *developmental increments;* there is only longitudinal prediction to the extent that the development at one age has already been attained at an earlier age. For example, while there are correlations between height in infancy and height in adulthood, there is no correlation between height in infancy and yearly *increments* in height (Bloom, 1964). The following discussion emphasizes one empirical approach to developmental transitions in performance during infancy and childhood that makes somewhat less restrictive conceptual assumptions concerning mental traits and their development than many previous orientations.

It is quite likely that the several skills that characterize a given stage in infancy will vary considerably in the extent to which they share common determinants. Thus, at any specific age there might be some skills that are highly related and others that are independent. This same proposition may apply when skills are viewed *developmentally*. Consequently, one way to approach the study of mental development in the first several years of life is to consider the enormous matrix of possible Skills × Skills × Ages (ideally, developmental level), and to ask not only which skills are related to or independent from other skills *within an age* (Skills × Skills) but which skills are related to which other skills *across ages*. The cross-age correlations mark one type of developmental transition.

The belief in an unchanging, pervasive general mental ability assumed that there was some constant determinant that governed the performance of a vast number of skills both within and across ages, and thus one should expect high within-age correlations among diverse behaviors and a single, unified, and continuous trend of relationship across age. The fact that many different abilities of childhood did show positive intercorrelations presumably testified to a single underlying dimension which then became reified under the rubric of intelligence (or g). Soon, intelligence was used to explain the very behavior that mothered its theoretical existence. The evidence for a single major mental ability either within an age (e.g., the independent "dimensions" of Guilford, 1967; or the "creativity" of Wallach & Kogan, 1965) or across age (see preceding review) is not very convincing. However, neither do these data argue for the conceptually opposite conclusion. It seems unlikely that there are no common processes underlying some mental activities, no hierarchical organization of skills, no generality from one task to another, and no predictability from one age to another for some processes. The Skills × Skills × Ages matrix of correlations is neither homogeneously 1.00 nor .00.

Consequently, one model of mental performance with heuristic value might fall somewhere between these two extremes (e.g., see Bayley, 1970). First, one would suppose that within any given age (or developmental level), one could discern subsets of skills that would be highly related within a set but the subsets would be independent from one another. Some of these skill sets might possess relationships with similar of qualitatively different skill sets at a future age; other might lead to a "dead end" in terms of their developmental significance. The matrix of developmental transitions and interactions might be quite complex.

The remainder of this essay is devoted to describing empirically such possible transitions during infancy and childhood with the purpose of illustrating this conceptual approach and generating hypotheses about the fabric of early development.

Developmental Transitions in the Fels Data

The responses of infants to individual items on Gesell tests at 6, 12, 18, and 24 months of age were subjected to principal component analyses separately at each age. The resulting components presumably represented independent skill areas within each age. Next, the component scores were correlated across age (and with childhood IQ scores) and the network of developmental transitions examined. A similar statistical model has been used provocatively by Livson (1965) to discern continuities in personality development in the Child Guidance Study data at Berkeley and by Bell, Weller, and Waldrop (1971) to observe transitions between the neonatal, preschool, and school periods.

Subjects and analyses. The subjects were all children from the Fels population who had at least one Gesell test at either 6, 12, 18, or 24 months,* and who had at least one of the following assessments in childhood: a Binet at 3½, 6, or 10 years; the WISC at 7 or 11 years; or the Wechsler-Bellevue at 13 years. Logically dependent items on the infant tests (e.g., "sits with slight support," "sits alone") were combined into a single item within each of the four Gesell assessments, leaving 32, 33, 34, and 28 items on each of the four Gesell tests, respectively. The subjects' responses to these were subjected to principal components analyses separately at each age (6, 12, 18, 24 months) on the combined-sex sample ($N = 158, 148, 145, 144$, respectively). Separate component analyses were performed for the two sexes, but no major sex differences were found. However, while the component structure within each age did not appear different for the sexes, the correlations between component scores across age did contain sex differences (see following results).

Results. The component scores at each age were correlated. The correlation matrix is depicted graphically for boys (Figure 1) and girls (Figure 2). In these figures, the boxes represent components, and the number within the box indicates whether it was the first, second, etc., component extracted at that age. Shaded boxes denote that at least one correlation between this component and a childhood IQ assessment (any Binet total score, or Wechsler verbal, performance, or total score for the tests indicated above) was significant ($p < .05$, two-tailed). The numbers placed above the lines connecting boxes indicate the correlation between these two component scores, with the asterisks indicating the significance of the correlation and the triangles denoting the significance of the difference between the sexes on this correlation (asterisk or tri-

---

* Only subjects having no ambiguous or missing item responses were included.

BOYS

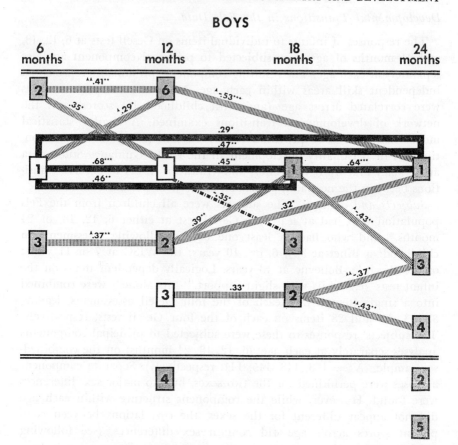

FIG. 1. Correlation matrix depicted graphically for boys. (See text for explanation.)

angle signifies $p < .05$, two-tailed). Boxes below the double line are components that predicted later IQ but were not involved in any significant pattern of continuity through the infancy period.

Figures 1 and 2 may be viewed as representing one estimate of the network of behavioral transitions that characterize infancy for boys and girls. Several general characteristics may be observed in these figures. First, each sex has a single *main developmental trend* consisting of the items loading on the first principal component at each age (connected by solid lines). The main trend was the only developmental pattern in which adjacent-age and non-adjacent-age correlations were both significant. While this major trend consisting of the first principal components

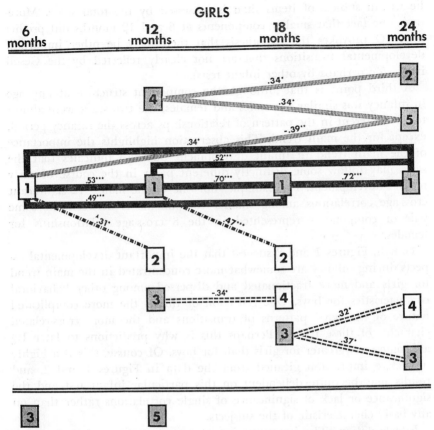

FIG. 2. Correlation matrix depicted graphically for girls. (See text for explanation.)

has the appearance of a g factor, none of the components accounted for more than 19% of the total test variance.

Second, at 6 months, the items in the main trend do not predict childhood IQ, though some smaller components do correlate with childhood IQ. This observation has several implications. Initially it suggests that precocity in certain skills characteristic of early infancy may not relate to later childhood IQ, even though such skills may be vital precursors of those childhood traits. Further, since the main trend was composed of the first principal component at each age and since that component is presumably the best single concentrated reflection of the test as a whole, a great deal more information and predictive power may lie within subsets of items than is possessed by the total score. More-over, the fact that smaller components at 6 and 12 months did predict later IQ provokes the hypothesis that there may be other important developmental transitions that are not clearly reflected by the Gesell items (or perhaps by other infant tests).

A third point is that although the component structure at any age in infancy was similar for males and females, the two sexes were almost totally different in the pattern of relationships across the infancy period, except for the main trend. This observation highlights the importance of the main trend in infant development but also indicates that the sexes may follow some distinctly different paths in the course of early mental development. For example, not one of the males' 12 significant cross-age correlations among smaller components is between the same pair of components represented in the 8 cross-age relationships for females.

Fourth, Figures 1 and 2 suggest that the important developmental aspects during infancy are somewhat more concentrated in the main trend for girls and more fractionated and dispersed among other behavioral characteristics for boys. One reflection of this is the more complicated nature of the boys' patterns of transitions and the more cross-related character of these trends. Perhaps this is why predictions to later IQ are sometimes greater for girls than for boys. Of course, this is a highly subjective impression gleaned from the data in Figures 1 and 2, and results may be quite dependent on this particular infant test and the significance or lack of significance of single correlations rather than on any basic characteristic of the subjects.

Interpretation. The interpretation of a component analysis is necessarily a subjective enterprise. One cannot be very confident about the reliability of component structures or of the ordering of items within a component. Still more subjective is discerning the common psychological link between the diverse items loaded on a single component. Consequently, the interpretation given below is offered for heuristic reasons and should be viewed as one of many possible implications of these descriptive data. Only the major developmental trend and a few subordinate transitions will be discussed, but a detailed set of tables may be obtained from the authors upon request.

Table 4 presents the items having loadings of .4 or greater for each component in the main trend. In addition, the significant correlations between each component and later childhood IQ are indicated separately for males and females at the bottom of the table.

The items loading on the main developmental trend at 6 months appear to incorporate visually guided manipulation of objects and gross and fine motor behavior. However, there is another more subtle and quite provocative interpretation that links several of the fine motor and manipulation items. Many of these behaviors involve the manipulation of objects that yield perceptual contingencies, behavior that has been called "the game" (Watson, 1972), or involve conjugate reinforcement (Rovee & Rovee, 1969). For example, the items "reaches for dangling ring," "lifts inverted cup," "bangs spoon on table," "splashes in tub," "conscious of fallen objects," and "pats table" all describe manipulation that produces a rather clear contingent perceptual consequence. With due interpretative caution noted, the "perceptual consequences" hypothesis is a particularly exciting one because of its relationship with other behaviors that are similar to it. For example, it has been shown that infants (e.g., Rovee & Rovee, 1969; Siqueland, 1969; Watson, 1972) as well as animals (e.g., McCall, 1965, 1966) will perform simple responses in order to produce a contingent perceptual event. Moreover, Watson (1972) has suggested that reciprocal behavior and social-perceptual contingencies may form the basis of early attachment in the human infant. In addition, the behaviors on this component are quite reminiscent of Piaget's (1952) secondary circular response in which the child repeatedly executes a simple behavior that produces an obvious perceptual consequence. Piaget observed this behavior and related activities between 3 and 8 months of life. Finally, one is tempted in this context to think of the concept of internal control found important in later intellectual, educational, and personality domains (Lefcourt, 1966; Rotter, 1966).

At 12 months, the items composing the main developmental trend still involve gross and fine motor skills, but the items reflecting visually guided manipulation and production of perceptual consequences seen at 6 months have been replaced by items requiring the imitation of fine motor behavior and the learning of rudimentary social skills. Many items on infant tests appear to reflect simple fine motor and prehensile skills. However, in many cases the examiner demonstrates the behavior and then waits for the child to imitate it. While a certain amount of fine motor skill is required to execute the behavior, passage of the item is equally dependent on the child's propensity to imitate the examiner. Consequently, the items "rings bell in imitation," "imitates rattle of spoon in cup," "builds tower of two to three cubes," "puts cube in cup," "performance box," and "scribbles in imitation" all require the child to imitate the examiner. The imitation interpretation is favored because some of these items (i.e., "rings bell," "rattles spoon," "scribbles") do not require a high degree of motor skill, and thus it may be inferred that

TABLE 4.—ITEMS, LOADINGS, AND CORRELATIONS WITH CHILDHOOD

6 months		12 months	
Component 1	Loading	Component 1	Loading
Reaches for dangling ring (5)	.66	Stands (3)	.63
Exploratory manipulations of spoon, cup, saucer	.62	Walks (4)	.60
Regards and accepts cube (3)	.62	Takes third cube without dropping	.55
Lifts inverted cup, secures cube (3)	.60	Waves bye-bye	.54
Inhibits head and one hand	.60	Rings bell in imitation	.54
Reaches directly for spoon	.58	Imitates rattle of spoon in cup	.49
Sits with support, alone (3)	.56	Creeps, climbs (3)	.48
Regards and secures pellet (4)	.56	Says 3 to 5 words (4)	.48
Plays with objects	.54	Builds tower of two–three cubes (3)	.47
Bangs spoon on table	.52	Puts cube in cup (4)	.46
Purposeful reaction to paper (3)	.47	Says bye-bye or hello	.45
Splashes in tub	.45	Performance box, rod in hole	.44
Shows consciousness of strangers	.42	Scribbles in imitation	.43
Conscious of fallen object (3)	.42	Tries to put on shoes	.42
Makes stepping movements	.42	Unwraps cube	.40
Pats table	.40	Plays peek or pat-a-cake	.40

Correlations with childhood IQ	
Males	
Females	S–B–3½ years: †.49***
	6 years: .46***
	10 years: .42***

Note.—See text for explanation of table.
* p <.05 for tests of the significance of a correlation.
** p <.01 for tests of the significance of a correlation.
*** p <.001 for tests of the significance of a correlation.
† p <.05 for tests of sex differences for these correlations.

passage of the item depends more on the child's propensity for imitation. Also loading on this component are several diverse behaviors that seem to reflect the learning of social behavior and simple verbal skills ("waves bye-bye," "says three to five words," "says bye-bye or hello," "plays peek or pat-a-cake"). The presence of these social-verbal behaviors on the same component with the imitation of fine motor behavior suggests that these are related behaviors, perhaps tied together in a social context. It seems reasonable that the child who develops the tendency to imitate probably imitates fine motor behavior first and later vocal-verbal skills in social contexts (e.g., saying hello or good-bye).

The importance of imitation in early mental development is highlighted by an analysis of mental test scores, nursery school ratings, and ratings of behavior in the home made by Virginia Crandall (personal communication, June 1972). A components analysis of these variables

IQ FOR THE MAIN TREND OF DEVELOPMENTAL TRANSITIONS

18 months	
Component 1	Loading
Pictures, names several (4)	.72
Pictures, points to several (3)	.72
Repeats things said	.64
Says five or more words	.60
Points to parts of body (3)	.59
Requests things at table (3)	.56
Names watch, 4th view	.52
Uses two or more words together	.47
Scribbles in imitation	.44
Throws ball in box	.43

24 months	
Component 1	Loading
Pictures, names five	.75
Pictures, points at several (3)	.73
Speaks in sentences	.66
Tells name (3)	.62
Tells experiences	.59
Names watch, many views (4)	.53
Listens to stories with pictures	.53
Drawing, imitates simple patterns (6)	.52
Uses pronouns, past, plural	.52
Asks for things at table by name	.51
Names five familiar objects	.51
Uses color names	.48
Knows prepositions (4)	.47
Puts cube in cup, plate, box	.44
Bowel control	.41

S–B—3½ years: .28* 6 years: .21 10 years: .20
W–B—13 years: V: .23 P: .41** T: .35*

S–B—3½ years: .42*** 6 years: .38* 10 years: .26
WISC—11 years: V: .46** P: .28 T: .42*
W–B—13 years: V: .34* P: .36* T: .37*

S–B—3½ years: .49*** 6 years: .51*** 10 years: .43**
WISC— 7 years: V: .43* P: .20 T: .37*
WISC—11 years: V: .46** P: .36* T: .44*

S–B—3½ years: .69*** 6 years: .59*** 10 years: .41**
WISC— 7 years: V: .43* P: .36 T: .46*
WISC—11 years: V: .56*** P: .17 T: .42*

revealed one component characterized by Gesell and Binet scores during the first 3 years. The only child behavior variable possessing a reasonably high loading on this component was "child imitates adults" as *independently* rated from prose descriptions of the child's behavior in an unstructured nursery school and at home.

Piaget (1951) has already seen the shift in emphasis from the production of perceptual consequences to imitation as being an important dynamic transition in the early development of sensorimotor intelligence. This begins as "pseudo-imitation, the child . . . apparently using the imitative schema to prolong a spectacle because it corresponds to what the child is already doing [Hunt, 1961, p. 133]." Later, when conceptions of object permanence, space, and causality are more mature, Piaget postulates a greater differentiation between imitative accommodation and playful assimilation, with genuine imitation as the result. Finally, the child appears to imitate "for its own sake" and begins to imitate vocal and verbal productions of the parent. Thus, the transition between the production of perceptual consequences through manipulation and the imitation of fine motor and social-vocal-verbal behavior observed in the Fels data was hypothesized long ago by Piaget as a major dynamic entity in the epigenic development in the first year.

By 18 months, the main developmental trend has become pervasively verbal in character. There are three general types of items loaded on the first principal component at 18 months. The first is verbal production ("names pictures," "repeats things said," "says five or more words," "requests things at table," "names watch," "uses two or more words together"), the second involves verbal comprehension ("points to several pictures." "points to parts of body"), and the third is an extension of the imitation of verbal and motor behavior ("repeats things said," "scribbles in imitation," "throws ball in box"). The propensity to imitate fine motor behavior and verbal skills in a social context at 12 months is related to the imitation of more complex verbal behavior and skill in verbal labeling and comprehension at 18 months.

At 24 months, the main trend has an even stronger verbal character. While there is still a hint of imitation ("imitates simple drawn patterns," "puts cube in cup, plate, box"), the predominant theme features the verbal skills of production and labeling ("names five pictures," "names watch," "asks for things at table by name," "names five familiar objects," "uses color names"), comprehension ("points at several pictures," "listens to stories with pictures"), and fluent verbal production and grammatical maturity ("speaks in sentences," "tells name," "tells experiences," "uses pronouns," "asks for things at table by name," "knows prepositions").

Although one must always be vigilant about overgeneralizations from such data and analyses, these results do provoke some hypotheses regarding the ontogeny of behavior in infancy. It is reasonable to speculate that the child who precociously develops the propensity to manipulate objects and appreciate their contingent perceptual consequences may soon apply this same strategy to the less consistent contingencies of social situations. A natural outgrowth of reciprocal social behavior is imitation, perhaps the parent imitating the child first and then the child imitating the parent. Early imitation will likely involve gross and fine motor behavior, but with development and the presence of a verbally fluent model the imitation of rudimentary language behavior subsequently emerges. Simplistically, the main behavioral trend emphasizes asocial and then social operant learning, followed by the propensity to imitate sensorimotor and then verbal behavior. Given adequate verbal models and encouragement, it is perhaps not surprising that a trend involving such basic learning processes should undergird a major developmental trend in infancy and predict later IQ.

However, there are alternative interpretations of the content of this developmental trend. The exploration of objects, imitation of adult behavior, and displays of verbal fluency all require the infant to possess a type of social extroversion that permits him to interact freely with a strange examiner. Thus, the major dimension underlying normal infant mental test performance may not be "mental" at all, but rather a social inhibition versus extroverted personality style. Another alternative is that the developmental trend observed in the infant behavior may actually reflect trends and consistencies in parental behavior that are then reflected in the child. A mother who plays contingently or provides toys with potential contingent effects during the first few months of her child's life may be the same parent who plays imitation games a few months later, and provides an adequate and encouraging language model for her child during the second year. It should be observed that these several alternatives are not mutually exclusive; all could operate in concert.

Prediction of childhood IQ. Does this major developmental trend during infancy, whatever its psychological interpretation, stretch into childhood? The significant correlations between the components of the infant trend with childhood IQ scores are given at the bottom of table 4. Notice first that there are no significant correlations from 6 months, yet the 6-month component is an integral part of the principal developmental trend in infancy. Perhaps it is in this sense that some (e.g., Ames, 1967; Bayley, 1970) have claimed that infant tests represent valid indexes of contemporary mental and neurological development, but nevertheless do not predict later IQ.

A second observation is that once verbal items appear on the principal components in the main trend (a few at 12 months, and more at 18 and 24 months), those component scores predict later IQ. Since it is known that females display more maturity in vocal-verbal behavior at younger ages than do males (e.g., perhaps even at 12 months), it may not be surprising that the main trend predicts childhood IQ for girls at 12 months but not until 18 months for boys.

Finally, the predictions for girls from the 12-month principal component to the Binet at $3\frac{1}{2}$, 6, and 10 years are nearly as high as the correlations for the 18-month and 24-month components. This is particularly clear when predicting the 10-year Binet where the correlations from 12, 18, and 24 months are nearly identical (.41, .43, and .41), respectively). In contrast, predictions to the Binet for males are infrequent and considerably lower than for the females. However, the picture is somewhat different when the Wechsler tests are used as the criterion measure of childhood IQ. Although these data confound age and specific childhood IQ test, sex differences in the prediction of childhood IQ may be dependent on the particular childhood IQ test as well as on the infant test and the nature of the sexes.

Minor Developmental Trends

Although the existence of smaller developmental trends may rest on the significance of a single correlation, it is also the case that minor trends in these data may be imperfect reflections by the Gesell test of major behavioral transitions that are actually quite important. Consequently, a few of the minor trends will be discussed briefly.

Males. One smaller trend for males (Figure 1) involves Component 2 at 6 months and Component 6 at 12 months, which relate to each other and to the main trend. It should be observed that some of the correlations in this trend are significantly larger for males than for females, and therefore this pattern may be unique for boys.

The items loading on components in this trend are listed in Table 5. The component at 6 months appears to emphasize the playful activity and social concern which is not part of the determination of perceptual-motor relations and contingencies. Similarly, the items on the 12-month component also have a social flavor and something of playful social activity. While this behavioral cluster relates positively to the main trend at 6 and 12 months (though within an age they are, of course, independent), it correlates negatively (—.53) with the main trend at 24 months (Figure 1). Further, while this social orientation at 6 months has at least one positive prediction (.39 for boys only) to a later Binet (at 6 years), the 12-month component of the trend shows negative relationships both with the verbally oriented principal component at 24 months (—.53), with the Binet at 3½ years (—.26), and with the verbal score on the WISC at 11 years (—.36).

Generally, this minor trend suggests that there is an inverse relationship, especially for boys, between social orientation and frolicsome play in the first-year test situation and later verbal skills. The importance of this observation derives from the fact that others have found grossly similar patterns (cf. McCall, 1971). For example, Bayley (1970) and Bayley and Schaefer (1964), using the Berkeley Growth Study data, reported that male infants who were rated as happy, positively responding, and calm in the infant test situation during the first year of life

TABLE 5

SMALL TREND FOR MALES

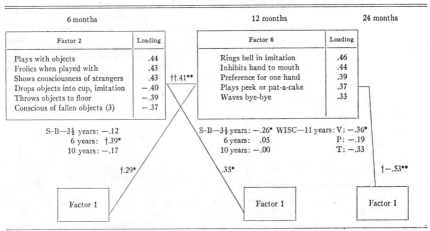

Note.—See text for explanation of table.
* p <.05 for tests of the significance of a correlation.
** p <.01 for tests of the significance of a correlation.
† p <.05 for tests of sex differences for these correlations.
†† p <.01 for tests of sex differences for these correlations.

had high mental test scores during infancy but low scores in early childhood. The shift in the direction of the relationship between this active social orientation and mental scores occurred at approximately 15 months, and these relationships were clearer for males than for females. These results conform nicely with this minor trend observed in the Fels data. An additional measure of support is offered by a longitudinal study involving neonatal physiological activity and mental and personality assessments at 2½ years of age (Bell et al., 1971). "Low-intensity" neonates, as reflected by low respiration rates, low tactile sensitivity, and minimum response to interrupted sucking, were described at 2½ years as being more advanced in speech development, verbal originality, geographic orientation, manipulative skill, and modeling of adults. Moreover, these relationships were observed more frequently for boys than for girls. At the risk of slighting important details and qualifications, these three studies concur in suggesting that males who are either physiologically high-intensity neonates, or who have a relatively strong social and playful nature during the infant test situation have relatively high concurrent infant test scores but relatively low standing on verbally oriented assessments later in early childhood. Thus, while early vocal-verbal behaviors have greater predictive salience for girls

TABLE 6

INDEPENDENT DEVELOPMENTAL TREND FOR FEMALES

18 months   24 months

Component 4	Loading
Drawing, imitates simple patterns (6)	−.45
Names five familiar objects	.38
Folds paper, makes square (3)	−.36

.32*

Component 3	Loading
Counts to two or three	.56
Throws ball in box	−.47
Walks alone	−.46
Builds tower of blocks (3)	−.41
Imitates vertical, horizontal lines (3)	.36
Names watch, 4th view	.35

.37*

Component 3	Loading
Knows own sex	.54
Uses spoon well	−.45
Form-board, no errors	.45
Shows affection	−.43
Form-board, solved in time	.34
Tells experiences	.28

S–B— 3½ years: .19   WISC— 7 years: V: .61***
       6 years: †.47**   P: .32
      10 years: †.47**   T: .54**
                 WISC—11 years: V: .63***
                            P: .33
                            T: .53**

S–B— 3½ years: .15   WISC— 7 years: V: .39*
       6 years: †.30*   P: .24
      10 years: ††.32*   T: .36
                 WISC—11 years: V: †††.55**
                            P: .21
                            T: ††.44*

Note.—Numbers in parentheses indicate number of Gesell items combined because of logical dependencies.
 * $p < .05$ for tests of the significance of a correlation.
 ** $p < .01$ for tests of the significance of a correlation.
 *** $p < .001$ for tests of the significance of a correlation.
 † $p < .05$ for tests of sex differences for these correlations.
 †† $p < .01$ for tests of sex differences for these correlations.
 ††† $p < .001$ for tests of sex differences for these correlations.

(see following discussion), early social and frolicsome acivity may have inverse predictability, especially for boys.

Females. Although the females showed several smaller trends (Figure 2), one pattern stands out because of its comparatively high predictions to later IQ and its relative uniqueness for females. The details of this trend are presented in Table 6. A common interpretation of these item sets is risky, but one theme is an emphasis on perceptual-verbal facility—one that is distinct from (a) gross and fine motor skills, (b) the imitation of fine motor behavior, and perhaps (c) perceptual-figural (as opposed to verbal) relations. These correlations between components forming this trend and childhood IQ are impressively high (some *rs* greater than .60) and are relatively unique to females (Table 6). One very tentative implication is that while the main trend represents advanced performance on a mixture of perceptual-verbal, fine motor, imitation, and perceptual-figural tasks, this smaller independent strain seems to highlight disproportionate skill in perceptual-verbal fluency relative to the other behaviors and emphasizes the special salience that vocal-verbal skills apparently have for females.

SUMMARY AND CONCLUSIONS

Several conclusions can be drawn from this review. First, until the second year of life there is relatively poor prediction from infant tests to IQ assessed in middle or late childhood. Infant tests may have some value in detecting neuromotor abnormalities, however, and a severely low score has somewhat greater predictive significance than average or high scores. Second, the low predictive correlations are not a function of poor test reliability. Third, while there are no pronounced sex differences on infant test total scores, girls may show higher correlations with later IQ than boys, especially for some infant tests and for relationships covering early infancy and childhood. Fourth, predictions from 12 to 24 months may be increased slightly by adding parental socioeconomic class into a multiple-regression formula with infant test score; prior to 12 months, parental socioeconomic status alone is the best single predictor. Fifth, infant tests administered in the first year of life have more predictive power in their item pool than the total score reflects, and early vocal-verbal behavior may have salience in predicting later IQ for girls and frolicsome social activity may have inverse predictability for boys. Sixth, despite the fact that correlations can be increased somewhat by the above procedures, for the most part the level of prediction from the total score for normal children remains modest and of minimum practical utility.

When specific skill areas were determined by subjecting Gesell items taken at 6, 12, 18, and 24 months to separate principal components analyses, the correlations of component scores across these ages as well as with childhood IQ indicated several patterns of developmental transitions. The most pronounced trend spanning the entire infancy period involved the manipulative exploration of objects that produced perceptual contingencies at 6 months, the imitation of simple fine motor and elementary verbal behavior particularly in a social context at 12 months, verbal labeling and comprehension at 18 months, and verbal fluency and grammatical maturity at 24 months. Tentatively, these data highlight the potential importance of early exploration and manipulation, especially the production of contingent perceptual and social consequences, and the role of imitation as the possible developmental mediator between exploration behavior in the first 6 months and verbal production and fluency in the second year of life. The fact that this major trend of development did not predict later IQ until 12 (females) or 18 months (males) illustrates how early behavior in infancy might form the basis out of which later childhood skills emerge without itself directly predicting those childhood performances. Parallels to the epigenic development of Piaget were illustrated. Another interpretation of these data suggested that a common factor underlying this major developmental pattern might be a socially uninhibited "extroversion" which moderates the behavior of infants in the test situation.

The overriding implication of this discussion is that a simple conception of a constant and pervasive g factor is probably not tenable as a model for "mental" development, especially for the infancy period. The data are strong in their denial of simple continuity of general precocity at one age with general precocity at another age during the infancy period, and emphatic in demonstrating marked qualitative shifts in behavioral dispositions. Moreover, to label as "mental" performances at every age perpetuates the belief in a pervasive and developmentally constant intelligence. Consequently, the term mental as applied to infant behavior or tests should be abandoned in favor of some conceptually more neutral label, perhaps Piaget's "sensorimotor," "perceptual-motor," or even more specific classes of behaviors (e.g., exploration of perceptual contingencies, imitation, language). The network of transitions between skills at one age and another is likely more specific and complex than once thought, and not accurately subsumed under one general concept.

REFERENCES

AMES, L. B.: Predictive value of infant behavior examinations. In J. Hellmuth (Ed.): *Exceptional Infant: The Normal Infant.* Vol. 1. New York: Brunner/Mazel, 1967.

ANDERSON, J. E.: The limitations of infant and preschool tests in the measurement of intelligence. *The Journal of Psychology,* 1939, 8, 351-379.

ANDERSON, L. D.: The predictive efficiency of infancy tests in relation to intelligence at five years. *Child Development,* 1939, 10, 203-212.

BAYLEY, N.: The consistency of mental growth during the first year. *Psychological Bulletin,* 1931, 28, 225-226.

BAYLEY, N.: Mental growth during the first three years: A developmental study of sixty-one children by repeated tests. *Genetic Psychology Monographs,* 1933, 14, 1-92.

BAYLEY, N.: The development of motor abilities during the first three years. *Monographs of the Society for Research in Child Development,* 1935, 1.

BAYLEY, N.: Consistency and variability in the growth of intelligence from birth to eighteen years. *Journal of Genetic Psychology,* 1949, 75, 165-196.

BAYLEY, N.: Some increasing parent-child similarities during the growth of children. *Journal of Educational Psychology,* 1954, 45, 1-21.

BAYLEY, N.: Comparisons of mental and motor test scores for ages 1-15 months by sex, birth order, race, geographical location and education of parents. *Child Development,* 1965, 36, 379-411.

BAYLEY, N.: Learning in adulthood: The role of intelligence. In H. J. Klausmeier & C. W. Harris (Eds.): *Analyses of Concept Learning.* New York: Academic Press, 1966.

BAYLEY, N.: Development of mental abilities. In P. H. Mussen (Ed.): *Carmichael's Manual of Child Psychology*. Vol. 1. New York: Wiley, 1970.

BAYLEY, N., & SCHAEFER, E. S.: Correlations of maternal and child behaviors with development of mental ability: Data from the Berkeley Growth Study. *Monographs of the Society for Research in Child Development*, 1964, 29, Serial No. 97.

BELL, R. Q., WELLER, G. M., & WALDROP, M. F.: Newborn and preschooler: Organization of behavior and relations between periods. *Monographs of the Society for Research in Child Development*, 1971, 36, Serial No. 142, 1-145.

BLOOM, B. S.: *Stability and Change in Human Characteristics*. New York: Wiley, 1964.

CALDWELL, B. M., & DRACHMAN, R.: Comparability of three methods of assessing the developmental level of young infants. *Pediatrics*, 1964, 34, 51-57.

CAMERON, J., LIVSON, N., & BAYLEY, N.: Infant vocalizations and their relationship to mature intelligence. *Science*, 1967, 157, 331-333.

CAVANAUGH, M. C., COHEN, I., DUNPHY, D., RINGWELL, E. A., & GOLDBERG, I. D.: Prediction from the Cattell Infant Intelligence Scale. *Journal of Consulting Psychology*, 1957, 21, 33-37.

DALES, R. J.: Motor and language development of twins during the first 3 years. *Journal of Genetic Psychology*, 1969, 114, 263-271.

DÉCARIE, T.: *Intelligence and Affectivity in Early Childhood*. New York: International Universities Press, 1965.

DRILLIEN, C. M.: A longitudinal study of the growth and development of prematurely and maturely born children: Part VII: Mental development 2-5 years. *Archives of Diseases in Childhood*, 1961, 36, 233-240.

ESCALONA, S. K., & MORIARITY, A.: Prediction of school-age intelligence from infant tests. *Child Development*, 1961, 32, 597-605.

FILLMORE, E. A.: Iowa tests for young children. *University of Iowa Studies in Child Welfare*, 1936, 11, 1-58.

FISH, B.: The detection of schizophrenia in infancy: A preliminary report. *Journal of Nervous and Mental Disease*, 1957, 125, 1-24.

FISH, B.: Involvement of the central nervous system in infants with schizophrenia. *AMA Archives of Neurology*, 1960, 2, 115-121.

FISH, B., SHAPIRO, F., HALPERN, F., & WILE, R.: The prediction of schizophrenia in infancy: III. A ten-year follow-up report of neurological and psychological development. *American Journal of Psychiatry*, 1965, 121, 768-775.

FURFEY, P., & MUEHLENBEIN, J.: The validity of infant intelligence tests. *Pedagogical Seminary and the Journal of Genetic Psychology*, 1932, 40, 219-224.

GOFFENEY, B., HENDERSON, N. B., & BUTLER, B. V.: Negro-white, male-female eight-month developmental scores compared with seven-year WISC and Bender test scores. *Child Development*, 1971, 42, 595-604.

GOLDEN, M., & BIRNS, B.: Social class and cognitive development in infancy. *Merrill-Palmer Quarterly*, 1968, 14, 139-140.

GOLDEN, M., BIRNS, B., BRIDGER, W., & MOSS, A.: Social class differentiation in cognitive development among black preschool children. *Child Development*, 1971, 42, 37-45.

GUILFORD, J. P.: *The Nature of Human Intelligence*. New York: McGraw-Hill, 1967.

HARMS, I. E., & SPIKER, C. C.: Factors associated with the performance of young children on intelligence scales and tests of speech development. *Journal of Genetic Psychology*, 1959, 94, 3-22.

HINDLEY, C. B. & MUNRO, J. A.: A factor analytic study of the abilities of infants, and predictions of later ability. Paper presented at the Symposium on Behavioral Testing of Neonates and Longitudinal Correlations, London, April, 1970.

HONZIK, M. P.: The constancy of mental test performance during the preschool period. *Journal of Genetic Psychology*, 1938, 52, 285-302.

HONZIK, M. P.: Developmental studies of parent-child resemblance in intelligence. *Child Development*, 1957, 28, 215-228.

HONZIK, M. P.: A sex difference in the age of onset of the parent-child resemblance in intelligence. *Journal of Educational Psychology*, 1963, 54, 213-237.

HONZIK, M. P., HUTCHINS, J. J., & BURNIP, S. R.: Birth record assessments and test performance at eight months. *American Journal of Diseases of Children*, 1965, 109, 416-426.

HUNT, J. V., & BAYLEY, N.: Explorations into patterns of mental development and prediction from the Bayley scales of infant development. *Minnesota Symposia on Child Psychology*, 1971, 5, 52-71.

HUNT, J. McV.: *Intelligence and Experience*. New York: Ronald Press, 1961.

ILLINGSWORTH, R. S.: The predictive value of developmental tests in the first year with special reference to the diagnosis of mental subnormality. *Journal of Child Psychology and Psychiatry*, 1961, 2, 210-215.

IRETON, H., THWING, E., & GRAVEM, H.: Infant mental development and neurological status, family socioeconomic status, and intelligence at age four. *Child Development*, 1970, 41, 937-946.

KAGAN, J.: On the meaning of behavior: Illustrations from the infant. *Child Development*, 1969, 40, 1121-1134.

KAGAN, J.: *Change and Continuity in Infancy*. New York: Wiley, 1971.

KAGAN, J. & MOSS, H. A.: Parental correlates of child's IQ and height: A cross-validation of the Berkeley Growth Study results. *Child Development*, 1959, 30, 325-332.

KNOBLOCH, H., & PASAMANICK, B.: An evaluation of the consistency and predictive value of the 40-week Gesell developmental schedule. *Psychiatric Research Reports of the American Psychiatric Association*, 1960, 13, 10-13.

KNOBLOCH, H., & PASAMANICK, B.: Predicting intellectual potential in infancy. *American Journal of Diseases of Children*, 1963, 106, 43-51.

KNOBLOCH, H. & PASAMANICK, B.: Prediction from the assessment of neuromotor and intellectual status in infancy. In: *Psychopathology of Mental Development*. New York: Grune & Stratton. 1967.

LEFCOURT, H. M.: Internal versus external control of reinforcement: A review. *Psychological Bulletin*, 1966, 65, 206-220.

LIVSON, N.: Developmental dimensions of personality: A longitudinal analysis. Paper presented at the meeting of the Western Psychological Association, Honolulu, Hawaii, June 1965.

MACRAE, J. M.: Retests of children given tests as infants. *Journal of Genetic Psychology*, 1955, 87, 111-119.

McCALL, R. B.: Stimulus-change in light-contingent bar-pressing. *Journal of Comparative and Physiological Psychology*, 1965, 59, 258-262.

McCALL, R. B.: The initial-consequent-change surface in light-contingent bar-pressing. *Journal of Comparative and Physiological Psychology*, 1966, 62, 35-42.

McCALL, R. B.: Discussion. In A. J. Sameroff (Chm.), Relations of newborn physiology and preschool verbal communication to intelligence, maturity, and pace of play in the school-age period. Symposium presented at the meeting of the American Psychological Association, Washington, D. C., September 1971.

MOORE, T.: Language and intelligence: A longitudinal study of the first eight years. Part I. Patterns of development in boys and girls. *Human Development*, 1967, 10, 88-106.

NELSON, V. L., & RICHARDS, T. W.: Studies in mental development: I. Performance on Gesell items at six months and its predictive value for performance on mental tests at two and three years. *Journal of Genetic Psychology*, 1938, 52, 303-325.

NELSON, V. L. & RICHARDS, T. W.: Studies in mental development: III. Performance of twelve-months-old children on the Gesell schedule, and its predictive value for mental status at two and three years. *Journal of Genetic Psychology*, 1939, 54, 181-191.

PIAGET, J.: *Play, Dreams, and Imitation in Childhood. [La formation du symbole chez l'enfant.]* (Trans. by C. Gattegno & F. N. Hodgson) New York: Norton, 1951.

PIAGET, J.: *The Origins of Intelligence in Children.* (Trans. by M. Cook) New York: International Universities Press, 1952.

RICHARDS, T. W. & NELSON, V. L.: Abilities of infants during the first eighteen months. *Journal of Genetic Psychology*, 1939, 55, 299-318.

ROTTER, J. B.: Generalized expectancies for internal versus external control of reinforcement. *Psychological Monographs*, 1966, 80 (1, Whole No. 609).

ROVEE, C. K. & ROVEE, D. T.: Conjugate reinforcement of infant exploratory behavior. *Journal of Experimental Child Psychology*, 1969, 8, 1-8.

RUTTER, M.: Psychological development—predictions from infancy. *Journal of Child Psychology and Psychiatry*, 1970, 11, 49-62.

SIQUELAND, E. R.: The development of instrumental exploratory behavior during the first year of human life. Paper presented at the meeting of the Society of Research in Child Development, Santa Monica, California, April 1969.

STECHLER, G.: A longitudinal follow-up of neonatal apnea. *Child Development*, 1964, 35, 333-348.

STOTT, L. H., & BALL, R. S.: Infant and preschool mental tests: Review and evaluation. *Monographs for the Society of Research in Child Development*, 1965, 30, Serial No. 101.

THOMAS, H.: Psychological assessment instruments for use with human infants. *Merrill-Palmer Quarterly*, 1970, 16, 179-224.

WACHS, T. D., UZGIRIS, I. C., & HUNT, J. McV.: Cognitive development in infants of different age levels and from different environmental backgrounds: An explanatory investigation. *Merrill-Palmer Quarterly*, 1971, 17, 283-318.

WALLACH, M. A., & KOGAN, N.: *Modes of Thinking in Young Children.* New York: Holt, Rinehart & Winston, 1965.

WATSON, J. S.: Smiling, cooing, and "the game." *Merrill-Palmer Quarterly*, 1972, in Press.

WERNER, E. E. & BAYLEY, N.: The reliability of Bayley's revised scale of mental and motor development during the first year of life. *Child Development*, 1966, 37, 39-50.

WERNER, E. E., HONZIK, M. P., & SMITH, R. S.: Prediction of intelligence and achievement at 10 years from 20 months pediatric and psychologic examinations. *Child Development*, 1968, 39, 1063-1075.

WILLERMAN, L., BROMAN, S. H., & FIELDER, M.: Infant development, preschool IQ, and social class. *Child Development*, 1970, 41, 69-77.

6

INFANTS AROUND THE WORLD: CROSS-CULTURAL STUDIES OF PSYCHOMOTOR DEVELOPMENT FROM BIRTH TO TWO YEARS

Emmy E. Werner, Ph.D.

University of California, Davis

Comparisons were made of the findings of fifty cross-cultural studies of psychomotor development, from birth to two years, of contemporary groups of infants on five continents. The effects of ethnicity, amount and type of caretaker stimulation, and nutritional status were discussed. African infants showed the greatest early acceleration, Caucasian infants the least, while Latin American and Asian Infants ranked intermediate. Within each ethnic group, "traditionally" reared, rural infants showed greater motor acceleration than "Westernized," urban infants in the first six to twelve months, and a greater decline, after weaning, in adaptive and language development, in the second year. Within both traditional and Westernized samples of the same ethnic groups, infants with higher birthweight were more accelerated.

In spite of a steady increase in cross-cultural studies during the past two decades, there have been relatively few concerned with the behavior of infants. Yet the study of infant development across cultural and ethnic boundaries is a line of research that could hold great promise. Child

---

Reprinted from JOURNAL OF CROSS-CULTURAL PSYCHOLOGY, Vol. 3, No. 2, June, 1972, pp. 111-134.

care practices during the first years of life are relatively open to systematic observation, and increasingly reliable methods of studying infant behavior have been developed. The present review provides a comparison, integration and evaluation of findings of cross-cultural studies of psychomotor development in infants, from birth to two years, and suggestions for the direction of future research.

Studies of infants' psychomotor development have had generally two aims: to describe general sequences in development, and to describe variations among infants as a result of environmental factors. The latter, *diagnostic* issue has attracted more recent attention due to an increasing concern with the assessment of the effects of perinatal stress, environmental deprivation and malnutrition, and the need to evaluate intervention efforts in social action programs for infants.

The most frequently used tests for these purposes are: the Gesell Developmental Schedule (1947) and its adaptations; the Cattell Infant Intelligence Scale (1940); and the Bayley Scales of Infant Development (1969), all standardized in the United States; the Griffith Developmental Scale (1954), standardized in Great Britain; the Brunét-Lézine Scale (1965), and the André-Thomas neo-natal examination (1960), standardized in France. The technical aspects (norms, reliability, validity) of these assessment instruments for human infants have been recently discussed by Hoben (1970).

In the age-range reviewed here, infant tests of psychomotor development satisfy several criteria that are commonly used to justify the assumption of "cultural equivalence" of a test measure: (a) the test situation is understandable *without* verbal instructions; (b) it *invites* action and the infant's response is judged *in terms of his actions*.

This report reviews studies which have used these tools with different cultural and ethnic groups in Europe, North, Central and South America, the Near East and Africa, Asia and Oceania. It includes both cross-sectional and longitudinal research. Although the literature is widely scattered, an attempt has been made to provide an extensive, if not exhaustive, coverage.

A comparison will be made between the findings of research undertaken in the developed countries of the West, reports from traditional, preindustrial communities, and from urban areas undergoing rapid modernization. Mean scores derived from the norms of the Western standardization groups will be reported for comparative purposes only, not as approximations to a universal standard of excellence. The results will be discussed in light of the possible effects of genetic potential, birthweight, patterns of adult-child interaction, especially handling, feeding and weaning practices, and the effects of malnutrition.

Recent European studies, one cross-sectional and five longitudinal, point to slight, but consistent, variations of psychomotor development, both in fine and gross motor skills, among infants in Western Europe.

Frances-Williams and Yule (1967) administered the Bayley Scales of Infant Development to a sample of 300 infants in Great Britain. Mean mental and psychomotor scores at ages 1-15 months were comparable to those obtained by United States infants. However, the British babies were between one and two months ahead of the United States infants on some fine motor skill items ("attempts to secure three cubes," "uncovers square box," "combines two spoons or cubes midline"). The authors speculate that the relative precocity of British babies in midline hand-skill and items involving eye-hand coordination may be due to the fact that English babies are rarely placed in the prone position in their cots, as is customary in the U.S., and their hands are relatively free to explore.

Hindley (1968), summarizing findings on the Griffiths Developmental Scale from five longitudinal studies in London, Paris, Brussels, Zurich and Stockholm, noted a significant difference in the age of "walking unaided" among his samples. Swedish and Belgian infants did so earlier than did the British, French and Swiss. They also weighed more at birth and at one year of age than the infants from France, Great Britain and Switzerland.

American Indians

Among the earliest cross-cultural observations of infant motor development is a study of the effect of cradling practices on the age of onset of walking among Indians in the southwestern United States. Dennis (1940) found no significant differences in the mothers' reports of age of onset of walking among Hopis who used the cradleboard for nine months, day and night, acculturated Hopi who no longer did so, and Tewa who used the cradleboard only for their infants' daytime naps. However, both Hopi and Tewa infants, on the average, walked two months later than a comparison group of white infants. Dennis suggests that the dietary practices of the Indians may contribute to their motoric retardation.

The average birthweight of American Indian babies exceeds that of both white and Negro infants (3.60 kg) but weight drops below these groups at year one (8.92 kg) (Meredith, 1970a, b).

U.S. Negroes

By far the largest number of cross-cultural studies of psychomotor development in the U.S. have been conducted with samples of Negro infants. The majority of the studies point to a general acceleration of Negro infants in gross and fine motor development during the first year.

Pasamanick (1946) and Knobloch and Pasamanick (1953) noted a definite acceleration in comparison with white norms in a group of 53 Negro infants, born in New Haven, Connecticut, during a period of high employment and good pre- and postnatal care. Developmental Quotients (DQ) on the Gesell Developmental Schedule for gross motor behavior increased from a mean of 109 at 26 weeks, to 114 at 50 weeks, and to 124 at 24 months, with a less pronounced acceleration in fine motor behavior.

Williams and Scott (1953) divided each of two socioeconomic groups (low/high) of Negro infants into a "permissive" and a "rigid" group, on the basis of information about child-rearing practices. Infants from the lower SES background came from homes where, comparatively, the atmosphere was more permissive and less exacting, but in *each* socioeconomic group, the *low* and the *high,* Negro infants from more permissive homes had a significantly larger mean gross motor score on the Gesell Developmental Schedule (114 vs. 100). Child-rearing practices which had a significant relationship to motor development were: a permissive attitude toward nonapproved habits; little area restriction; freedom to experiment and reach out; and a "causal" attitude toward motor development.

The most comprehensive set of data on Negro-white differences in psychomotor development was obtained in the standardization of the Bayley Scales of Infant Development (Bayley, 1965, 1969). Included were 1,262 infants, ages 1-30 months, approximately 55% of whom were white, 42% Negro, and the remainder Puerto Rican. The sample represented all socioeconomic and educational levels and all geographical regions of the U.S. mainland. While no differences were found between Negro and white infants on the mental scale, the mean psychomotor scores for Negro infants were higher at every age from one to 14 months, and significantly so at 3, 4, 5, 7, 9, and 12 months. For eleven items (out of 60) on the motor scale, the median age placement was at least .7 of a month younger for the Negro infants than for the white babies.

Two items in which Negro infants were relatively advanced were indicators of *midline handskill* and *eye-hand coordination* ("combines spoons or cubes midline," and "pat-a-cake"). The others were behaviors which require muscular strength and tonus. Four of these relate to *anti-gravity* ("holds head steady," "balances head when carried," "sits alone steadily," and "stands alone"). The other five deal with *locomotion* ("turns from side to back," "raises self to sitting position," "stepping movements," "walks with help," and "walks alone"). In a study of the reliability of the Bayley Scales of Infant Development it was found that these items have a high degree of tester-observer and test-retest reliability (Werner & Bayley, 1966).

ORIENTAL AND POLYNESIAN INFANTS IN HAWAII

A recent longitudinal study of a cohort of 635 infants of Oriental and Polynesian descent on the island of Kauai (Werner, Simonian & Smith, 1968; Werner, Bierman & French, 1971) found significant ethnic differences among infants of Japanese, Filipino, Hawaiian, Portuguese and "haole" descent on the Cattell Infant Intelligence Scale.

At 20 months, Japanese infants obtained the highest mean scores on the Cattell (mean 103) regardless of social class; Filipino and Hawaiian infants had the lowest, with means of 95 and 96 respectively. Portuguese and Anglo-Caucasian infants occupied an intermediary position with mean scores of 99 and 98.

The results of the infant test appeared to reflect the early effects of differential expectations and child-rearing practices among the different subcultures on the island. Kitano (1961), in a comparison study of child-rearing attitudes, found significant differences between first and second generation Japanese-Americans, with the Nisei putting less stress on fostering dependency and excluding outside influences, and more stress on the approval of activity and acceleration of development than the Japan-born parents. In contrast, the child-rearing attitudes of the Filipinos are characterized by indulgence and few demands on the infant (Whiting, 1963). There is no specific encouragement of walking, talking, or other skills. Maturation is seen as a leisurely process, one that adults do not accelerate.

ASIA AND OCEANIA

Japan

A recent cross-cultural study of maternal care and infant behavior by Caudill and Weinstein (1969) found significant differences in early motor behavior between urban, middle-class Japanese infants (from Tokyo and Kyoto) and American infants, which appear to be mediated by the maternal style of caretaking. Time-sampled observations of mother-child interaction at home indicated that American infants at ages 3-4 months appeared to be more physically active and vocal, and more involved in the exploration of their bodies and their environment than Japanese babies of the same age. The Japanese infants were, in contrast, much more subdued in their motor and vocal activity.

These differences in infant behavior showed a significant positive correlation ($r = .80$) with the customary caretaking style of the mother, both during waking and sleeping states of the infant. American mothers seemed to have a more lively and stimulating rapport with their infants, positioning the babies' bodies more frequently, and looking at and chattering with the infants more. The Japanese mothers, in contrast, were more often present with the baby, even when he was asleep, and had a more soothing and quieting rapport, as indicated by more lulling, carrying in arms, and rocking. The results of a study by Arai, Ishikawa, and Toshima (1956) of the development of a cross-sectional sample of 776 urban and rural Japanese infants, aged 1-36 months, from the northern part of the main island (Tohoka area), are in agreement with Caudill's observations.

Japanese infants showed a rate of motor and language development comparable to that of U.S. infants on the Gesell Developmental Schedule from the fourth to the twelfth week. From the sixteenth week on there was a steady decline in motor scores, clearly apparent by 20-24 weeks. Both gross motor development (movements of hands and feet) as well as fine motor development diminished. The authors ascribed the slowing down in the rate of gross and fine motor development to the limited stimulation provided by the Japanese mothers.

After the twentieth to twenty-fourth week, motor development improved, as the infants now spent most of their time on their mother's backs. From the forty-fourth to the fifty-second week, motor development slowed down again, for lack of opportunity to practice walking skills. Finally, between the ages of 18 and 36 months the children were freed from motoric constraint and were able to practice newly acquired walking skills.

Indonesia

Mead and MacGregor (1951) analyzed some 4,000 photographs of a longitudinal sample of eight Balinese children, reared in a traditional mountain village, and interpreted their psychomotor development in terms of Gesell categories. In the process they raised some interesting questions about linkage between adult handling and infant motoric activity. Balinese infants seem to go through the same general stages of motor behavior as U.S. infants, but significant and consistent differences could be identified. Where the American children go from frogging to creeping on all fours, then to standing and walking, with squatting coming after standing, the Balinese infants who do much less creeping (and spend most of the period when American babies are moving actively about, either sitting or being carried) combine frogging, creeping, and all-fours behavior simultaneously in a flexible state, from which they go from sitting to squatting to standing. A second area of contrast is found in the Balinese emphasis upon extension and outward rotation, and use of the ulnar side of the hand, as opposed to the greater inward rotation, inversion, and use of the thumb with good opposition between thumb and forefinger of American children. A third area of contrast is found in the persistence in Balinese children of a type of meandering tonus, characteristic of the fetal infant, with a very high degree of flexibility, and a capacity for the maintenance of positions of great discrepancy, in which parts of the whole body and of the hand or foot are simultaneously partly in flexion and partly in extension.

Mead and MacGregor also found the low tonal organization of the Balinese infant reinforced by the way Balinese adults carry and handle children. A sling permits the child to be attached to the mother or child nurse, resting on her hip, without either person making an active effort, once the sling is fastened. When the sling is absent, the carrier's arm appears equally relaxed. This light tie between child and carrier, touching close but without grasping by either one, allows peripheral responsiveness to predominate over grasping behavior or purposeful holding. The habitual method of handling the child is passive and involves minimal child-adult interaction.

One may note that Indonesian infants have one of the lowest birthweights (mean 2.89 kg) of all the samples studied, and are the smallest babies at age one year, with a mean weight of 7.52 kg and a mean body length of only 67.6 cm (Meredith, 1970a, b).

The low tonal organization of the Balinese infants, regardless of its origin, whether genetic or nutritional, appears constantly reinforced by the pattern of adult care and handling.

INDIA

Phatak (1970a, b) completed an extensive study of the mental and motor development of Indian infants on the Bayley Scales of Infant

Development. Her findings were based on three samples: 4,141 longitudinal records of upper-class urban babies in Baroda, with subsamples ranging from 60 to 178, at 1-30 months; 1,090 cross-sectional records of lower-class urban babies, with subsamples ranging from 59 to 78, at 1-15 months; and 633 cross-sectional records of rural infants from surrounding villages in the state of Gujarat, with subsamples ranging from 25 to 52, at 1-15 months.

The analysis of both the mean mental and psychomotor scores and of item placements seems to indicate that Indian infants, regardless of social class or urban-rural upbringing, are advanced in comparison with U.S. infants in both fine and gross motor skills during the first six to nine months of their lives.

The more traditionally reared rural infants showed the greatest acceleration, followed closely by the poorest urban infants. The motor development of the more Westernized upper-class urban infants (whose parents enroll their preschool age children in the University Nursery School) was less accelerated than that of the poor urban and rural infants, though superior to that of U.S. infants in the first half of the first year.

However, there was a gradual slowing down of the motor competence of the Indian babies as they approached year one, with the rural and lower-class urban infants falling behind the upper-class urban infants in the second year. In the latter part of the second year of life, even the more privileged urban infants in Baroda had psychomotor scores that were lower than those of U.S. infants of comparable age.

On the *mental* scale, the upper-class urban babies tended to score consistently higher than the lower-class urban and rural samples at *all* age levels studied, with mean scores comparable to or slightly above those of U.S. infants. The mean mental scores of the urban and rural poor declined steadily from a normal level at two months to a below average level at fifteen moths. By the time they had passed their first birthday, their mean scores were 15 points lower than those of the upper-class urban infants.

It is interesting to note the differences in the type of *motor* items on which Indian babies were *advanced* in comparison with U.S. infants. They included items that deal with fine motor skills, eye-hand coordination, anti-gravity and locomotion—all finished products of maturation, involving independent control of head, hand, wrist, upper and lower extremities.

Items on the *mental* scale which showed Indian babies ahead of U.S. infants also involved eye-hand coordination, manipulation of objects and spatial relationships, reflecting well-developed fine motor skills. In contrast, *motor* items on which even the upper-class urban infants *lagged behind* U.S. infants required a certain amount of risk-taking, self-reliance and independence as well as getting used to unfamiliar equipment (walking-board, tape measure).

The acceleration of the Indian infants in the first part of the first year, followed by a drop in performance in the latter part of year one and in year two, may be explained with reference to several factors: (1) birthweight: Indian babies have the lowest birthweight of all samples studied (mean 2.74 kg) and the next to lowest mean weight at year one (8.00 kg) (Meredith, 1970a, b); (2) a warm, tropical climate that requires little or no restriction by clothing; (3) a permissive child-rearing philosophy in an extended family of several caretakers that results in a combination of great freedom to explore, but also great dependency on adults for the immediate satisfaction of the infant's needs.

Interviews with most of the mothers who participated in the Baroda study indicated that they were still largely influenced by traditional child-rearing practices. Because they lived in a joint family system— grandparents, aunts, uncles, cousins—they were helped by several caretakers. During the first two to three months, both the mother's and the infant's activities were confined, with the mother spending much time feeding the baby on demand, and resting. After the third month, the mother assumed her usual responsibilities, but took her child with her wherever she went, and breast-fed him on demand. Since the baby slept with the mother, breast-feeding was no problem. There was no set sleeping, waking or toilet routines. The infants did not have playpen, or a special room for themselves, and roamed freely about in the house and yard. Most of the sample mothers did not feel anxious if their infants were late in attaining certain developmental milestones, such as sitting, standing, walking, bowel and bladder control, speech, regular sleep and eating habits, and made no special efforts to help their children attain these skills.

Adult interaction with babies was generally aimed at producing a cessation of a response rather than a stimulation. The period of undivided attention ended usually when the mother was pregnant again or when she stopped breast-feeding. After weaning, and especially after the birth of a new baby, a combination of protein-calorie malnutrition, a dearth of educational toys, and lack of verbal stimulation appeared to contribute jointly to a steady slowing down in the developmental rate of the urban and rural poor infants.

Phatak's findings with the Bayley Scales of Infant Development in

West India have been confirmed with smaller samples and other developmental tests in other parts of the Indian subcontinent. Venkatachan (in Phatak, 1970) found Mysore children in South India to be superior to U.S. infants on Gesell test items of pursuit and manipulation of objects up to the age of six months. Uklenskaya, Pari, Caudharai, Dang and Raj Kumari (1960) studied the development of static and psychomotor functions in a cross-sectional sample of 900 New Delhi children in North India, at the ages of one to twelve months, and found them to be on a par with Russian infants up to seven months, but noted a slowing down of their psychomotor development thereafter. Recently, Abhichandani (1970) confirmed these findings in a longitudinal study of 80 New Delhi babies from one to eighteen months of age, using both the Bayley Scales of Infant Development and the Denver Developmental Screening Test. In a longitudinal study of infants from the poorest section of Bombay in East India, the infants of a sweeper community appeared on a par with the New Delhi babies *until* they reached the age of standing and walking. After that, they appeared retarded in both gross motor skills and vocabulary (Tha in Phatak, 1970).

MIDDLE EAST

Lebanon

Dennis and Najarian (1957) were among the first to test hypotheses about the detrimental effects of stimulus deprivation on infants reared in institutions in a cross-cultural context. They contrasted the psychomotor development of 49 Lebanese children, residing in a Beirut foundling home, with a control group of 41 home-reared infants, from the poorest section of Beirut, drawn from the well-baby clinic of the American University Hospital.

The infants in the "Crèche" were adequately nourished and healthy, but there was severe understaffing—a ratio of one attendant to ten children. During the first two months, infants were taken out of their cribs only for their daily bath and change of clothing. They were not held while they were fed, but instead were given a bottle propped on a small pillow from which they drank as they lay on their backs. Cribs had a covering around the sides so that the infants could see only the ceiling while lying supine.

Results on the Cattell Infant Intelligence Test indicated that in comparison with the development of the home-reared Lebanese babies (mean 101), the mean quotients of the Crèche infants dropped from 100 at two months to a mean of 63 between three and twelve months. While

Cattell test items at two months are given in a supine position, to which the Crèche infants were accustomed, test items from three to twelve months required that they be tested in a sitting position to which they were unaccustomed. As a group, they had a poor record on test items which involved holding the head erect and steady, and items requiring eye-hand coordination and manipulation of objects.

In an attempt to modify the usual institutional environment and to test the hypothesis that appropriate supplementary experiences can result in rapid increases in the psychomotor development of environmentally restricted infants, Sayegh and Dennis (1965) gave a one-hour practice session for five days a week to five 7-12 months old institutionalized infants in the Beirut Crèche, whose initial developmental age was only four months. The supplementary experiences stressed sitting, watching, and manipulating objects. This extra stimulation resulted in significant gains on the Cattell Infant Intelligence Test one month later.

In a similar study of 174 children, aged 1-3 years, in three institutions in Teheran, Dennis (1960) contrasted the psychomotor development of children reared in two public orphanages with a group reared in a private institution. All children were healthy and well-fed. In the public orphanage, because of a lack of attendants (8 children to one adult), there was a paucity of handling, including the failure of the attendants to place the children in the sitting and in the prone position. The absence of experience in these positions retarded these children in regard to sitting alone (fewer than half did so by age two) and to the onset of locomotion (none walked by age two). The lack of experience in the prone position prevented the children from creeping; prior to walking most locomoted by scooting.

In contrast, infants in the private orphanage, where there was a ratio of one attendant to three or four children, were frequently handled, propped in the sitting position, and placed prone. Their motor development in the first two years of life resembled closely that of home-reared children in Teheran and that of Western babies. Thus the motor retardation of the infants in public institutions appeared to be due to a restriction of specific kinds of perceptual learning.

Israel

One of the features of institutional care is that it provides interaction with many caretakers. Even if an institution provided adequate opportunity for perceptual-motor stimulation and the learning of social behavior, the diffusion of attachment over a number of individuals could be detrimental to the optimal behavioral development of infants. Studies of children raised in the Israeli kibbutz are relevant here.

Kibbutz infants, although fed, handled and cared for by their mothers, are brought up in small groups (4-8) lodged in premises separated from the living quarters of the parents, from the time the mother returns from the hospital after delivery. In these "infant houses" two or three professional caretakers, in addition to the mother, are in charge of day and night routine care of the infants, thus exposing the children to "concomitant mothering" (Rabin, 1958). The mother gradually turns over more and more child-rearing duties to the "metapelet" in the latter part of the first year, as she returns to her regular job. Weaning from the bottle or breast occurs at about 6-8 months. At about one year the smaller group of children is merged with another group and moves to the "toddler house" where a new metapelet looks after a group of four to six toddlers. The toddler sees his mother less (she begins to work full-time about one year after delivery) and is expected to undergo toilet-training and to cooperate with his peers.

Kohen-Raz (1967, 1968) contrasted the mental and psychomotor development of kibbutz, institutionalized, and home-reared infants on the Bayley Scales of Infant Development. The sample consisted of 405 babies, ranging in age from one to twenty-seven months, belonging to three subpopulations: 166 infants reared in middle-class homes in Jerusalem and Rehovoth, 151 babies, born in collective settlements, selected as a representative sample of the kibbutzim in Israel, and 88 institutionalized infants from five large Baby Homes in Jerusalem, Tel-Aviv and Haifa, who had resided in the institution for at least one month.

There is a striking similarity between the results of the Kohen-Raz study on institutionalized Israeli babies and the findings reported by Dennis (1960, 1963) from institutions in Lebanon and Iran: The institutionalized infants were significantly retarded in relation to Israeli non-institutionalized samples and to samples of U.S. infants. Their mean scores dropped from 99 at age two months to a mean score of 60 on the mental scale by age twelve months, and they also slowed down in their motor development, though not quite as drastically. There was a continuous leveling off of performance in the second year of life on both the mental and motor scales. Institutionalized infants performed significantly lower than kibbutz and private home babies on all subscales, except the eye-hand scale.

In contrast, kibbutz infants maintained a high average to superior performance on *both* mental and motor scales in the first half of the first year of life. This performance was consistently (though not significantly) superior to the private home babies, except for items on the "vocalization-social contact" scale, where private home babies excelled. However, in the latter part of the first year, at around 10 months, there was an abrupt drop in the performance of the kibbutz infants on the mental scale (from a mean of 105 at six months to a mean of 94 at ten months) and an ever sharper decline on the psychomotor scale (from a mean of 100 at six months to a mean of 84 at ten months). Mean scores of kibbutz infants on both the mental and motor scales picked up again around 15 months, though motor scores were consistently lower than mental scores at ages 15, 18, 21, and 24 months. There was no such drop in mean scores for private home infants in the same age range.

Kohen-Raz's findings at ages 10 and 12 months are quite similar to those of an earlier study by Rabin (1958), who compared a group of 24 infants from five kibbutzim with a group of 20 infants reared at home in the Moshave noncollective rural settlement. Around year one (mean age 13 months, range 9-17 months), the kibbutz babies obtained a mean score of 82 on the Griffiths Developmental Scale, while the Moshave infants obtained a mean score of 90.

One might speculate that the "temporary" drop in the performance of the kibbutz infants at ages 10 and 12 months is related to weaning practices, and the transfer, around 12 months, of the children from the "infant house" to the "toddler house" and the care of a new metapelet. Golan (1958) in a discussion of some of the potential problem areas of collective education points out that the most stressful period in the life of kibbutz children appears to be the one immediately after being weaned, from 9 to about 15 months. There is a tendency for many caretakers to treat weaned children as though they were still infants. Sometimes children are kept in playpens, isolated or together, with little freedom of motion, and with little opportunity to crawl or make attempts at walking. Golan also comments on the fact that at this age fewer provisions have been made for suitable toys or sensorimotor activities that encourage exploration. Most of the items on the mental scale on which Israeli babies appeared to be slower than U.S. babies of comparable age are placed somewhere in the age range between 10 and 20 months and deal with eye-hand coordination, manipulation of objects and the comprehension and initiation of actions that require an adult model and a one-to-one adult-child relationship. Kohen-Raz's study demonstrates, however, that there appears to be no lasting "retardation" among kibbutz-reared infants. By the time they reach the second half of their second year of life, mean mental and motor scores of kibbutz infants are comparable, if not slightly superior, to the home-reared infants of middle-class parents.

AFRICA

A fairly extensive literature has accumulated on the precocity of African babies in psychomotor development, drawn from different tribal groups, both in traditional rural and Westernized urban areas of Uganda, Cameroun, Congo, Nigeria, Senegal, and South Africa.

Uganda

Geber (1956, 1958a, b, 1960, 1961) and Geber and Dean (1957a, b, 1958, 1964) have published a series of studies that report the results of developmental tests on several hundred infants and preschool children, predominantly from the Ganda tribe, in and around Kampala in Uganda, East Africa. Children were examined both cross-sectionally and longitudinally at birth with the André-Thomas neonatal examination, and from ages 1-6 months, 7-12 months, 1-2 years, and 2-3 years with the Gesell Developmental Schedules. Ainsworth (1967) and Akim, McFie and Sebigajju (1956) have studied smaller samples of Ganda and Luo infants with the Griffiths Developmental Scale and reported similar results.

Data on the psychomotor development of Uganda infants are now available for a group of 216 that were traditionally reared in families of small landholders and agricultural laborers, and for a group of 86 infants from a Westernized urban milieu, where the parents were professionals and well-educated. Comparison samples of Caucasian and Indian infants were also tested.

The newborn examination showed a considerable precocity of African infants; much of the activity corresponded to that of 4-6-week-old European infants. The advance was shown chiefly by a lesser degree of flexion of the African babies and low tonicity, by a remarkable control of head and trunk, and by the absence of primitive reflex activity (Moro, grasping, marching reflexes) (Geber & Dean, 1957). Subsequently, Nelson and Dean (1959) reported that the encephalograms of African newborns were suggestive of a greater degree of maturity than is usually found in the European newborn child. Vincent and Hugo (1962) confirmed these findings in a sample of low birthweight infants from the Congo.

Consistent with the newborn findings, there was a remarkable precocity of both gross and fine motor development in the first six months, putting the traditionally reared Ganda babies between two and three months ahead of Western infants. Their mean fine motor score was 130; mean adaptive and language scores were 125 and 120, respectively. Mean gross motor scores between 7 and 12 months were about 135; fine motor scores about 125; mean adaptive and languages scores ranged from 125 to 120.

In the age range 1-2 years, the motor precocity tended to be lost among the traditionally reared children. Their rate of development slowed down, so that only nine months' progress by European standards was made in the second year. The slight progress made in language and the great dependence of the infant on the mother were especially notable in the testing situation. At 18 months, mean gross and fine motor scores were about 120; adaptive scores, 105; and language scores about 100.

After two years, the traditionally reared children needed the constant encouragement and approval of their mothers to initiate the test. Their interest in the test materials flagged and their adaptive and language development appeared quite impaired. This trend was continued after age three, when the developmental quotients for the traditionally reared children dropped below 100, with the lowest mean scores in adaptive (95) and in language development (90).

Geber interprets her findings in terms of the pattern of adult care and handling of infants in traditional villages and contrasts this with the differential effect of a "Westernized" regime in urban families.

In the traditional Ganda family, as in most other African tribes, there is a great deal of physical contact in the mother-child relationship. In the first year the child is inseparable from his mother who carries him on her back when she goes to the field to work or to visit neighbors, and feeds him on demand, day and night. Geber speculates that the continual carrying on the back by the mother may strengthen the child's ability to hold his head firmly, by forcing him to compensate for her various movements. In the same way, his sitting position on her back, with his back straight, and his legs pressed against her waist, may help him to sit earlier than the European child. Since he is taken everywhere, his life in the changing scene is more stimulating than that of the child who remains in the cradle, crib or cot. From time to time he is held by some other member of the extended family and offered to neighbors and visitors with a greeting. The child becomes easily accustomed to sorties into strange arms, with varying degrees of contact-comfort, security and reinforcing pressure.

The mother begins to offer supplementary food besides her breast milk at about six months of age, but continues to give the breast on demand, and to sleep with the child. The first birthday is often chosen for complete weaning, unless the mother is pregnant earlier. This decision made, not only does the mother stop breast feeding, but she no longer carries the infant on her back, and no longer sleeps with him. She teaches him to stay quiet and passive; the assumption is that the child is now old enough to fend for himself. In some traditional Ganda villages it is still the custom to reinforce weaning by physical separation. The child may be sent to a grandmother or aunt for several months. His new diet is low in animal protein and consists mostly of bananas, sweet potatoes, yams and cassavas. Thus, in the second year of life and thereafter, the withdrawal of protection and proper nourishment is not balanced by an enlargement of opportunity. There is little in the home and rural surroundings that would stimulate and foster cognitive development—a few mats, no books, pictures or ornaments, no toys, no kitchen utensils, and hardly any tools.

In a contrasting study of 86 children from Westernized homes of the same Ganda tribe, Geber and Dean (1958, 1964) found a somewhat different pattern of psychomotor development. Up to the age of two years, motor development, although precocious in comparison with Western infants, was not quite so remarkable as that previously found among infants in the poorer rural families; but after two years the falling off in language and adaptive development found so consistently among the traditionally reared Ganda did not occur. Mean developmental quotients for the African infants from a privileged urban milieu (their parents were government officials, doctors, teachers, journalists) ranged from 115 at 6 months to 110 at 18 months, and rose after age two years steadily to a level between 115 and 120—results comparable to those found among Western children of the same socioeconomic status.

The slight, but constant, failure of the privileged children to match the early development of the traditionally reared infants was also explained in terms of upbringing. Instead of being fed on demand, the wealthier infants were usually fed at more or less regular intervals, and spent much of their time lying in their cots. More of the "Westernized" urban mothers bottle-fed, or if they breast-fed their babies, were less successful in lactation. The partial failure of lactation occurred more frequently as sophistication increased. However, in contrast with the traditionally reared village children, the opportunities for cognitive stimulation and self-education afforded by the parents, and the relative extensive equipment of the well-to-do homes were much greater.

The findings of Geber and Dean in East Africa have been confirmed with other tribal groups in Central, Equatorial, West, and South Africa.

Senegal

Falade (1955, 1960) and Bardet, Masse, Moreigne and Sénécal (1960) examined more than a hundred infants in Dakar with the Gesell Developmental Schedule and the Brunét-Lézine scale. They found three distinct stages that characterized the psychomotor development of Senegalese infants of the Wolof tribe: The first stage extended from birth to about one year of age when the infant walked alone. During this time there was a remarkable precocity that put the Wolof infants 2-3 months ahead of European infants. In the second stage, from about 12-18 months, psychomotor development was less rapid, and performance was comparable to that of European babies. In the third stage, around 24 months, development slowed down considerably. Both Falade and Bardet ascribe this arrest in development to weaning practices and profound changes in the affective relationship between mother and child.

Cameroun

Vouilloux (1959a, b) reports comparable results from a study of 48 healthy infants of the Doula Bassa, Bamilieke and Ewondo tribes in Doulas, Cameroun. Postural, locomotor and eye-hand coordination of the home-reared infants was extremely accelerated in the first three months, and remained superior to that of Western infants throughout the first 18 months, with gross motor development somewhat ahead of fine motor development. This psychomotor acceleration was more pronounced for children from low socioeconomic status homes (mean 131) than for children from higher SES homes (mean 115) and was not apparent among orphans (mean 97). Scores for the home-reared infants were comparable to those of Western children between 20 and 36 months of age, after a rather late weaning (between 18 and 35 months) and the end of a period of demand feeding. Vouilloux, like Geber, favors an environmental explanation for the observed changes over time and the differences between poorer and richer homes.

Nigeria

In an attempt to test the hypothesis that Westernization is accompanied by a retarding of psychomotor development among African children, Poole (1969) measured the attainment of 90 Yoruba infants in two equal-sized samples drawn from urban and rural homes. At each month, from 5 to 15 months, five infants from traditional rural homes were compared with five infants from Westernized urban homes. The average yearly income of the rural group was below $300, that of the urban group $2,000 and upward. None of the rural mothers had any formal education; all of the urban mothers had elementary education to age 14, and some secondary education or more. Most of the urban mothers had terminated breast-feeding far earlier than the traditional mothers, who tended to breast-feed for between one and two years.

Poole results are somewhat inconclusive: Both the rural and urban groups were somewhat advanced on most of the developmental milestones of the Griffiths Scale, with the rural babies more advanced than the urban ones at age 2-3 months. The trend of the difference was in the predicted direction, but did not achieve statistical significance because of the very small samples at each age. This study also excluded the age range (birth to 5 months) where motor acceleration has been most pronounced in other African samples.

South Africa

In a study of 480 healthy urban infants in Johannesburg, with 40 infants at each age level from one to 12 months, Bantu babies appeared to be generally one to one-and-a-half months in advance of 210 white infants on all major locomotor milestones in the first year of life (Liddicoat, 1969).

On the average the birthweight of the different African samples studied is between 300 and 400 g below that of Caucasian babies in Europe and the United States (means between 2.92 and 3.08 kg) and similar to that of U.S. Negroes (3.10 kg) (Meredith, 1970a). The weight of African babies increases rapidly during the first six months, until the European and Caucasian growth curves intersect. After that, weight gain tends to decrease, so that African babies, on the average, are between 2.2 and 1.2 kg lighter than Caucasian babies at age one year (Meredith, 1970b). Apparently the maternal milk provides adequate nourishment in the first six months, but is not sufficient thereafter. After weaning, generally between one and two years, protein-calorie malnutrition is making major inroads, as is vividly shown in a comparison of mean Gesell Developmental Quotients of 21 malnourished Capetown children who were matched with 21 adequately nourished controls of the same age, sex, and socioeconomic status (Stoch & Smythe, 1963). The children were first examined at about one year of age and subsequently at six to twelve month intervals thereafter, throughout the preschool years. At final testing the mean developmental quotients of the undernourished group (71, range 45-80) differed from that of the adequately nourished control group (93, range 85-110) by 22 points.

LATIN AMERICA

Results of several cross-cultural studies of the psychomotor development of infants in Central and South America (Jamaica, Mexico, Guatemala, Peru, Chile, and Brazil), using the Gesell Developmental Schedules and the Bayley Scales of Infant Development, seem to vary, depending on whether infants lived in traditional, preindustrial, or transitional urban communities.

Jamaica

Two studies of gross motor development conducted in Kingston, Jamaica, 36 years apart (Curti, Marshall & Steggerda, 1935; Granthan-McGregor & Back, 1971) found infants of predominantly Negroid extraction to be accelerated over white children on the Gesell Developmental Schedules. The early cross-sectional study of 26 infants reported earlier ages of creeping, standing and walking. The recent study, in which 300 infants were followed longitudinally throughout the first year of life and tested every month, found the majority of Jamaican infants from predominantly working-class and lower-middle class homes to be significantly accelerated on items that dealt with control of the head; supported and unsupported sitting; standing; pulling self to standing position; creeping; walking with and without support.

Among the Jamaican children large numbers were sleeping with their mothers and were being fed on demand. A lack of physical restrictions, such as cribs and playpens, gave the impression of great permissiveness in handling the children. No socioeconomic status differences were noted in this predominantly lower and lower-middle class sample. However, a greater weight at one year had a beneficial effect on age of walking. Children of low birthweight (below 2.5 kg) were significantly slower than children with birthweights above 2.5 kg, but were equal to normal Caucasian children in their performance on the Gesell Developmental Schedules.

Guatemala and Mexico

This finding was replicated by Cravioto (1967) in a study of 95 Guatemalan infants with birthweights between 1,450 and 2,490 g, drawn from a hospital in Guatemala City, and was presented as indirect evidence of precocity in motor development among full-term infants in preindustrial settings of Latin America.

Infants from two rural communities in Guatemala (Cakchiquel Indians) and from four preindustrial communities in Mexico (two mestizo, one Zapotec Indian, one Nahoa Indian), after acceleration in motor development in the first 12 months, began to show a steady decline in the second year, so that by the age of 18-24 months their performance was below that shown by their Caucasian counterparts (Robles, 1959; Wug de Leon, Licardie & Cravioto, 1964). Mean scores in motor development declined from a high of 155 and 137 for Mexican and Guatemalan infants respectively (age one year) to mean scores of 77 after year two (Cravioto, 1966).

The advanced motor status of newborn infants found in Jamaica and Guatemala has recently also been documented in two preindustrial communities in Mexico. In a longitudinal study of 300 infants in a semi-tropical village in southwestern Mexico undergoing a slow transition to mixed economy, Cravioto, Birch, DeLicardie, Rosales and Vega (1969) examined motor competence at birth with selected items from the Gesell Developmental Schedules, and found a median performance among the newborn comparable to that of two-week-old U.S. infants. The distribution of birthweights in this cohort bore a clear resemblance to African and Asian samples, with an excess of birthweights below 2,500 g. Items on which the newborn infants appeared precocious were similar to those noted by Geber and Dean in Uganda (1957a). There was no such precocity in adaptive performance. The level of motor competence at birth appeared to be directly related to birthweight. The most motorically competent infants were in the upper quartile of birthweights.

Brazelton, Robey and Collier (1969) gathered twelve neonatal observations and 93 tests of psychomotor development during the first nine months of life among the Zinacanteco Indians of southwestern Mexico who lived in scattered mountain villages in relative isolation. Although the newborns were small, weighing only about five pounds, their limb movements were free and smooth and of low tonicity. The infants showed a striking sensory alertness, turning to voices and following a visual stimulus when they were but a few hours old. Their Moro and grasping reflexes were more subdued than those of U.S. infants. Their high organization of response, their adaptation to repeated stimuli, and their maturity in sucking were superior to U.S. newborns. However, while the output of spontaneous motor activity gradually increased from day to day in U.S. infants of like age, the Zinicanteco infants maintained a relatively low output of spontaneous movement that seemed to reflect the nature of mother-child interaction.

The infants, throughout the first year, were clothed in a long heavy skirt, extending beyond their feet, held in place by a wide belt or cinch wrapped firmly around the abdomen. They were then wrapped in additional layers of blankets which swaddled the baby and acted as a constant suppressor of motor activity. The infants were carried in a "rebozo," a shawl large enough to hold and enclose them on their mother's back when not feeding. Infants' faces were covered except during feeding, especially in the first three months, to ward off illness and the effects of the evil eye.

During the first year, infants were never propped up to look around, were not talked to or put on the floor in the prone position to explore on their own. Their mothers rarely attempted to elicit social responses from their babies by looking at their faces or talking to them. The primary purpose of the frequent breast-feeding (up to nine times in four hours) was to quiet the infant's restlessness when he would not be lulled back to sleep in the rebozo. The most striking feature of the mother's caretaking style was the paucity of vocalization and active stimulation of the infant. The Zinacanteco mothers seemed to establish and maintain a kinesthetic communication with their infants which reinforced the suppression of extraneous motor activity. This caretaking style produced quiet, non-exploratory infants who developed in a slightly delayed (about one-and-a-half months) but parallel fashion to infants in the U.S. as judged by their performance on the Gesell Developmental Schedules and the Bayley Scales of Infant Development.

Brazil, Peru and Chile

Studies of infants' psychomotor development in the large urban areas of Latin America failed to show the motor precocity noted among infants growing up in traditional rural communities.

Schmidt, Maciel, Boskovitz, Rosenberg and Cury (1971) published a large-scale pediatric social survey of 762 infants living in an industrial city near Sao Paulo, Brazil, with nearly 150,000 inhabitants. On major milestones of psychomotor development, the children from poor homes, and of illiterate parents, were more precocious in head control during the first three months. On all other major psychomotor milestones (sitting, standing, walking) they were retarded in comparison with infants from homes where parents had some education.

Among the illiterate families there was a significantly larger percentage of infants with a birthweight below 2,500 g, and a larger number of children with short periods of breast feeding.

Using the Bayley Scales of Infant Development and the Gesell Developmental Schedules, studies in Lima, Peru (Pollitt & Granoff, 1967) and in Chile (Moenckeberg, 1968) have graphically demonstrated the presence of retarded levels of psychomotor and adaptive development in infants at different stages of rehabilitation from severe malnutrition. Cravioto and Robles (1965) found greater persistence of low performance scores in adaptive and motor behavior on the part of infants who experienced the onset of protein-calorie malnutrition *prior* to six months of age than in infants whose onset of malnutrition came at a later age. Their numbers are rapidly increasing with the process of "modernization" and social change in the developing countries.

CONCLUSIONS

Comparisons have been made of the findings of some fifty cross-cultural studies of the psychomotor development of contemporary groups of infants in Africa, Asia and Oceania, Latin America, Europe, and the United States. The following conclusions are presented.

1. There was a distinct acceleration of psychomotor development among samples of infants reared in traditional, preindustrial communities in Africa, Asia and Latin America, with the African samples (from Uganda, Cameroun, Congo, Nigeria, Senegal and South Africa) showing the greatest acceleration, followed closely by Latin American infants (from Jamaica, Mexico and Guatemala) and samples from different parts of the Indian subcontinent (Baroda, Mysore, New Delhi, Bombay).

2. The acceleration was most pronounced at birth and during the first six months of life. Neonatal observations of samples of infants in Africa (Uganda, Congo) and in Latin America (Mexico, Guatemala) indicated a precocious sensorimotor development, equalling that of European and U.S. infants 3-4 weeks old. EEG examinations of newborn African babies were suggestive of greater maturity of the central nervous system, and even "premature" babies in Africa and Latin America, weighing less than 2,500 g, showed adequate motor development.

3. In spite of a great deal of cultural and geographical diversity, all of the infants drawn from preindustrial communities shared certain common experiences during the first year: membership in an extended family system with many caretakers; breast-feeding on demand, day and night; constant tactile stimulation by the body of the adult caretaker who carried the infant on her back or side, and slept with him; participation in all adult activities, with frequent sensory-motor stimulation; lack of set routines for feeding, sleeping and toileting; and lack of restrictive clothing in a (semi) tropical climate. On the average, birth-weights of these infants were below 3.0 kg.

4. Beginning in the second half of the first year, when volume of

breast milk is no longer adequate if taken alone, or when supplementary food was low in animal protein or contaminated by a high dose of bacteria, there was a steady downward trend in the psychomotor scores of infants reared in traditional rural communities of Africa, Asia and Latin America. This downward trend became accentuated at and after the age of weaning, sometime in the second year of life, and the restrictions in sensory-motor and affective stimulation associated with it. After age two, mean scores of infants from traditionally reared samples in the developing countries were significantly lower than those of Western children in gross and fine motor development, with the lowest scores in adaptive and language development.

5. Samples of "Westernized," upper-middle class urban infants from the same ethnic groups in Africa (Uganda, Cameroun, Nigeria) and India (Baroda) who were breast-fed less frequently and for a shorter duration, and who lived in nuclear families, sleeping alone in cots or cribs, were not as accelerated as traditionally reared, rural infants but were still superior to Western infants in their psychomotor development during the first year of life. Their development in the second year of life proceeded on an accelerated level, comparable to that of Western infants of the same socioeconomic status.

6. Among home-reared infants in non-Western cultures, there were some samples that did not show a discontinuity between early acceleration and later decline. These were infants brought up in settings where the mother-infant interaction was quiet and passive, and where infants tended to be somewhat restricted by heavy clothing (Zinacanteco Indians in Mexico, Japanese infants in urban and rural Japan). In these samples there was a psychomotor development comparable to that of Western infants in the first two to three months, which then leveled off and lagged a steady one to one-and-a-half months behind the rate of Western infants until year two.

7. The sharpest early decline in psychomotor development was found among infants in the urban slums whose period of breast-feeding was consistently shorter than that of the rural communities, and among institutionalized children with few caretakers in the Middle East (Lebanon, Iran, Israel). After a normal development in the first two months, their psychomotor scores dropped abruptly below the mean of home-reared babies, and remained on a severely retarded level from three months on.

8. Among infants in the developed countries, accelerated psychomotor development was noted among samples of U.S. Negro infants, reared in permissive homes, Japanese-American infants, reared in homes which

stressed acceleration, and kibbutz infants in Israel, reared in a system of "concomitant mothering." This acceleration, however, was not as pronounced as that of traditionally reared infants in the developing countries of Africa, Asia and Latin America, and resembled more the rate of "Westernized" urban samples in Africa and Asia.

9. While the Japanese-American infants maintained their acceleration until age two, the scores of kibbutz infants dropped temporarily, after the age of weaning and transfer to the toddler house, with another caretaker and peer group at ages 10-15 months, but then climbed up to an above average level. In contrast, the acceleration in psychomotor development of U.S. Negro samples leveled off by year one. In the second year of life, they began to fall behind the norms of Caucasian babies in the U.S. due to perceptual and cognitive restrictions, not unlike their "traditional" counterparts in Africa.

10. The rate of psychomotor development appeared essentially the same for infants in the U.S. and in Europe (France, Great Britain, Switzerland, Sweden, Belgium). All of these samples had mean birthweights above 3 kg, approaching 3.5 kg. Heavier infants tended to walk earlier.

Frijda and Jahoda (1966) in a thoughtful article on the scope and method of cross-cultural research have raised the question whether there is not perhaps an unduly exclusive emphasis on the so-called "culture-fair" or "culture appropriate" test. As this review has illustrated, a good deal can be said in favor of using the *same* test (s) in various cultures and attempting to tease out the causes of such differences as are found. Thus the finding of cross-cultural studies of infants' psychomotor development, both cross-sectional and longitudinal, appear quite consistent, in spite of some methodological shortcomings due to the nature of the assessment instruments used. They seem to point to a significant interaction between ethnicity, amount and type of caretaker stimulation, and nutritional status of the infant.

Of all the *ethnic* groups studied, the Negroid samples, both in Africa and in the U.S., showed the greatest early acceleration of psychomotor development, the Caucasian samples showed the least, with the Latin American Indian and Mestizo and the Asian samples occupying an intermediary position—even if they live in the *same ecological* setting (Africans, Gujaradi Indians, and Caucasians in Uganda; Negro and Caucasian in the West Indies; Mestizo and Caucasian in Latin America; Caucasian, Negro and Indian samples in the U.S.).

However, *within* each ethnic group, whether in Africa (Uganda, Cameroun, Nigeria), Asia (Gujarati Indian) or the U.S. (high and low SES Negro samples), consistent differences were found between samples of infants brought up in a "traditional" *permissive* manner with much stimulation by many caretakers, and more privileged, but also more *restrictive*, "Westernized" samples. In each case, the more permissively reared samples of the *same ethnic stock* showed the greatest acceleration in early psychomotor development, and the greatest decline, after weaning, in adaptive and language development. In turn, *within* traditional and Westernized samples of the same ethnic stock, infants with a *higher birthweight* showed a greater early motor acceleration.

The abrupt termination of both breast-feeding *and* stimulation at the time of weaning appears to have a devastating effect, that reverses the earlier course of precocious development among infants from traditionally reared preindustrial communities. There is some indication from recent studies that deficits in sensorimotor development will appear even earlier among the illiterate poor in crowded city slums of the developing countries where breast-feeding has become less frequent and of shorter duration. Feeding by bottle of tinned and diluted milk is nutritionally inadequate and conducive to infective diarrhea and earlier appearance of marasmus (Jelliffe, 1962; Winick, 1969).

Failure to lactate, and it is beginning to spread in developing countries with rapid social change, will increase the number of infants weaned before six months who face permanent irreversible central nervous system damage (Winick, 1969; Harfouche, 1970). The need for better maternal and child health care, feeding of lactating mothers, and better nutrition and day care services for the infants of poor working mothers in the city slums of the developing countries has never been so urgent.

Even in the developed countries, such as the U.S., recent intervention programs for infants from underprivileged homes have come to the sobering recognition that *prevention* needs to start *before* the infant's first birthday, since social class differences in sensorimotor development have been reported as early as seven months and the greatest gains through intervention (feeding, day care, stimulation) in developmental quotients have been reported in the period from seven to eleven months (Starr, 1971).

There remain other questions that only future cross-cultural research with infants can answer:

1. What associations can be demonstrated between fetal activity and early sensorimotor development among cross-cultural samples, varying in quality of prenatal care and maternal nutrition? A study by Walters (1965) has shown a significant correlation between fetal activity in the seventh month of pregnancy and psychomotor activity at 12, 24, and

26 months, and a study by Sontag (1940) has shown a negative correlation between *fetal activity* and *birthweight*. Both studies were conducted on middle-class Caucasian samples in the U.S. Can these findings be replicated with other ethnic groups in the developing countries?

2. Can neonatal precocity be demonstrated in other cross-cultural samples besides the African and Latin American populations studied so far? Studies need to be undertaken that take a look at the behavior of the newborn in the developing countries of Asia and Oceania. One such study is now in progress among the Central Australian aborigines (Francis *et al.*, in press).

3. What important *changes* in the reciprocal interaction of mothers' caretaking styles and infants' psychomotor behavior take place with increasing industrialization and urbanization in the developing world?

4. What are the effects of recent international intervention programs (feeding of lactating mothers, infant nutrition, crèches and day-care centers) on the development of infants in Asia, Latin America and Africa?

REFERENCES

ABHICHANDANI, P.: A study of growth and development in the first eighteen months of life. Unpublished doctoral dissertation, All India Institute of Medical Sciences, 1970.

AINSWORTH, M. D. S.: *Infancy in Uganda: Infant Care and the Growth of Love.* Baltimore: The Johns Hopkins Press, 1967.

AKIM, B., McFIE, J., & SEBIGAJJU, E.: Developmental level and nutrition: A study of young children in Uganda. *Journal of Tropical Pediatrics*, 1956, 2, 159-165.

ANDRÉ-THOMAS, C. Y., CHESNI, Y., & SAINT-ANNE DARGASSIE, A.: *Neurological Examination of the Infant.* London: National Spastics Society Publications, 1960.

ARAI, S., ISHIKAWA, J., & TOSHIMA, K.: Developpement psychomoteur des enfants Japonais. *Revue de Neuro-psychiatrie infantile et d'Hygiene Mentale de l'Enfance,* 1958, 5-6, 1-8.

BARDET, C., MASSE, G., MOREIGNE, F., & SÉNÉCAL, M. J.: Application du test de Brunét-Lézine à un groupe d'enfants Oulofs de 6 mois à 24 mois. *Bulletin Société Médicine d'Afrique Noire,* 1960, 5, 334-356.

BAYLEY, N.: Comparisons of mental and motor test scores for ages 1-15 months by sex, age, birth order, race, geographical location, and education of parents. *Child Development*, 1965, 36, 379-411.

BAYLEY, N.: *Bayley Scales of Infant Development: Manual.* New York: Psychological Corporation, 1969.

BRAZELTON, T. B., ROBEY, J. S., & COLLIER, G.: Infant development in the Zinacanteco Indians of Southern Mexico. *Pediatrics,* 1969, 44, 274-290.

BRUNÉT, O. & LÉZINE, I.: *Le développement psychologique de la première enfance.* Paris: Presses Universitaires de France, 1965.

CATTELL, P.: *The Measurement of Intelligence in Young Children.* New York: Psychological Corporation, 1940.

CAUDILL, W., & WEINSTEIN, H.: Maternal care and infant behavior in Japan and America. *Psychiatry,* 1959, 32, 12-43.

CRAVIOTO, J. & ROBLES, B.: Evolution of adaptive and motor behavior during rehabilitation from kwashiorkor. *American Journal of Orthopsychiatry*, 1965, 35, 449-464.

CRAVIOTO, J.: Malnutrition and behavioral development in the preschool child. In *Preschool Child Malnutrition*. Washington, D. C.: National Academy of Sciences, 1966. Pp. 74-84.

CRAVIOTO, J.: Motor and adaptive development of premature infants from a preindustrial setting during the first year of life. *Biologia Neonatorum*, 1967, 11, 151-158.

CRAVIOTO, J., BIRCH, H., DELICARDIE, E., ROSALES, L., & VEGA, L.: The ecology of growth and development in a Mexican preindustrial community. Report I: Method and findings from birth to one month of age. *Monographs of the Society for Research in Child Development*, 1969, Ser. No. 128.

CURTI, M., MARSHALL, F. B., & STEGGERDA, M.: The Gesell schedules applied to one, two and three year old Negro children of Jamaica. *Journal of Comparative Psychology*, 1935, 20, 125-156.

DENNIS, W.: The effect of cradling practices upon the onset of walking in Hopi children. *Journal of Genetic Psychology*, 1940, 56, 77-86.

DENNIS, W.: Causes of retardation among institutional children: Iran. *Journal of Genetic Psychology*, 1960, 96, 47-59.

DENNIS, W., & NAJARIAN, P.: Development under environmental handicap. In W. Dennis (Ed.): *Readings in Child Psychology* (2nd ed.). Englewood Cliffs: Prentice-Hall, Inc., 1963. Pp. 315-331.

FALADE, S.: Le développement psycho-moteur du jeune Africain originaire du Sénégal au cours de sa première année. Paris: Foulon, 1955.

FALADE, S.: Le développement psycho-moteur de l'enfant Africain du Sénégal. *Concours Médical*, 1960, 82, 1005-1013.

FRANCIS, S. H., MIDDLETON, M. R., PENNEY, R. E. C., & THOMPSON, C. A.: Social factors related to aboriginal infant health. *Report to the Minister of Interior, Commonwealth of Australia* from the Department of Psychology, Australian National University, Canberra. (In preparation.)

FRANCIS-WILLIAMS, J. & YULE, W.: The Bayley infant scales of mental and motor development: An exploratory study with an English sample. *Developmental Medicine and Child Neurology*, 1967, 9, 391-401.

FRIJDA, N. & JAHODA, G.: On the scope and methods of cross-cultural research. *International Journal of Psychology*, 1966, 1, 110-127.

GEBER, M.: Développement psycho-moteur de l'enfant Africain. *Courrier*, 1956, 6, 17-29.

GEBER, M. & DEAN, R. F. A.: The state of development of newborn African children. *Lancet*, 1957, 1, 1216-1219. (a)

GEBER, M. & DEAN, R. F. A.: Gesell tests of African children. *Pediatrics*, 1957, 20, 1055-1065. (b)

GEBER, M.: Tests de Gesell et de Termann-Merrill appliqués en Ouganda. *Enfance*, 1958, 10, 63-67. (a)

GEBER, M.: The psycho-motor development of African children in the first year and the influence of maternal behavior. *Journal of Social Psychology*, 1958, 47, 185-195. (b)

GEBER, M. & DEAN, R. F. A.: Psychomotor development in African children: The effect of social class and the need for improved tests. *Bulletin of the World Health Organization*, 1958c, 18, 471-476.

GEBER, M.: Problèmes posés par le développement du jeune enfant africain en fonction de son milieu social. *Le Travail Humain*, 1960, 23, 99-108.

GEBER, M.: Développement psycho-moteur des petits Baganda de la naissance à six ans. *Schweizerische Zeitschrift für Psychologie*, 1961, 20, 345-357.

GEBER, M. & DEAN, R. F. A.: Le développement psychomoteur et somatique des jeunes enfants africains en Ouganda. *Courrier*, 1964, 14, 425-437.

GESELL, A., & AMATRUDA, C. S.: *Developmental Diagnosis.* (2nd ed.) New York: Hoeber, 1947.

GOLAN, S.: Collective education. *American Journal of Orthopsychiatry,* 1958, 28, 553-554,

GRANTHAN-McGREGOR, S. M., & BACK, E. H.: Gross motor development in Jamaican infants. *Developmental Medicine and Child Neurology,* 1971, 13, 79-87.

GRIFFITHS, R.: *The Abilities of Babies: A Study in Mental Measurement.* New York: McGraw-Hill, 1954.

HARFOUCHE, J. K.: The importance of breast-feeding. *Journal of Tropical Pediatrics and Environmental Child Health,* 1970, 16, 134-175.

HINDLEY, C. B.: Racial and sexual differences in age of walking: A reanalysis of the Smith *et al.* (1930) data. *Journal of Genetic Psychology,* 1967, 111, 161-167.

HINDLEY, C. B.: Growing up in five countries: A comparison of data on weaning, elimination training, age of walking and IQ in relation to social class from five European longitudinal studies. *Developmental Medicine and Child Neurology,* 1968, 10, 715-724.

HOBEN, T.: Psychological assessment instruments for use with human infants. *Merrill-Palmer Quarterly of Behavior and Development,* 1970, 16, 179-223.

JELLIFFE, D. B.: Culture, social change and infant feeding: Current trends in tropical regions. *American Journal of Clinical Nutrition,* 1962, 10, 19-43.

KITANO, H.: Different child-rearing attitudes between first and second generation Japanese in the United States. *Journal of Social Psychology,* 1961, 53, 13-19.

KOHEN-RAZ, R.: Scalogram analysis of some developmental sequences of infant behavior as measured by the Bayley Infant Scale of Mental Development. *Genetic Psychology Monographs,* 1967, 76, 3-21.

KOHEN-RAZ, R.: Mental and motor development of kibbutz, institutionalized and home-reared infants in Israel. *Child Development,* 1968, 39, 489-504.

KNOBLOCH, H. & PASAMANICK, B.: Further observations on the behavioral development of Negro children. *Journal of Genetic Psychology,* 1953, 83, 137-157.

KNOBLOCH, H. & PASAMANICK, B.: The relationship of race and socio-economic status to the development of motor behavior patterns in infancy. *Psychiatric Research Reports,* 1958, 10, 123-133.

LEVINE, S.: Stimulation in infancy. *Scientific American,* 1960, 202, 80-86.

LIDDICOAT, R.: Development of Bantu children. *Developmental Medicine and Child Neurology,* 1969, 11, 821-822.

MEAD, M. & MACGREGOR, F. C.: *Growth and Culture: A Photographic Study of Balinese Childhood.* New York: G .P. Putnam's Sons, 1951.

MEREDITH, H. V.: Bodyweight at birth of viable human infants: A world-wide comparative treatise. *Human Biology,* 1970, 42, 218-264. (a)

MEREDITH, H. V.: Body size of contemporary groups of one year old infants studied in different parts of the world. *Child Development,* 1970, 41, 551-600. (b)

MOENCKEBERG, F.: Effect of early marasmic malnutrition on subsequent physical and psychological development. In N. Scrimshaw and J. E. Gordon (Eds.): *Malnutrition, Learning and Behavior.* Cambridge: M.I.T. Press, 1968.

NELSON, G. K. & DEAN, R. F. A.: The electroencephalogram in African children: Effects of Kwashiorkor and a note on the newborn. *Bulletin of the World Health Organization,* 1959, 21, 779-782.

PASAMANICK, B.: A comparative study of the behavioral development of Negro infants. *Journal of Genetic Psychology,* 1946, 69, 3-44.

PHATAK, P.: Mental and motor growth of Indian babies: 1-30 months (Longitudinal growth of Indian children). Department of Child Development, Faculty of Home Sciences, M.S. University of Baroda, India, 1970. (a)

PHATAK, P.: Motor growth patterns of Indian babies and some related factors. *Indian Pediatrics,* 1970, 7, 619-624. (b)

POLLITT, E., & GRANOFF, D.: Mental and motor development of Peruvian children treated for severe malnutrition. *Revista Interamericana de Psicologica,* 1967, 1, 93-102.

POOLE, E.: The effect of westernization on the psychomotor development of African (Yoruba) infants during the first year of life. *Journal of Tropical Pediatrics,* 1969, 15, 172-176.

RABIN, A. I.: Behavior research in collective settlements in Israel: Infants and children conditions of "intermittent" mothering in the Kibbutz. *American Journal of Orthopsychiatry,* 1958, 28, 577-584.

ROBLES, B.: Influencia de ciertes factores ecologicos sobra la conducta del niño en el medio rural Mexicano. IX. *Reunion de le Sociedad Mexicana de Investigacion Pediatrica.* Cuernavaca, Morales, Mexico, 1959.

SAYEGH, Y., & DENNIS, W.: The effect of supplementary experiences upon the behavioral development of infants in institutions. *Child Development,* 1965, 36, 81-90.

SCHMIDT, B. J., MACIEL, W., BOSKOVITZ, E. P., ROSENBERG, S., & CURY, C. P.: Une enquête de pédiatrie sociale dans une ville brasilienne. *Courrier,* 1971, 21, 127-133.

SMITH, D. E. & STERNFIELD, J.: The Hippie communal movement: Effects on childbirth and development. *American Journal of Orthopsychiatry,* 1970, 40, 527-530.

SONTAG, L. W.: Effect of fetal activity on the nutritional stage of the infant at birth. *American Journal for Diseases of Childhood,* 1940, 60, 621-630.

STARR, R. H.: Cognitive development in infancy: Assessment, acceleration and actualization. *Merrill-Palmer Quarterly of Behavior and Development,* 1971, 17, 156-186.

STOCH, M. B. & SMYTHE, P. M.: Does undernutrition during infancy inhibit brain growth and subsequent intellectual development? *Archives of Diseases of Childhood,* 1963, 38, 546-552.

UKLENSKAYA, R., PURI, B., CHAUDHARAI, N., DANG, N., & RAJ KUMARI: Development of static and psychomotor functions of infants in the first year of life. *Indian Journal of Child Health,* 1960, 9, 596.

VINCENT, M. & HUGO, J.: L'insufficiance ponderale Africaine au point de vue de la santé publique. *Bulletin of the World Health Organization,* 1962, 26, 143-174.

VOUILLOUX, P.: Tests moteurs et reflexe plantaire chez les jeunes enfants camerounais. *Presse Medicale,* 1959, 67, 1420-1421. (a)

VOUILLOUX, P.: Etude de la psycho-motricité des enfants africains au Cameroun. Test de Gesell et reflexes archaiques. *Journal de la Société d'Africanistes,* 1959, 29, 11-18. (b)

WALTERS, C. E.: Prediction of post-natal development from fetal activity. *Child Development,* 1965, 36, 801-808.

WALTERS, C. E.: Comparative development of Negro and white infants. *Journal of Genetic Psychology,* 1967, 110, 243-251.

WERNER, E., & BAYLEY, N.: The reliability of Bayley's revised scale of mental and motor development during the first year of life. *Child Development,* 1966, 37, 39-50.

WERNER, E., SIMONIAN, K., & SMITH, R.: Ethnic and socioeconomic status differences in abilities and achievement among preschool and school-age children in Hawaii. *Journal of Social Psychology,* 1968, 75, 43-59.

WERNER, E., BIERMAN, J., & FRENCH, F.: *The Children of Kauai: A Longitudinal Study from the Prenatal Period to Age Ten.* Honolulu: University of Hawaii Press, 1971.

WHITING, B. (Ed.): *Six Cultures: Studies of Child Rearing.* New York: John Wiley and Sons, 1963.

WILLIAMS, J. R. & SCOTT, R. B.: Growth and development of Negro infants: IV. Motor development and its relationship to child rearing practices in two groups of Negro infants. *Child Development,* 1953, 24, 103-121.

WINICK, M.: Malnutrition and brain development. *Journal of Pediatrics,* 1969, 74, 667-679.

WUG DE LEON, E., LICARDIE, E., & CRAVIOTO, J.: Desarrollo psicomotor del niño en una poblacion rural de Guatemala. *Guatemala Pediatrica,* 1964, 4, 92.

Part II

DEVELOPMENTAL ISSUES

These papers survey issues in development from the early infancy period through adolescence. Connolly questions the emphasis placed on the concept of "critical periods." He feels that attention should be paid to events and processes within sensitive periods of early development rather than to their temporal characteristics. Mahler expands further on her well-known formulation of the separation-individuation process in the first two years of life and on the three sequences that she postulates during this period. Briggs' cross-cultural study of an Eskimo community challenges the validity of generalizing as universally significant certain developmental concepts drawn from studies in our culture. Hertzig and her colleagues contribute another significant epidemiologic study of the relationship between severe malnutrition in early childhood and levels of intellectual functioning at school age. Thomas and Chess use data from the middle childhood period of youngsters in their New York Longitudinal Study to question the familiar concept of the "latency period." King reviews a number of studies on coping and growth in adolescence and contributes data from his own sample of college students. He concludes that the capacity of most adolescents to cope is greater than we would be led to expect from theories based primarily on clinical data and suggests the possibility that alternatives to the "crisis" model of adolescence are in order.

7

LEARNING AND THE CONCEPT OF CRITICAL PERIODS IN INFANCY

Kevin Connolly, Ph.D.

Department of Psychology, University of Sheffield (England)

INTRODUCTION

The notion of development concerns a directional pattern of changes in structure and function associated with growth and with aging processes. The terms "growth," "maturation" and "development" have sometimes been used synonymously and this can be seriously misleading. Growth emphasizes changes which are due to tissue accretion; a further and related term, that of "differentiation," refers to variations and changes in structural aspects with increasing age. The concept of development encompasses both of these plus behavior, and places emphasis on progressive changes in the organization of an individual considered as a functional adaptive system throughout its life history.

Gesell's (1954) notion of human ontogeny, in which early behavior emerges through the innate processes of growth (which he termed maturation), implies a process of gradual unfolding. Development is neither a process of unfolding, directed solely by intrinsic forces, nor is it a moulding process directed only by extrinsic forces—it is a combination of both (Connolly, 1970). Behavioral development was ascribed by Coghill

Reprinted with permission from DEVELOPMENTAL MEDICINE AND CHILD NEUROLOGY, 1972, Vol. 14, No. 6, pp. 705-714. Copyright © Spastics International Medical Publications.

This article is based on a paper presented to a colloquium on Recent Advances in Knowledge of Bladder Control in Children, Department of Psychological Medicine, University of Newcastle upon Tyne, July 1971.

(1929) to the maturation of central nervous system tissues, the nervous system being represented as a carrier of the innate determinants of behavioral patterns presumed to arise through passive development. A preformationist theory, or a theory of genetic predetermination, cannot readily account for data now available to us from developmental genetics (Connolly, 1971).

The problem of development is one of understanding what changing integrations underlie the successive functional stages which are characteristic of a given species. In order to deal with this problem, Schneirla (1966) postulated two concepts which stand for the complex system of intervening variables. They are: *maturation,* which he defined as "the contributions to development of growth, and of tissue differentiation together with their organic trace effects surviving from earlier development"; and *experience,* which he defined as ". . . the contributions to development of stimulation from all available sources (external and internal) including their functional trace effects surviving from earlier development." Trace effects refer to organic changes which affect further development. The developmental contributions of these two complexes must be viewed as fused at all stages of ontogenesis. Schneirla's definition of experience is extremely broad-ranging, from the stimulative effects of biochemical and physiological processes to the ideas of learning and conditioning as used by psychologists.

EARLY LEARNING AND EARLY EXPERIENCE

At one level we all know what is meant by the term "learning," and yet it is astonishingly difficult to define adequately. When we speak of learning we refer to relatively permanent changes in behavior which are a consequence of the organism's experience and commerce with its environment. However, the inadequacy of this definition is apparent on reflection. Let us take an extreme example to illustrate the point. Consider a bipedal animal which loses its legs in an accident. Its behavior will certainly be changed by this experience, but we should not consider such a change to be an example of learning, though it may learn to adapt its behavior to its new circumstances. Defined in this way, learning is too crude and too general an entity. What we imply by the term is a set of dynamic processes concerned with the formation of structures and modes of operation. We are concerned with the ways in which an organism constructs and modifies models of its world in order to adapt to the demands made upon it by its environment. The processes can and are being analyzed at many levels—biochemical, physiological, behavioral and cognitive.

Early experience has been considered as particularly important by many developmental psychologists because they argue that it lays the foundations of an individual's characteristic behavior. In this paper I propose to discuss some of the recent work in the field of early learning and early experience, with particular emphasis on the concept of critical periods of behavioral development.

Early experience refers to all effects of stimulation in infancy, both immediate and long-lasting. In contrast, early learning has a narrower connotation, because certain kinds of early experience involve no learning but all learning implies early experience. Whether early learning differs from learning which occurs later in life has been the subject of some controversy. Hebb (1949) believed that later learning builds upon, rather than replaces, initial learning, and this in itself would make the characteristics of the two different. He argued that much early learning was foundational in that it provided the organism with essential perceptual and motor skills and formed the framework within which subsequent learning took place. If you consider an animal as a self-organizing system, then early inputs will be responsible for determining the basic organizational structure.

Work reported since Hebb published his extremely influential theory has tended to modify but, in general outline, support his conception.

EFFECTS OF EARLY EXPERIENCE ON LATER BEHAVIOR

In the course of the past fifteen years, a very extensive literature has grown up on the effects of early experience on later behavior (Newton and Levine, 1968). We now know that genetically based characters may be extensively modified by early experience, and we know also that early experiences are one of the principal sources of individual differences in behavior. We know, too, that early experiences have multiple effects and that the age at which they are administered is crucial. Let me illustrate these points by citing some experiments.

It is a common characteristic of most strains of mice that two adult males will fight when placed together in a restricted environment. Strain differences are well known and provide evidence of a genetic component. Dennenberg and co-workers (1964) fostered four day-old mice pups on to lactating rats until weaning. Mice so reared show an almost zero incidence of fighting during adulthood.

Cooper and Zubeck (1958) reported important findings on the effects of early experience in lines of rats selectively bred for maze brightness and maze dullness. At weaning, rats from these two strains were placed in one of three environments: normal, enriched, or restricted. The normal environment was the usual laboratory arrangement; the restricted environment was a cage containing only food and water receptacles; and the enriched environment contained ramps, mirrors, swings, balls, barriers, slides, tunnels and so on, in addition to food and water containers. The animals were maintained from weaning at day 25 to day 65 in these conditions and were then tested in a Hebb-Williams maze. The results, i.e., number of errors made in learning the maze, are startling. In the normal environment, the maze dull rats made a little over 30 per cent more errors than the maze bright animals. When reared in an enriched environment, the number of errors made by the two groups did not differ significantly. Similarly, no differences were obtained between animals reared in restricted environments.

Harlow's (1962) studies of monkeys raised in social isolation from birth to adulthood showed that these animals had great difficulty in performing the basic steps involved in copulation. Females coached by Harlow to mate did become pregnant but turned out to be very bad mothers (Arling and Harlow, 1967).

A study by Landauer and Whiting (1964) revealed an interesting correlation between stress in infancy and the adult height of males. They compared boys subjected to two stressors with control subjects who were not so treated. The stressors were piercing of the nose, lips or ears and moulding of the arms, legs or head. Their results revealed that in societies where the infants were subjected to stress during the first two years of life, the average height of males was over two inches greater than boys who did not experience this stress. A similar pattern was found by Whiting and colleagues (1968) when they compared the adult height of American children inoculated before the age of two years with children not inoculated. In this study it proved possible by various statistical procedures to correct for parental height. It is possible, of course, that those parents who have their children inoculated early differ in many ways from those who do not; for example, they may practice other forms of medical care more assiduously.

These studies and many others point to the long-term and, in some cases, dramatic effects which may be brought about in an animal's behavior by appropriate intervention in early life. Dennenberg (1969) has suggested that the human analogue of pre-weaning stimulation in the rat (handling) is represented by the first 4-24 weeks of the baby's life, and that the analogue to successful use of an enriched environment in the case of the rat begins at roughly six months in the human.

DEVELOPMENTAL CHANGES IN LEARNING

The way in which an organism's learning capacity develops with age is by no means fully understood, and it is difficult to decide whether there are developmental changes in learning over and above the effects of growth, neuromuscular maturation, experience and motivation. Some studies by Vince (1958, 1959) on the learning of young and adult passerine birds (finches and titmice) are illuminating in this context. Vince trained birds on tasks involving the pulling of string and lifting the lids of pots, etc. Basically, the author considered two features of the learning process: the acquisition of the appropriate response when reinforced, and the suppression of the tendency to respond in the absence of reinforcement. On the whole, she found that juvenile birds were more generally responsive and capable of acquiring the correct response more rapidly than mature birds. However, adult birds were found to be better able to inhibit incorrect responses, that is, to learn not to respond inappropriately. Depending on the exact nature of the task, the young or old birds could learn more quickly. What is important is not that early learning is less or more important than later learning, but that early and later learning may differ in certain features. A single criterion of learning efficiency may, in fact, be seriously misleading.

Luria (1932) has made similar observations on the development of certain simple reactions in young children. The tasks with which the children were faced involved such things as pressing a button when a signal was received and making delayed movements. On testing children from two to seven years of age he found that the capacity to make these responses develops slowly. A child aged four to five years could produce a reaction to a signal but each signal tended to produce many movements, so that gaps between signals were filled with extra responses. In some cases, the extra responses could be inhibited in children aged three to four years, but this might disrupt the habit so that the occurrence of a signal inhibited the reaction. Delayed movements were found by Luria to be almost impossible in children up to the age of seven. Luria maintained that the excitatory aspects are no problem for the young child and that the difficulty lies in controlling the excitation. Paramenova (1955) reported that 3-year-old children can learn to press a key in response to a signal, such as a red lamp, but usually give the same response to other signals, such as a blue or a green lamp. It appears that at this age it is extremely difficult for the child to refrain from making a generalized response even though he well understands the instructions. The problem of inhibiting responses is not usually overcome until the child had reached the age of six or so.

These studies of young birds and children do suggest that different aspects are important in the young as compared with the adult organism.

CRITICAL PERIODS IN THE DEVELOPMENT OF BEHAVIOR

The concept of critical periods is not new either to biology or to psychology. The origins of the idea are to be found in experimental embryology. From his experiments on the effects of various inorganic compounds on the development of *Fundulus* eggs, Stockard (1921) originally thought that the production of one-eyed monsters was caused specifically by the magnesium ion. However, further experiments showed that almost any substance would produce the same effect if administered at the appropriate time during development. In embryology, therefore, the concept refers to time periods of maximum sensitivity or indifference to chemical forces acting on the cellular mass.

Freud's ideas about the origin of human neurosis relied heavily upon the importance of early childhood experiences and implied that certain periods or stages in the life of an infant are times of particular sensitivity. The concept of critical periods in behavioral development was emphasized by Lorenz (1935) in his work on the formation of primary social bonds in precocial birds—the following and approach behaviors which he called "imprinting." Lorenz commented upon the similarity of these behavioral phenomena to the critical periods in the development of the embryo. Following this, McGraw (1946) argued that there was a critical period for the optimal learning of motor skills in the human infant. The all-embracing notion of educational readiness and stage-dependent theories of development, such as that elaborated by Piaget, are implicitly related to the critical period hypothesis. Relating as it does to the learning process, the idea of readiness differs very little from the hypothesis advanced by many working on imprinting.

Three principal kinds of critical period phenomena have been described in behavioral studies: optimal periods of learning, for infantile stimulation and for the formation of basic social relationships. Dealing first with the establishment of social relationships, there is now an extensive literature on imprinting which has been reviewed by Sluckin (1964) and by Bateson (1966). I do not propose to discuss this in any detail; suffice to say that there is good evidence for the existence of sensitive periods for the establishment of primary social bonds in many species. The dog has been studied from the viewpoint of socialization more extensively than any other mammal (Scott, 1958). From 3 weeks up to about 10 weeks, the puppy is susceptible to socializing influences. During this time, primary socialization determines to what living things, including humans, the animal will become attached. Work on humans has explored the question of whether there are periods during which the human infant is maximally sensitive to social contacts with its mother—contacts which will lead to the cementing of an affectional bond. For obvious reasons this is a difficult problem to tackle experimentally, and most of our knowledge comes from clinical cases where the mother-infant relationship either did not develop or where it was disrupted. However, the work of Bowlby (1951, 1958, 1969), Yarrow (1960), Ambrose (1963), Scott (1963) and Klaus, et al. (1972) all provide evidence in support of the basic contention for sensitive periods.

Turning to infantile stimulation, Levine (1956) found that handling rats after weaning did not have the same consequences as handling during the first three weeks of life. In a subsequent study, Levine and Otis (1958) report differential effects of pre- and post-weaning stimulation on adult resistance to deprivation. Dennenberg and co-workers (1968) found that the enhanced free-environment experience during the second three weeks of life had a greater effect on learning than did the same experience during the first three weeks. Levin and Mullins (1966) have suggested that early experience may serve to set or "tune" the neuroendocrine system, so that later in the organism's life history, the threshold and duration of emotional stress reactions are altered. There is evidence, too, of early stimulation having morphological and physiological consehuences. Shapiro and Vulovich (1970) investigated the effects of a wide range of sensory stimulation on the development of cortical pyramidal cell synaptic loci in rats. Stimulation given 3-5 times per day was found to increase the number of dendritic spines measured at days 8 and 16. This effect of early afferent input on brain development may provide a neuroanatomical basis for the influence of early experience.

From her now famous studies on the twins Jimmy and Johnny, McGraw (1935, 1946) concluded that there are critical periods for learning which vary from activity to activity. To one member of the twin pair, McGraw gave extra training. The results showed that some activities, such as walking, were not affected. Others, notably roller skating, showed a substantial effect in the trained twin. In some activities, performance was actually worsened by the acquisition of inappropriate responses.

Forgays and Forgays (1952) have demonstrated that pet rats, raised in the rich environment of a home, performed much better on learning tasks than rats reared in laboratory cages.

Bernstein (1957) provided evidence indicating that discrimination learning could be improved by gentle handling beginning at 20 days. In this context, the effects may well be on fear, which affects the capacity for future learning.

Thorpe (1961) has described a critical period for song learning in the chaffinch. If the young male is isolated three or four days after hatching, it produces an incomplete song only. However, if, as a fledgling of two to three weeks old, or in early juvenile life before he himself sings, the young bird hears adult chaffinches singing, he will, during the following year, produce the song characteristic of the species even if he has been kept in isolation. In nature, the fine details of the song are added in the time of competition over territory, within a period of 2-3 weeks when the bird is about a year old. At this time, the bird learns the "local song" and never learns any others in subsequent years. The critical period for song learning is thus quite long but is certainly over by the end of a year.

Money and his colleagues (1957) studied the development of hermaphroditic children who had been reared as one sex and then changed to the other. They found that if this occurred before the age of two-and-a-half years very little emotional disturbance resulted. On the basis of this data it has been suggested that there is a critical period for learning the sex role.

THE NATURE OF THE PERIOD

The critical period concept has been used in two quite distinct ways (Caldwell, 1962). Some authors have spoken of a critical period *beyond* which a given phenomenon will not appear, that is, a point in time which marks the onset of total indifference or resistance to certain patterns of stimulation. Another way in which the term has been used is to refer to a period of time *during* which the organism is especially sensitive to various developmental modifiers which, if introduced at a different point in the life-cycle, would have little or no effect. In other words, a period of maximum sensitivity.

At the embryological level there are data to support both versions of the critical period hypothesis. Cell transplants done prior to a particular critical time will develop in conformity with the region into which they are transplanted. Beyond this terminal point, transplantation will result in the misplaced development of the organ. The "during" version of the hypothesis has also been demonstrated by embryologists in the experimental production of congenital abnormalities. The teratogen used may vary, but, in order to produce an effect, the timing must be precise. Periods exist, therefore, in which organisms are vulnerable, while, at other times, they are relatively immune to external factors. From the embryological studies we know that organ systems are particularly sensitive during their period of maximum cellular proliferation (Hamburger and Habel, 1947).

The "beyond" version of the hypothesis, with respect to the development of social behavior, is considered by Scott (1958) to be an established generalization. From his studies with dogs, Scott has provided a great deal of evidence supporting the contention that there is a period early in the animal's life during which primary social relationships become established and after which they rarely do so. Clear evidence relating to human behavior is lacking, and for obvious reasons is very difficult to obtain, though Bowlby (1951) has asserted that there is a parallel between the "during" version of the chemical organizer and maternal care.

The basic timing mechanisms for developmental periods are biological processes ongoing through time. Time as such does not explain the changes which have been described. For various reasons these processes are not precisely correlated with age from birth. For example, birds often retain newly formed eggs in their bodies overnight, thus incubating them for several hours before laying. Gottlieb (1961) chilled duck eggs prior to incubating them (this process kills embryos except those in the earliest stages of development) and found that the critical period for imprinting in these birds showed a much reduced variance.

Studies investigating critical periods for imprinting in precocial birds have shown that there is not so much a *critical* as a more extended *sensitive* period during which the animal is particularly sensitive to forming a primary social bond. The period for imprinting, claimed by Hess (1959) to be between 13 and 16 hours post-hatch, can be extended by administering tranquilizer drugs such as chlorpromazine (Hess, 1960), or shortened by social rearing (Guiton, 1959). Freedman and co-workers (1961) have shown that although the optimum period for socializating dogs is seven to nine weeks, adequate socialization is possible up to thirteen weeks. The distinction between the terms "critical" and "sensitive" in speaking of periods of development is very largely semantic. Whilst not wishing to imply categorically that critical periods do not exist, on the basis of our present knowledge it would be more prudent to use the slightly weaker term "sensitive period."

In searching for causal mechanisms, we should ask whether a period is sensitive because of the events which occur within it, because of the organism's physiological state at that time, and because of the sequence in which developmental events occur. In one child the boundary may occur at χ months whilst in another it may occur at $\chi + 1$ months. This suggests that there is a danger of emphasizing the period too strongly. Sensitive periods for attachment behavior would be expected to show a general uniformity from one child to another in much the same way as most children learn to walk at twelve to eighteen months or to talk at about two years. A similar uniformity might also be expected for children becoming dry at night, and indeed there is evidence to support this (Mac Keith, 1968). Here, of course, parental expectation will play a part, as is clear from the cross-cultural studies of Whiting and Child (1953). However, it is important to remember that wide individual differences exist both in maturation and in learning significant life functions.

Those of us who study the behavior of children often tend to assume that what we are currently observing is crucial for that child. A child who lacks a warm relationship during infancy will not necessarily become an affectionless psychopath. There may well be adaptive characteristics which come into play later and, on the whole, evolution has built many modifying mechanisms into the processes of ontogeny. Feeding, which is initially sucking and swallowing, must be replaced by chewing and swallowing and eventually will involve using tools. Similarly, intense filiative behavior must give way to other attachments. The failure of an intense mother-infant relationship to weaken and change (Harlow and Harlow, 1965) is maladaptive ontogenetically and phylogenetically, as shown by studies on mother-infant bonds in monkeys.

To speak of a critical or a sensitive period is in essence to describe certain temporal characteristics of a phenomenon. Mac Keith's (1964), 1968) hypothesis regarding a sensitive period for learning nocturnal bladder control provides a relevant example. Whilst this is a useful generalization it is not in itself an explanation. It is essential that we pursue our enquiries further in order to uncover the causal mechanisms involved in behavioral change. From a knowledge of the mechanisms involved and important factors affecting these, more effective diagnosis and treatment programs will be possible.

CONCLUSIONS

(1) Development is an extremely complex set of processes which are often oversimplified.

(2) Learning is difficult to define adequately.

(3) Early experience has far reaching consequences for an organism's development.

(4) Learning does take place in very young animals and in the human newborn.

(5) There are significant developmental changes in the nature of learning.

(6) Certain periods in an organism's life history appear to be specifically sensitive for the development of certain behaviors.

(7) We should concentrate less on "critical periods" and more on critical events in trying to understand the mechanisms involved in the so-called "sensitive periods."

SUMMARY

The importance of early experience in the development of behavior is amply documented by empirical research. This paper discusses learning in infancy and the critical period hypothesis as an explanation of behavioral development. The use of the term "sensitive period" is advocated rather than "critical period" and examples of such sensitive periods associated with quite different behavioral parameters are given. Two quite separate ways in which the term "critical period" has been used are distinguished and examples given of each. The view is advanced that attention should be devoted primarily to the events and processes occurring within the sensitive period rather than to its temporal characteristics.

REFERENCES

AMBROSE, J. A. (1963): The concept of critical periods for the development of social responsiveness. In B. M. Foss (Ed.), *Determinants of Infant Behavior*, Vol. 2. London: Methuen, p. 201.

ARLING, G. L. & HARLOW, H. F. (1967): Effects of social deprivation on maternal behavior of rhesus monkeys. *Journal of Physiological and Comparative Psychology*, 64, 371.

BATESON, P. P. G. (1966): The characteristics and context of imprinting. *Biological Reviews*, 41, 177.

BERNSTEIN, L. (1957): The effects of variations in handling upon learning and retention. *Journal of Physiological and Comparative Psychology*, 50, 162.

BOWLBY, J. (1951): *Maternal Care and Mental Health*. London: H.M.S.O.

BOWLBY, J. (1958): The nature of the child's tie to his mother. *International Journal of Psycho-Analysis*, 39, 350.

BOWLBY, J. (1969): *Attachment and Loss. Vol. 1. Attachment.* London: Hogarth.

CALDWELL, B. M. (1962): The usefulness of the critical period hypothesis in the study of filiative behavior. *Merrill-Palmer Quarterly of Behavior and Development*, 8, 229.

COGHILL, G. E. (1929): *Anatomy and the Problem of Behavior*. New York: Hafner. (Reprinted 1963).

CONNOLLY, K. (1970): Skill development: Problems and plans. In K. Connolly (Ed.), *Mechanisms of Motor Skill Development*. London: Academic Press.

CONNOLLY, K. (1971): The evolution and ontogeny of behavior. *Bulletin of the British Psychological Society*, 24, 93.

COOPER, R. M. & ZUBEK, J. P. (1958): Effects of enriched and restricted early environments on the learning ability of bright and dull rats. *Canadian Journal of Psychology*, 12, 159.

DENNENBERG, V. H. (1969): Animal studies of early experience: Some principles which have implications for human development. In J. P. Hill (Ed.), *Minnesota Symposia on Child Psychology*, Vol. 3. Minneapolis: University of Minnesota Press.

DENNENBERG, V. H., HUDGENS, G. A., & ZARROW, M. X. (1964): Mice reared with rats: Modification of behavior by early experience with another species. *Science*, 143, 380.

DENNENBERG, V. H., WOODCOCK, J. M., & ROSENBERG, M. K. (1968): Long-term effects of preweaning and postweaning free environment experience on the rat's problem solving behavior. *Journal of Physiological and Comparative Psychology*, 66, 533.

FORGAYS, D. G., FORGAYS, J. W. (1952): The nature of the effect of free-environmental experience in the rat. *Journal of Physiological and Comparative Psychology*, 45, 322.

FREEDMAN, D. G., KING, J. A., & ELLIOTT, O. (1961): Critical period in the social development of dogs. *Science*, 133, 1016.

GESELL, A. (1954): The ontogeny of infant behavior. In L. Carmichael (Ed.), *Manual of Child Psychology*. New York: John Wiley.

GOTTLEIB, G. (1961): Development age as a baseline for determination of the critical period in imprinting. *Journal of Physiological and Comparative Psychology*, 54, 422.

GUITON, P. (1959): Socialization and imprinting in Brown Leghorn chicks. *Animal Behavior*, 7, 26.

HAMBURGER, V. & HABEL, K. (1947): Teratogenic and lethal effects of influenza-A and mumps viruses on early chick embryos. *Proceedings of the Society for Experimental Biology and Medicine*, 66, 608.

HARLOW, H. F. (1962): The heterosexual affectional system in monkeys. *American Psychologist*, 17, 1.

HARLOW, H. F. & HARLOW, M. K. (1965): The affectional systems. In A. M. Schrier, H. F. Harlow & F. Stollnitz (Eds.), *Behavior of Nonhuman Primates*, Vol. 2. London: Academic Press.

HEBB, D. O. (1949): *The Organization of Behaviour*. London: John Wiley.

HESS, E. H. (1959): Two conditions limiting critical age for imprinting. *Journal of Physiological and Comparative Psychology*, 52, 515.

HESS, E. H. (1960): Effects of drugs on imprinting behavior. In L. Uhr & J. G. Miller (Eds.), *Drugs and Behaviour*. London: John Wiley.

KLAUS, M. H., JERAULD, R., KREGER, N. C., McALPINE, W., STEFFA, M., & KENNELL, J. H. (1972): Maternal attachment. Importance of the first post-partum days. *New England Journal of Medicine*, 286, 460.

LANDAUER, T. K. & WHITING, J. M. W. (1964): Infantile stimulation and adult stature of human males. *American Anthropologist*, 66, 1007.

LEVINE, S. (1956): A further study of infantile handling and adult avoidance learning. *Journal of Personality*, 25, 70.

LEVINE, S. & OTIS, L. S. (1958): The effects of handling before and after weaning on the resistance of albino rats to later deprivation. *Canadian Journal of Psychology*, 12, 103.

LEVINE, S. & MULLINS, R. F. (1966): Hormonal influences on brain organization in infant rats. *Science*, 152, 1585.

LORENZ, K. (1935): Der Kumpen in der Umwelt des Vogels. *Journal of Ornithology*, 83, 137, 289.

LURIA, A. R. (1932): *The Nature of Human Conflicts*. New York: Liveright.

McGraw, M. B. (1935): *Growth: A Study of Johnny and Jimmy*. New York: Appleton-Century.

McGraw, M. B. (1946): Maturation of behavior. In L. Carmichael (Ed.), *Manual of Child Psychology*. New York: John Wiley.

Mac Keith, R. (1964): A new concept in development. *Developmental Medicine and Child Neurology*, 6, 111.

Mac Keith, R. (1968): A frequent factor in the origins of primary nocturnal enuresis: Anxiety in the third year. *Developmental Medicine and Child Neurology*, 10, 465.

Money, J., Hampson, J. G., & Hampson, J. L. (1957): Imprinting and the establishment of gender role. *Archives of Neurology and Psychiatry*, 77, 333.

Newton, G. & Levine, B. (Eds.) (1968): *Early Experience and Behavior*. Springfield, Ill.: Charles C Thomas.

Paramenova, M. P. (1955): On the question of the development of the physiological mechanism of movement. *Vaprosy Psichologii*, 1, 51.

Schneirla, T. C. (1966): Behavioral development and comparative psychology. *Quarterly Review of Biology*, 41, 283.

Scott, J. P. (1958): Critical periods in the development of social behavior in puppies. *Psychosomatic Medicine*, 20, 42.

Scott, J. P. (1963): The process of primary socialization in canine and human infants. *Monographs of the Society for Research in Child Development*, No. 85.

Shapiro, S. & Vukovich, K. R. (1970): Early experience effects on cortical dendrites: A proposed model for development. *Science*, 167, 292.

Sluckin, W. (1964): *Imprinting and Early Learning*. London: Methuen.

Stockard, C. R. (1921): Developmental rate and structural expression: An experimental study of twins, "double monsters" and single deformities and their interaction among embryonic organs during their origins and development. *American Journal of Anatomy*, 28, 115.

Thorpe, W. H. (1961): *Bird-song*. Cambridge: Cambridge University Press.

Vince, M. A. (1958): String-pulling in birds. 2. Differences related to age in greenfinches, chaffinches and canaries. *Animal Behavior*, 6, 53.

Vince, M. A. (1959): Effects of age and experience on the establishment of internal inhibition in finches. *British Journal of Psychology*, 50, 136.

Whiting, J. W. M. & Child, I. L. (1953): *Child Training and Personality*. London: O.U.P.

Whiting, J. W. M., Landauer, T. K., & Jones, T. M. (1968): Infantile immunization and adult stature. *Child Development*, 39, 59.

Yarrow, L. J. (1960): Maternal deprivation: Toward an empirical and conceptual re-evolution. *Psychological Bulletin*, 58, 459.

8

ON THE FIRST THREE SUBPHASES OF THE SEPARATION-INDIVIDUA- TION PROCESS

Margaret S. Mahler

I have based this presentation upon two thoughts of Freud—two pillars of psychoanalytic metapsychology. The first is that, at the time of his biological birth, the human being is brought into the world in an immature state. (This is due to the fact that the over-development of his CNS requires a large cranial cage.) Hence he is *at first absolutely,* and remains later on—even "unto the grave"—*relatively* dependent on a mother.

The second Freudian tenet, which is probably a result of the first, is his emphasis that *object relationship*—i.e., one person's endowing another with object libido—is the most reliable single factor by which we are able to determine the level of mental health on the one hand and, on the other, the extent of the therapeutic potential.

Object relationship develops on the basis of, and *pari passu* with, differentiation from the normal mother-infant dual unity, which Therese Benedek (1949) and I, independently of each other, have designated as the *normal phase of human symbiosis* (Mahler & Goslinger, 1955).

"Growing up" entails a gradual growing away from the normal state

Reprinted from INTERNATIONAL JOURNAL *of* PSYCHO-ANALYSIS (1972) 53, pp. 333-338.

This paper was originally presented as the first introductory contribution to a series of three panels: "The Experience of Separation-Individuation in Infancy and Its Reverberation through the Course of Life" (jointly sponsored by the Association for Child Psychoanalysis and the American Psychoanalytic Association) on 19 December, 1971.

of human symbiosis, of "one-ness' with the mother. This process is much slower in the emotional and psychic area than in the physical one. The transition from lap-babyhood to toddler-hood goes through gradual steps of a separation-individuation process, greatly facilitated on the one hand by the autonomous development of the ego and, on the other hand, by identificatory mechanisms of different sorts. This growing away process is—as Zetzel, Winnicott and also Sandler & Joffe indicate in their work—a lifelong mourning process. *Inherent in every new step of independent functioning is a minimal threat of object loss.*

Following my work with a few psychotic latency children, whom I tried to help with the traditional child analytic method in Vienna back in the 1930s—and on the basis of engrams left in my mind as a pediatrician and head of a well-baby clinic, after having studied tics and early infantile psychosis from the early 1940s on—I decided to look more closely at the *fountainhead*—to examine the phenomena that those two Freudian thoughts I mentioned earlier entail. I decided to study the earliest average mother-infant and mother-toddler interaction *in situ.*

The biological birth of the human infant and the psychological birth of the individual are not coincident in time. The former is a dramatic and readily observable, well-circumscribed event; the latter, a slowly unfolding intrapsychic process.

For the more or less normal adult, the experience of being both fully "in" and at the same time basically separate from the "world out there" is among the givens of life that are taken for granted. Consciousness of self and absorption without awareness of self are the two polarities between which we move, with varying ease and with varying degrees of alternation or simultaneity. This too is the result of a slowly unfolding process. In particular, this development takes place in relation to (a) one's own body, and (b) the principal representative of the world, as the infant experiences it, namely the primary love object. *As is the case with any intrapsychic process, this one reverberates throughout the life cycle. It is never finished;* it can always become reactivated; new phases of the life cycle witness new derivatives of the earliest process still at work (cf. Erikson, 1968). However, the principal psychological achievements in this process take place, as we see it, in the period from about the fourth or fifth to the 30th or 36th month of age, a period that we refer to—at Dr. Annemarie Weil's helpful suggestion (personal communication)—as the *separation-individuation phase.*

In the course of our rather unsystematic naturalistic *pilot study,* we could not help but take note of certain *clusters of variables* at certain crossroads of the individuation process, insofar as they *repeated them-*

selves. This strongly suggested to us that it would be to our advantage to subdivide the data that we were collecting on the intrapsychic separation and individuation process, in accordance with the *repeatedly observable, behavioral and other surface referents of that process.* Our subdivision was into four subphases: differentiation, practising, rapprochement, and "on the way to libidinal object constancy." (The timing of these subphases is still inaccurate, and we are still working on the timetable as we go along with the processing of our data.)

I should also mention in passing that I have described an objectless phase: *the phase of normal autism,* and the phase corresponding to Anna Freud's "need-satisfying" and Spitz's "pre-object" phase—which I like to call *the symbiotic phase.* Both these precede the first subphase of separation-individuation—that of *differentiation.*

DIFFERENTIATION

At about four to five months of age, at the peak of symbiosis, the behavioral phenomena seem to indicate the beginning of the first subphase of separation-individuation—called *differentiation.* It is synonymous in our metaphorical language with "hatching from the mother-infant symbiotic common orbit." During the symbiotic months, through that activity of the pre-ego, which Spitz has described as *coenaesthetic receptivity,* the young infant has familiarized himself with the mothering half of his symbiotic self, indicated by the unspecific social smile. This smile gradually becomes the specific (preferential) smiling response to the mother, *which is the supreme sign that a specific bond* between the infant and his mother has been established.

When inner pleasure, due to safe anchorage within the symbiotic orbit—which is mainly entero-proprioceptive and contact perceptual—continues, and pleasure in the maturationally increasing outer sensory perception stimulates outward-directed attention cathexis, these two forms of attention cathexis can oscillate freely (Spiegel, 1959; Rose, 1964). The result is an optimal symbiotic state, out of which smooth differentiation—and *expansion beyond the symbiotic orbit*—can take place. This "hatching" process is, I believe, a gradual ontogenetic evolution of the sensorium—the perceptual-conscious system—which leads to the infant-toddler's having a more *permanently alert* sensorium, whenever he is awake (cf. also Wolff, 1959).

In other words, the infant's attention—which during the first months of symbiosis was in large part *inwardly* directed, or focused in a coenesthetic and somewhat vague way *within the symbiotic orbit*—gradually gains a considerable accretion through the coming into being of a perceptual activity that is outwardly directed during the child's increasing periods of wakefulness. This is a change of degree rather than of kind, for during the symbiotic stage the child has certainly been highly attentive to the mothering figure. But gradually that attention is combined with a growing store of memories of mother's comings and goings, of "good" and "bad" experiences; the latter were altogether unrelievable by the self, but were predictably relieved by mother's ministrations.

Six to seven months is the peak of the child's hair-pulling, face-patting, manual, tactile and visual exploration of the mother's mouth, nose, face, as well as the covered (clad) and unclad *feel* of parts of the mother's body; and furthermore the discovery of a brooch, eyeglasses or a pendant attached to the mother. There may be engagement in peek-a-boo games in which the infant still plays a passive role. This later develops into the cognitive function of checking the unfamiliar against the already familiar—a process that Sylvia Brody termed "customs inspection."

It is during the first subphase of separation-individuation that all normal infants achieve their first tentative steps of breaking away, in a bodily sense, from their hitherto completely passive lap-babyhood—the stage of dual unity with the mother. They stem themselves with arms and legs against the holding mother, as if to have a better look at her as well as at the surroundings. One was able to see their individually different inclinations and patterns, as well as the general characteristics of the stage of differentiation itself. They all like to venture and stay just a bit away from the enveloping arms of the mother; if they are motorically able to slide down from mother's lap, they tend to remain or to crawl back as near as possible and play at the mother's feet.

Once the infant has become sufficiently individuated to recognize the mother, visually and tactilely, he then turns, with greater or less wonderment and apprehension (commonly called "stranger reaction"), to a prolonged visual and tactile exploration and study of the faces of others, from afar or at close range. He appears to be comparing and checking the features—appearance, feel, contours and texture—of the stranger's face with his mother's face, as well as with whatever inner image he may have of her. He also seems to check back to her face in relation to other interesting new experiences.

In children for whom the symbiotic phase has been optimal and "confident expectation" has prevailed (Benedek, 1938), curiosity and wonderment are the predominant elements of their inspection of strangers. By contrast, among children whose basic trust has been less than optimal, an abrupt change to acute stranger anxiety may make its appearance;

or there may be a prolonged period of mild stranger reaction, which transiently interferes with pleasurable inspective behavior. This phenomenon and the factors underlying its variations constitute, we believe, an important aspect of and clue to our evaluation of the libidinal object, of socialization, and of the first step towards emotional object constancy.

THE BEGINNING PRACTICING PERIOD

The period of differentiation is followed—or rather, is overlapped—by a practicing period. This takes place usually from about seven to ten months, up to 15-16 months of age. In the course of processing our data we found it useful to think of the practicing period in two parts: (1) the early practicing phase—overlapping differentiation—characterized by the infant's earliest ability to move away physically from mother by crawling, climbing and righting himself, yet still holding on; and (2) the practicing period proper, characterized by free, upright locomotion.

At least three interrelated, yet discriminable, developments contribute to and/or, in circular fashion, interact with the child's first steps into awareness of separateness and into individuation. They are: the rapid *body differentiation* from the mother; establishment of a *specific bond* with her; and the *growth and functioning of the autonomous ego apparatuses in close proximity to the mother.*

It seems that the new pattern of relationship to mother paves the way for the infant to spill over his interest in the mother on to inanimate objects—at first those provided by her—such as toys which she offers, or the bottle with which she parts from him at night. The infant explores these objects visually with his eyes, and their taste, texture and smell with his contact perceptual organs, particularly the mouth and the hands. One or the other of these objects becomes a transitional object. Moreover, whatever the sequence in which these functions develop in the beginning practicing period, the characteristic of this early stage of practicing is that, while there is interest and absorption in these activities, interest in the mother definitely seems to take precedence. We also observed in this early period of practicing that the "would-be fledgling" likes to indulge in his budding relationship with the "other than mother" world.

For instance, we observed one child, who during this period had to undergo hospitalization of a week's duration. During that period, it seems, he was frustrated *most* by his confinement to a crib, so that he welcomed *anyone* who would take him out of it. When he returned from the hospital, the relationship to his mother had become less exclusive, and he showed no clinging reaction or separation anxiety; his greatest need now in the Center and at home was to be taken for walks, with someone holding his hand. While he continued to prefer his mother to do this—with and for him—he would readily accept substitutes.

Mark was one of those children who had the greatest difficulty in establishing a workable distance between himself and mother. His mother was ambivalent as soon as Mark ceased to be part of herself, her symbiotic child. At times she seemed to avoid close body contact; at other times she might interrupt Mark in his autonomous activities to pick him up, hug him and hold him. She did this, of course, when *she* needed it, not when *he* did. This ambivalence on mother's part may have been what made it difficult for Mark to function at a distance from his mother.

During the early practicing subphase, following the initial push away from mother into the outside world, most of the children seemed to go through a brief period of increased separation anxiety. The fact that they were able to move independently, yet remain connected to mother— not physically, but through the distance modalities, by way of their seeing and hearing her—made the successful use of these distance modalities extraordinarily important for a while. The children did not like to lose sight of mother; they might stare sadly at her empty chair, or at the door through which she had left.

Many of the mothers seemed to react to the fact that their infants were moving away by *helping* them move away, i.e., by giving them a gentle, or perhaps less gentle, push. Mothers also became interested in and sometimes critical of their children's functioning at this point; they began to compare notes, and they showed concern if their child seemed to be behind. Sometimes they hid their concern in a pointed show of non-concern. In many mothers, concern became especially concentrated in eagerness that their children should begin to walk. Once the child was able to move away some distance, it was as if suddenly these mothers began to worry about his being able to "make it" out there, in the world, where he would have to fend for himself. In that context, walking seemed to have great symbolic meaning for both mother and toddler: it was as if the walking toddler had proved by his attainment of independent upright locomotion that he had already graduated into the world of fully independent human beings. The expectation and confidence that mother exudes that her child is now able to "make it out there" seems to be an important trigger for the child's own feeling of safety and perhaps also for his exchanging some of his magical omnipotence for autonomy and developing self-esteem (Sandler, et al., 1963).

THE PRACTICING SUBPHASE PROPER

With the child's spurt in autonomous functions, especially upright locomotion, the "love-affair with the world" (Greenacre, 1957) is at its height. During these precious six to eight months (from 10-12 to 16-18 months), for the junior toddler the world is his oyster. Libidinal cathexis shifts substantially into the service of the rapidly growing autonomous ego and its functions; the child seems intoxicated with his own faculties and with the greatness of his world.

At the same time, we see a relatively great imperviousness to knocks and falls and other frustrations, such as a toy being grabbed by another child. As the child, through the maturation of his locomotor apparatus, begins to venture farther and farther away from the mother's feet, he is often so absorbed in his own activities that for long periods of time he appears to be oblivious of the mother's presence. However, he returns periodically to the mother, seeming to need his physical proximity and refuelling from time to time.

It is not at all impossible that the elation of this subphase has to do not only with the exercise of the ego apparatuses, and the body feeling of locomotion in the upright position like the bipedal grown-up dashing through the air, but also with the elation of escape from absorption into the orbit of mother. From this standpoint, we might say that, just as the infant's peek-a-boo games seem to turn from passive to active—the losing and then regaining of the love object—the toddler's constant running off, to be swooped up by mother, turns his fear of re-engulfment by mother from passive to active. This behavior also, of course, guarantees that he *will* be caught, i.e., it confirms over and over again that he is connected to mother, and still wishes to be. We need not assume that the child's behavior is intended to serve these functions when it first makes its appearance; but it is necessary to recognize that it produces these effects, which can then be repeated intentionally.

Phenomena of mood are of great importance at this stage. Most children in the practicing subphase appeared to have major periods of exhilaration, or at least of relative elation; they became *low-keyed* only when they became aware that mother was absent from the room. At such times, their gestural and performance motility slowed down; their interest in their surroundings diminished; and they appeared to be preoccupied once again with inwardly concentrated attention, with what Rubinfine (1961) called "imaging."

LOW-KEYEDNESS

Our inferences about the low-keyed state start from two recurrent phenomena: (1) if a person other than mother actively tried to comfort the child, he would lose his emotional balance and burst into tears; and (2) the visible termination of the child's "toned-down" state, at the time of his reunion with the briefly absent mother, both these phenomena heightened our awareness that, up to that point, the child *had been* in a special "state of self." This low-keyedness and inferred "imaging" of mother are reminiscent of a miniature anaclitic depression. We tend to see in the child's effort to hold on to a state of mind that Joffe & Sandler (1965) have termed "the ideal state of self," what Kaufman & Rosenblum (1967) have termed "conservation withdrawal" in monkeys.

THE SUBPHASE OF RAPPROCHEMENT

The third subphase of separation-individuation (from about 16 to 25 months) begins hypothetically by *mastery* of upright locomotion and consequently less absorption in locomotion *per se.*

By the middle of the second year of life, the infant has become a toddler. *He now becomes more and more aware, and makes greater and greater use of his awareness of physical separateness.* Yet, side by side with the growth of his cognitive faculties and the increasing differentiation of his emotional life, there is a noticeable warning of his previous imperviousness to frustration, as well as of his relative obliviousness to the mother's presence. Increased separation anxiety can be observed—a fear of object loss inferred from the fact that when he hurts himself he discovers, to his perplexity, that his mother is not automatically at hand. The relative lack of concern about the mother's presence that was characteristic of the practicing subphase is now replaced by *active approach behavior,* and by a seemingly constant concern with the mother's whereabouts. As the toddler's awareness of separateness grows—stimulated by his maturationally acquired ability physically to move away from his mother, and by his cognitive growth—he now seems to have an increased need and wish for his mother to *share with him* every new acquisition on his part of skill and experience. We call this subphase of separation-individuation, therefore, *the period of rapprochement.*

The earlier "refuelling" type of contact with mother, which the baby sought intermittently, is now replaced by a quest for constant interaction of the toddler with mother (and also with father and familiar adults) at a progressively higher level of symbolization. There is an increasing prominence of language, vocal and other intercommunications, as well as symbolic play.

In other words, when the junior toddler grows into the senior toddler of 18 to 24 months, a most important emotional turning point is reached. The toddler now begins to experience, more or less gradually and more or less keenly, the obstacles that lie in the way of his anticipated "conquest of the world." Side by side with the acquisition of primitive skills and perceptual cognitive faculties, there has been an increasingly clear differentiation between the intrapsychic representation of the object and the self-representation. At the very height of mastery—towards the end of the practicing period—it has already begun to dawn on the junior toddler that the world is *not* his oyster; that he must cope with it more or less "on his own," very often as a relatively helpless, small and separate individual, unable to command relief or assistance, merely by feeling the need for them, or giving voice to that need.

The quality and measure of the wooing behavior of the toddler during this subphase provide important clues to the assessment of the normality of the individuation process.

Incompatibilities and misunderstandings between mother and child can be observed even in the case of the normal mother and her normal toddler, these being in part specific to certain seeming contradictions of this subphase. Thus, in the subphase of renewed, active wooing, the toddler's demand for his mother's constant participation seems contradictory to the mother: while he is now not as dependent and helpless as he was six months before, and seems eager to become less and less so, nevertheless he even more insistently expects the mother to share every aspect of his life. During this subphase some mothers cannot accept the child's demandingness; others cannot face the fact that the child is becoming increasingly independent and separate.

In this third subphase, while individuation proceeds very rapidly and the child exercises it to the limit, he also becomes more and more aware of his separateness and employs all kinds of mechanisms to resist separation from the mother.

But no matter how insistently the toddler tries to coerce the mother, she and he no longer function effectively as a dual unit; that is to say, he can no longer participate in the still maintained delusion of parental omnipotence. Verbal communication becomes more and more necessary; gestural coercion on the part of the toddler, or mutual preverbal empathy between other and child, will no longer suffice to attain the goal of satisfaction, of well-being (Joffe & Sandler, 1965). The junior toddler gradually realizes that his love objects (his parents) are separate individuals with their own individual interests. He must gradually and painfully give up his delusion of his own grandeur, often with dramatic fights with mother—less so, it seemed to us, with father.

This is the crossroad that my co-workers and I termed the rapprochement crisis.

According to Annemarie Weil's suggestion, at this point the three basic anxieties of early childhood so often coincide. There is still a fear of object loss, more or less replaced by a conspicuous fear of loss of love and, in particular, definite signs of castration anxiety.

Here, in the rapprochement subphase, we feel is the mainstring of man's eternal struggle against both fusion and isolation.

One could regard the entire life cycle as constituting a more or less successful process of distancing from and introjection of the lost symbiotic mother, an eternal longing for the actual or fantasied "ideal state of self," with the latter standing for a symbiotic fusion with the "all good" symbiotic mother, who was at one time part of the self in a blissful state of well-being.

REFERENCES

BENEDEK, T. (1938): Adaptation to reality in early infancy. *Psychoanal. Q.*, 7, 200-215.

BENEDEK, T. (1949): The psychosomatic implications of the primary unit mother-child. *Am. J. Orthopsychiat.*, 19, 642-654.

ERIKSON, E. H. (1968): The life cycle: Epigenesis of identity. In *Identity, Youth and Crisis*. New York: Norton.

GREENACRE, P. (1957): The childhood of the artist: Libidinal phase development and giftedness. *Psychoanal. Study Child*, 12.

JOFFE, W. G. & SANDLER, J. (1965): Notes on pain, depression, and individuation. *Psychoanal. Study Child*, 20.

KAUFMAN, I. C. & ROSENBLUM, L. A. (1967): The reaction to separation in infant monkeys: Anaclictic depression and conservation-withdrawal. *Psychosom. Med.*, 29, 648-675.

MAHLER, M. S. (1963): Thoughts about development and individuation. *Psychoanal. Study Child*, 18.

MAHLER, M. S. (1965): On the significance of the normal separation-individuation phase: With reference to research in symbiotic child psychosis. In M. Schur (Ed.), *Drives, Affects, Behavior*, Vol. 2. New York: Int. Univ. Press.

MAHLER, M. S. (1968): *On Human Symbiosis and the Vicissitudes of Individuation*, Vol. I: *Infantile Psychosis*. New York: Int. Univ. Press.

MAHLER, M. S. & GOSLINGER, B. J. (1965): On symbiotic child psychosis: Genetic dynamic and restitutive aspects. *Psychoanal. Study Child*, 10.

MAHLER, M. S. & L. PERRIERE, K. (1965): Mother-child interaction during separation-individuation. *Psychoanal. Q.*, 34, 483-498.

ROSE, G. J. (1964): Creative imagination in terms of ego "core" and boundaries. *Int. J. Psycho-Anal.*, 45, 75-84.

RUBINFINE, D. L. (1961): Perception, reality testing, and symbolism. *Psychoanal. Study Child*, 16.

SANDLER, J., HOLDER, A., & MEERS, D. (1963): The ego ideal and the ideal self. *Psychoanal. Study Child*, 18.

SPIEGEL, L. A. (1959): The self, the sense of self, and perception. *Psychoanal. Study Child*, 14.

WOLFF, P. H. (1959): Observations on newborn infants. *Psychosom. Med.*, 21, 110-118.

9

THE ISSUES OF AUTONOMY AND AGGRESSION IN THE THREE-YEAR-OLD: THE UTKU ESKIMO CASE

Jean L. Briggs, Ph.D.

Associate Professor, Department of Anthropology,
Memorial University of Newfoundland

The purpose of this paper is to raise questions concerning some widely accepted generalizations about normal growth sequences and crises in childhood. Much of our current thinking about the emotional development of children is based on the foundations laid by Freud and Erikson, and rightly so, as they have perceptively described many of the processes that characterize the growth of middle class children in Western cultures. It seems possible, however, that if one were to observe non-Western, non-middle class children, a different picture might emerge. This paper is an exercise in such observation. It will present data from a Canadian

Reprinted by permission of Grune and Stratton, Inc. and the author from SEMINARS IN PSYCHIATRY, Vol. 4, No. 4 (November), 1972, pp. 317-329.

Fieldwork was supported by the Wenner-Gren Foundation, the Northern Coordination and Research Centre of the Department of Northern Affairs and National Resources (now the Northern Science Research Group of the Department of Indian Affairs and Northern Development) of the Canadian Government, NIMH Pre-doctoral Research Fellowship 5 Fl MH-20, 701-02 BEH with Research Grant Attachment MH-07951-01, and the Canada Council (award from Isaak Walton Killam bequest to the Department of Sociology and Anthropology of the Memorial University of Newfoundland). The author is grateful to Ronald Schwartz for his comments on the draft of this paper.

Eskimo group and will examine the extent to which Eskimo patterns of development conform to the expectations that we have derived from our observation of Western children. In particular, it will deal with the events characteristic of ages two to three.

ERIKSON'S LIFE STAGES

As a basis of comparison for the Eskimo data, I shall take Erikson's account of the significant psychosocial events in the life of a 2-3-year-old. Erikson, like Freud, assumes that the emotional development of a child depends on his biologic maturation, and that the child's libidinal attention is focused on a different part of his body at each stage of his development. In the orthodox Freudian view, of course, the child goes through three stages, oral, anal, and genital. In each of these stages, he derives erotic pleasure from the corresponding part of his body and directs his libido toward a different object: himself, one of his parents, other children, and ultimately, a spouse. Erikson accepts Freud's biologically based psychosexual stages, characterized by different modes of experiencing one's body; but he introduces sociologic variables as well into his view of human emotional development. He correlates each stage of sexual development with a different social experience or "task," which a person masters, or fails to master, before moving on to the next stage. There are eight such tasks in Erikson's scheme: the acquisition of trust, autonomy, initiative, industry, identity, intimacy, generativity, and ego integrity. Each of these is a mode of experiencing oneself in relation to others, and each is thought to be systematically related to the others, such that each "depends on the proper development in the proper sequence of each (preceding) item" (3). The sequence is thought to be predetermined by biologic maturation and by the individual's "readiness . . . to interact with a growing social radius" (3). The role of society is to "meet and invite this succession of potentialities for interaction and . . . to encourage the proper rate and the proper sequence of their enfolding [sic]" (3). The child's attempt to meet the demands of society and to make them consonant with his inner biologic needs produces a characteristic learning crisis or "critical period," which, hopefully, culminates in a new level of integration at each life stage. However, for various reasons, a person may fail to develop one or many of these potentialities, and in Erikson's scheme the experience of failure is characteristically different in each stage: mistrust, shame and doubt, guilt, inferiority, role confusion, isolation, stagnation, and despair.

In this paper we will be concerned primarily with the second crisis, that which Erikson labels "autonomy vs. shame and doubt," but the questions to be raised relate to the conceptual framework as a whole, not to this stage alone.

The eight psychosocial tasks that Erikson postulates are certainly intrinsic to social relationships generally, and therefore it seems very likely that in some form or other they are encountered by members of all societies. It may be questioned, however, whether they are necessarily encountered in the same order, or are necessarily associated with the same modes of experiencing one's body. More fundamentally, we may ask whether experiences with organ modes are in fact prototypical of social experiences. It may be questioned also whether psychosocial development always proceeds by critical steps, that is, by periods of relative quiescence followed by "turning points," or "moments of decision between progress and regression, integration and retardation" (3). And finally, I wonder whether the particular kind of failure experience that Erikson associates with each stage is necessarily associated with that stage. Are shame and doubt always associated with the learning of autonomy? Is guilt necessary associated with initiative?

Obviously, these questions cannot all be addressed in a paper concerned with just one life stage; and none of them can be conclusively answered in a paper that deals with just one culture. Nonetheless, it is hoped that thoughts concerning some of them may be sparked by the Eskimo data that follow.

THE AUTONOMY CRISIS

Let us look now at the autonomy crisis. I will first summarize what Erikson says about this stage, and then compare the Eskimo data, to see what light they throw on the questions raised above.

Erikson says that "muscular maturation sets the stage for experimentation with two simultaneous sets of social modalities: holding on and letting go. . . . To hold can become a destructive and cruel retaining or restraining, (or) it can become a pattern of care: to have and to hold. To let go, too, can turn into an inimical letting loose of destructive forces, or it can become a relaxed 'to let pass' and 'to let go' " (3). Erikson concludes that at this stage the infant must have the reassuring experience of being firmly controlled by others, so that his "basic faith in existence . . . will not be jeopardized by . . . this sudden violent wish to have a choice, to appropriate demandingly, and to eliminate stubbornly. Firmness must protect him against the potential anarchy of his as yet untrained sense of discrimination, his inability to hold on and to let go with discretion" (3). If he is not so protected, he will experience "meaningless and arbitrary . . . shame and . . . doubt," and will attempt to compensate, to gain power over the environment, by compulsive self-control (3).

Erikson describes shame as a feeling that "one is completely exposed and conscious of being looked at. . . . One is visible and not ready to be visible. . . . [It] exploits an increasing sense of being small, which can develop only as the child stands up and as his awareness permits him to note the relative measures of size and power. . . ." "Where shame is [related to] the consciousness of being upright and exposed, doubt . . . [is related to] a consciousness of having a front and a back—and especially a 'behind.'" The invisible behind is subject to magical domination by those who threaten one's autonomy and label "evil" the products of one's body. Doubt, in other words, relates to the child's feelings about the value of what he produces, bodily and, by extension, socially (3).

Erikson concludes: "This stage . . . [is] decisive for the ratio of love and hate, cooperation and willfulness, freedom of self-expression and its suppression. From a sense of self-control without loss of self-esteem comes a lasting sense of good will and pride; from a sense of loss of self-control and of foreign overcontrol comes a lasting propensity for doubt and shame" (3).

CRISES OF THE UTKU 3-YEAR-OLD

Utku children do have a "holding on or letting go" crisis at about the age of three, but it is not related to toilet training. It is connected with three other lessons that they have to learn at about this age: to give up nursing, to walk instead of being backpacked by the mother, and to control their feelings.

The Utku, until recently, have tended to space their children about 3 years apart, and until the younger child is born, the elder is indulged and gratified as completely as possible. He is the center of affectionate attention, cuddled, played with, and cooed at by everybody. He is nursed on demand, except on the very rare occasions when his mother is doing something that cannot be interrupted; and he sleeps when he is sleepy, either on his mother's back or lying under a quilt on the sleeping platform, surrounded by other members of the family. He is never alone, awake or asleep, and most of the time, he is in physical contact with someone else. Until he can walk, and even afterwards, his mother carries him on her back for long periods of the day. She does this partly to keep him warm, partly to keep him soothed and happy, occasionally to restrain him—to keep him safe or out of mischief—and sometimes because it is convenient to carry him with her as she moves about the camp. At night he sleeps between his mother and his father, under the same quilts.

The Utku believe that a child's mind, his mental faculties, and understanding grow only gradually, so there is no point in trying to discipline a small child; he is incapable of learning or remembering. The fact that a small child has no mind also means to the Utku that he is incapable of understanding, and reconciling himself to, deprivations. Consequently, adults pity his tears. Both for this reason and because they believe him incapable of learning anyway, they give him what he demands, if at all possible. If it is necessary to refuse—because, for example, there is no more of what he asks for—it is done in the gentlest possible way, often by offering a substitute, or by distracting his attention.

Toilet "training" is begun at birth. The baby wears no diapers or other clothing but is carried naked against the mother's naked back. The mother can thus be sensitive to the child's slightest sign of restlessness, and as soon as she suspects that he is about to evacuate, she shakes herself rapidly to inhibit his impulse, quickly pulls him out of her parka and holds him over a can, which she grasps between her knees. She may also hold him over a can before putting him into her parka or before laying him down for the night. Usually, she will try to encourage urination on these occasions by tapping the baby's genitals and humming in a monotone: "Olo-olo-olo-olo-olo. . . ." In general, very few accidents seem to occur, at least after the mother has accustomed herself to the baby's rhythms. Eventually, the child learns to ask for the can, himself, though I never heard anyone directly coaching him to do so. I was told that a child learns to signal by imitating children slightly more advanced than himself, and this seems quite in line with the freedom to regulate his own growth that is granted to the child in many other areas of his development, too. Adults and older children may, however, ask him occasionally, when he seems restless: "Do you feel like peeing?" Or when they put him on the can before packing him or laying him down, they may say, in the tender tone of persuasion that is regularly used with small children: "Pee." Thus, it is likely that the child is not only imitating older children when he learns to signal his desire to eliminate, but is also picking up verbal and other cues from his caretakers concerning what is expected of him. There seems to be no pressure placed on a 2-3-year old to use the can or to signal for it to be brought. If an older child, say a 5- or 6-year-old, accidentally soils himself or wets the family bed at night, he may be "mooed" at, that is, spoken to in a disapproving tone of voice and told that he is not using his mind. But in the case of smaller children, the onus is on the caretaker to watch for the child's nonverbal signals or to respond to his verbal ones. The child is not scolded if he has an accident; the caretaker simply wipes him off if he is wet and wrings out whatever else (her parka or the child's pants) may have gotten wet. If the child's clothes are very wet, she may hang them up to dry; otherwise she will allow them to dry by body heat. If he is dirty, she will wash the clothing, and will clean the child's skin by taking water into her mouth, spitting it onto the child and wiping him with a rag or bit of hide. It is not often that he gets his clothes wet or dirty, however, because, first, as I have said, he is carried for long periods naked on his mother's back, and second, because even after he is old enough to be dressed and running around, his clothing is adapted to his state of development. If the weather is warm, both boys and girls may go naked from the waist down; otherwise their pants will be slit at the crotch, so that when they squat, the pants automatically open and are not soiled.

In many ways, Utku show much less revulsion toward bodies and body products than we do. There are no areas of the body that are considered intrinsically dirty or repulsive. Small children are often patted and kissed on the genitals or anus; in fact one has the impression that these areas are considered especially charming. A parent picking up a child or cuddling him will often put his arm through the child's crotch and lift him up that way. And a mother nursing her small son may rest her hand affectionately on his genitals, as he lies in her lap. Attitudes toward some body products, too, seem much more relaxed than our own. A mother cleans her baby's nose by sucking out the mucus, then spitting it out of her mouth. She may also blow her own nose into her fingers, suck off the fingers, and spit out the mucous. Before the baby has teeth, she may pre-chew food and feed it to him, mouth-to-mouth; adults, too, pass chewing gum from mouth to mouth, without regard for the saliva mixed with it. A mother taps her baby's genitals to encourage him to urinate, and when the flow begins, she allows it to run over her hand without sign of revulsion, merely wiping her hand afterward on the skirt of her parka. Similarly, if a child accidentally urinates into a cup or dish, it is emptied and wiped out, but not necessarily washed, before being used again. The attitude toward urine seems to be quite matter-of-fact: it will dry. To be sure, mothers do say that urine is disgusting, but it is hard to find behavioral evidence that bears this out. Children are removed with haste from laps and backs when they start to urinate, but this may be as much because the wetness is cold and uncomfortable as because it is disgusting.

The same is not true of attitudes toward feces. Here, too, the cleaning-up is always done in a very matter-of-fact manner, but it is done immediately, and it is in a voice of some alarm or revulsion that the child is warned: "Don't touch!" One young mother admitted that she felt nauseated by her child's feces.

A child surely picks up cues to adult attitudes toward urine and feces from the speed with which he is removed from a person's lap or back when he starts to evacuate; from tones of voice; and from the manner in which his mother holds him while she cleans him. He learns them also by virtue of the fact that feces of carnivorous animals in general are spoken of as disgusting and not to be touched or eaten. If a caretaker wants to persuade a child to avoid an object or an activity, she will pretend that there are feces in the vicinity and will point them out to the child in a tone of exaggerated disgust. In fun, she may also pretend that there are feces on the child—but never when he is really soiled. By the time the child is two or three, he has come to share the adult reluctance to touch feces, but I think the fact that the child learns these attitudes partly in play and partly in relation to sources of dirt other than himself, rather than exclusively in the context of his own soiling, may have a significant influence on his attitude toward himself. At no time in the process of acquiring these attitudes toward body products has his own soiling or wetting been made an issue. Moreover, the child is by no means the only one who soils in the environment. Daily, he comes into contact with other feces: those of dogs, other people, and the animals whose carcasses he eats. In our own antiseptic world, the child's own feces—and those of an occasional pet that is not yet house-broken—are the only ones the child encounters. But the Utku child need not single himself out as "dirty," in contrast to other "clean" people and animals. He can, rather, see himself as sharing in a pervasive aspect of the environment, perhaps more or less the way our own children feel about being earth-stained. He is never made to feel that his self is contaminated by the dirtiness of his product: it will wash off; the apertures from which feces and urine come are lovable; and there is nothing "naughty" about producing inedible, untouchable material, even if one does it in an awkward place. The dirtiness of the feces and the wetness of the urine are not used to shame the child. His soiling behavior is simply taken as evidence that he is still lacking in mind, and it is assumed that when he acquires sufficient mind, he will produce his feces and his urine in a more appropriate spot. Moreover, the interest a child shows in his productions—"look, mother, feces!"—is also regarded as natural, and his mother shares his pleasure with an affectionate smile even as she prevents him from touching it. Thus, toilet training is not made a battleground. The child is taught the appropriate attitudes toward his products and shown the appropriate place to deposit them, but the decision as to when to start imitating other people is up to him. Since no one is going to challenge him, there is no reason for him to utilize bodily modes of holding on and letting go as symbolic expressions of independent will. And I see no evidence that he does so.

Nonetheless, as I have mentioned, Utku children do undergo lessons in "holding on" and "letting go" at about the age of three. And interestingly enough, though negative attitudes toward the body and its products are not directly utilized in teaching the child physically to hold on, to keep himself clean, they are used to teach him the other lessons associated with retentive modes of interaction: letting go of his mother and holding on to his feelings. Consequently, it is in the latter contexts, too, that he learns shame. We shall see, however, that the content of these negative attitudes is quite different from our own, and that they are not primarily focused on the anus and its product.

The crisis occurs, as I have said, at the time that the next child is born. Then the period of almost total gratification comes to an end, and the 3-year-old has to learn to stop nursing, to walk and to play independently of his mother, and to control his demandingness, his temper, and his selfishness.

Weaning is begun while the mother is pregnant with the next child, but it progresses very gradually and is often not accomplished until after the baby is born. The mother's first step in weaning is to stop offering the breast voluntarily, and when the child demands it, she will try to postpone giving it. She may offer a substitute food or activity— always in an affectionate, persuasive voice—or she may simply ignore the demand and try to discourage the child by passive resistance until he gives up and turns his attention elsewhere, of his own accord. After the baby is born, however, the mother combines these techniques with stronger measures. She says to the child in a tone of exaggerated but always sympathetic disgust: "You don't want to nurse; ugh, the breast is all covered with feces; the baby has shit all over it; it tastes terrible." If the child still insists, she may give in briefly, let him have a suck, then try again to distract his attention, with the help of others present. In the case I observed most closely, weaning was completely accomplished within a month of the baby's birth (1). However, in other cases, the displaced child may continue to cry at night for some months. One child was still having occasional temper tantrums over nursing when her younger sister was well over a year old.

The second lesson that has to be learned when the baby is born is to relinquish one's place on mother's back. This, too, is taught by degrees, beginning probably when the mother is pregnant. A fawnskin suit is made for the child, and he is encouraged—again in an affectionate, persuasive voice—to put it on and "run run" around the iglu, "go visit" his grandfather next door, or play with the older children outdoors. But again, more threatening techniques may be used as well to encourage the child to want to get dressed. During the years when the child is carried naked on his mother's back, or passed naked from hand to hand for others to cuddle and play with, a great deal of affectionate attention is focused on his body. He is kissed and patted and admired, and various games are played with his body. Children of both sexes are encouraged to posture in various ways and to present specific parts of their bodies to be kissed, patted, poked, and admired: "Let me kiss your navel, your breast, your armpit, your nose. . . ." But eventually, these games become a means not of gaining attention and affection but of learning modesty.

Modesty is not phrased as a matter of decency. The child is not taught that it is "sinful" or "improper" to expose his body, but that it is dangerous. Now, instead of *inviting* the child to present his armpit to be kissed or his navel to be poked, the mother *warns* him that if he doesn't quickly cover up, his uncle or his grandmother or, worse, the visiting stranger will see, kiss, or poke him. And the uncle, the grandmother, or the stranger cooperate by laughingly pretending to do just that. The situation—naked child playing with affectionate adults—is the same as it was, but the mother's tone of voice has changed to one of "alarm" and "protectiveness," and the demonstrative overtures of others quickly become reinterpreted as threatening attacks. Similar methods of making the child self-conscious are utilized also in other situations in which the parents want him to become unobtrusive, for example, when they are going to bed and want him to settle down, or when he is having a tantrum and they want him to be quiet.

After the baby is born, efforts to get the child dressed and physically separated from the mother are reinforced, as in the case of weaning, by passive resistance on the part of the mother. She simply sits still and fails to help the child in his attempts to climb into her parka. Sometimes she laughs at his screams and tears, at other times she pretends not to notice him at all. This lesson, too, took a month or so to learn in the case I knew best (1).

Self-restraint and self-subordination, the third lesson that Utku 3-year-olds have to learn, are probably the hardest, judging both from the length of time it takes and from associated signs of conflict, such as nightmares and depressions. This lesson is not physically related to the birth of a sibling, as are weaning and walking, but it is related in other ways. I have mentioned that children are not considered teachable until they have minds; and one of the milestones that Utku watch for in the development of mind is the ability to speak. Thus, it often happens that, about the time the next child is born, the older sibling is beginning to show signs that he is capable of learning, and the baby's birth provides the occasion for instruction. There are at least two reasons for this. In the first place, it is difficult to cope with two children who are crying for instant attention, and therefore, it would be convenient if the older child were not so demanding. Secondly, the baby provides an object on whom to practice the virtues of generosity, patience, and helpfulness.

These qualities are intrinsic to the concept of *naklik-,* protective concern, which is one of the cardinal virtues of the Utku. As one woman defined it, it means wanting to feed those who are hungry, warm those who are cold, and protect those who are in physical danger. In practice, however, the naklik concept is far broader than this. It is invoked to describe all "good" behavior, and above all, perhaps, unaggressive behavior. It is said that a person who feels naklik will never express hostility in any form toward human beings. Ways in which the Utku actually do express hostility toward humans and others are described elsewhere (2).

Logically, it is toward the weak and helpless above all that Utku feel and behave in a naklik manner. Children are trained to share these feelings as soon as they begin to demonstrate understanding, and, of course, a younger sibling is a most appropriate object. From the time the baby is born, the older child is taught to kiss him, to hold him gently, and never to hurt him. As the baby grows stronger and more active, these instructions are followed by others: to give up one's playthings to the younger, not to be angry when the youngest interferes in one's activities, and to wait for attention until the youngest has been seen to.

Aggression control is one area of behavior in which Utku adults have little tolerance for deviance. Training in this area, as in others, is delayed until the child shows signs of developing mind, and, as usual, it is believed that the child will gradually conform, of his own accord, as his mind grows; thus it is not necessary to enforce good behavior on every occasion or to punish misbehavior.

Nonetheless, once training is started, considerable pressure is brought to bear on the child to encourage him to remember. Every opportunity is taken to tell him what the proper behavior is, even when he is playing happily and is not misbehaving in any way. When he is patient, generous, and affectionate toward the baby, he is praised and hugged; and when he is angry or demanding, he is "mooed" at in a disapproving voice. Threats of imaginary dangers may also be used to motivate the child, and, as usual, the mother presents herself in the role of protector, rather than threatener. She may tell her crying child that strangers will hear him and will come to adopt him, because they love noisy children; he had better be quiet so that she can hide him. Fear of aggression is inculcated by teaching the child that he is omnipotent and that his anger can have disastrous consequences. For example, if he throws a pebble at his mother, she may ask him in a solemn voice: "Do you want to kill me? Do you want me to die?" Or she may tell him that the reason the sky gets dark at night is that he is noisy and disobedient.

Any of the child's natural fears may be utilized in this way, and other fears are instilled. Among the latter are fears of what one's body may do to one. The child is told, sympathetically: "Don't cry, look, your eyes are bleeding because you're crying so much"; or "Your tears will wet your feet, and they will freeze." Thus, negative attitudes toward the body are instilled, both in the context of learning to separate from the mother and in the context of learning aggression control; only in the former case, it is a fear of what others will see or do to one's body that is taught, and in the latter, a fear of what the body itself may do, either to itself or to others.

CONCLUSION

We have seen that, more or less simultaneously, the Utku 3-year-old experiences several interrelated "crises" or turning points in his psychosocial development: He must give up nursing and being carried, must learn to subordinate his wishes to those of others, and finally, he must learn to control the feelings of anger and distress generated by these conflicts.

Let us now examine the ways in which this situation is related to the autonomy crisis described by Erikson. It is clear that there are conflictual turning points in the lives of Utku children, as in our own children's lives, and that autonomy is one of the issues involved.

In a sense, all of the crises experienced by the Utku 3-year-old have to do with autonomy. They can also be seen as symbolically related to holding on and letting go, in both positive and negative senses. Moreover, it is true for Utku children as for Western children that negative attitudes toward the physical and social self, including feelings of shame, are taught in the context of the autonomy crisis.

If one looks more closely at this crisis, however, it appears that there are fundamental differences between the shape it takes in the two cultures. First, and most importantly, in Utku society it is not associated with toilet training. The Utku theory of psychic development supports a very gradual, relaxed training and places no importance on winning battles, so toilet training never becomes an issue. One wonders whether, under these circumstances, we are justified in assuming, as Erikson does, that the child's relationship to his body products necessarily provides a model for less tangible social attitudes and relationships. Is it the first experience of a certain mode of interaction, or is it the creation of such a crisis around an experience that makes it memorable and leads to the accumulation of social meanings centering on it? If the latter, then in the Utku case, the child's attitudes toward his body products presumably do not provide a prototype either for social holding on and letting go, or for attitudes toward the self. It is not urine and feces that one has to learn to hold on to and to let go appropriately; it is one's loving mother, and secondarily other objects associated with affection—toys and food— that one has to relinquish, and anger and disappointment that one has to control. Demands are also made on the child to begin to "hold on" to other people in a positive, valued sense of taking care of them. One has to begin to let go of the desire to be nurtured, to some extent, and instead begin to nurture.

It is interesting that some of these conflicts—those associated with separation from the mother—are associated with a prior trust crisis in Erikson's scheme, rather than with the autonomy crisis. In Utku society, I am not sure that there is a *trust* crisis, in Erikson's sense of a conflict, which comes to a head and is then resolved. Limitations of space preclude a full discussion of Utku infancy, but, in brief, it can be said that the baby never needs to fear that its biting will make the mother withdraw the breast or leave, because she does not withdraw when bitten; she just laughs slightly at the pain and says, tolerantly: "The baby has no mind." Moreover, she is almost always within sight, sound, or touch of the baby. So, to use Erikson's phrase, the paradise is forfeited only after the child has had a long, secure, and highly gratifying symbiotic relationship with his mother. Up to the moment of separation, neither trust nor autonomy has been an issue. The child has had his own way without having to fight for it and has not really been aware that the possibility of defeat exists. His mother has been there, as an extension of himself, to serve him. Now, suddenly, he loses a large measure of the control he has exerted over others, at the same time that he is required to gain control over himself as a separate being.

What the effects of this late separation and its conjunction with the autonomy issue are, I am not sure. On the one hand, the separation occurs at a time when the child has a more mature understanding of what is happening to him, and is thus, perhaps, better (or at least differently) able to cope with feelings of abandonment, as compared with our own children. On the other hand, he may have acquired a much stronger (or more conscious) desire that mother should always be with him, which could intensify the conflict attendant on separation (4). It is possible that the association between separation and autonomy is one of the reasons why the latter is so jealously guarded by Utku throughout their lives. In other words, the value placed on autonomy may in part be compensation for a desire to remain dependent. Elsewhere (2), I have also related it to certain aggressive ways of expressing affection toward small children and to the rejections experienced by the child who is being taught to control his demandingness and his desire for demonstrative affection. Affection comes to be seen as both desirable and dangerous, and a certain distance from others is maintained as a defense.

There are, however, other considerations that may counteract the negative aspects of the separation experience and, consequently, lessen the intensity of the autonomy crisis. One of these is the Utku policy of not making issues out of daily disagreements between parent and child. The effect of this policy is that even though the 3-year-old is made aware that some of his behavior is undesirable, he is rarely frustrated by being physically prevented from engaging in these unwelcome activities. Occasionally, a caretaker may backpack him again briefly to restrain him—which, incidentally, may contribute to the ambivalence about affection that has been posited. In general, however, the Utku child is granted a great deal of autonomy in his activities without having either to ask for it or to fear that he will be forcibly deprived of it. Indeed, autonomous judgment is required of him in many circumstances in which Western children are told what to do and are restrained or "protected": "Don't touch that"; "don't go there." The Utku child who hurts himself is merely told: "I warned you," or "you weren't using your mind."

One might wonder about possible deleterious effects of the lack of firm control on the part of caretakers, which Erikson considers necessary in order to prevent the child from making socially dangerous mistakes in his search for legitimate autonomy (3). I think, however, that what seems to us a lack of "firmness" on the part of Utku caretakers—their failure to insist on winning every battle—is not experienced as anarchical by the Utku child. Their permissiveness is rationalized very consistently: it is seen as the most appropriate way of helping a child to encounter learning situations, situations in which he can find out for himself the consequences of various courses of action and can discover that the advice that adults give him is often good. Utku believe that only in this way will he remember. This is not at all the same situation that Erikson had in mind when he recommended firmness; the Utku child never has to worry that his wrong choices will destroy his social relationships. Under the circumstances, the permissiveness that characterizes Utku child-rearing—the fact that both adults and children have considerable freedom to act autonomously, to make choices that they perceive as independent—may be a source of great satisfaction and may have the effect of lessening the potential for conflict regarding autonomy.

One of the other important implications of the conjunction of separation with autonomy is that feelings of shame are taught not in the context of toilet training but in connection with separation from the mother. As Erikson says, "shaming exploits an increasing sense of being small, which can develop only as the child stands up and as his awareness permits him to note the relative measure of size and power" (3). This statement seems even truer in the Utku case than in our own, since the Utku child is standing down off his mother's back, where he was big and powerful, whereas the Western child stands up from a crawling position, where he was even smaller and more helpless than he is now. The experience of smallness, then, should be more vivid for the Utku child, since for him it is contrasted with his former bigness. It is also contrasted with his former powerfulness, since, as we have seen, it is when the child is put down that he loses his control over his mother and other caretakers. This physical "put down" is, then, a most appropriate setting for the teasing to which the child is subjected now, as a means of teaching him to control himself. This ridicule, gentle as it seems to our Western eyes, is strongly experienced by the Utku child as a symbolic "put down." As one man said to me: "It [criticism] makes me feel very small."

In both cultures, then, the experience of autonomy is accompanied by that of shame, and feelings of exposure, vulnerability, and smallness seem to be components in the latter experience. Though it is not clear to me why the negative side of autonomy should *necessarily* be shame, it seems logical that it should be so in Utku culture where autonomy is the result of separation from the protective, enfolding mother.

The fear of being seen implies negative attitudes toward the body, and here again Erikson accurately describes the Utku case, to a point. However, the content of the "shame"and the context in which it is taught are both different from our own culture, and it seems to me likely that these differences significantly affect the meaning of "shame" and the role that it plays in personality structure.

First of all, since autonomy is not taught in the context of toilet training, bodily shame does not focus on body products, but rather on nakedness in general. If specific parts of the body are singled out, it is most likely to be parts that are considered "sexy," such as the genitals, the navel, the armpit, or the face. It is true that one of the teasing remarks sometimes made about these sexy parts of the body is: "It stinks! It smells like feces!" But I think it is important that these remarks are made with affectionate smiles and never when the child is actually dirty or wet. The children enter into the jokes, laughingly, and sometimes even solicit the remarks in play. Shame does not seem to be associated with them, and my impression is that they form part of quite a different syndrome than our own derogatory remarks about the body and its products. Being "shitty" seems to be much less threatening to Utku children than to our own, perhaps partly because revulsion toward feces is not taught primarily when the child has, *himself*, soiled, and because, as I have said, he is not the only one who soils in his world.

Moreover, the Utku experience of "shame" is, in part, derived not from a feeling that the body is somehow worthless but from the reverse: a feeling that it is too lovable, dangerously lovable. As we shall presently see, the notion that affection can be physically dangerous is associated also with the other bodily fears that are engendered. So, the body is, in general, perceived as too desirable, rather than not desirable enough, and is therefore to be protected. Positive attitudes toward the body and, more pervasively, toward the self are encouraged also by the Utku view that "bad" behavior is not symptomatic of a "bad" personality but only of a temporary and expectable lack of understanding.

The second kind of negative feeling about the body that Erikson associates with the autonomy crisis is self-doubt, the consciousness of having a "behind" that can be dominated by the will of others (3). Here, too, there is a partial parallel with the Utku case, in the fears that are engendered concerning the possibility of bleeding or freezing to death. But there is also a fundamental difference. The Utku child's fear of the unseen body is a fear that his own acts may injure him, not a fear that others may dominate or hurt him. And again, the danger is not associated with bad feces but with bad temper.

This is not to deny that Utku children fear physical attack, but these fears concern the whole body (or, later, the penis, in the case of boys), not the anal area. The fears are of being eaten, or bitten, in an access of affection; and I am not sure how pervasive or profound they are in the Utku case. The violent expression of affection is much more evident among certain Baffin Islanders (2); I was only rarely aware of it in the Central Arctic. On the contrary, I was impressed by the respect that Utku adults show for the physical integrity of children. Even if a child is interfering with an adult, he is not physically removed, but rather asked to move. The only physical "insults" commonly suffered by an Utku child are being backpacked as a means of restraint and being teasingly held in a tight grip until he protests and struggles free.

Let us see now how the Utku data relate to the questions posed at the beginning of the paper. It seems clear that Utku 2-3-year-olds, like their Western counterparts, do experience a crisis that has to do with "holding on" and "letting go," and with autonomous decision-making in these areas. Moreover, this crisis seems to follow a period in which trust is learned through long and intimate association with the mother.

However, we have seen that the Utku autonomy crisis is different from that of Western children in several ways; and had space allowed, I should like to have argued in more detail that the learning of trust is also different. I think that trust does not become an issue until the same moment when autonomy becomes an issue: when the child is separated from the mother at about the age of three. And perhaps it does not become an issue even then, because it has already been thoroughly learned, without a "crisis." In any case, I do not see the learning of trust associated with the mastery of biting impulses, since the mother does not withdraw when bitten. And I think it is clear that the learning of autonomy is not primarily associated with mastery over the bowels.

These data show that the specific content of Erikson's eight psychosocial lessons—the meaning that "trust" and "autonomy" have within the whole structure of affective relationships—is not universally the same. The lessons are not always associated with the same organ modes, and the fears engendered by failure are not the same.

I think we also have grounds for asking more fundamental questions about the organization and structure of psychosocial development. The first question concerns the idea that experiences with organ modes always and necessarily provide the models on which modes of social experience are based. In the Utku case, the learning of autonomy is *directly*—not just secondarily, by association—related to the social task of controlling one's temper. It is also directly related to the physical experiences of being put down and weaned, and these experiences may well become an intrinsic part of the meaning of autonomy for an Utku child, and symbolic of being socially "put down" (ridiculed) and "weaned" (rejected). But this is quite different from the proposition that mastery over the bowels is prototypical of the social modes of restraint and relaxation. It means that the learning of specific "social tasks" is not so inextricably bound to specific stages of biologic maturation as Erikson thought. Though it is likely that social experiences are very commonly, if not always, cognitively associated with physical experiences, the specific associations—what social experience is related to what physical one—may vary widely across cultures. And if this is so, perhaps a broader survey may show that the tasks are not encountered in a predetermined order that is the same in all societies.

Most fundamentally of all, one may ask whether detaching the social tasks from specific, biologically determined experiences with the body leaves room for the possibility that the lessons that Erikson singles out as central issues of psychosocial development are not *focal* in the sense that he thought them—are not, in other words, issues on which "successful" development hinges at given life stages—but are merely lessons, albeit important ones, like a multitude of others that the child encounters in the course of growing up.

REFERENCES

1. BRIGGS, J. L.: *Never in Anger: Portrait of an Eskimo Family.* Cambridge, Harvard University Press, 1970.
2. BRIGGS, J. L.: *The Origins of Non-Violence: Eskimo Aggression Management.* To be published in Muensterberger (Ed.), *The Psychoanalytic Study of Society.* New York: International Universities Press, 1972.
3. ERIKSON, E. H.: The eight stages of man. Reprinted in C. B. Stendler (Ed.), *Readings in Child Behavior and Development* (ed. 2). New York: Harcourt, Brace & World, 1964, pp. 245-253.
4. LUBART, J. M.: *Psychodynamic Problems of Adaptation—MacKenzie Delta Eskimos.* Ottawa, Department of Indian Affairs and Northern Development, 1970, p. 36.

10

INTELLECTUAL LEVELS OF SCHOOL CHILDREN SEVERELY MALNOURISHED DURING THE FIRST TWO YEARS OF LIFE

Margaret E. Hertzig, M.D., Herbert G. Birch, M.D., Ph.D.,

Stephen A. Richardson, Ph.D., and Jack Tizard, Ph.D.

ABSTRACT. Intellectual functioning at school age was studied in boys who had been severely malnourished during the first 2 years of life (index cases). IQ in these index cases was compared with that of male siblings closest in age and unrelated classmates or neighbors matched for sex and age (comparisons). Full Scale, Verbal and Performance IQs were lowest for the index cases. All IQ measures were significantly lower in the index cases than in the comparisons. Full Scale and Verbal IQ were significantly lower in the index cases than in the siblings. Siblings differed from comparison children only in Performance IQ. No association

---

Reprinted with permission from PEDIATRICS, Vol. 49, No. 6, pp. 814-824, June 1972. Copyright © The C. V. Mosby Co., St. Louis, Mo.

This paper is one of a series exploring the consequences for growth and development of severe malnutrition in infancy. The studies were carried out in Jamaica in the Tropical Metabolism Research Unit of the Medical Research Council. The investigations also received active support from the Epidemiology Research Unit of the Medical Research Council in Jamaica. Though most patients had been treated initially in the Tropical Metabolism Research Unit, additional patients, particularly in the younger age group at hospitalization, were obtained with the help of the Department of Pediatrics, University of West Indies. The follow-up studies included anthropometric, pediatric, neurological, psychological, educational, and social evaluations. Different aspects of the inquiry will be considered in separate reports.

was found between the intellectual level of index cases and the ages at which they had been hospitalized for the treatment of severe malnutrition during the first 2 years of life.

This is a report of a study conducted in Jamaica, West Indies, on the long-term consequences of severe malnutrition during the first 2 years of life. In it we have studied school children who, during their first 2 years of life, had been hospitalized for severe clinical malnutritian (marasmus, kwashiorkor, or marasmic-kwashiorkor). They have been compared with two groups of school-aged children of like sex. The first comparison group consisted of siblings of these cases. The sibs chosen were children in the sibship closest in age to the index case. The second comparison group was composed of unrelated classmates or neighbors closest in age to the index child. In later reports we will deal with the physique, neurologic characteristics, social and school functioning, as well as with the social and biologic background characteristics of these children. The present report, however, is restricted to a consideration of measured intelligence.

The concerns and design of the study stem from problems in interpretation and questions which have arisen in the course of previous investigations of the effects of early malnutrition upon physical and mental development. Until recently few children who were severely malnourished in infancy survived to reach school age. Research in malnutrition quite properly was focused primarily on its physiological effects and on the development of treatment and management procedures which would prevent death and maximize recovery. As Champakam, et al. (1) have put it, "survival was the main concern. Awareness and knowledge of the biochemical pathology of malnutrition and the availability of more efficient means for better diagnosis and treatment have reduced the immediate mortality among malnourished children. In direct proportion to the success in this regard is the clear possibility of increasing pools of survivors who may be handicapped in a variety of ways and for variable periods of time."

These changed circumstances have, over the past decade, resulted in a growing number of investigations exploring the long-term consequences of both severe acute malnutrition and "chronic subnutrition" (2) on growth and intellectual development. In addition, numerous experimental animal models for studying such consequences have been employed (3).

In studies of human subjects where controlled experiment could not be undertaken, follow-up studies have been conducted in children for whom both direct or indirect evidence of malnutrition is available. Two types of study designs have been used to explore the consequences of malnutrition for cognitive functioning in children. In some studies the presence of antecedent malnutrition in school-aged and preschool children has been inferred from differences in height for age. In communities where the risk of malnutrition is endemic, short children have been judged to have been a greater nutritional risk than taller agemates. Groups of tall and short children have then been compared for IQ level and intersensory competence (4, 5). The absence of direct evidence of severe malnutrition and the wide range of variables other than nutritional ones which differentiate the families of tall children from those of short ones (6, 7) have made it difficult directly to attribute the differences between the tall and short groups to malnutrition *per se*.

In the second type of study children with known histories of severe malnutrition have been compared with children in their communities without such histories (1, 8-17). While the fact of antecedent malnutrition has been clearly established in such studies, other factors limit the degree to which they can be interpreted as indicating a direct association between antecedent malnutrition and intellectual outcome. Children who are severely malnourished early in life come from families which are at greater risk for disorganization, cultural limitation, social and economic disadvantage, poor housing, excessively frequent and short-spaced reproduction, maternal and child ill-health, and so forth, than are other families even of the same social class (6). These additional factors themselves are capable of influencing intellectual development (18-20). In all instances the children with whom index cases have been compared could not be sufficiently well matched on these non-nutritional variables to meet the requirements of rigorous experimental design. The most thorough attempt is that of Champakam, et al. (1). in which age, sex, religion, caste, socioeconomic status, family size, birth order, and parental education were taken into consideration. However, in that study it was possible that the families of children hospitalized for kwashiorkor were either genetically different, or provided less adequate experiential opportunities for intellectual development than the comparison families (6, 18).

Another tactic is to use siblings of the malnourished children as comparisons. Such sib studies, though admittedly imperfect, provide different opportunities for interpreting findings. Only two such sib studies have thus far been carried out (21, 22). In one of these (21), sibs without a history of hospitalization for severe nutritional illness were found to be significantly superior in IQ to their hospitalized brothers or sisters.

However, the conclusions from this study are limited by the facts that the sample studied was relatively small, the sibs not like sexed, and no general population comparison group examined. In the other sib study (22), age at which malnutrition was experienced ranged from 10 months to 4 years with only 10 of the children in the group under 18 months of age. Moreover, gross differences in IQ in different segments of the kwashiorkor sample as well as in their siblings make the data difficult to interpret.

In conducting a sibling comparison study it must be recognized that while sibs may have many background characteristics in common, a number of differences must be considered in the analysis of findings. Sibs, unless they are twins, are necessarily different in age and in ordinal position, both of which factors may affect child-rearing practices as well as intellectual outcome (23). Moreover, in a community such as Jamaica, sibs not infrequently have different fathers and experience different conditions of child-rearing. These factors must all be taken into account in designing and interpreting a sib comparison study.

A second question with which the present study is concerned has emerged both from reports of animal investigation and from studies of recovery in children who have been hospitalized for severe malnutrition at different ages in early life. The evidence of the animal investigations indicates that the risk of defective myelination, reduced cell replication, and delayed biochemical maturation are greatest when malnutrition coincides with particular periods of rapid brain growth (24-27). In the human organism the period of most rapid growth of brain extends from about the beginning of the last trimester of pregnancy to the last 3 months of the first postnatal year. Moreover, during this period cellular replication in the central nervous system is completed.

These facts have led to speculation that severe malnutrition during the first 9 months after birth would have more severe consequences than severe malnutrition experienced later in infancy and early childhood. Some support for these expectations have derived from the study of Cravioto and Robles (12) in which children admitted to hospital with severe malnutrition in the first 6 months of life were found during convalescence to recover behavioral competence less fully than children hospitalized for the same illness later in infancy. However, for several reasons, these data are by no means conclusive. Although cell replication is completed at an early age, other aspects of growth and differentiation in the nervous system such as dendritic proliferation, exonal branching, and synapse formation, all of which may be more important for integrative organization than cell number, continue to develop at very rapid rates throughout early childhood. Moreover, the Cravioto and Robles study (12) did not follow the children in order to evaluate later aspects of development and their conclusions cannot be extended for outcomes beyond the immediate recovery period.

An additional issue requires consideration. Though animal experimental data have indicated that particular vulnerabilities to nutritional stress exist in the brain in relation to the age at which the stress is experienced, our knowledge is incomplete. At present, we cannot with certainty identify a specific age after which such vulnerability ceases to exist. However, since many aspects of neuronal growth and differentiation continue to occur throughout the first years of life (28, 29), it is unlikely that vulnerability is restricted to the prenatal period and to early infancy. Since interference with brain development would be reflected in altered IQ, a first step in exploring this issue is the determination of the degree to which intellectual functioning at school age is differentially depressed in children who have experienced severe clinical malnutrition at different ages in the first years of life.

Therefore, in the present report we are concerned with two issues:

1. The degree to which children malnourished before 2 years of age differ from their sibs and classmates in intellectual competence at school age.

2. The degree to which malnutrition at different times during the first 2 years of life is differentially associated with intellectual outcome at school age.

SUBJECTS AND STUDY DESIGN

The 74 severely malnourished children (hereafter referred to as index cases) studied were all boys who had been treated in hospital for severe infantile malnutrition during the first 2 years of life. Sixty of these children had been inpatients on the metabolic ward of the Tropical Metabolism Research Unit of the British Medical Research Council, Mona, Jamaica, W.I. The remaining 14 cases were added in order to have fuller representation over the entire first 2 years of life. These were obtained from the Pediatrics ward of the University Hospital, University of the West Indies, Mona. All children were suffering from severe malnutrition at the time of hospitalization, reflected variously in syndromes of marasmus, kwashiorkor, or marasmic-kwashiorkor. In all cases detailed clinical and metabolic records were available. Children on the average received 8 weeks of inpatient care. In general, follow-up visits in the homes were conducted for 2 years following discharge.

Sixty-four male infants had been treated on the metabolic ward of the Tropical Metabolic Research Unit in the years relevant to the study. At follow-up two of these children and their families had moved and could not be traced. Two additional children were found but not included in the study, one because he was a mongoloid and the other because of the presence of infantile hemiplegia, most probably of perinatal origin. The remaining 60 children were all included in the follow-up study. The 14 cases deriving from the pediatrics ward were the first 14 to be located from an initial pool of 50 cases. Approximately half of these lived in the city of Kingston and the remainder in other towns, villages and rural districts, in some cases more than 100 miles from Kingston.

At the time of the study the index cases were 5 years, 11 months through 10 years of age. These ages were selected in order to be far enough removed from the time of acute illness to eliminate the effects of immediate sequelae and for the children to be at an age where intelligence testing has predictive validity for later life.

Wherever there was a male sibling of the index case between 6 and 12 years of age and nearest in age to the index case, and without a history of severe clinical malnutrition, he was included in the study. Because of widely varying patterns of family composition in Jamaica, a sib was defined as having the same biologic mother as the index case and having shared a home residence with the index child for most of his life. Thirty-eight such sibs were available and studied. Because of the selection criteria used, the sibs were somewhat older than the index cases.

In addition to the sibs, a classmate or neighbor comparison was selected for each index case. For index children attending school, two classmates of the same sex closest in age to the index case were selected. If the first comparison child was not available for examination, the second comparison was used. Some of the index boys, though of school age, were not going to school. For these cases, a comparison case was chosen by finding the nearest neighboring child who was not a relative and who was of an age within six months of the index case. For some index cases at small schools no classmate was within 6 months of age. For these cases neighbor children were also used as comparisons. Of the 74 comparison cases, 63 were classmates and 11 were yardmates who met all criteria of selection. As would be expected from the method of selecting comparison children, index and comparison children lived in the same general neighborhood from which the school drew its pupils. In three cases comparison children could not be brought in for study.

TABLE I

AGES OF INDEX, SIBLING, AND COMPARISON BOYS
AT TIME OF IQ TESTING

Age in yr-mo	Number of		
	Index	Sib	Comparison
5–0 to 5–11	1		5
6–0 to 6–11	19	3	16
7–0 to 7–11	16	6	14
8–0 to 8–11	15	10	13
·9–0 to 9–11	19	4	20
10–0 to 10–11	4	9	3
11–0 to 11–11		4	
12–0 to 12–11		2	
Total	74	38	71

This resulted in 71 matched pairs of index and comparison children. Table I summarizes the ages at testing of the children studied.

The comparison children should not be considered as controls but rather children who were identified because of their geographical proximity and their closeness in age to the index children. Detailed interviews were conducted on the background histories of all children. These indicated that eight of the comparison children had been sick either with malnutrition or with symptoms that could have been associated with malnutrition between the ages of 1 month and 2 years of life. Only one of these was hospitalized during this age interval. The reason was diarrhea and vomiting. The hospitalization was for 2 weeks.

Each child's intellectual level was individually evaluated by means of the WISC. Although this intelligence test has not been standardized for Jamaican chidren, its use in the present study is appropriate. It contains subtests which broadly sample cognitive abilities, both verbal and nonverbal, and standardized forms of administration of test items together with well-defined scoring criteria. As a standardized test it also provides scores across age groups which may be combined for meaningful group comparisons. Clearly the IQs obtained for Jamaican children are not directly comparable with those of children in the cultures for which the test has been standardized. However, as Vernon (30) has pointed out, comparisons of children *within* a culture on a test standardized in another setting are entirely appropriate so long as the test is not so difficult or so easy as to produce scores which do not discriminate among individuals and groups in the population tested. In the present study the test discriminated across groups; individual differences were equally great at all ages; no trend in mean IQ by age was shown. Thus the test provides a useful basis for comparing relative levels of competence among groups of Jamaican children.

All testers were experienced examiners from the United States or England. All children were examined without the examiners being aware of the study group to which the child belonged. Cases were scheduled for examination by a public health nurse who provided coded information on the group to which the child belonged (sib, index, or comparison) which was decoded after all examinations had been completed.

The characteristics of the groups selected would lead us to anticipate that the index cases having suffered acute malnutrition would be most severely impaired in intellectual functioning, that their sibs, some of whom would have experienced chronic subnutrition but not an acute severe episode, would have been intermediately impaired, and that comparison children, not identified by belonging to a family having a child with a history of severe clinical malnutrition, would be least impaired. The first set of analyses provide tests of these hypotheses by comparing Full Scale, Verbal, and Performance IQ in the three study groups. In the second set of analyses intellectual ability in the index children is related to the age of acute nutritional illness.

RESULTS

The Group as a Whole

For the Full Scale, Verbal, and Performance IQ measures the index cases have the lowest mean scores, the sibs occupy an intermediate position, and the comparison children have the highest scores (Table II). These differences are in accordance with expectation. The three IQ measures are seven to nine points lower for the index children than for the comparisons. Each of the differences is statistically significant at less than the 0.001 level of confidence (Table III).

That these mean differences in IQ score are not the result of a few cases of extreme competence in the comparison group or of extreme incompetence in the index cases, but represent differences over the whole range, is clearly indicated in Figure 1. As may be seen from this figure, the groups, in general, differed from one another in Full Scale IQs over the whole range of measures. The cumulative frequency percent curves for Performance and Verbal IQ in the two groups are almost

TABLE II

INTELLECTUAL LEVELS OF INDEX CASES, SIBLINGS,
AND COMPARISON CHILDREN

		Index	Sib	Comparison
	N	71	38	71
	Full Scale IQ	57.72	61.84	65.99
Mean Score	Verbal IQ	64.92	71.03	73.70
	Performance IQ	56.30	58.03	63.69
	Full Scale IQ	10.75	10.82	13.59
S.D.	Verbal IQ	11.80	12.87	14.55
	Performance IQ	11.85	10.47	13.30

TABLE III

LEVELS OF SIGNIFICANCE OF DIFFERENCE IN IQ OF THE INDEX, SIBLING, AND COMPARISON GROUPS*

	Index vs. Comparison		Index vs. Sib		Sib vs. Comparison	
N	71	71	38	38	38	71
	t	p	t	p	t	p
Full Scale IQ	5.25	<0.001	2.08	<0.025	1.83	<0.10
Verbal IQ	4.78	<0.001	2.95	<0.005	1.08	NS
Performance IQ	3.57	<0.001	0.45	NS	2.47	<0.02

* All p values are one-tailed in view of the directional nature of the hypotheses. All t tests are matched pairs dependent t tests.

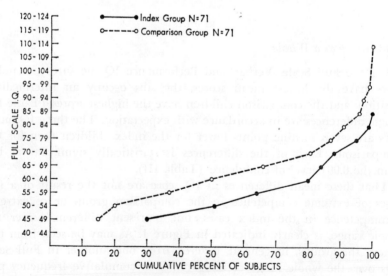

FIG. 1. IQ Distributions of index and comparison cases.

identical in form and indicate that the comparison group is also superior on these measures.

Sibling Comparison

The index children also have lower scores on the three IQ measures than their sibs. The Full Scale and Verbal IQ differences are statistically significant ($p < 0.025$). Differences in Performance IQ are not significant. When the sibs are contrasted with the comparison children they are found to differ from them significantly only in Performance IQ.

Before the results can be interpreted two further analyses are required. In the first place, sibs tend to be older than index and comparison cases and the differences between the sibs and the other two groups could have derived from this age difference. Moreover, since ordinal position can affect IQ within a sibship, differences between sibs and index cases could have been the result of differences in ordinal position. To deal with the first question, the relation of IQ level to age was analyzed in each of the groups. No age trends for IQ were found. To deal with the second question, older sibs were separately compared with younger index cases and younger sibs with older index cases. Identical trends and directions of difference were found when the sibs were respectively in lower or higher ordinal positions in the sibship. These analyses indicate clearly that the differences among groups were not artifacts either of age or of ordinal position.

TEST LIMITATIONS

The structure of the intelligence test and its scoring result in the artificial inflation of mean IQ levels in groups having members where functioning is very poor. As a result of scoring convention, children who answer no questions correctly will receive IQs of 46 for Full Scale and Verbal Scale and of 44 on the Performance Scale. Therefore, if a significant number of individuals in the index group was functioning at the very lowest level, the arbitrary floor value for the scale would artificially inflate the mean for the group and thus alter the size and significance of group differences. Because the index cases have the lowest scores, the effect of this artifact of scoring is to provide an excessively conservative estimate of the size of the differences in intellectual level between the index cases and comparison children and between index cases and sibs.

One can obtain a more accurate appreciation of the differences by comparing the groups with respect to the number of individuals who

TABLE IV

Numbers of Children in Index and Comparison Groups Performing At or Below
the Floor Scoring Level of the Test Scales

Full Scale IQ			Verbal IQ			Performance IQ		
Index	Comp.		Index	Comp.		Index	Comp.	
$\leq$46 17	5	X^2=7.69	$\leq$46 3	1	X^2=1.03	$\leq$46 17	4	X^2=9.38
>46 57	69	p<0.01	>46 71	73	p N.S.	>46 57	70	p<0.01

perform at or below the floor level. The number of children in the index and comparison groups who scored at the floor of the test are presented in Table IV. For Full Scale IQ 23% of the index cases as compared with 7% of the comparison children performed at or below the floor of the test. This difference is significant at less than the 0.01 level of confidence. A similar set of findings is obtained for the Performance Scale but not for the Verbal Scale. Sibs fall in an intermediate position and in no comparison are significantly different in proportion of minimally functioning cases from either the index or comparison group. These findings indicate that mean differences we have found between the index cases and other groups are minimal differences and do not fully reflect the low level of IQ in the severely malnourished children.

Age of Severe Malnutrition

The age distribution of the children when admitted for the treatment of severe malnutrition ranged from 3 to 24 months, with admissions at almost every month between these ages.

If the age at which a child is hospitalized for severe malnutrition is systematically related to the severity of his intellectual impairment, we would expect a significant positive correlation to exist between age at admission and IQ at school age. When IQ and age at hospitalization are correlated, Full Scale, Verbal, and Performance IQs do not correlate significantly with age of hospitalization for severe nutritional illness. The respective Pearson correlations obtained are —0.13, —0.13, and —0.14, and indicate a random relationship between age of the severely malnourished child at hospitalization and IQ at school age.

Because the replication of cells in the central nervous system tends to be completed before the age of 9 months, it has been suggested that children experiencing severe malnutrition before this age are at particular risk of brain damage and lowered intellectual level. Therefore, we

TABLE V

ANALYSIS OF VARIANCE OF IQ LEVELS IN CHILDREN HOSPITALIZED FOR SEVERE
MALNUTRITION AT DIFFERENT AGES IN THE FIRST TWO YEARS OF LIFE

	IQ Full Scale			IQ Verbal			IQ Performance		
Age at Admission in Months	0–7	8–12	13–24	0–7	8–12	13–24	0–7	8–12	13–24
N	15	26	33	15	26	33	15	26	33
Mean	57.93	59.27	55.42	64.93	66.15	62.73	56.93	58.54	54.18
SD	9.08	11.66	10.69	12.62	12.54	11.27	9.33	13.15	11.76
F Ratio	0.96			0.61			1.01		
p	ns			ns			ns		

considered it desirable to compare those children who had been hospital-ized before the age of 8 months with those admitted to hospital for severe malnutrition at later ages. When children admitted before 8 months of age, between 8 and 12 months, and between 13 and 24 months are compared, no significant differences are found between groups for Full Scale, Verbal, and Performance IQ (Table V). The data, therefore, provide no support for the hypothesis that systematic differences in intellectual outcome at school age attach to severe malnutrition ex-perienced at different ages during the first 2 years of life.

DISCUSSION

In this report we have presented two sets of findings. The first indi-cates that children who have experienced severe malnutrition in the first 2 years of life have lower levels of intelligence at school age than their sibs and classmates. The second finding shows no association be-tween the intellectual level of cases and the ages at which the children were hospitalized for the treatment of severe malnutrition during the first 2 years of life. Each of these findings has a bearing on the relation between antecedent malnutrition and mental development and their implications for this issue will be considered.

The lower level of intelligence of the index children compared with classmates or neighbors of the same sex and age is a result which agrees with the findings of previous studies (1, 8-11, 16). The method used for selecting the comparison cases has constricted the range of social, eco-nomic, and familial characteristics in the index and comparison groups but has by no means fully controlled them. Thus, we have found that our ability to interpret the differences between index and comparison children is subject to the same limitations as those which characterize prior studies. Since the index and comparison children may also differ in other attributes which may influence intellectual level (6, 18, 31), the obtained differences in IQ cannot be directly attributed to differences in nutritional status during the first 2 years of life. Thus it is possible that the index children could have been subjected to stresses other than malnutrition either pre- or postnatally. However, a consideration of this issue will be presented in future reports dealing with this study. We have examined in detail these and other biological and social factors which may contribute to intellectual differences in the children studied and will report on these findings in subsequent papers. However, many of the difficulties in interpretation are reduced when the index children age differences between the sibs or of their different ordinal positions social circumstances but do differ in antecedent exposure to malnutrition. Though a sib comparison does not control all nonnutritional factors influencing mental growth, it goes far toward doing so.

In the present study we have found that like-sexed sibs as a group have scores which are significantly higher for Full Scale and Verbal IQ than their brothers who experienced severe malnutrition during the first 2 years of life. These differences in level are not the result of the age differences between the sibs or of their different ordinal positions in the families. The findings which agree with and extend those of one other sib comparison study carried out (21) indicate that the early experiences of severe malnutrition and the attendant hospitalization contribute to depressed intellectual development. Comparison of the findings with those of the other sib study (22) is not possible because of the gross differences in age at which severe malnutrition and hospitalization occurred and because of the peculiarities of the reported mean IQs.

The tendency of the sibs to have somewhat lower IQs than the comparison groups can either derive from the experience of chronic undernutrition (2), from differences in familial environment, or from a combination of these factors. Although the likelihood is high that children reared in a family in which one child has been severely malnourished have also been chronically malnourished, one cannot with confidence attribute the differences in IQ between the sibs and the comparison group to nutritional factors alone because of differences in familial characteristics of the groups. However, the gradient of intellectual level obtained ranging from the index cases at the lowest end to the comparison group at the highest may parsimoniously be considered as reflecting a gradient of nutritional experience across groups. It is of special interest to note that these findings occurred under circumstances in which the severely malnourished children received excellent care in hospital through a long convalescence and were followed by public health nurses who advised the caretaker on feeding for a 2-year period after discharge.

Our failure to find a systematic association between the age during the first 2 years of life at which severe malnutrition was experienced and the degree of intellectual impairment, does not support the hypothesis that brain vulnerability is limited to the first year of life. Although it is true that cell number and enzyme levels may be altered by severe malnutrition, especially when it occurs prior to the end of the first postnatal year, the relations between damage to such systems and the functional integrity of the nervous system is by no means clearly defined. It must be recognized that other aspects of nervous system growth such as dendritic proliferation, axonal branching, and synapse formation, all of which are potentially of great functional significance, have a developmental course which is not restricted to early infancy (28, 29). It can be argued, also, that whereas cell number is most affected by early nutritional stress, these other, less readily measured, features of central nervous system development remain vulnerable to malnutrition at considerably later ages. If this is the case, continued vulnerability of the nervous system to malnutrition after cell replication has been completed should not be surprising. The results indicate a need for further and detailed studies of populations of children who experience malnutrition at even later ages than those we have been able to study.

Alternatively, it should be recognized that children experiencing severe malnutrition at different times of life are hospitalized at different ages. There is evidence (32-34) to indicate that the effects of hospitalization on adaptive development are least great in children under 6 months of age and grow increasingly more severe thereafter. Consequently, if subsequent psychological development is being conjointly affected by the influences of nutritional illness on the nervous system and by hospitalization, the effect of the latter at later ages may compensate for possible diminution in the effects of the former. This, too, could result in the absence of a systematic relationship between degree of mental impairment and the age of severe malnutrition. Finally, it is possible that nutritional illnesses are systematically more severe in the older infants. All of these questions require further investigation and in view of the complexities noted we see the present study as one step in the exploration of a complex issue.

REFERENCES

1. CHAMPAKAM, S., SRIKANTIA, S. G., & GOPALAN, C.: Kwashiorkor and mental development. *Amer. J. Clin. Nutr.*, 21:844, 1968.
2. BROCK, J.: *Recent Advances in Human Nutrition.* London: J. & A. Churchill, 1961.
3. SCRIMSHAW, N. S. & GORDON, J. E. (Eds.): *Malnutrition, Learning and Behavior,* Part 4. Cambridge: MIT Press, pp. 168-248, 1968.
4. CRAVIOTO, J., DELICARDIE, E. R., & BIRCH, H. G.: Nutrition, growth and neurointegrative development: An experimental and ecologic study. *Pediatrics* (Suppl.), 38:319, 1966.
5. CRAVIOTO, J. & DELICARDIE, E. R.: Intersensory development of school-age children. In N. S. Scrimshaw and J. E. Gordon (Eds.), *Malnutrition, Learning, and Behavior.* Cambridge: MIT Press, pp. 252-269, 1968.
6. CRAVIOTO, J., BIRCH, H. G., DELICARDIE, E. R., & ROSALES, L.: The ecology of infant weight gain in a pre-industrial society. *Acta Paediat. Scand.*, 56:71, 1967.
7. POLLITT, E. & RICCIUTI, H. N.: Biological and social correlates of stature among children living in the slums of Lima, Peru. *Amer. J. Orthopsychiat.*, 39:735, 1969.
8. BARRERA-MONCADA, G.: *Estudios sobre alteraciones del crecimiento y del desorrollo psicologico del sindrome pluricarencial (kwashiorkor).* Caracas, Editora Grafos, 1963.
9. BOTHA-ANTOUN, E., BABAYAN, S., & HARFOUCHE, J. K.: Intellectual development relating to nutritional status. *J. Trop. Pediat.*, 14:112, 1968.
10. CABAK, V., & NAJDANVIC, R.: Effect of undernutrition in early life on physical and mental development. *Arch. Dis. Child.*, 40:532, 1965.
11. CHASE, H. P., & MARTIN, H. P.: Undernutrition and child development. *New Eng. J. Med.*, 282:933, 1970.
12. CRAVIOTO, J. & ROBLES, B.: Evolution of adaptive and motor behavior during rehabilitation from kwashiorkor. *Amer. J. Orthopsychiat.*, 35:449, 1965.
13. MONCKEBERG, F.: Effect of early marasmic malnutrition on subsequent physical and psychological developments. In N. S. Scrimshaw and J. E. Gordon (Eds.), *Malnutrition, Learning and Behavior.* Cambridge: MIT Press, pp. 269-277, 1968.
14. POLLITT, E.: Ecology, malnutrition, and mental development. *Psychosom. Med.*, 31:193, 1969.
15. POLLITT, E. & GRANOFF, D.: Mental and motor development of Peruvian children treated for severe malnutrition. *Revista Interamericana de Psicologia*, 1: (2), 93, 1967.
16. STOCH, M. B. & SMYTHE, P. M.: Does undernutrition during infancy inhibit brain growth and subsequent intellectual development? *Arch. Dis. Child.*, 38:546, 1963.
17. STOCH, M. B. & SMYTHE, P. M.: The Effect of undernutrition during infancy on subsequent brain growth and intellectual development. *S. Afr. Med. J.*, 41: 1027, 1967.
18. BIRCH, H. G. & GUSSOW, J. D.: *Disadvantaged Children: Health, Nutrition and School Failure.* New York: Harcourt Brace and World, and Grune and Stratton, Inc., pp. 322, 1970.
19. Perspectives on Human Deprivation: Biological, Psychological and Sociological. NICHD National Institutes of Health. Public Health Service, U.S. Dept. of HEW, 1968.
20. RICHARDSON, S. A. & GUTTMACHER, A. F. (Eds.): *Childbearing: Its Social and Psychological Aspects.* Baltimore: Williams and Wilkins Co., 1967.
21. BIRCH, H. G., PINEIRO, C., ALCALDE, E., TOCA, T., & CRAVIOTO, J.: Kwashiorkor in early childhood intelligence at school age. *Pediat. Res.*, in press, 1971.

22. HANSEN, J. D. L., FREESEMANN, C., MOODIE, A. D., & EVANS, D. E.: What does nutritional growth retardation really imply? *Pediatrics*, 47:299, 1971.
23. ANASTASI, A.: Intelligence and family size. *Psychol. Bull.*, 53:187, 1956.
24. CHASE, H. P., DORSEY, J., & McKHANN, G. M.: The effect of malnutrition on the synthesis of a myelin lipid. *Pediatrics*, 40:551, 1967.
25. DAVISON, A. N. & DOBBING, J.: Myelination as a vulnerable period in brain development. *Brit. Med. Bull.*, 22:1-40, 1966.
26. DOBBING, J.: The influence of early nutrition on the development of myelination of the brain. *Proc. Roy. Soc.*, B 159:503, 1964.
27. WINICK, M.: Nutrition and cell growth. *Nutr. Rev.*, 26:195, 1968.
28. CONEL, J. L.: *The Postnatal Development of Human Cerebral Cortex*. Cambridge: Harvard University Press, 1963.
29. ALTMAN, J., DAS, G. D., & SUDARSHAN, K.: The influence of nutrition on neural and behavioral development. *Develop. Psychobiol.*, 3: (4) 281, 1970.
30. VERNON, P. E.: *Intelligence and Cultural Environment*. London: Methuen, 1969.
31. RICCIUTI, H. N.: Theoretical and methodological issues in the study of nutrition and mental development: Malnutrition in infants. Unpublished manuscript, 1970.
32. BOWLBY, J.: Separation anxiety. *Int. J. Psychoanal.*, 41:89, 1960.
33. AINSWORTH, M. D. (Ed.), Deprivation of maternal care; a reassessment of its effects. Geneva, World Health Organization (W.H.O. Public Health Papers No. 14), pp. 165, 1962.
34. BAKWIN, H. & BAKWIN, R.: *Clinical Management of the Behavioral Disorders in Children*. Philadelphia: W. B. Saunders, 1960.

ACKNOWLEDGMENT

Many persons contributed to the study. We thank in particular Professor J. C. Waterlow, Director of the Tropical Metabolism Research Unit; Dr. W. E. Miall, Director of Epidemiology Research Unit, Professor Eric Back, Department of Paediatrics, University of the West Indies; Mrs. Caroline Ragbeer, Mrs. Patricia Desai, and Mr. V. A. Morris. Members of the research team included Dr. Ira Belmont, Dr. Morton Bortner, Mrs. Juliet Bortner, and Dr. Barbara Tizard.

Support for this study was provided by the Association for the Aid of Crippled Children; the Nutrition Foundation, Inc., New York; The National Institutes of Health, NICHD (HD 00719); NICHD (NIH 71-2081); from the program support to the Child Development Research Unit, University of London, Institute of Education; and from the Medical Research Council. Dr. Hertzig received support from a Research Scientist Development Award, National Institutes of Health Type 1 (KI-38832).

11

DEVELOPMENT IN MIDDLE CHILDHOOD

Alexander Thomas, M.D.

Professor of Psychiatry, New York University Medical Center

and

Stella Chess, M.D.

Professor of Child Psychiatry, New York University Medical Center

Much attention has been paid to many of the general adaptational issues confronting children between the ages of 6 and 12. To Freud this was a period of "latency" between the passing of the Oedipal stage and the beginning of adolescence. During this period, the energy of infantile sexuality is turned away either wholly or partially from sexual utilization and directed toward other aims (7). More specifically in psychoanalytic thinking, the latency child "transfer(s) libido to contemporaries, community groups, teachers, leaders, impersonal ideals and aim-inhibited, sublimated interests" (6).

While the Freudian use of latency implies a kind of "psychosexual moratorium in human development" (5), it "does not mean that changes do not occur during this period. In the psychoanalytic view, it is primarily a period of acquisition of culturally valued skills, values and roles" (1). However, latency has sometimes been used in the literature as an all-encompassing concept denoting the absence of change during this age period without recognition that Freud restricted its meaning to

Reprinted from SEMINARS IN PSYCHIATRY, Vol. 4, No. 4 (November), 1972, pp. 331-341, by permission.

issues of sexuality. As a result, Shaw calls it "an unfortunate term since it suggests that nothing really important is happening and that the child is simply waiting for puberty to begin" (21).

The concept of latency arising from the emphasis on classical Freudian theory on the vicissitudes of sexual development has led even some writers with a psychoanalytic orientation to question the usefulness of this theory for understanding the 6-12-year age period. Thus, Lidz states that "psychoanalytic psychology has relatively little to offer concerning the critical aspects of the period" (14). Even the concept of latency in sex is open to question. Jersild, a leading student of child development, states that "when viewed in the light of empirical studies of children's interest and actions during this period, 'latency' can not be taken literally. For many children, interest in sex during this period is not latent or inactive or held in abeyance but is distinctly manifest and active. In normal development, sex never takes a holiday" (8).

Erickson calls this age period the "age of industry." Having "mastered the ambulatory field and the organ modes [and having] experienced a sense of finality regarding the fact that there is no workable future within the womb of his family, the child becomes ready to apply himself to given skills and tasks. . . . To bring a productive situation to completion is an aim which gradually supercedes the whims and wishes of his autonomous organism" (4). For the child, "this is socially a most decisive stage," during which the dangers to identity development are a sense of inadequacy and inferiority. These may arise if the child's family life has not "prepared him for school life, or when school life . . . fail (s) to sustain the promises of earlier stages" (4).

Sullivan considers these years in terms of a child's interpersonal relationships. He refers to a "juvenile era" that follows childhood and precedes preadolescence (which he puts at 8½ or 9½ to 12 years of age) (25). The juvenile is marked by the "maturation of a need for compeers," even an "urgent need for compeers with whom to have one's existence." School becomes "the great new arena for experience," and the "talents for cooperation, competition and compromise" are developed. For this author, a child's developing a relationship to a social environment and peer groups is crucial in that stage. It is the beginning of the end of a youngster's "egocentristic" outlook and the start of the true social orientation he develops in preadolescence.

While these investigators have focused on the motivational and psychodynamic aspects of personality development, Piaget has highlighted factors of cognitive functioning that are crucial in the middle years of childhood (18). He has found that 6-11-year-olds are in the stage of concrete operations, during which they develop the concept of conservation and the notion of invariance upon which rest the later acquisition of complex reasoning.

Lidz has presented a thoughtful summary of the work of these investigators and has, in addition, suggested "other character traits that appear to have their roots in this period of life" (14). These are a "sense of belonging" and a "sense of responsibility" both of which are basic to the trait of "leadership." He notes, too, that "adapting to . . . new environments and finding his place in them has required a substantial reorganization of the personality" of the school-age child.

The above authors have made major contributions to our understanding of the general developmental tasks facing youngsters in middle childhood. However, they have, for the most part, not paid much attention to how individual children characteristically meet these new demands. They have also focused on broad theoretical issues rather than on the particular dynamics of specific interactive processes.

THE NEW YORK LONGITUDINAL STUDY

The New York Longitudinal Study, in which the behavioral development of 136 children has been followed from the first months of infancy onward, has provided data of a number of features of development during the 6-12 year age period. These have included the specific nature of behavioral attributes that characterize this stage of development, the frequency of new behavior disorders and symptoms as compared to earlier ages, the followup of behavior disorders first manifested in the preschool and early school periods, and the dynamics of the child-environment interactional process.

In our longitudinal study, data has been gathered anterospectively at sequential age levels on the nature of each child's individual characteristics of functioning at home, in school, and in standard test situations; on special environmental events and the child's reactions to them; and on parental attitudes and child-care practice (5). Parent and teacher interviews, as well as direct observation of the youngsters, have been the source of most data. In addition, each child has been tested by a staff psychologist at 3 and 6 years and at some time during his middle childhood years. The staff child psychiatrist has done a psychiatric evaluation of each child presenting symptoms. Wherever necessary, neurologic examination or special testing (such as perceptual tests) has been done.

A major focus of the longitudinal study has been on the delineation of temperamental characteristics in the early years of life and their relationship to later functioning, to the development of behavior disorders and to academic achievement and school functioning. The definition of temperamental characteristics, methods of data collection and analysis, and findings have been reported extensively in the literature (2, 3, 26-28).

Our theoretical framework from the beginning has involved an interactionist approach that views development as a constantly evolving process of interaction between the child and his environment from the very first days of life onward (and even prenatally). We have attempted to avoid simplistic environmentalist or constitutional approaches and any adherence to a "heredity" versus "environment" dichotomy. The concept of a continuous evolving organism-environment interaction has been formulated in various ways in the work of Pavlov (17), Stern (24), and Lewin (13), among others, and has been precisely stated by Schneirla and Rosenblatt (20):

> Behavior is typified by reciprocal stimulative relationships. . . . Behavioral development[,] because it centers on and depends upon reciprocal stimulative processes between female and young, is essentially social from the start. Mammalian behavioral development is best conceived as a unitary system of processes changing progressively under the influence of an intimate interrelationship of factors of maturation and of experience—with maturation defined as the developmental contributions of tissue growth and differentiation and their secondary processes, experience as the effects of stimulation and its organic traces on behavior.

An interactionist approach to individual development, therefore, involves the simultaneous scrutiny and analysis of responses of the organism and of the objective circumstances in which these responses occur. Individual differences in the degree and even quality of response to stimuli and demands must be considered as well as the specific nature of these environmental influences. Furthermore, the crucial factors in this dynamic interplay will vary both from one child to another and in the same child at different age periods. New behavioral attributes and abilities emerge as the child grows older, and fresh environmental demands and expectations replace or supplant those of earlier years. At the same time, previous patterns of interaction may persist and continue to influence the child's reactions to what is new.

BEHAVIORAL CHARACTERISTICS

As indicated above, Erikson, Sullivan, and Lidz, among others, have defined in general terms some of the behaviors that characterize the

middle childhood period. The specific traits through which industriousness, peer relations, and a sense of belonging are manifested have, however, not been spelled out by these authors.

We have started to examine the protocols of our study population in
the 6-12-year age period to identify specific behavioral characteristics that
appear ubiquitous and prominent and capable of differentiating the
children from each other. Our initial effort has been in the 6-8-year
period, for which we have parent reports, teacher reports, and school
observations. (Also available are detailed descriptions of each child's behavior during I.Q. testing at 6 years, but these data have not as yet
been utilized for the present analysis.) The protocols of ten children
were selected at random, and an inductive content analysis of the behavioral data was done. Fifteen categories were defined, each of which
could be rated on a three-point scale. These categories are: (1) Spontaneity (high vs. low): the child's initiation of an activity or the injection of his own ideas without overt instruction to do so. (2) Autonomy
vs. interdependence: the child's requests for or rejection of help when
unable to perform on his own. (3) Degree of organized activity (high
vs. low). (4) Frequency of interaction with other children (high vs.
low): the frequency with which a child interacts with others and the
number of children he prefers. (5) Social assertiveness, positive (high vs.
low): refers to whether or not the child stands up for his own rights
and has leadership abilities. (6) Social assertiveness, negative (high vs.
low): refers to the degree to which the child is disruptive, abusive, or
domineering. (7) Popularity (high vs. low): how other youngsters respond to the child. (8) Frequency of initiation of interaction with
others (high vs. low): how frequently the child initiates interaction with
others. (9) Coping ability in disagreements with other children (high vs.
low): how the child settles disagreements. (10) Independence vs. Dependency: absence or presence of demands for help when the child is
capable of performing on his own. (11) Cooperation with rules, regulations, and routines (high vs. low). (12) Degree of participation and interest in various activities (high vs. low). (13) Decisiveness vs. indecisive-
ness: the child's ability to make up his own mind and stick to his
decisions. (14) People vs. tasks: refers to the child's preference for activities (tasks) or people. (15) Emotional expressiveness (clear vs. unclear):
can an observer tell what the child is feeling by his expression or
verbalization?

Categories 1, 2, and 3 appear to relate primarily to the way in which
a child undertakes activities and may be related to Erikson's overall
category of industriousness. Categories 4 through 9 relate to the character

of the child's social relationships. Categories 10 through 14 relate to both issues inasmuch as each describes both how the child goes about an activity and the way he relates to people. Category 15, the clarity of the youngster's emotional expressiveness, does not appear related to either his industry or his social relations, although it may indirectly affect the reactions of others to him.

The scoring of the protocols of the study sample as a whole is currently in progress. While the results are as yet incomplete, they appear to indicate that these categories can reliably differentiate these children in the 6-8-year period. When this analysis is completed, we plan to extend it to the older age periods, to determine the correlations between these behavioral traits and temperamental characteristics in the first 5 years of life, and to examine their relationship to the development and course of behavior disorders.

A number of these 15 behavioral characteristics can be identified in some of the children at ages earlier than 6 years. It is in the school-age period, however, that these traits appear to become prominent and ubiquitous.

These characteristics, of course, are not the only ways to describe school-age children. Other important aspects of their functioning—temperament, cognitive level, perceptual abilities, special talents—remain influential in determining the child-environment interaction, as was the case in the preschool period.

An additional new factor in psychologic development in the middle childhood years has been the transition from action to ideation that characterizes the course of development from infancy to adulthood. This transition was clearly evident in the sequential analysis of the characteristics of symptom expression and evolution in some of the children who developed behavior disorders in the preschool period that continued into the middle childhood years. In the earlier period, their symptoms were expressed primarily on an overt behavioral level. As they grew older, the symptoms became more and more ideational in character and reflected complex subjective states, attitudes, distorted self-images, and psychodynamic patterns of defense.

A typical example of this shift in symptom expression was found in a child, Diana, who as an infant had organic bowel symptoms, the result of a defect in anal structure. These symptoms did not respond satisfactorily to either physical or pharmacologic treatment. Her difficulties in evacuation became over time a source of tension and stress because of marked inconsistency in the mother's approach. The child also met disapproval in nursery school when teachers complained about having to clean up her intermittently huge and odorous evacuations. An avoidance mechanism developed in the 3-4-year period, which Diana expressed primarily in behavioral terms: she withheld bowel movements, hid in corners to evacuate, and refused to use the toilet. As Diana grew older, her mother continued to be inconsistent in handling the issue and began to exhibit an overall tendency to minimize the extent of the problem. Diana herself also began to use this denial mechanism and tried to avoid acknowledging the existence of a problem. By 8½ years of age, she developed a neurotic denial mechanism in which she insisted that she had not soiled herself even when it was evident that she had and denied having to evacuate while wiggling to hold back a bowel movement. Although she persisted in denying having a bowel problem, she showed no overt or indirect manifestations of anxiety extending to other areas of functioning. However, at age 9 years, the reaction of disapproval by others in her environment became so sharp and frequent that her denial mechanism became ineffective. Diana became aware that her disguise was not perfect and finally requested help for her bowel problem.

Another example is a child with explosive tantrum-type behavior that led repeatedly to disapproval, condemnation, and punishment. As he grew older, he began to conceptualize the meaning of his behavior in terms of a derogatory self-image that was fated to endure forever and then developed the defense mechanism of avoidance. Another boy with quick adaptability as a prominent temperamental characteristic showed two periods of disturbance, at 4 and 8 years, with markedly different symptoms at each age. In both instances, the disturbance resulted primarily from inappropriate imitation of selected aspects of his father's behavior and attitudes. At age four, the symptoms were basically behavioral, and, at age 8, ideational in character.

These three cases, among others, illustrate the shift in psychologic organization from action to ideation that becomes increasingly evident in the middle childhood years, both in normal development and in symptom formation.

BEHAVIOR DISORDERS

It is possible to divide the children in the longitudinal sample in the 6-12-year age period into five groups with regard to behavior disorder. First, there were those youngsters who had coped successfully with the demands of previous age periods and continued to do so in their school years. These children, a majority of those in the study, maintained a steady course of healthy development.

Second were those children who had behavior difficulties in earlier age periods, which now were resolved, either because the stress on the child was diminished or eliminated or the child's maturation gradually enabled him to cope successfully with previous excessive stresses. This change occurred spontaneously in some cases, in others through therapeutic intervention. In these cases, the original excessive stress had not produced any structural psychologic changes in the child, such as fixed neurotic personality characteristics, so that the youngster could begin to cope successfully with his environment and develop in a healthy direction with no significant neurotic residue.

Third, there were children whose behavioral difficulties in earlier age periods had been resolved, either spontaneously or following therapy, but who later developed new maladaptive behavior patterns or were confronted by a recurrent or new environmental demand or expectation that was excessively stressful for their capacities. In these cases, there was a recurrence of behavior disturbance. When this happened, the symptoms shown by a child might be similar to those found earlier, or they might be quite different, due to the youngster's higher level of psychologic functioning.

Fourth, there were those children whose behavior disorders at earlier age periods continued into their school years, either because there had been no lessening of the excessive stress with which they were confronted, or because structural psychologic change had developed, or both.

Finally, there were a few youngsters, whose earlier development had been normal, who developed problems *de novo* during middle childhood. In these instances the new demands and expectations of this period were not consonant with the child's capacities even though there had been no such dissonances earlier.

In this last group the analysis of the anterospective longitudinal data, as well as the clinical psychiatric evaluation, indicated that the behavior disorder did not reflect the repetition of conflicts of earlier age periods with new symptoms or symbolic representation but rather new conflicts, excessive stresses, and maladaption arising in the middle childhood period.

The children who have developed normally from early childhood onward are not drawn from any special group regarding temperament, intellectual ability, sociocultural background of the family or hierarchal position (firstborn vs. second, third or fourth child). Thus, even though the children with the "difficult child" temperamental constellation—slow adaptability, initial negative responses to many new situations, intense and frequently negative reactions to stimuli, and irregularity of sleep and feeding patterns—show a significantly higher percentage of behavior problem development than do children with other temperamental patterns (28), some difficult children did cope successfully with the demands of each stage of development without developing symptoms. Furthermore, the children with normal development included some with special environmental stresses in their lives, such as divorce of the parents, death of a parent, hospitalization in early childhood, etc. Whether the mother worked outside the home or not also seemed irrelevant as such. The basic issue determining normal development appeared to be the existence of a consonance or "goodness of fit" between the child with his individual characteristics and the demands and expectation of the intra- and extra-familial environments.

An example of a child with earlier behavior disorder and complete resolution in the school-age period—of whom we have seen a number —is a girl with the difficult child temperament pattern, which made her care in the early years stressful to the parents. The mother responded with uncertainty and inconsistency in handling, the father with antagonism, hostility and punitiveness. The youngster developed multiple symptoms at 5 years of age, including explosive anger, fear of the dark, difficulty in relating to groups of children, and an insatiable desire for attention. At psychiatric evaluation 3 months later, the diagnosis of neurotic behavior disorder was made. Psychotherapy for the child was recommended and instituted. In the following few years her symptoms improved gradually. Also she blossomed out with artistic talents in a number of directions, was intellectually bright and did well in school. These combinations of talents and success in school so impressed her father that his attitude toward her changed dramatically and radically. His hostility changed to affection and his criticism to praise and admiration. The change in child and father gave the mother increasing confidence in her handling of the girl, which was positively reinforced by her progressive improvement. This combination of help provided by psychotherapy, the success in school and the increasingly positive interaction with both parents resulted in progressive improvement to the point where psychiatric evaluation at age 10 years showed no evidence of psychopathology. Followup over the next five years showed continued normal development.

The sequence of a behavior disorder in the preschool period that was resolved and then recurred in the school years is illustrated by the two boys cited above, the one with explosive tantrum-type behavior in a frustrating school situation at age five, and the other with inappropriate imitation of selected aspects of his father's behavior at age four. The first youngster's symptoms disappeared after a change more appropriate to his needs, and the second after a change in parental attitudes and behavior. Both boys experienced a recurrence of disturbance in the middle childhood years, due to child-environment interactions similar to those of the earlier age period. The new symptoms were different, however, and reflected the new age-stage level of development.

Diana, the girl with bowel symptoms cited previously, illustrates the sequence of behavior disorder starting in the preschool years and continuing into the school years.

The youngsters with the development of a behavior problem *de novo* in middle childhood showed variations on two themes: (1) excessive stress resulting from new or altered demands or traumatic situations, leading to symptom formation, or (2) stress that had been present earlier, due to a dissonant child-environment interaction, but which did not crystallize in the form of behavior disorder until this age. These two sequences are illustrated by two cases.

During early childhood, Margie had a habitual pattern of ritualizing routines. For example, before she would go to bed each night she had to have a special story, a snack, some water, a certain song, a kiss on her nose, be tucked in just so and then given a special doll. Each one of these had been gradually added into the routine, which was now the ritual of getting to sleep. However, with this situation, as with others with similar rituals, she would easily give up specific aspects when requested to do so by her parents. This tendency, therefore, to organize routine activities in a compulsive manner, was not a pathologic defense, nor was it a problem for the parents, as she would give up her rituals following suggestions that she do so. Furthermore, she showed no other indications of tension or maladaptive functioning.

At age 10, Margie was confronted by a series of traumatic experiences. She had to have warts removed from her feet, and this became an extremely painful procedure since the local anesthetic did not work despite multiple injections. Following this surgery, there were frequent dressing changes and her physician insisted that she be "super clean" to prevent the recurrence of the warts. Then, a few months later, she developed a severe sore throat that necessitated medication. However, Margie went into shock following the penicillin injection and required emergency treatment; for several days afterwards there was considerable apprehension about her condition.

In the wake of these experiences, Margie developed a series of fears with regard to the dangers of wastes (cat droppings) and poisons (lead paint) that she picked up from the passing comments of others and warnings on television. She included menstruation among the things she considered poisonous. In addition, she showed a number of symptoms related to the need to be clean—excessive handwashing, fear of dirt and animal excretions—and developed rituals around these as well as a general state of tension.

Margie was seen by the staff psychiatrist, who diagnosed her as having a reactive behavior disorder. It was felt that her obsessional behavior was situationally determined and that in the absence of further trauma she could be talked out of these new rituals as she had been talked out of others in the past. On the psychiatrist's recommendation, the parents brought each set of behavioral compulsions and obsessive ruminations into the open and discussed them with Margie clearly and compassionately. In this way, her grave fears were reduced to nonproblem issues, and her rituals were easily ended.

In Tina's case, by contrast, the behavioral disorder was not precipitated suddenly but crystallized slowly, after several years of a negative child-parent interaction. Tina was a slow-to-warm-up and persistent child, who reacted negatively to her initial exposures to new people or new situations. She had a twin sister, an easily adaptable child, with whom the mother frequently compared Tina—and the latter always came out on the bottom. Tina came to see herself as less loved than her sister, and this was a realistic reaction in view of her mother's obvious favoritism for her twin.

Over the years, this negative interaction between mother and child continued to build up. When she was seven, symptoms of disturbance began and finally, at age nine, the parents brought her for evaluation. Their major concern was what they saw as her learning problem: she often did things wrong, "avoided" using her mind, and had poor achievement grades. In addition, she frequently showed negative mood, behaved immaturely and was easily frustrated if her wishes were not immediately granted. The parents' concern at this time was the result not of her problems (as all had been present for quite some time) but of their worries about her academic achievement. By this stage, Tina was in third grade and often had homework assignments. The parents felt they had to help her, but her reaction was to dawdle, not to work quickly and to stick to what she was doing when they wanted to move on to something else. This additional negative interaction between child and mother, over and above the latter's obvious favoritism for and special attention to her other daughter, was sufficiently stressful to result in Tina's developing a behavior disorder.

The initial therapeutic recommendation was for parent guidance, and

TABLE 1

AGE AT ONSET AND REFERRAL OF BEHAVIOR DISORDER

	0-3 Yr.	3-6 Yr.	6-9 Yr.	9-12 Yr.
Onset, males	4	16	7	0
Onset, females	4	10	5	1
Onset, total	8	26	12	1
Referral, males	0	16	11	0
Referral, females	1	10	6	3
Referral, total	1	26	17	3

the mother, especially, was advised as to specific ways in which to modify her approach with Tina. At this writing, too little time has elapsed for a followup study.

INCIDENCE AND SYMPTOMATOLOGY

Table 1 shows the distribution in our study population of age of onset of behavior disorder as well as age at which symptoms became severe enough for the child to be referred for psychiatric evaluation.

As can be seen from Table 1, the great majority of cases, 34 out of 47, had the onset of their behavior disorders before the age of six. Only one new case developed between the ages of 9 and 12 years.

The total number of cases, 47, is a cumulative number. At any one time the actual number was less because of recovery in some cases. The great majority of the cases were milder disturbances, diagnosed as reactive behavior disorder (28), and this was true for all the age periods of onset covered in this report. The high incidence of mild disorders in children has been reported by others (10, 11, 19). Some authors have emphasized the transient nature of the behavior disorder and the tendency to spontaneous improvement in many children (22), others have advocated the need for professional help for school-age children with behavioral difficulties (23). Our own followup of the first 42 cases in the longitudinal sample, with onset ranging from 2 to $8\frac{1}{2}$ years of age, showed that eventually (4-11 years after initial evaluation) 14 children had recovered and 19 others displayed either marked or moderate improvement (29). There was therapeutic intervention in all cases—simple parent guidance in all cases, supplemented by psychotherapy in seven children—so that we cannot estimate the possibilities of spontaneous recovery in the sample.

The low incidence of behavior onset in the middle childhood years has also been reported by MacFarlane et al. in the Berkeley Study (15). Lapouse and Monk in their extensive epidemiologic study (9-12) confirmed the finding that "increased age is associated with a decreased prevalence of behavior disorder in school-age children." This finding is most likely related to the lesser number of new environmental demands and expectations in this age period, at least for middle class children. The demands for routinization and socialization—toilet-training, regular sleep and feeding patterns, adaptation to rules and regulations, etc.—had been made in the preschool years. Most of the children attended nursery school, so that the demands for adaptation to a new structured extrafamilial situation, for adaptation to a peer group, and for working with educational materials all came early in life.

By contrast, the incidence of behavior disorders in a population of working class Puerto Rican children was relatively higher during the school years as compared to the preschool years than in the middle class children in the New York Longitudinal Study. The difference in age period occurrence of behavior disorders in the two groups appears related to the fact that the Puerto Rican parents were very permissive and nondemanding with their preschool children. They did not pressure them to modify sleep or feeding irregularities or other types of mild behavioral deviations. Their typical attitude was "he's a baby—he'll outgrow it."

With the start of school, however, there was a sudden increase in the number of new demands made of Puerto Rican children. And whereas the preschool years presented more stresses to the middle class children, the school years were more stressful for the Puerto Rican youngsters. The latter did not have the experience of going to nursery school and it was only at age 5 or 6 that demands for regularity of sleep, discipline, learning, and obedience to safety regulations began to be made (29).

A review of the kinds of presenting symptoms in the 47 middleclass children with behavior disorders showed that, in the younger children, sleep disturbances, temper tantrums, and maladaptation to the rules of social living were predominant. During the school years, symptoms associated with peer relations and learning came to the fore. This age-level distribution of symptoms corresponds in general to the findings of other studies (11, 15, 16, 30).

Masturbation was observed and reported by many parents in their preschool and school-age children, but with the statement that, since they knew it was "harmless and normal," they did not interfere with it. Many parents also reported increasing sexual interest and curiosity in their school-age children, and this, too, they said, did not worry them and was not considered a problem. It was the impression of the staff interviewers that some parents were not fully at ease with this stated attitude toward their child's masturbation, and that they might have intervened were it not for the influence of child-care authorities. However, independent evaluation of the children by the staff indicated that neither the masturbation nor sexual curiosity of these children was a problem indicative of psychopathology in any case.

CONCLUSIONS

The findings of our longitudinal study indicate that the middle childhood period is one of continued development and psychologic change. New behavioral characteristics emerge and become influential in determining the nature of the child-environment interaction. Of those children earlier diagnosed as having behavior problems, some showed improvement or recovery where others showed worsening. Several children who were without problems earlier first developed disorders at school age. In the vast majority of the school-age children, sexual interest and activity were evident throughout the age period but were without any pathologic significance.

The term latency, therefore, would appear to be a confusing and inappropriate way to designate and characterize children between the ages of 6 and 12. We would suggest that this term be abandoned and that simple descriptive designations, such as middle childhood and elementary school age, which imply no *a priori* assumptions or theories about the dynamics and course of psychologic development, be used in its place.

REFERENCES

1. BALDWIN, A. L.: *Theories of Child Development.* New York: Wiley & Sons, 1967.
2. CHESS, S.: Temperament and learning ability in school children. *Amer. J. Public Health,* 58:2231, 1968.
3. CHESS, S. & THOMAS, A.: Differences in outcome with early intervention in children with behavior disorders. In M. Roff, L. N. Robins, and M. Pollack (Eds.): *Life History Research in Psychopathology,* Vol. II. Minneapolis: University of Minnesota Press, 1972.
4. ERIKSON, E.: *Childhood and Society.* New York: Norton, 1950.
5. ERIKSON, E.: *Identity: Youth and Crisis.* New York: Norton, 1968.
6. FREUD, A.: *Normality and Pathology in Childhood: Assessments of Development.* New York: International Universities Press, 1965.
7. FREUD, S.: *Collected Papers II.* London: Hogarth, 1924.
8. JERSILD, A. T.: *Child Psychology.* Englewood Cliffs, N. J.: Prentice-Hall, 1968.
9. LAPOUSE, R.: The relationship of behavior to adjustment in a representative sample of children. *Amer. J. Public Health,* 55:1130, 1965.
10. LAPOUSE, R., & MONK, M. A.: An epidemiologic study of behavior characteristics in children. *Amer. J. Public Health,* 48:1134, 1958.
11. LAPOUSE, R. & MONK, M. A.: Fears and worries in a representative sample of children. *Amer. J. Orthopsychiat.,* 29:803, 1959.

12. LAPOUSE, R. & MONK, M. A.: Behavior deviations in a representative sample of children: Variation by sex, age, race, social class and family size. *Amer. J. Orthopsychiat.*, 34:436, 1964.
13. LEWIN, K.: *Dynamic Theory of Personality.* New York: McGraw-Hill, 1935.
14. LIDZ, T.: *The Person.* New York: Basic, 1968.
15. McFARLANE, J. W., ALLEN, L., & HONZIK, M. P.: *A Developmental Study of the Behavior Problems of Normal Children Between Twenty-one Months and Fourteen Years.* Berkeley: University of California Press, 1962.
16. MENSH, I. N., KANTOR, M. B., DOMEK, W. R., GILDEA, M. C.-L., & GLIDEWELL, J. C.: Children's behavior symptoms and their relationships to school adjustment, sex and social class. *J. Social Issues*, 15:8, 1959.
17. PAVLOV, I. P.: *Conditioned Reflexes.* G. V. Anrep (Editor & Translator). London: Oxford University Press, 1927.
18. PIAGET, J.: *The Origins of Intelligence in Children.* New York: International Universities Press, 1952.
19. RUTTER, M., TIZARD, J., & WHITMORE, K.: *Education, Health and Behavior.* New York: Wiley & Sons, 1970.
20. SCHNEIRLA, T. C., & ROSENBLATT, J. S.: Behavioral organization and genesis of the social bond in insects and mammals. *Amer. J. of Orthopsychiat.*, 31:223, 1961.
21. SHAW, C. R.: *The Psychiatric Disorders of Childhood.* New York: Appleton-Century-Crofts, 1966.
22. SHEPHERD, M., OPPENHEIM, A., & MITCHELL, S.: Childhood behavior disorders and the child guidance clinic: An epidemiological study. *J. Child Psychol. Psychiat.*, 7:9, 1966.
23. STENNET, R. G.: Emotional handicap in the elementary years: Phase or disease. *Amer. J. Orthopsychiat.*, 36:444, 1966.
24. STERN, W.: *Psychologie der frühen kindheit, biz zum sechsten lebensjahre.* Leipzig: Quelle and Meyer, 1927.
25. SULLIVAN, H. S.: *Conception of Modern Psychiatry: The First William Alanson White Memorial Lectures.* Reprinted from *Psychiatry: Journal of the Biology and Pathology of Interpersonal Relations*, Volume 3, February, 1940 and Volume 8, May 1945.
26. THOMAS, A.: Significance of temperamental individuality for school functioning. In J. Hellmuth (Ed.): *Learning Disorders.* Seattle: Special Child Publications, 1968.
27. THOMAS, A., BIRCH, H. G., CHESS, S., HERTZIG, M. E., & KORN, S.: *Behavioral Individuality in Early Childhood.* New York: New York University Press, 1963.
28. THOMAS, A., CHESS, S., & BIRCH, H. G.: *Temperament and Behavior Disorders in Children.* New York: New York University Press, 1968.
29. THOMAS, A., CHESS, S., SILLEN, J., & MENDEZ, O.: Crosscultural Study of Behavior in Children with Special Vulnerabilities to Stress. In M. Roff and M. Pollack (Eds.): *Life History Research in Psychopathology*, Vol. III. Minneapolis: University of Minnesota Press. In press.
30. WERRY, J. S. & QUAY, H. C.: The prevalence of behavior symptoms in younger elementary school children. *Amer. J. Orthopsychiat.*, 41:136, 1971.

12

COPING AND GROWTH IN ADOLESCENCE

Stanley H. King, Ph.D.

Director of Research, Harvard University Health Services

Recent years have witnessed subtle and important shifts in the study and understanding of adolescents, marked primarily by less emphasis on data obtained from the consulting room and by more emphasis on studies of nonclinical groups. The effect of the change is still minimal because of limitations in the studies of normals, as well as the recency of the research, yet because of the potential impact on theory, it is an appropriate time to review current positions.

The most prominent view of personality development during adolescence and young adulthood might be characterized as the crisis or psychiatric orientation. In simple terms, conflict, turmoil, and rebellion are expected to some degree in adolescence as part of the process of growing up. Some writers imply that, without turmoil, development is in some way impaired, and the achievement of maturity is delayed. This view finds support from various writers through the centuries, as Kiell (11) has demonstrated; and certainly within this century the crisis theme has been expounded by novelists and other observers of contemporary life. The strongest support in recent years, however, has come from the clinical literature, especially that written by psychoanalysts.

Reprinted by permission of Grune and Stratton, Inc. and the author, from SEMINARS IN PSYCHIATRY, Vol. 4, No. 4 (November, 1972), pp. 355-366.

This article is based on a longer article, which appeared under the title, "Coping Mechanisms in Adolescents," in *Psychiatric Annals*, Vol. I, No. 3, November, 1971, pp. 10-46.

One respected theorist, Anna Freud, has described the adolescent years as a "developmental disturbance" (5). The task of the adolescent is to learn how to handle increased sexual and aggressive drives and to find new ways of relating to parents and peers. She does not feel these can be accomplished without upheaval because the ego is not strong enough at that time to handle the increased drives in an integrated, harmonious way.

Another writer, Erik Erikson (3), has described the major task of the adolescent years as the establishment of a stable identity. As the individual questions his values and ponders what kind of person he is, there may be conflict with parents and other authority figures. There may be rebellion and anger, lack of communication with adults, and even apathy and depression. The identity crisis may extend into the young adult years. Although Erikson does not state that an identity crisis is part of normal development, his term has become part of the common parlance of the day.

Although the crisis model is useful in understanding the behavior of many adolescents, it does have a serious bias if used as a general explanation of adolescent development. The data on which it is based are drawn primarily from the consulting room, with the assumption that an accurate picture of healthy functioning can be obtained from a study of disturbed functioning. There is another assumption that health is the absence of disease, and that health does not involve any new conceptions of functioning that are absent in illness. Both these assumptions are questionable. By so questioning, I would not deny that adolescence is a time of substantial physical and emotional change, nor that the adolescent is particularly vulnerable to stress. Rather, I would suggest that a review of recent studies suggests that turmoil and conflict are not necessarily the hallmark of adolescent development.

One of the more interesting studies of recent years is that by Offer (16) of a group of high school boys who were the "modal" group of a range between psychopathology and superior adjustment, as determined by psychologic tests. The subjects were interviewed at intervals from their freshman through senior years.

In the *handling of drives and affects,* few of the subjects had difficulty controlling impulses; as a group they were poised, well-mannered, and did not show any strongly deviant behavior. Mood swings were not dramatic, nor depression prolonged. When the latter occurred the cause was usually exogenous and the boys worked out of it by turning attention to other activities. As for anger, they had adequate controls and outlets. They never had chronic rage reactions toward their parents and usually were able to sublimate anger in physical activity.

There was some conflict about the sexual drive, especially in the early years, and the boys did not feel they could communicate openly with parents or teachers about sex. However, their curiosity about girls enabled them to overcome their unease and by senior year most of them were enjoying relationships with girls.

Anxiety and fear were present at times, but the effect was facilitative, a prelude to action, rather than inhibiting or disabling.

The major reason for effective handling of drives was the use of good *coping mechanisms*, particularly the recourse to physical action. Sports offered the opportunity for controlled and socially approved aggression but other kinds of social activities offered outlets for energy and achievement motivation. Offer's subjects were primarily "doers" rather than introspective or brooding teenagers, and appeared to have a limited fantasy life.

At the same time, the subjects were able to deal openly with painful affect, confronting conflict or trauma and talking with others about the feelings involved. They also searched for interpretation of their behavior and Offer commented that they were good amateur psychologists. Thus, they sought reassurance about themselves and often found it.

They could also be appropriately critical of themselves, but when they evaluated their faults they did not dwell on guilt or lose self-esteem. Their self-criticism was, therefore, constructive rather than denigrating, and led to changes in behavior. This was one other way of being open and direct.

One coping mechanism that they used was humor, not often seen in clinical patients. This helped self-criticism because they could laugh at themselves and thus reduce guilt and anxiety to manageable proportions. But humor also provided a release of negative affect and provided a feeling of enjoyment of life, and a way of sharing pleasurable experiences with others.

The idea of sharing leads us to a third area of results: *interpersonal relations* with parents, teachers, and peers. Although the boys were often critical of their parents, the communication was generally good, and most of them felt that the ideal parent was very much like the one of their own parents to whom they felt closer. Basically, they shared their parents' values, and the vast majority said that their parents were fair and reasonable in discipline. There was rebellion, most often in the early adolescent years, and it appeared in the form of chronic disagreements with parents and teachers. Rules of the home or school were broken, which produced annoyance, but this rebellion almost never involved major differences in values or life style and was not flagrantly antisocial or illegal. The rebelliousness led to individuation from parents without losing love and respect for parents, and without loss of the ego ideal that had been drawn from parents. The rebelliousness and negative behavior decreased in the later years of high school when the subjects became more involved in activities outside the home.

Much of the professional literature stresses a breakdown in family communication and a generation gap, but in Offer's study family life for most subjects was well integrated. There was a division of family roles that closely followed the traditional middle class pattern, with mother as warm and understanding, while father was more likely to be viewed with respect and distant admiration.

Offer concluded that the adolescent years do present a challenge on many fronts, but that his subjects were able to cope successfully with these growth tasks. They did not show the turmoil that we might expect from the crisis model of growth, because their egos were strong enough to withstand the pressures.

Additional data come from a study by Masterson (15), in which he compared a group of adolescent patients with a group of matched controls, with a focus on the diagnostic category of adolescent turmoil. Although both groups had painful affect and limited functioning, these were more severe in the patient group. Fewer controls had severe depression or patterns of acting out behavior. When Masterson compared the "healthiest" of the control group with the patients, he found some striking differences in family relationships. In the healthy group, parents accepted their offspring and felt and acted toward them in constructive ways, and, in turn, the adolescents were accepting of parents and siblings. But within the patient group, family members were more often engaged in chronic conflict, and father was absent more often from the home. The healthy subjects were action-oriented, much like Offer's subjects, while the patients more often had restricted interests and much more limited interaction with the environment. Masterson concluded by urging modification of current pathology-based theories.

MIDDLE THROUGH LATE ADOLESCENCE

The bulk of data on the functioning of healthy adolescents comes from this later age span and information in these studies about the early adolescent years depends on retrospective accounts by the subjects. This is a limitation on the conclusions that can be drawn, but it is a limitation that applies equally well to data based on studies from the consulting room where reconstruction of events also depends on retrospective accounts.

The first study to be cited was conducted by an interdisciplinary group at the National Institute of Mental Health (1, 2, 7, 17, 18), who followed a group of high school seniors into college. Although the group was small, 15 subjects, the findings are provocative.

The subjects were "competent adolescents." By this term, the researchers meant that their subjects had demonstrated the ability to carry out academic work, and form close relationships with a peer(s) and have active participation in social groups.

In their behavior these subjects sought out and dealt with manageable levels of challenge in the environment. They regarded the new as exciting and desirable, a problem to be solved and something to be mastered. Thus, they demonstrated White's (21) concept of *competence* or *effectance striving*. As one illustration, they assumed much of the responsibility in making preparations for college and went about this task with a sense of purpose and autonomy. The reader should note that the crisis model of adolescence stresses self-doubt and conflict more than competence and pleasurable engagement with the environment, yet for many adolescents this latter emphasis may be more accurate.

The coping strategies that these competent adolescents used were numerous. In planning for college, they referred to analogous past experiences, especially ones they had mastered, and thus could transfer to the new situation a sense of familiarity and probable success. They carried out an anticipatory socialization before leaving home by thinking through separation from parents and contemplating the kinds of behavior that would be expected of them as young adults. They learned as much as they could about the college they were to attend and in a sense went through a role rehearsal, or "dry run," of what was to come. Even though they made mistakes, they built a framework within which new experiences could be fitted. They lowered their level of aspiration as a cushion against disappointment, but not to the point of an adverse effect on self-image. They focused on the encouraging aspects of the new situation rather than on dangers or unpleasant aspects. They were aware of discouraging elements but elected not to dwell on them. Like subjects in other studies, they were anxious at times but used this feeling as a facilitator of action, and also reduced the anxiety by sharing their feelings with others.

When they moved into college their anticipatory or planning mechanisms enabled them to look ahead and see clearly what was expected in terms of academic and other requirements. They could distinguish short-term and long-term goals and distinguish between primary and secondary demands on their time, yet find activities that provided some sense of immediate satisfaction.

From a cognitive point of view they had good power of concentration, for long stretches or under difficult conditions. When they started a task they could sort out extraneous material and quickly come to the central issue. Another aspect of this was a sensitivity to environmental demands, what I have referred to elsewhere as "polling the environment" (13).

They reached out for new friends, sought information from upperclassmen, and were ready and open in sharing feelings and experiences with peers.

The competent adolescents were also compared with a matched group of patients by using a college-oriented Thematic Apperception Test. Of interest is the finding that the competent group projected a view of college where problems were manageable and peers were viewed optimistically, whereas the patients saw problems as yielding few solutions, people were passive in the face of obstacles, and peers were seen as malevolent.

Subjects in a similar situation, that is, moving from high school to college, were studied by Westlake and Epstein (20) in Montreal. The writers drew subjects from white, Anglo-Saxon, Protestant families, and by interviews and tests they selected ten healthy and ten disturbed students and their families. The disturbed were defined by presence of structured psychiatric symptoms, social and occupational maladaptation, and moderate or severe psychopathology with moderate or severe anxiety.

The two groups were distinguished from each other in a variety of ways. The healthy students and families were more willing to cooperate in the study, welcoming new experience as a way of deepening and enriching their lives. They also responded with a full range of human emotions. The disturbed students, correspondingly, felt threatened and attempted to withdraw, and had problems in the expression of rage. All subjects had some anxieties in the sexual area but the problem was greater for those who were disturbed. The healthy subjects were more aware of the demands of the future while the less healthy were more confused and vague about goals and occupational future. Much of the difference could be summarized by saying that the healthy students had developed a sense of inner self that was congruent with their social group and the world around them, while the disturbed students had not.

Differences were also observable among the families of the two groups, particularly in the area of problem solving and communication. Families with emotionally healthy children recognized and talked about things that were emotionally important, while those with disturbed offspring seemed largely unaware of emotional problems. In other ways also, the families of healthy students showed positive coping. They dealt with threats to the family's physical and emotional well-being directly and in ways that did not damage family equilibrium. They felt they could meet and solve problems, yet were sensitive to the needs of individual family members. Families with disturbed children more often showed negative coping, and had difficulty in identifying and dealing with problems, or did so at the expense of a family member.

Families were most effective when the parents seemed to satisfy each other's needs and were secure with each other. This was the "emotional thermostat" of family life. Westlake and Epstein noted that psychopathology in the parents was not necessarily associated with disturbed children if parents did not project their difficulties onto the children or use the children as objects of anxiety or contained rage. They also noted that the balance of power between parents had important effects and that the healthiest children were found in families that were "father led" and had a balanced division of labor, in contrast to egalitarian families or those where one parent was dominant.

There are limitations to the conclusions that can be drawn from the Westlake and Epstein data, due to the small size of the sample, its social and ethnic narrowness, and the difficulty in getting families of disturbed children to cooperate with the study. However, the data suggest hypotheses to be tested under more rigorously controlled conditions; to wit, that active engagement with the environment is associated with effective coping, that openness of communication within the family and identification of problems aids in the development of healthy children, and that a balance of power between parents is more often associated with satisfaction in the family and healthy offspring.

LATE ADOLESCENCE INTO YOUNG ADULTHOOD

The most vigorous research has come in this age span, and within the last two decades. Of the many studies there are four that are particularly relevant to the argument being presented in this paper.

As Grinker, et al. (6) were looking for subjects for psychosomatic research they "discovered fortuitously" a group of healthy young men at George Williams College. As in many other studies, the subjects came primarily from white, middle and lower middle class, Protestant backgrounds. In this particular group there was also the factor of a rather strict and rigorous religious training.

On the basis of responses to psychologic tests, 65 of the students were classified as healthy. As a group they were not given much to introspection and were not bothered by internal anxiety. They were action-oriented, like the subjects in studies previously cited here, and used physical activity as a way of dissipating tension or anger. Although they felt anxiety or depression at times, the sources were usually exogenous, and the feelings were not generally severe or prolonged.

The typical home environment of these students was stable, with love from both parents and consistency in discipline. The division of labor in the family seemed much like the balanced power in the Westlake and Epstein study; responsibilities and interests between parents were shared. In general, mother was viewed by the students as warmer, and father more as the disciplinarian, though not a harsh one.

Grinker found no evidence of identity crises as the young men went through adolescence. There was some rebelliousness and conflict in early adolescence, but like Offer's subjects, it seemed to be in the service of individuation. The students were conventional in social outlook, not especially creative in fantasy, nor showing much use of abstraction, but they were solid in personality functioning and integration.

Further insight into development comes from a comparison Grinker made of a group of very-well-adjusted (VWA) students with a group of marginally-adjusted (MA). In the VWA group, parental relationships were more positive in terms of agreement about child-rearing and in expressed affection. In the MA group, father was more often dominant. There was for this group more conflict between children and parents in early adolescence and the subjects more often felt that their parents did not understand them. They were less socially involved during adolescence than the VWA group, less focused and less able to specify goals. They more often used fantasy in their attempts to solve problems. They often became bored and depressed; they inhibited anger rather than used it in some kind of constructive engagement with the environment.

Haverford College was the setting for the next study to be cited, where Heath (8, 9) has conducted some extended research on the topic of maturity. Although his subjects might be classified as intellectually élite, his conclusions can also provide the basis for hypotheses to be tested in further research. Subjects were divided into groups of more mature and less mature. The mature person was defined as stably organized in both a cognitive and emotional sense, as consistent and integrated, as allocentric and adjusted to reality (but without repressing autocentric trends when they are appropriate), and as less burdened by more primitive and unsocialized material in thought and fantasy. Yet the mature person can regress in the service of the ego.

Test batteries and observer ratings were used to form the study groups. The more mature group had higher academic achievement, were less depressed, and less impaired by self-centered trends. They described their siblings as effective and stable people, while every student in the immature group subtly derogated at least one sibling in some manner. Also, among the immature, achievements were more sporadic and often directed toward some capricious part of themselves, rather than toward some aspect of the external world.

From a set of adjectival statements by the two groups, Heath concluded that the less mature group showed less stability and control, were more labile in emotions, were more introspective, and evidenced more painful affect. Although individuals like these could not be characterized as showing structured psychiatric symptoms they might be subject to a more stormy adolescence.

A final point of interest: the immature group used the medical clinic more frequently and reported more headaches, fatigue, localized pain, and accidental injuries. This finding is comparable to King's (12) finding that students who visited a psychologist or psychiatrist also used the medical and surgical clinics more frequently than did other students.

The last two studies to be cited are longitudinal, following large samples of subjects through the four years of college.

Our study at Harvard (4, 13) utilized a 25% random sample of students who matriculated in the fall terms of 1960 and 1961. The subjects were given an extensive battery of tests and questionnaires and were retested each year. In addition a subsample of 50 students were also interviewed regularly.

We observed four major patterns of personality change, *progressive maturation, delayed maturation, crisis and reintegration,* and *deterioration.* The majority of students were characterized by the first of these patterns and showed a strong feeling of continuity between past and present. Like students in the NIMH study, our students found experiences in the past in which they had coped and could transfer aspects of these experiences to present problems. They also brought forward the satisfying aspects of interpersonal relationships with parents, other adults, siblings, or peers and used these experiences in forming new relationships. These students were successful at adapting.

Change over four years of college occurred mainly in six areas for students in the progressive maturation pattern. In *object relations,* students worked out their feelings about parents and by graduation had formed reciprocal and rewarding relationships with peers. They learned to accept ways they were like father, and to be free of guilt in their uniqueness from him, which seemed to release emotional energy that could be invested in relationships with others. Many students described the most important part of their Harvard experience in terms of interpersonal rewards, rather than academic gains.

There was an increase in *self-esteem* and in a sense of competence, and by graduation students knew better where their strengths lay. They knew they could have an effect on people and events, and thereby had an increase in the sense of power.

Stabilization of mood also occurred, and when shifts in mood did take place they were more likely to result from changes in the environment than from changes in internal states. Students became more adept at recognizing reasons for depressive shifts and found ways of modifying the depressed feelings. Like the other studies cited previously, the healthy adolescent and young adult is not necessarily at the mercy of his moods but can alter them by turning to other activities.

Interests did not often change in direction, but there was a deepening of them, a process of discrimination and synthesis, and greater recognition of the way in which interests fitted in with needs and values.

We noted a rise in the level of aspiration and in *good-directed activity*. By the senior year, students more often selected careers on the basis of status and prestige. Students also were moving away from absolute value positions, and by the senior year they were emphasizing a life style that allowed personal freedom in moral decisions. We may have seen in, our data an underlying shift in value positions that preceded many of the striking life style changes of recent years.

Under changes in *ego control* there was both a freeing of impulse expression and of greater impulse control. Though a seeming paradox, in reality students became easier with their impulse life and brought more rationality and selectivity into it. In the directing of energy, students learned to handle the environment more effectively, to take account of contingencies, and to plan ahead with ease and comfort. There was also an increased tolerance for painful feelings by the senior year. In some cases there appeared to be more anxiety, but we saw it not as a sign of disturbance but as a growing ease in allowing anxiety to surface.

These changes were less evident among students in the pattern of delayed maturation, where there was a discontinuity with past experience that was heightened by being in college. Such students sensed a disjunction between their personality characteristics and those of their parents, and between themselves and their background. Most often it took place in students who lacked solid identification with individuals or with a racial or ethnic group. Few of our black students were in this group, because their sense of racial identification was strong, and they felt a keen sense of continuity with their cultural background.

Students in the delayed maturation group were sometimes unhappy and depressed and seemed to be more at the mercy of the environment than engaging and transforming it. They seemed to be searching and waiting.

A more classic picture of late adolescent disturbance came in the crisis and reintegration pattern. Often there was anxiety of sufficient severity to interfere with sleep or study, or depression that at times included suicidal ideation, psychosomatic disorders, and confusion. Some of these students dropped out of college while others remained in a state of reduced effectiveness. Although these crises were severe, most students moved into a reintegrative phase by the senior year, and showed some of the changes characterized by students in the progressive maturation pattern, but the changes were less consistent. Looking back, these students had not learned how to deal with people effectively, often had problems with anger, and could not share their feelings easily. They were often hostile to key identification figures in childhood. There were negative feelings about the self, and, as a result, these students felt overwhelmed by the pressures in college. Resolution of the crisis involved coming to terms with their feelings of guilt, anger, and helplessness.

A few students showed a deterioration pattern, with an impairment in reality testing that led to unrealistic fantasies about their ability and their future achievement. With an increase in environmental stresses they relied more on fantasies and retreated into primitive defenses rather than using coping mechanisms.

The final study to be cited was conducted by Katz, et al. (10) at Stanford and Berkeley. They too did not find turmoil and identity crisis among as many students as they had expected; for most students adaptation to the role demands of college and to the expectations of their future roles in society took place without conscious conflict. Students changed toward more adequate self-conceptions and improved in their ability to relate to others in mutually gratifying ways. The data from this study and the Harvard study emphasize the developmental tasks of achieving intimacy and its overriding importance in cognitive and social concerns.

Although there was little evidence of crisis, many students showed an incompleteness of identity by graduation, and deferred an occupational life commitment till later years. Yet, the students continued to move within the life space of their families. They showed a strong sense of continuity with their families in values, occupational preferences, and social expectations. Once again, evidence supports the existence of close ties rather than a gap between parents and offspring.

We might wonder from these studies if the changes that occur are due to the college experience or are universal and would be found in a cross section of the 18-22-year-old group. Data are sparse, but there is a study by Trent and Medsker (19) of nearly 5000 high school graduates who were studied over a 4-year period. Subjects who persisted in college were more likely than the others to move toward an open-minded, flexible, and autonomous disposition, whereas those who went to work or into full-time homemaking were more constricted, had less intellectual curiosity, less interest in new experiences, and a lower tolerance for ambiguity. The authors concluded that those who go to college can learn more about themselves, their potential, and their desires. College students seemed to have more awareness of their environment and to be more open to it.

We must be careful not to conclude that those who went to college were healthier than those who went to work or married immediately after high school. Psychologists and psychiatrists have a bias that open-mindedness, autonomy, and creativity are necessary for successful coping and emotional health, but we cannot confirm that conclusion without obtaining much more systematic data than we currently have available.

COMMON FINDINGS

In one way or another the following findings appear in most or all of the studies that have been cited.

(1) Turmoil and conflict are limited in adolescence and the identity crisis is not common. A developmental disturbance is not necessary for successful progress through adolescence. (2) There is little evidence for a generation gap, and although there is rebellion in adolescence, the relations between parents and offspring are generally good. (3) Healthy adolescents have good relations with peers, are able to share feelings, and are not generally shy and withdrawn. (4) Although adolescents at times have doubts about themselves, self-esteem and a sense of competence are high; depression is limited; and most adolescents have ways of working out of depressed states. (5) Adolescents cope by dealing directly with painful affect and sharing such feelings with others. They also cope by turning away from painful feelings to other topics and activities, often of a physical nature. They can sublimate sexual and aggressive energy in social activities and sports, and find thereby a sense of satisfaction

as well as a release of tension. They also use humor in coping, to blunt feelings of anxiety, limit guilt, and to provide a sense of perspective on their problems. They use role rehearsal and cognitive planning for new situations, and utilize anxiety as a facilitator in action rather than an inhibitor. Finally, they are able to integrate new experiences with past ones where they have felt satisfaction and success.

These common findings are not typical of all adolescents, nor of any adolescent all the time, but they do suggest that the capacity to cope is greater than we would be led to expect from theories based primarily on data from the consulting room. These findings also suggest the possibility that alternate models to the crisis model of adolescence are in order.

TYPES OF DEVELOPMENT IN ADOLESCENCE

Most of the readers of this article, at least those in clinical practice, will be familiar with adolescents who are *seriously impaired,* who show anti-social behavior, who cannot control their impulses, who are overcome by anxiety or depression, and who show abundant evidence of crisis and turmoil. This is one kind of adolescent development, and there is good reason to believe that the waning of adolescence still leaves these individuals vulnerable and subject to adjustment problems throughout their lives.

A second group has been described in this article—the *normal and competent.* Although numbers are not available, this group may constitute a majority of adolescents. These individuals are successful in coping, begin to develop a sense of identity, and show strong continuity with past experiences.

There is reason to believe that this second group is actually two subgroups: the modal or average, and the highly competent. The former cope successfully but are not dreamers or exciting innovators, and their fantasy is limited. The highly competent are more likely to be innovators, leaders, and generally more exciting people. Both subgroups are well integrated in personality functioning but different in a creative sense.

A third group is composed of the *sensitive and vulnerable,* for whom adolescence may be a time of some distress. They may show some combination of an active fantasy life, sudden and extensive swings of mood, painful questioning about self-esteem, difficulty in sharing feelings with others, periods of strong depression, unrealistically high idealism, and active rebellion. They can be characterized by identity concerns and will often say that they are desperately trying to find out who they are. Often they tend to be loners, and cannot talk easily with adults. They may be sent to counselors, or psychologists, or psychiatrists for help, or may seek it out themselves.

Adolescents in this group are different from the emotionally disturbed in that they have a basic capacity to form meaningful relationships with others, and can share feelings if they are helped to do so. They do need support and advice but they are able to utilize that help. Most importantly, the upheaval these people experience is limited in time, and in most cases they become well-integrated and mature as adults.

The third group may well be the source of many of our ideas about adolescent development. They are often the ones who are described in novels or autobiographic accounts, or who are seen in the consulting room. They are puzzling and frustrating to adults, and their very actions draw our attention as if to demand the need for explanation. We can't help but notice them, but it is questionable if they are in the majority and if their lives provide the most reliable conceptual model for understanding adolescence and young adulthood.

ADOLESCENT DEVELOPMENT IN HISTORICAL PERSPECTIVE

Many people feel that the third type of development just described occurs with greater frequency today than in other generations, and indeed some historical perspective is useful in understanding adolescence. The key is the interrelationship between psychologic development and social processes (14).

Passage through adolescence is relatively smoother under certain social conditions. One of these is the presence of *meaningful adult roles,* with appropriate rewards for their fulfillment, which are accepted by all members of the society. Another is the utilization of *clearly defined transition points* from child to adult status, which are important in the formation of firm identity. Also, there must be *stability and consensus in the value system* of the society so that daily activities make sense in terms of those values. These conditions are most often met when a society is stable, cohesive, and has a well-defined set of traditions and life style.

When there is instability and social change, or upheaval in the social order, there is more likely to be upheaval in adolescent development. When there is confusion about adult roles, and when transition points between statuses become fuzzy, and when value systems are changing, then the adolescent may feel pulled in two directions at once. These social conditions are characteristic of most industrialized countries today, and, as a consequence, we might expect more adolescents to fall into the sensitive and vulnerable category of development that was outlined above.

The situation is further complicated by two other factors that are particular to the United States. In the past few decades we have seen a change in child-rearing practices in this country. This change has been brought about by the admonitions of educators, psychologists, and psychoanalysts, who felt that development could be hampered by over-rigid control. Many parents have responded by rearing their children in a more permissive manner, but in the process some have lost a sense of direction in child-rearing. In these families, children have often grown up with a vague uneasiness that their parents did not really care for them.

The other factor comes from the "American Dream," which leads us to believe that the manner in which we were born does not prevent us from attaining social prestige or from making some kind of significant contribution to our society. The "Dream" has been a significant factor in the history of the United States, but in the present situation of rapid technologic advances, an adolescent or young adult may feel that infinite potentialities are open to him. As a consequence, there may be a reluctance to limit options on the future, but such reluctance can make more difficult the attainment of goals and direction in life.

Not all adolescents will be affected adversely by these social conditions, but the potential for a sense of crisis and turmoil will be increased. The effect will probably be felt most acutely by children of the professionals, the intellectuals, and the managers in the social system, because they are very aware of the social changes taking place but can do little to change their own lives. It is no surprise that many of our contemporary alienated youth come from such upper middle class families, and fewer from middle and lower middle groups where social change comes more slowly.

It is easy in the present day to feel that the majority of adolescents are in crisis, or turmoil, or active rebellion, or withdrawal, and to feel that what we see around us confirms the crisis model of adolescent development. Yet, that view may be misleading. The studies that have been reviewed here certainly suggest that a significant proportion of the younger generation are able to come to grips with the problems that arise in a changing society and to cope successfully with problems in their own lives. They can do this because they have had successful experiences in the past with coping, because they feel secure, and because they can share their feelings of anxiety and of confidence with others. If this is true, some revision of our views of adolescent and young adult development is in order.

REFERENCES

1. COELHO, G. V., SILBUR, E., & HAMBURG, D. A.: Use of the Student-T.A.T. to assess coping behavior in hospitalized, normal and exceptionally competent college freshmen. *Percept. Motor Skills,* 14:355, 1962.
2. COELHO, G. V., HAMBURG, D. A., & MURPHEY, E. B.: Coping strategies in a new learning environment. *Arch. Gen. Psychiat.* (Chicago), 9:433, 1963.
3. ERIKSON, E.: *Childhood and Society.* New York: W. W. Norton, 1963.
4. FINNIE, B.: The statistical assessment of personality change. In J. M. Whitely and H. Sprandel (Eds.), *The Growth and Development of College Students.* Washington, D. C.. Student Personnel Series No. 12, American Personnel and Guidance Association.
5. FREUD, A.: Adolescence as a developmental disturbance. In G. Kaplan and S. Lebovici (Eds.), *Adolescence: Psychosocial Perspectives.* New York, Basic Books, 1969.
6. GRINKER, R. R.: "Mentally healthy" young males (homoclites). *Arch. Gen. Psychiat.* (Chicago), 6:405, 1962.
7. HAMBURG, D. A. & ADAMS, J. E.: A perspective on coping behavior. *Arch. Gen. Psychiat.* (Chicago) 17:277, 1967.
8. HEATH, D. H.: *Explorations of Maturity.* New York: Appleton-Century-Crofts, 1965.
9. HEATH, D. H.: *Growing Up In College.* San Francisco: Jossey-Bass, 1968.
10. KATZ, J., ET AL.: *No Time for Youth.* San Francisco: Jossey-Bass, 1968.
11. KIELL, N.: *The Universal Experience of Adolescence.* New York: International Universities Press, 1964.
12. KING, S. H.: Characteristics of students seeking psychiatric help during college. *J. Amer. Coll. Health Ass.,* 17:150, 1968.
13. KING, S. H.: *Lives of Harvard Men: Personality Change during College.* In press.
14. KING, S. H.: Youth in rebellion: An historical perspective. In *Drug Dependence: A Guide for Physicians.* Chicago, Ill.: American Medical Association, 1969.
15. MASTERSON, J. F., JR.: *The Psychiatric Dilemma of Adolescence.* Boston, Little, Brown, 1967.
16. OFFER, D.: *The Psychological World of the Teen-ager.* New York: Basic Books, 1969.
17. SILBER, E., ET AL.: Adaptive behavior in competent adolescents. *Arch. Gen. Psychiat* (Chicago), 5:359, 1961.
18. SILBER, E., ET AL.: Competent adolescent coping with college decisions. *Arch. Gen. Psychiat.* (Chicago), 5:517, 1961.
19. TRENT, J. W. & MEDSKER, L. L.: *Beyond High School.* San Francisco: Jossey-Bass, 1968.
20. WESTLAKE, W. A. & EPSTEIN, N. B.: *The Silent Majority.* San Francisco: Jossey-Bass, 1969.
21. WHITE, R. W.: Motivation reconsidered: The concept of competence. *Psychol. Rev.,* 66:5, 297, 1959.

Part III

PARENT-CHILD SEPARATION

The papers in this section take up an issue of great theoretical and practical importance, namely, the consequence of separating child and parent as well as the mechanisms determining such consequences. They all challenge the global characterization of maternal separation as tantamount to maternal deprivation with inevitable pathological effects on the young child.

Rutter provides his usual comprehensive and authoritative critical review. In this case, he offers a tight summary of the material covered in his recent volume, *Maternal Deprivation Reassessed*. He concludes that the concept of "maternal deprivation" is a complex one which includes a number of quite different experiences with quite different outcomes. Unless careful distinctions are made between these, it is unlikely that any progress will be made in disentangling the various psychological mechanisms involved.

Hinde and Davies' study on the rhesus monkey underscores this conclusion by suggesting that separation as such may not be the issue. Rather, the consequences of separation, such as its effect on the mother which may then lead to altered mother-infant interaction, may be crucial.

Caldwell's study on the consequences of day-care for both child and parent shows consistent findings as to its positive effect. Kaffman's paper is of special interest because of the great attention paid by many centers to the Kibbutz experience. The author enters a caveat, which is pertinent for all cross-cultural studies, against foreign observers making broad generalizations regarding psychological phenomena after only a brief visit to a different culture.

13

MATERNAL DEPRIVATION RECONSIDERED

Michael Rutter, M.D.

The Institute of Psychiatry, University of London (England)

The concept of "maternal deprivation" is one that rapidly caught the imagination of both the general public and professional workers. It became widely accepted that severe distortions in a child's early family life could have long-lasting effects on his later development, and "maternal deprivation" has been thought to be the cause of conditions as diverse as mental subnormality, delinquency, depression, dwarfism, acute distress and affectionless psychopathy (1, 2). Most writers have recognized that the experiences covered by the term "maternal deprivation" are diverse and complex, but nevertheless there has been a tendency to regard both the experiences and the outcomes as one syndrome which can be discussed as a whole (3). Thus, in Ainsworth's critical review of the topic in 1962 (1), the term "deprivation" was repeatedly used in the summary of findings as if it were a single entity, although earlier in the paper she had indicated that it was not. Furthermore, in recent years theorists have been inclined to the view that most of the ills of deprivation are accountable for in terms of lack of an attachment to a mother-figure (1, 4, 5).*

The purpose of this paper is to question these assumptions. It will be suggested that "maternal deprivation" includes many different types

---

Reproduced from the JOURNAL OF PSYCHOSOMATIC RESEARCH, Vol. 16, 1972, pp. 241-250 with the permission of Microforms International Marketing Corp., licensee. © Pergamon Press Journal back files.

* Nevertheless, Bowlby has been careful to point out on several occasions that other factors are also important.

of experiences involving lack, loss and distortion; that little progress is likely to occur until the separate effects of each experience are determined (6); that different psychological mechanisms account for different types of outcome; and finally that the term "maternal deprivation" is misleading in that in most cases the deleterious influences are not specifically tied to the mother and are *not* due to deprivation. Reference to the Shorter Oxford English Dictionary shows that deprivation means "dispossession" or "loss." While loss is probably an important factor in one of the syndromes associated with "maternal deprivation" a review of the evidence suggests that in most cases the damage comes from "lack" or "distortion" of care rather than from any form of "loss."

As there are several reviews (1, 2, 6-12) which summarize the findings on the various effects of deprivation and several critiques (6, 13-15) which discuss the assets and deficits of the many studies of maternal deprivation, these aspects of the topic will not be considered here. Instead attention will be focused on *"why"* and *"how"* children are adversely affected by those experiences included under the term "maternal deprivation"; I shall take for granted the extensive evidence that many children admitted to hospital or to a residential nursery show an immediate reaction to acute distress; that many infants show developmental retardation following admission to a poor-quality institution and may exhibit intellectual impairment if they remain there for a long time; that there is an association between delinquency and broken homes; that affectionless psychopathy sometimes follows multiple separation experiences and institutional care in early childhood; and that dwarfism is particularly seen in children from rejecting and affectionless homes. The evidence on factors which modify the effects of deprivation has been discussed elsewhere (7) and this evidence will be used to analyze the psychological mechanisms which might account for the six main syndromes of childhood associated with maternal deprivation.* Depression will not be discussed as this has mainly been studied in adults (16). The important evidence that children differ in their response to stress (7, 11, 16) will also not be considered.

Acute Distress

Largely as a result of Bowlby's emphasis on the value of studying children's immediate responses to separation experiences (17) there is

---

* It is not suggested that any of these syndromes is entirely explicable in terms of "deprivation." Genetic and biological factors are also important but will not be discussed here. Rather, possible mechanisms will be discussed only with respect to that part of the variance which is due to "deprivation."

now a substantial body of evidence on what happens in these circumstances (7). Nowhere is this better illustrated than in the Robertsons' films. Most work has been concerned with the effects on children of their admission to hospital or to a residential nursery. It is well established that many (but not all) young children show an immediate response of acute distress and crying (the period of "protest"), followed by misery and apathy (the phase of "despair") and finally there is a stage when the child becomes apparently contented and seems to lose interest in his parents ("detachment" in Robertson's and Bowlby's terms).

There is considerable individual variation in how children respond and not all children are upset by the experience. Nevertheless the pattern as described is a common one in children between six months and four years of age.

It is evident that several factors must be operative. One of these is the type of care provided during the separation. Experimental studies have shown how distress may be reduced by provision of toys, and clinical investigations have demonstrated how measures designed to make hospital admission less traumatic can help alleviate children's unhappiness while away from their parents. The Robertsons' films have also illustrated how children looked after in a good family setting adapt to separation much better than children in hospital or in a residential nursery. All these findings indicate that quite apart from the experience of separation, what happens to the child during separation can make a big difference to whether or not he reacts by showing severe distress.

On the other hand, there is a good deal of evidence to suggest that, in some circumstances, separation itself can be a disturbing influence. For example, experimental studies with toddlers have shown how very brief departures of mothers may lead to immediate distress. Perhaps the most convincing evidence that separation is one key variable is the finding that the presence of sibs or other familiar persons greatly reduces children's distress following admission to hospital or in some other stress situation. Distress seems to be less even though the accompanying person neither provides nor improves maternal care. A further pointer to the importance of separation is the fact that distress is rarely seen in infants under six months. It is significant that children show most distress at an age just after they are beginning to show attachment to their parents. Separation is probably stressful then just because it is interrupting an important bond at a time when children have difficulty maintaining a relationship through an absence.

It may be concluded that the syndrome of acute distress following hospital admission is due in considerable part to a child's separation from his family, although poor care and unpleasant experiences also play an important role. But, is separation *per se* the crucial factor? Recent evidence suggests that probably it is not.

So far as rhesus monkeys are concerned this has been well demonstrated in Hinde's very important studies (18-20). He has emphasized three findings all of which point toward the conclusion that the basic variable is disturbance in the mother-infant interaction, not separation as such. First, infants' distress is a function of the characteristics of both the pre-separation and the contemporaneous mother-infant relationship, Second, changes in the mother-infant interaction following reunion largely depend on the mother. Third, infants who have been temporarily removed from their usual living group show *less* distress on their return than do infants who have remained "at home" but whose mothers have been removed for a period. Accordingly, in rhesus monkeys separation seems to have its deleterious effects by virtue of its alteration of the mother-infant interaction. When separation is *not* associated with any disturbance in this interaction, then ill-effects are minimal. When separation *is* associated with a disturbed relationship ill-effects are maximal.

Does the same apply to human infants? The evidence is meager but what findings there are are certainly consistent with Hinde's view. The role of the mother in mother-infant interaction may well be different in humans, but disturbance in the relationship still seems to be the crucial variable. For example, in the two cases studied, the Robertsons' films show that children separated from their family and placed in the private home of people they had only met for the first time a few days ago did *not* exhibit the acute distress of similar children placed in a residential nursery. In both situations the children's physical needs were well met and there was a probably adequate provision of toys and activities. What differentiated the private home from the nursery was the provision of an intense individual interaction between the child and *one* person (the same person throughout the separation experience).

It is suggested that the syndrome of acute distress occurs when there is a lack of opportunity for the infant to manifest attachment behavior or where the mother-infant interaction associated with attachment is distorted or disrupted for some reason. However, the evidence that distress in hospital or some other stressful situation is much reduced by the presence of a sib or friend, even though the mother remains absent, strongly suggests that there is nothing specific about *mother*-attachment.

In summary, the syndrome of distress is probably due in part to a disruption of the bonding process, but the bonding is not necessarily with the mother. Thus, so far as this syndrome is concerned, the description "deprivation" is correct, as "loss" is a key variable. The adjective "maternal" is somewhat misleading as it appears that it is loss of a person to whom the child is attached which matters. Nevertheless, it is only slightly inaccurate because the person to whom infants are usually most attached is the mother.

Developmental Retardation

Do the same mechanisms apply to the other syndromes associated with "maternal deprivation?" "Developmental retardation" will be considered first as the only other short-term consequence of much importance. The findings here are quite different. First the association with age differs in that there is no lower age limit. Infants under the age of six months in institutions where there is little stimulation vocalize little and become socially unresponsive (7). Deviations in language, social and motor development have been reported as early as the second month. Severe retardation has been found in children born in, or admitted to institutions in the first month of life at a time when they have yet to develop any attachments and when they have a very limited ability to differentiate between the adults providing care. This stands in sharp contrast to the syndrome of distress which is rare before six months.

Secondly, developmental retardation seems to be completely reversed by increasing social, tactile, and perceptual stimulation without altering any other aspect of institutional life and without altering the child's separation from his family. Furthermore this reversal occurs even though the stimulation is given by someone who is not providing maternal care. There are now some half-dozen independent studies all producing closely similar results which provide evidence for this conclusion (7). Thirdly, some institutions do not give rise to developmental retardation in spite of the fact that the children in them have all experienced separation from their parents.

Developmental retardation, then, is due to a *lack* of stimulation and not to a *loss* of stimulation. Accordingly, privation is a more correct description than deprivation. Moreover, it is a lack of stimulation which matters and not mother's presence, so that "experiential" is a more appropriate adjective than "maternal." Altogether, the psychological mechanisms appear quite different to those operating in the case of the syndrome of distress.

Intellectual Impairment

In turning to the long-term consequences of "maternal deprivation" it is appropriate to start with intellectual impairment, which may follow on from developmental retardation if the infant remains in a poor-quality institution. As one might expect, comparable mechanisms seem to be operative.

The main findings to be taken into account are as follows—parent-child separation and broken homes are *not* associated with mental retardation; an institutional upbringing is often accompanied by intellectual impairment but this effect is found only with some institutions; similar effects stem from depriving circumstances in the child's own home; and retardation is more evident with respect to language and verbal skills, while perceptuo-motor skills seem less susceptible to the retarding effect of privation.

If we focus on institutions first, it is apparent from several studies that if the provision of child-care is improved then the children's intellectual growth also increases. It follows from these findings that really good institutions should not cause any intellectual retardation and indeed that seems to be the case. It appears that it is not whether you are brought up at home or in an institution which matters for cognitive growth but rather the type of care you receive. It is more difficult to provide adequate opportunities for intellectual development in institutions but it can be done.

If it is the quality of care which matters, then mental retardation should also be apparent in children who remain with their own family but whose home life provides little stimulation: that *is* the case. For example, the early studies of canal boat children and of children from isolated mountain communities all showed that verbal abilities were seriously retarded and were more so in older children than in youngsters, suggesting progressive impairment due to deprivation of some aspect of experience. The importance of experiential factors is also demonstrated by the many studies which have shown that children in large families have a poor verbal intellectual development compared with children in small families (6). Whereas the exact mechanism involved remains uncertain, the effect seems to be environmental rather than genetic.

The conclusion that "stimulation" is necessary for intellectual growth does not take us very far unless we can specify what sort of stimulation is needed. Is it social, sensory or linguistic stimulation which matters and is it the quantity or quality of stimulation which is relevant?

There are numerous animal studies which have shown that a lack of sensory stimulation can have a profound effect on development. For example, animals reared in darkness show later deficiencies in perceptual discriminations and visual learning. These animals also show defects in the retina and visual cortex so that the effects are neural as well as behavioral. However, these experiments are concerned with highly specific effects of highly specific sensory restriction and so are of very limited relevance to the question of "maternal deprivation" in man. Casler (22) has nevertheless suggested that pure perceptual restriction plays a crucial role in the retardation of institutional children. This may well be the case in conditions of severe global retardation (as in the worst types of old-fashioned institution) but it appears less likely to be the main factor in more ordinary circumstances of privation.

Perhaps the two key findings are (1) that environmental privation leads largely to an impairment in *verbal* intelligence and (2) that the effects are similar in this respect for children reared in their own homes and for those brought up in institutions. Consideration of the situation of children reared in large families (one of the circumstances associated with verbal impairment) makes it clear that a mere reduction in the *amount* of sensory, social or linguistic stimulation is unlikely to provide an explanation, although impairment in the quality of any of these might. It has been suggested that children in large families show impaired verbal intellectual development because their contacts are more with children than with adults with the result that their language environment is less rich and complex than in smaller families. However, it may be the *clarity* of the language environment rather than its complexity which is the key variable. Preliminary studies of family conversations by Friedlander (20) suggest that the presence of several children tends to lead to a tumultuous clamor in which several people speak at once at several different levels.

Much the same conclusions stem from an examination of environmental influences on language development (21). In babies the main stimulus to vocalization is provided by non-social *verbal* stimulation rather than by non-verbal *social* stimulation—in other words a tape-recorded voice has more effect than a silent person. But to be effective the words must be meaningful to the child—a mere repetition of words is not enough. The same applies to the effects on language development in older preschool children. If deprived children are given extra play sessions with an adult this has no significant effect on language unless there is also talking. But the special provision of sessions when adults deliberately engage children in conversation has been shown to have a significantly beneficial effect on language development.

In summary with respect to mental retardation, the evidence suggests that an absolute restriction of any type of stimulation can have deleterious effects but probably the single most important factor concerning verbal intellectual development is the child's language environment.* How much he is talked with is important, but the content of the conversational interchange he experiences is more important. Because it is necessary that adults develop and respond to the child's speech, in all ordinary circumstances it is necessary for the verbal stimulation to be provided by people. Nevertheless, it is the conversation that matters, the mere presence of an interested adult is not enough. Probably with all forms of stimulation the distinctiveness and meaningfulness of stimuli are more important than the absolute level of stimulation. So again the effect is explicable in terms of "privation" which is "experiential" (especially linguistic) rather than "maternal deprivation."

Dwarfism

The next syndrome to consider is "deprivation dwarfism," a condition found in children who have experienced extreme and long-standing emotional deprivation (9). It has usually been assumed that *emotional* deprivation can lead to dwarfism even when nutritional intake remains adequate. I suggest that this is probably wrong and that inadequate food intake is usually the correct explanation.

Possible mechanisms include endocrine dysfunction, anorexia following depression, distortion of diet, and malabsorption. There is not time to consider the evidence on these in detail. Suffice it to say that although each may play a part in individual cases the evidence is against any constituting the main mechanism (7). In contrast, there are two recent studies which both point to the importance of underfeeding. First, confirming Davenport's earlier study with chimpanzees, Kerr et al. (24) showed that when infant rhesus monkeys are reared under conditions of total social isolation but normal opportunities for dietary intake they developed gross behavioral abnormalities but their growth rates were entirely normal.

The importance of undereating has been shown more directly in a well-controlled study by Whitten and his colleagues (25). Thirteen maternally deprived human infants with height and weight below the third percentile were investigated. The inadequate mothering at home was simulated in hospital by solitary confinement for two weeks in a windowless room, but the infants were offered a generous diet. In spite of the continuing emotional and sensory deprivation all but two showed accelerated weight gain. Following this period of understimulation, the

---

* Other aspects of the environment may well be more important for the growth of other types of cognitive functions.

infants were given a high level of mothering and sensory stimulation but the diet remaining as before. This caused no change in rate of weight gain.

Following this study, three other infants were investigated. They were not admitted to hospital nor were the parents told of the suspected diagnosis of maternal deprivation. Instead, under the guise of investigation of caloric intake, feeding was carried out by mothers in the presence of an observer, no attempt being made to alter maternal handling or social circumstances. All infants gained weight at a markedly accelerated rate and the mothers subsequently admitted that the infants ate more food during the experimental period than previously, although the diets were duplicates of what the mothers *claimed* that they fed the infants. Other evidence also suggested that the mother's dietary histories were often grossly inaccurate.

The findings are not conclusive in that short-term weight gain was studied rather than a long-term increase in height and the infants were younger than most cases of "deprivation dwarfism." In individual children a variety of mechanisms may operate but the balance of evidence suggests that, overall, impaired food intake is the most important factor. The impaired food intake may be due to either the child being given insufficient food or to his eating too little because of poor appetite.

Again "privation" needs to be the term rather than "deprivation" and in this case the adjective should be "nutritional" rather than "maternal."

Delinquency and Antisocial Disorder

The strong association between "broken homes" and delinquency has commonly been held to demonstrate the seriously deleterious long-term effects of disruption of affectional bonds (4). However recent evidence suggests that this view is probably mistaken and that the harm comes from distortion of family relationships (16).

The relative importance of bond disruption and distorted relationships may be assessed by comparing homes broken by death (where family relationships are likely to have been fairly normal prior to the break) and homes broken by divorce or separation (where the break is likely to have been preceded by discord or a lack of affection). Several independent studies have all shown that the delinquency rate is much raised when the parents divorce but it is only slightly above expectation when one parent dies.

This suggests that it may be the discord and disharmony *preceding* the break (rather than the break itself) which led to the children's delinquency. If that is correct, parental discord should be associated with antisocial disorder in children even when the home is unbroken. There is good evidence that this is indeed the case. In children from unbroken homes there is a strong association between parental marital disharmony and antisocial disorder in the sons. Antisocial disorder seems to be a function of a tense unhappy and quarrelsome home—only incidentally is it associated with family break-up as such.

The same conclusion applies to temporary separations. In our own studies we examined the issue with respect to separations of at least one month's duration (16). Separations which had occurred as a result of family disorder or disharmony (usually break-up following a quarrel) were associated with antisocial disorder in the children. On the other hand, separations for other reasons (mainly hospital admission or a convalescent holiday) were *not*. Transient separations as such were unrelated to the development of antisocial behavior; they only appeared to be so when separation occurred as a result of family discord.

As to the type of discord or disturbed relationships which predisposes the child to delinquency only very limited evidence is available. Our own studies suggested that both active discord and lack of affection were associated with the development of antisocial disorder but the combination of the two was particularly harmful. Any type of prolonged family discord was associated with an increased risk of antisocial disorder but a good relationship with one parent went some way towards mitigating the harmful effect of a quarrelsome home. In short, the findings emphasized the importance of good relationships in personality development but did not suggest that any one specific type of defect in relationships was of predominant importance. Furthermore, the harm appears to come from disturbed family relationships in general and *not* specifically from a distorted relationship with the mother.

In the case of delinquency, then, neither "maternal" nor "deprivation" seems an appropriate term. Rather, the association is explicable in terms of some type of "family discord" or "disturbed relationships."

Affectionless Psychopathy

The last syndrome to be discussed is that of "affectionless psychopathy." In spite of this being the condition first associated with maternal deprivation (26), it is the one on which there is the least satisfactory evidence. At first it was regarded as a common consequence of prolonged separation experiences but it is now clear that this is not generally so. This is shown, for example, by Bowlby's follow-up study of young children admitted to a T.B. sanitorium (27). However, an examination of the findings of different studies suggests that the child's *age* is a key variable in this connection. Bowlby's original study of forty-four thieves suggested that affectionless psychopathy was particularly associated with frequent changes of mother-figure during the first two years. Perhaps the damaging experience is failure to form bonds or attachments, rather than any breaking of bonds. To examine this possibility it is necessary to search for environments which lack what is required for attachments to develop—this is provided by the old-style large long-stay institutions —and then to see what happens to children who spend a prolonged period in this environment during the phase of development when attachments normally form—namely the first two or three years of life.

There is surprisingly little known about children with such an experience but what little there is supports the suggestion that this may be the crucial factor leading to affectionless psychopathy (7).

Thus, Pringle and her colleagues found that emotionally stable institutional children had generally remained with their mothers until well after the first year and so had had the opportunity of forming bonds prior to admission. Similarly, the stable children had more often experienced a dependable and lasting relationship with a parent or parent-substitute after going into care. The results of a failure to form bonds may also be examined by studying children reared in an institution from infancy and then comparing those placed in homes before three years when bonds may develop more readily, and those not placed until after three years when bond-formation may not occur for the first time so easily. This comparison is provided by Goldfarb's studies which showed that the children who remained in an institution until after three years were especially characterized by an inability to keep rules, a lack of guilt, a craving for affection and an inability to make lasting relationships.

Further evidence is provided by Wolkind's recent study of children in care (28). Psychiatric disturbance in these children took several forms but the characteristics of indiscriminate friendliness and lack of social inhibitions were a special feature of children admitted before the age of two years. This suggests that a failure to form bonds may lead to a particular type of disturbance.

No firm conclusions are yet possible from the patchy findings of these diverse studies. Nevertheless, the evidence is certainly compatible with the view that a failure to form bonds in early childhood is particularly likely to lead to attention-seeking, uninhibited indiscriminate friendliness and finally to a personality characterized by a lack of guilt and an inability to form lasting relationships. As a sub-issue it may be asked whether the bonds have to be with the mother or whether any bonds will serve to prevent this harmful outcome. There is no evidence on this point but circumstantial evidence strongly suggests that it is bond formation which matters and that in this context the bonds do *not* have to be with any particular person.

So with respect to "affectionless psychopathy," the term "maternal deprivation" is again rather inaccurate. It is a question of "privation" rather than "deprivation" and in so far as it is bonding which is crucial, rather than the mother, "bond privation" might be the best description.

CONCLUSION

In the time available it has not been possible to consider all the various alternatives to the suggestions put forward here, nor has it been possible to outline in any detail the evidence upon which the arguments have been based. These have been discussed at some length elsewhere (7). However, it should be evident that the concept of "maternal deprivation" is a complex one which includes a number of quite different experiences with quite different outcomes. Unless we make careful distinctions between these we are unlikely to make any progress in disentangling the various psychological mechanisms which are involved. Further research is required but it is suggested that the evidence to date indicates that the syndrome of acute distress is probably due in part to a disruption of the bonding process (not necessarily to the mother); developmental retardation and intellectual impairment are both a consequence of experiential privation; dwarfism is usually due to nutritional privation; delinquency follows family discord; and affectionless psychopathy may be the end-product of a failure to develop bonds or attachments in the first three years of life.

REFERENCES

1. AINSWORTH, M. D.: The effects of maternal deprivation: A review of findings and controversy in the context of research strategy. In *Deprivation of Maternal Care: A Reassessment of Its Effects*. Public Health Papers No. 14. W.H.O. Geneva (1962).
2. BOWLBY, J.: *Maternal Care and Mental Health*. W.H.O. Geneva (1951).
3. JESSOR, R. & RICHARDSON, S.: Psychosocial deprivation and personality development. In *Perspectives on Human Deprivation: Biological, Psychological and Sociological*. United States Department of Health, Education and Welfare (1968).
4. BOWLBY, J.: Effects on behavior of disruption of an affectional bond. In J. M. Thoday and A. S. Parkes (Eds.), *Genetic and Environmental Influences on Behaviour*. Edinburgh: Oliver and Boyd (1968).
5. BOWLBY, J.: *Attachment and Loss*. Vol. 1. Attachment. Hogarth, London (1969).

6. YARROW, L. J.: Maternal deprivation: Toward an empirical and conceptual re-evaluation. *Psychol. Bull.*, 58, 459-490. (1961).
7. RUTTER, M.: *Maternal Deprivation Reassessed.* Penguin Books, Harmondsworth (1972).
8. YARROW, L. J.: Separation from parents during early childhood. In M. L. Hoffman and L. W. Hoffman (Eds.), *Review of Child Development Research*. Vol. 1. Russell Sage Foundation, New York (1964).
9. PATTON, R. G. & GARDNER, L. I.: *Growth Failure in Maternal Deprivation*. Chas. C Thomas, Springfield, Ill. (1963).
10. VERNON, D. T. A., FOLEY, J. M., SIPOWICZ, R. R., & SCHULMAN, J. L.: *The Psychological Responses of Children to Hospitalization and Illness.* Chas. C Thomas, Springfield, Ill. (1965).
11. BERGER, M. & PASSINGHAM, R. E.: Early experience and other environmental factors: An overview. In H. J. Eysenck (Ed.), *Handbook of Abnormal Psychology*. 2nd edition (in press) (1972).
12. THOMPSON, W. R. & GRUSEC, J. E.: Studies of early experience. In P. H. Mussen (Ed.), *Carmichael's Manual of Child Psychology.* 3rd edition. Wiley, New York (1970).
13. ORLANSKY, H.: Infant care and personality. *Psychol. Rev.*, 46, 1-48 (1949).
14. O'CONNOR, N.: The evidence for the permanently disturbing effects of mother-child separation. *Acta Psychol.*, 12, 174-191 (1966).
15. WOOTTON, B.: *Social Science and Social Pathology.* Allen & Unwin, London (1959).
16. RUTTER, M.: Parent-child separation: Effects on the children. *J. Child Psychol. Psychiat.*, 12, 233-260 (1971).
17. BOWLBY, J.: Childhood bereavement and psychiatric illness. In D. Richter, J. M. Tanner, Lord Taylor, and O. C. Zangwill (Eds.), *Aspects of Psychiatric Research*. Oxford University Press, London (1962).
18. HINDE, R. A. & SPENCER-BOOTH, Y.: Individual differences in the responses of rhesus monkeys to a period of separations from their mothers. *J. Child Psychol. Psychiat.*, 11, 156-176 (1970).
19. HINDE, R. A. & SPENCER-BOOTH, Y.: Effects of brief separtion from mother on rhesus monkeys. *Science*, 173, 111 (1971).
20. HINDE, R. A.: Maternal deprivation in rhesus monkeys. *J. Psychosom. Res.*, 16, 227-228 (1972).
21. RUTTER, M. & MITTLER, P.: Environmental influences on language development. In M. Rutter and J. A. M. Martin (Eds.), *Young Children with Delayed Speech*. S.I.M.P./Wm. Heinemann, London (in press).
22. CASLER, L.: Perceptual deprivation in institutional settings. In G. Newton & S. Levine (Eds.), *Early Experience and Behaviour*. Chas. C Thomas, Springfield, Ill. (1968).
23. FRIEDLANDER, B. Z.: Listening, language and the auditory environment: Automated evaluation and intervention. In *The Exceptional Infant*. Vol. 2 Studies in Abnormalities. Brunner/Mazel (1971).
24. KERR, G. R., CHAMOVE, A. S., & HARLOW, H. F.: Environmental deprivation: Its effect on the growth of infant monkeys. *J. Pediat.*, 75, 833-837 (1969).
25. WHITTEN, C. F., PETIT, M. G., & FISCHOFF, J.: Evidence that growth failure from maternal deprivation is secondary to undereating. *J. Am. Med. Assoc.*, 209, 1675-1682 (1969).
26. BOWLBY, J.: *Forty-four Juvenile Thieves: Their Characters and Home-Life.* Bailliere, Tindall & Cox, London (1946).
27. BOWLBY, J., AINSWORTH, M., BOSTON, M., & ROSENBLUTH, D.: The effects of mother-child separation: A follow-up study. *Brit. J. Med. Psychol.*, 29, 211 (1956).
28. WOLKIND, S. N.: Children in care: A psychiatric investigation. Thesis submitted for M.D. degree, University of London (1971).

14

REMOVING INFANT RHESUS FROM MOTHER FOR 13 DAYS COMPARED WITH REMOVING MOTHER FROM INFANT

Robert A. Hinde and Lynda Davies

*MRC Unit on the Development and Integration of Behaviour,
Madingley, Cambridge (England)*

INTRODUCTION

A number of studies have shown that temporary separation from the mother may affect the behavior of infant rhesus monkeys for some time after reunion with her (refs. in Hinde and Spencer-Booth, 1971). In most of these experiments the separation involved temporary removal of the mother, the infant remaining in the same physical and social environment in which it had lived previously: in this way, any additional effects which might arise if the infant were moved temporarily to a strange environment were avoided. In the present experiment the procedure was reversed, the infant being removed to a strange cage and the mother left in her familiar environment. It was predicted that the effects on the infant of this treatment involving both separation from the mother and the trauma of a strange environment, would be more severe than those of mere removal of the mother.

Reproduced from the JOURNAL OF CHILD PSYCHOLOGY AND PSYCHIATRY, Vol. 13, 1972, pp. 227-237 with the permission of Microforms International Marketing Corp., licensee. © Pergamon Press Journal back files.

Subjects

The experiments were performed with rhesus monkeys living in small captive groups. Each group consisted of an adult male, 2-4 females and their young. Five mother-infant pairs were used, the infants (3 female and 2 male) being 30-to-32 weeks-old at the time they were removed from their mothers. Data on these "infant-removed" infants are compared with those from 6 (4 female and 2 male) "mother-removed" infants as published previously (Spencer-Booth and Hinde, 1971).

Accommodation

Each group occupied an outside pen (5.50 × 2.44 × 2.44 m) connecting with an indoor room (2.29 × 1.83 × 1.37 m) (see also Hinde and Rowell, 1962). While separated from their mothers, the infants were kept in a cage (1.13 × 1.00 × 1.18 m) in an indoor room about 50 m from and out of sight of the group: they were visually but not auditorally isolated from other monkeys in the room. The latter were caged singly or in pairs, and were not undergoing separation at the time.

Methods

Each infant was removed from its mother when between 30- and 32-weeks-old and placed in the indoor cage for 13 days, after which it was returned to its mother in the group cage. The data used in this analysis were concerned only with 3-4 days before the infant's removal, the separation period, and 4 weeks after the infant's return.

At 10.00 hours on 3 of the 4 days before the separation, routine data on mother-infant interactions and the infant's activity while off its mother were recorded (see Spencer-Booth and Hinde, 1967). These watches were continued until the infant has been off its mother for two hours or until 14.30 hours, whichever was earlier.

At 10.00 hours on day 4, the infant was caught in the outside pen and taken to the indoor room, where data on activity and vocalizations were recorded for 2 hours. These watches were repeated on days 5, 9, 12, 15 and 16. At 10.00 hours on day 17, the infant was returned and data collection began immediately as on days 1-3. Similar data were collected on days 18, 19, 21, 23, 30, 37 and 44.

For observations in the home pens the observer was in a small hut, 7.7 m from the end of the pen, and was visible to the monkeys through a window. The monkeys were thoroughly habituated to this procedure, and there was no reason to believe that the observer's presence influenced their behavior in any way. For observations in the indoor cage the observer was seated about 2 m from and in full view of the infants: in this case the animal's behavior could be affected by sudden movements by the observer.

More limited data on the mothers were also collected. On one of the four pre-separation days, and on days 4 and 15 within the separation period, the mother's locomotor activity and vocalizations were recorded from 10.00 to 12.00 hours.

Measures

The following were used in this analysis:

Time off. The percentage of half min watched in which the infant was off the mother and all other animals.

The relative frequency of rejections $(R/(A + M + R))$. Every time the infant got on or tried to get on the mother's nipple we recorded whether it was through the mother's initiative (M) or the infant's: in the latter case the infant could be accepted (A) or rejected (R). From this was calculated the proportion of the number of times the infant got on the nipple, or attempted to do so, which were rejected.

Infant's role in making successful nipple contacts. This is given by the ratio $A/(A + M)$.

Infant's role in breaking nipple contacts. When the infant came off the nipple we recorded whether it was the infant's initiative (I'), the mother's initiative (M') or mutual. The ratio $I'/(I' + M')$ gives a measure of the infant's role.

Time at a distance from mother (> 60 cm). The percentage of half min in which the infant was off in which it was recorded more than 60 cm from the mother (60 cm is roughly the distance a mother can reach in a hurry, and was assessed in relation to the 120 cm divisions of the wire netting).

Infant's role in maintaining proximity ($\%Ap - \%L$). The percentage of occasions that the distance between mother and infant decreased from more than 60 cm to less than 60 cm (approaches) or increased from less to more (leavings), that were due to movements by the infant, were calculated. The difference between the proportions of approaches and of leavings which were due to movement by the infant gives a measure of the infant's role in maintaining proximity which is relatively independent of the absolute levels of activity of the two animals (Hinde and Atkinson, 1970).

Whoo calls. The mean number of whoo calls per hundred half min in which the infant was off its mother (infant) or per hundred half min (mother).

Locomotor activity. The outside pen was subdivided into 16 "boxes" (upper and lower sections and eight equal floor areas) and the indoor cage into six. Locomotor activity was assessed in terms of the number of boxes entered per half min watched for the mother, and per half min off the mother for the infant.

Activity when active (> 5/> 1%). The number of half min in which the infant or mother enter > 5 boxes, as a percentage of the number in which it entered more than one.

Sitting (%S). The number of half min in which the animal was recorded sitting still and not engaged in any obvious activity, as a percentage of the number in which it was off its mother (infant) or the number watched (mother).

Rough-and-tumble social play (%R&T). The number of half min in which the infant engaged in rough-and-tumble social play, as a percentage of the number it was off its mother.

Approach/withdrawal social play (%A/W). The number of half min in which the infant engaged in approach/withdrawal social play, as a percentage of the number it was off its mother.

Method of Analysis

Data were analyzed separately for each animal for each watch, and were grouped as follows. The mean of the data was determined for days 1-3, days 18-23 and days 30-44, for each infant. The effects of the separation period were assessed by analyzing the data for each day of that period (days 4, 5, 9, 12, 15, 16) separately. For changes between periods, Sign tests (two-tailed) were used, while for comparisons between groups, Mann-Whitney *U* tests (two-tailed) were employed.

It must be emphasized that comparisons of infants or of mothers between infant-removed and mother-removed groups during the separation period are limited by the difference in size between the outside runs and the indoor cages.

RESULTS

Comparison of Groups Before Separation

The mother-removed and infant-removed groups did not differ significantly on any of the measures of mother-infant interaction, or of infant behavior when off mother.

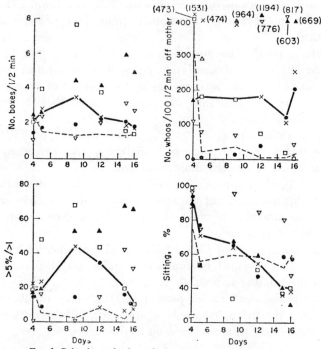

Fig. 1. Behaviour of infants during the separation period.

The symbols indicate individual infant-removed infants, the closed circle and the inverted triangle representing the data for the two males. The continuous line shows the medians for the infant-removed infants, the discontinuous one those for mother-removed infants obtained in the earlier study. Top left—locomotor activity, measured by the number of "boxes" entered per half min. Top right—whoo calling. Bottom left—activity when active. Bottom right—percentage of half min sitting doing nothing .

Behavior of the Infants During Separation (Fig. 1)

Initial hypoactivity was shown by the two males (Whisky and Matthew). On release into the indoor cage they immediately climbed into a top corner and stayed there for most of the 2 hour watch. They first moved only after 1 hour 21 minutes and 1 hour 45 minutes respectively, and when they did so their movements were slow and cautious. Matthew did not call at all, while Whisky only gave soft whoo calls when other animals in the room called. By the next day, Matthew had just started to call, while Whisky's calling had decreased from that of the previous day. They were both moving around more. On day 9, Whisky seemed to be suffering from exhaustion: his activity and calling had decreased, and although he was still whooing fairly often, he was eating very little, moving around slowly and sometimes falling over. Matthew's activity and calling continued to increase steadily. By day 12, Whisky had recovered considerably; he was more active and his calling had increased markedly, but he still spent much time inactive. Matthew showed a further increase in activity and calling. By day 15, the calling of both had increased again, but Matthew's activity had decreased very slightly. On day 16, Whisky's calling had decreased considerably but he was still quite active. He clung to the cage bars and flung his head back. Matthew's calling had increased, but his activity had decreased slightly and he was nail-biting and thumb-sucking.

Although one of the females was immobile for 20 minutes after release into the indoor cage, the others became active immediately. All three thereafter whooed frequently, and were active for much of the time, though they also frequently sat inactive. They sometimes growled at the observer. One made frantic scrabbling movements along the sides of the cage and another frequently ground her teeth. On days 5 and 9 all three showed a progressive increase in locomotor activity, accompanied in two cases by some decrease in calling. By day 12, activity was decreasing and they spent longer periods eating. The activity of two of these females decreased further by days 15 and 16, and they showed signs of depression. One sat huddled to the wall for much of the time. All three were noticeably unresponsive to the observer and to room noises. One, however, still scrabbled intermittently at the sides of the cage, and thus had a high activity score, and still called often. All three showed some stereotyped pacing of the cage. By this time all five infants had the typical depressed physical appearance of separated infants. Their coats were raised and matted, their cheeks sunken and bodies hunched.

The individual differences in the pattern of responding over the separation period, as well as the differences in cage-size, limit the usefulness of comparisons with infants of the mother-removed group during the separation period. In general the sorts of behavior shown were qualitatively similar in the two groups, but the fear and associated immobility of some of the infant-removed infants were more marked than anything seen in the mother-removed infants. Furthermore, the searching behavior and/or hyperactivity was more marked and longer-lasting in the infant-removed group: perhaps for this reason the onset of depression was delayed.

To be more specific, the initial median frequency of whoo calling was somewhat higher in the mother-removed group, owing largely to the hypoactivity of the two males in the infant-removed group. However the difference was not significant: indeed, one of the infant-removed infants called over twice as often as any other infant in either group on day 4. Subsequently the situation was reversed, the medians for the mother-removed group being lower (day 12, $p = 0.03$; day 15, $p = 0.004$; days 5, 9 and 16, *n.s.*).

Comparisons of locomotor activity between the two groups are especially liable to be influenced by the differences in cage size, but it is noteworthy that, while the median number of boxes entered was (not-significantly) higher for the mother-removed infants on the first day of separation, it was lower on all subsequent days (days 5 and 12, $p = 0.004$; day 15, $p = 0.03$; days 4, 9 and 16, *n.s.*; Mann Whitney U test, two-tailed).

The proportion of minutes in which the infants were recorded sitting showed, as might be expected, opposite trends. At first it was higher for the infant-removed group (day 4, $p = 0.02$; days 5 and 9, *n.s.*), but subsequently non-significantly lower. The decrease in %S with time was not due merely to the increase in locomotor activity of the two males, but was characteristic of all individuals (Spearman rank order correlation with serial order of observation negative in all cases, $p < 0.05$ in two).

In conclusion, although individual differences amongst the infant-removed infants were marked, their behavior during separation involved the same sort of changes as were found in the mother-removed group, but with considerable differences in degree. In particular, two animals showed initial fear and immobility, all later showed hyperactivity, and symptoms of depression appeared rather later.

Behavior of Mother During Separation (Fig. 2)

Data were collected from four mothers on day 4 and from all five before separation and on day 14. While none gave whoo-calls during the pre-separation watch, all four watched on day 4 did so. They seemed extremely restless, alternating periods of sitting (%S was higher than pre-separation in all four) with periods of activity. (No. of boxes entered higher than before separation in 3 out of 4 animals, and activity when active in all 4).

On day 14 whoo-calling had decreased virtually to zero. The frequency with which they were recorded sitting tended to be lower than on day 4 (3 out of 4 animals), but still higher than before separation (4 out of 5). Similarly, locomotor activity tended to be less than on day 4 (3 out of 4 animals) but still higher than before separation (4 out of 5).

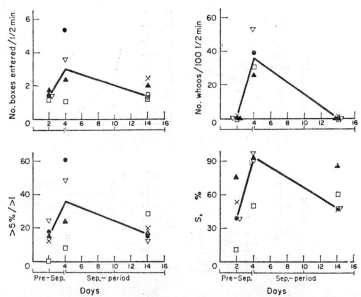

Fig. 2. Behaviour of mothers of infant-removed infants before and during separation. Symbols used for mothers are those used for their own infants in Fig. 1. Measures as in Fig. 1.

Comparison with mothers from the mother-removed group are possible only on day 4. The mother-removed mothers were recorded sitting more than the infant-removed mothers ($p = 0.03$), tended to be less active (n.s.), and were less active when active ($p = 0.01$). However the frequency of calling showed no clear difference between the groups. In general, in so far as the differences in cage size permit comparison, the mother-removed mothers appeared to be more disturbed during separation than were the infant-removed mothers.

Infant Behavior After Reunion (Fig. 3)

After reunion the behavior of the infant-removed infants differed from their pre-separation behavior in ways similar to, but less marked than, that seen in mother-removed infants. In no period did whoo-calling differ significantly from the pre-separation level. Locomotion activity was at first slightly lower, the difference for both the mean number of boxes entered per half min and for activity when active being significant for days 18-23 ($p = 0.06$, Sign test): this difference had disappeared by days 30-44. The percentage of minutes in which they were recorded sitting tended to be similar to that before separation in all periods. Although

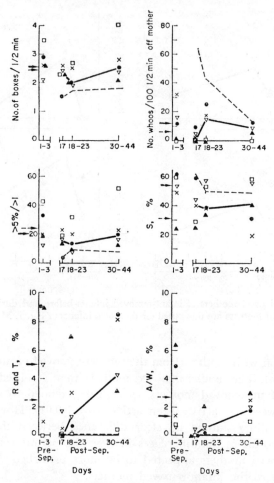

FIG. 3.   Behaviour of infants before and after the separation period.
Symbols as in Fig. 1. Measures in top 4 graphs as in Fig. 1. Bottom left—percentage of half
min in which rough-and-tumble play occurred. Bottom right—percentage of half min in which
approach/withdrawal play occurred. The thick arrow indicates the preseparation Median for the
infant-removed infants and the thin arrow that for the mother-removed infants.

social play was somewhat depressed in the early post reunion periods in
most individuals, again in no period (except for approach/withdrawal
on day 17) was the difference from preseparation level significant.

The mildness of the effects of separation on the infant-removed infants
represents a marked contrast to the mother-infants. The former whoo-
called less than the mother-removed infants in all three post re-union

periods ($p = 0.004$, $p = 0.03$ and *n.s.* respectively). They also showed more locomotor activity in all three periods (No. boxes, $p = 0.04$, 0.03 and 0.01; activity when active, *n.s.*, *n.s.* and $p = 0.004$). There were no significant differences in the percentage of minutes in which they were recorded sitting, but the infant-removed infants played significantly more than the mother-removed ones (approach-withdrawal play, *n.s.*, $p = 0.004$ and 0.004; rough and tumble play, *n.s.*, $p = 0.008$ and 0.02).

Mother-Infant Interaction After Reunion (Fig. 4)

After reunion the mother-infant relationship at first differed from that obtaining before separation in ways similar to, but less marked than, that seen in mother-removed infants. The proportion of time off the mother was lower on the day of reunion than before separation in all five cases ($p = 0.06$, Sign test, two-tailed), but the median was near or above pre-separation levels in the two later post reunion periods. The median proportion of time off which the infant spent more than 60 cm from the mother remained near the pre-separation level throughout, though it tended to be low in two individuals on days 18-23. The mothers rejected few of the infants' attempts to gain the nipple, the relative frequency of rejections being below pre-separation levels ($p = 0.06$, 0.06 and *n.s.*), but the relative responsibility of infant and mother for nipple contact was little changed. On the day of reunion the infants played a smaller role in maintaining proximity to the mothers ($p = 0.06$), though subsequently the median value of this measure returned to close to its pre-separation level.

In a number of respects the post-reunion mother-infant relationships of the infant-removed infants differed from those of the mother-removed ones. The infant-removed infants tended to spend more time off their mothers (*n.s.*, *n.s.*, and $p = 0.052$) and more of that time at a distance from them (*n.s.*, *n.s.* and $p = 0.008$). These differences could have been due to differences between the mothers of the two groups, to differences between the infants, or both (Hinde, 1969). Some measures relevant to the relative roles of mothers and infants in determining time off the mother are given in table 1. The initial reduction in time off the mother after reunion in the infant-removed infants was associated with a decrease in the relative frequency of rejections, but no significant change in the infant's role in making or breaking nipple contacts. It was thus due primarily to greater receptiveness by the mothers to the infants' demands for nipple contacts. By contrast, in the mother-removed group the frequency of rejections and the infants' role in making nipple

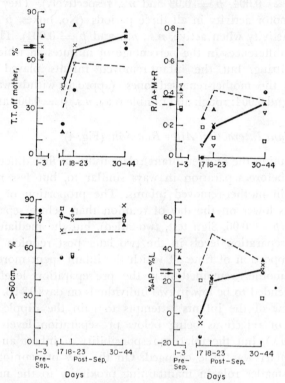

FIG. 4. Mother–infant interaction after reunion.

Symbols as in Figs. 1 and 3. Top left—total time off mother. Top right—relative frequency of rejections. Bottom left—proportion of time off mother spent at a distance from her. Bottom right—infants' role in maintaining proximity to mother when off her.

TABLE 1. RELATIVE ROLES OF MOTHER AND INFANTS IN NIPPLE CONTACTS

		Period (days)			
		Pre-separation	17	18–23	30–44
$R/(A + M + R)$	Infant-removed	0·38	0·08*	0·30*	0·34
	Mother-removed	0·33	0·26	0·42	0·31
	Sig. of inter-group difference, p	n.s.	<0·06	<0·01	n.s.
$A/(A + M)$	Infant-removed	0·94	0·90	0·92	1·0
	Mother-removed	0·89	0·92	0·93	0·92
	Sig. of inter-group difference, p	n.s.	n.s.	n.s.	<0·01
$I'/(I' + M')$	Infant removed	0·58	0·95	0·47	0·55
	Mother-removed	0·52	0**	0·06**	0·20**
	Sig. of inter-group difference, p	n.s.	<0·09	<0·01	<0·02

Median values for Infant-removed and Mother-removed groups. * and ** indicates difference from pre-separation value with $p < 0·06$ and $p < 0·02$ respectively (Sign test).

contacts changed little, but there was a marked decrease in the infants' role in breaking nipple contacts. Here, therefore, the decrease in time off was due primarily to a decrease in the role of the infants in breaking contact once they were on the nipple: the mothers did not become more receptive in the face of the infants' demands and played a greater role in terminating nipple contacts.

Similar arguments can be applied to the time spent at a distance from the mother. The non-significant change in the infant-removed group was associated with a decrease in the infants' role (i.e., increase in the mother's role) in maintaining proximity. The slight decrease in the mother-removed group was associated with a (non-significant) tendency for the infants' role in maintaining proximity to increase. However, the differences between the two groups in the infants' role in maintaining proximity did not reach significance.

In summary, the post-reunion behavior of the infant-removed group was characterized by fewer maternal rejections and a greater maternal role in maintaining proximity, while that of the mother-removed infants was characterized by a smaller maternal role in nipple contact and (non-significantly) in maintaining proximity. The lesser degree of disturbance in the infant-removed group was thus associated with a more positive role by their mothers in mother-infant interaction after reunion.

DISCUSSION

Infants removed from both their mothers and the environment with which they were familiar showed changes in behavior which were rather different from those shown by infants left in their familiar environment when their mothers were removed. While the latter showed a reduction in locomoter activity, some of the former tended to show first hyperactivity, and in association with this the onset of depression was delayed. Although differences in environmental conditions during separation make direct comparisons between the two groups difficult, it is probable that, in the absence of reunion, the infant-removed infants would have been the more profoundly disturbed.

However after reunion the reverse was the case. While the mother-removed infants continued to show obvious signs of disturbance for at least several weeks, the behavior of the infant-removed infants soon returned to levels similar to those seen before separation. At least three types of explanation could be suggested for this difference:

(i) The effects of the experience on the infants are different in *kind* in the two groups, and produce more enduring effects in the mother-removed than in the infant-removed infants. While this possibility cannot be ruled out, it seems improbable in that both groups experienced separation from the mother and the infant-removed infants experienced the strange pen as well. A difference in the opposite direction would therefore be predicted, except as indicated in (ii) below.

(ii) Apart from the trauma associated with catching, the infant-removed infants had no unpleasant experience in the home pen, while the mother-removed infants lived there throughout the separation period. The latter could therefore have become adversely conditioned to the home environment, while the former did not and therefore behaved normally as soon as they were returned to it. This possibility cannot be ruled out by our data: if it does represent an important issue, it indicates at least that the trauma of separation can be largely overcome by suitable subsequent experience.

(iii) Post-reunion behavior could depend primarily on the degree of disturbance suffered by the mothers. This was almost certainly much less in the infant-removed group. In harmony with this view are the findings that (a) the smaller degree of disturbance shown by the infant-removed infants after reunion was associated with a more rapid restoration of mother-infant relations, and (b) this involved a greater maternal role in mother-infant interaction.

Thus these findings strongly suggest that the effects sometimes produced on infant behavior and development by a period of separation from the mother may be due not (or not only) to separation *per se,* as has often been suggested for both human and subhuman primates, but (also) to the associated disturbance of the relationship between the infant and the individual who has hitherto formed the most important part of its environment.

SUMMARY

In a previous experiment, 6 rhesus monkey mothers were removed from their infants for 13 days, the infants being left in their familiar environment. Here the procedure was reversed—5 infants were removed to an isolation cage in a strange room, the mothers staying in their familiar environment. Contrary to expectation these infant-removed infants were less disturbed than the mother-removed infants. This difference was associated with, and was probably due to, a more positive role by the mothers of the infant-removed group in mother-infant interaction after reunion. It is suggested that the effects of a separation experience may be mediated in part by the disturbance to the mother-infant relationship which results.

Acknowledgments—This work was supported by the Medical Research Council and the Royal Society. We are grateful to C. Perkis for help in collection of the data, to F. Jolley for his daily care of the animals, and to members of the Department of Veterinary Clinical Studies, Cambridge, especially A. R. Jennings and D. E. Bostock, for their help.

REFERENCES

HINDE, R. A. (1969): Analyzing the roles of the partners in a behavioral interaction—mother-infant relations in rhesus macaques. *Ann. N.Y. Acad. Sci.*, 159, 651-667.

HINDE, R. A. & ATKINSON, S. (1970): Assessing the roles of social partners in maintaining mutual proximity, as exemplified by mother-infant relations in rhesus monkeys. *Anim. Behav.*, 18, 169-176.

HINDE, R. A. & ROWELL, T. E. (1962): Communication by postures and facial expressions in the rhesus monkey (*Macaca mulatta*). *Proc. Zool. Soc. Lond.*, 138, 1-21.

HINDE, R. A. & SPENCER-BOOTH, Y. (1971): Effects of brief separation from mother on rhesus monkeys. *Science*, 173, 111-118.

SPENCER-BOOTH, Y. & HINDE, R. A. (1967): The effects of separating rhesus monkey infants from their mothers for six days. *J. Child Psychol. Psychiat.*, 7, 179-197.

SPENCER-BOOTH, Y. & HINDE, R. A. (1971): The effects of 13 days maternal separation on infant rhesus monkeys compared with those of shorter and repeated separations. *Anim. Behav.*, 19, 595-605.

15

WHAT DOES RESEARCH TEACH US ABOUT DAY CARE: FOR CHILDREN UNDER THREE

Bettye M. Caldwell, Ph.D.

Director, University of Arkansas Center for Early Development and Education (Little Rock)

Until very recently research could tell us very little about day care for the child under 3, for the simple reason that there was no such research. Furthermore, there was almost no day care—that is, no officially sanctioned day care—for such young children.

By definition, day care involves separation of a child from its mother for all or part of the day. For at least two decades in this country maternal separation was considered tantamount to maternal deprivation. And, as documented in numerous clinical studies, maternal deprivation was most damaging and appeared to have the most toxic long-range effects if it occurred during the first 3 years of life. Thus, at the policy level, day care for the child under 3—and by inference, employment for his mother—was discouraged. No resources were allocated to the planning of facilities and programs for infants.

But the need for infant day care did not go away simply because neither public nor private agencies officially sanctioned it. We know that in June 1958 there were 883,000 children under 3 years of age whose mothers were employed full time. By March 1967, the number had increased to 1,024,000; of these children, 471,000 were cared for in their

---

Reprinted from CHILDREN TODAY, Vol. 1, No. 1, January-February 1972.

own homes, 427,000 were cared for in someone else's home, 77,000 were in other arrangements, and 49,000 were in group care center programs.

The Women's Lib movement had not yet been officially launched, but more and more women were entering the work force and social censure for such entry was diminishing. While maternal employment at that time was not regarded as a patriotic act, as had been the case two decades earlier, it often meant the difference between financial dependence and independence for a family. Each mother choosing to work had to find some type of day care for her very young child or children.

In addition to mothers in the work force, another group of mothers began to seek infant care. These were mothers in their teens, who benefitted from a little noticed—but dramatic—change in the attitudes and programs of public school systems toward them. Until the mid-1960's the pregnant school-age girl and the young mother were invariably excluded from continuing their education. Then demonstration projects initiated by the Children's Bureau developed special programs or classes for the continuing education of the young girl during pregnancy and the period following the birth of her baby. As a result of the rapid acceptance of this concept, about 50,000 pregnant girls today attend classes in more than 200 programs in the United States.

The encouragement and support of the mother's return to school created a new demand for infant day care during school hours. Once the demand was created, public and private community agencies began to give some thought to the provision of day care and to the development of standards. And a recent survey of 67 infant care programs showed that one-third was primarily concerned with the needs of the school-age parent.

Almost simultaneously a number of people whose original interests were far from the day care arena published descriptive studies suggesting that many children were being deprived of essential experiences in their early years in terms of sensory input, consistency of response from adults, and even emotional warmth and support. These workers saw the need to plan and arrange environments for young children that would provide favorable experiences without producing any of the deleterious byproducts associated with institutionalization. Day care for infants offered the possibility of such enrichment in a planned setting and, at the same time, a much needed service to the family.

Recognizing the potential importance of both these social currents— the desire for more day care for children under 3 and the interest in developmental environments for young children, the Child Welfare Research and Demonstration Grants program of the Children's Bureau initiated several demonstration projects in infant day care between 1964 and 1967.

Enriching Experience

On the research front, accumulating evidence suggested that during the first 3 years a child needs a certain amount and quality of experience for an optimal rate of intellectual development. Stimulated largely by the writings of Hunt (1), Bruner (2), and Bloom (3), researchers in the field of human development began to give serious consideration to whether the environments available to many young children—especially the children of the poor—adequately provided these experiences. Projects were conducted in centers in Syracuse, N. Y.; New Haven, Conn.; and Chapel Hill and Greensboro, N. C.

Although these research-based projects are still relatively young—so young that the oldest children who participated in day care from early infancy are only now reaching public school, they all have produced important information about day care for children under 3.

Of course, these were not the only centers offering infant day care. In 1967, the Parent-Child Center program, a component of Headstart, was launched in 36 cities. Planning for this project reflected, in part, the concern of many professional workers and parents that infant day care could conceivably weaken the basic ties between parent and child. Therefore, these programs concentrated on the parent-child dyad rather than the child as an individual. Several parent-child centers, however, offered infant day care.

Intellectual Development

What are the effects of day care in infancy on a child's intellectual development? This is probably the question answered most frequently by research workers concerned with early childhood because it is easier to answer than the other questions we ask. That is, there are virtually no appropriate research instruments for use with very young children, except in the area of intellectual—or more aptly, pre-intellectual—development. Of course, all the scales for assessing infants' progress touch upon all aspects of the child's development, no matter what they might be labeled. Furthermore, it can be argued that a child's rating on a developmental scale gives a valid indication of his overall social and emotional functioning.

Studies relating to the effects of day care on intellectual or cognitive development show that in general children are not harmed by experiences in a day care environment at an early age as many researchers had feared and, in fact, many young children benefit significantly from such exposure.

For example, the progress of children in the Syracuse infant development project between 1965 and 1968 has recently been summarized (4). During that time 86 children who had entered day care prior to age 3 and had remained in the program for at least 6 months were compared to a control group of 34 children from comparable social backgrounds without day care experience. Each child was rated twice, the first time on either the Cattell Infant Intelligence Scale or the Stanford-Binet test, and near the end of the study period on the Stanford-Binet test. Scores for children who had been in day care showed an increase of about 17 points while those of children in the control group showed a decrease of about 6 points.

Another study supports the finding that young children in day care were in no way cognitively harmed by their experience. Data from an infant center in Greensboro, funded as a Children's Bureau demonstration project, did not show cognitive gains associated with day care experience, however (5).

The difference between the findings of these two studies can perhaps be explained by the fact that they served different types of populations. Approximately two-thirds of the children in the Syracuse project represented economically and socially disadvantaged families, whereas those in the Greensboro sample came from middle-class families.

Social and Emotional Development

The effects of day care on a child's social and emotional development is the special interest of the infant care project conducted at the Yale Child Study Center under the direction of Sally Provence. Sensitive, detailed descriptions of the psychosocial development of a small group of children in day care are being studied to discover the way a young child internalizes the social experiences inherent in early group activities and integrates them with other significant social, emotional, and developmental tasks.

My associates at Syracuse and I have dealt with one extremely important aspect of social and emotional development—the attachment of children to their own mothers, and the reciprocal attachment of the mothers to their children (6). Primary maternal attachment is considered an essential foundation to all other social attachments that a child forms in later life (7). In order to obtain some information on how infant day care affects this basic attachment, the Syracuse staff compared two groups of mother-child dyads.

Children in one group of 18 mother-child pairs had been involved in the Syracuse day care program from the time they were approximately 1 year old. Children in the other group of 23 mother-child pairs had remained in the exclusive care of their mothers during that same period. All assessments were made when the children were approximately 30 months of age. Based on observations of interaction between the mothers and the children in a 3-hour session, interviews about the child's behavior at home, and discussions of the mother's own child-rearing patterns, a cluster of ratings pertaining to attachment behavior was made for each mother and child.

Findings of the study should be very reassuring to all persons concerned with infant day care. In terms of the attachment of the children to their own mothers, there were no significant differences between the day care and the home-reared infants. That is, the children who had been enrolled in day care and had been exposed to several adults daily since before their first birthday were just as attached to their own mothers as were the children who had remained at home during this same period.

The children were also rated on breadth of attachment, in terms of their attachment to people other than their mothers. The day care infants enjoyed interaction with other people more than the home-reared infants. This finding is compatible with data from the Schaffer and Emerson study, which showed that infants who had had extensive contacts with other people tended to develop attachment to more people than infants who had been isolated (8).

In regard to strength of attachment of the mothers for their children, there were again no major differences between the groups. One factor may affect the conclusion that "infant day care does not affect attachment": all infants in the Syracuse project were at least 6 months old when they were enrolled. This policy was adopted to permit the primary child-mother attachment to develop before the child was placed in a situation that might conceivably weaken it.

Other findings in this Syracuse study which, while not directly answering our question about the effects of day care upon social and emotional functioning, demonstrate the informational byproducts that can generally be expected from broad-based research. For example, when the day care and home-reared samples were combined, we found that strength of attachment of a child for his mother was correlated with developmental level. That is, children whose development was most advanced usually were rated as the most attached to their mothers. Similarly, there was some evidence that the most advanced babies tended to have the most attached mothers. Both of these findings corroborate the point made earlier that one cannot effectively separate intellectual development from other aspects of development.

Several other projects are continually monitoring the social and emotional development of infants whose early experience has included day care. Within the next 5 years a great deal of information on this topic should be available.

Health

The question of the effects of day care for children under 3 on their health is a major one. Because of the associated health hazards, it would have been folly until just a few years ago to advocate bringing large numbers of infants together in groups—epidemics of measles or polio could have been the disastrous consequences. Now, however, such illnesses can be controlled by immunization and, provided a family receives good medical care, they no longer need to pose a serious threat to the presence of infants in groups.

What about the array of less serious, but still troublesome, illnesses that beset infants in any environment? Specifically, what effect will infant day care have on the incidence and severity of colds and other respiratory illnesses? Will infants in groups have perpetual runny noses and will one infant in a group so spread his illness that no one will be safe?

Several infant centers are currently collecting data on this subject, but to date only the Chapel Hill research group has published preliminary results (9). Over a 5-year period, this research group studied respiratory illnesses among approximately 100 preschool children who had attended the Frank Porter Graham Child Development Center for some length of time. Most of the children entered day care before their first birthday. The average incidence of respiratory illness for this group was 8.9 illnesses per child per year. The highest incidence rate, 10 per year, was found among children under 1 year, with the figure dropping below 8 per year among the 3-year-olds.

The Chapel Hill data were compared to data from a large metropolitan community, which showed an average of 8.3 illnesses per year for 1-year-old children and 7.4 per year for those from 2 through 5.

Glezen and his associates concluded that day care might be associated with a slightly higher rate of respiratory illnesses in children under 1 year of age than for older ones but that after that age the incidence figures were very similar to those reported for home-reared children.

Data from the Chapel Hill study should be very reassuring to those who are interested in operating infant day care programs. In the Chapel Hill Center, no attempt was made to isolate the ill children unless this appeared necessary for the ill child's own well-being. Of course, high standards of cleanliness were maintained by the staff. Also, all children received excellent medical care through the program and, by 1967, a nurse and part-time pediatrician were part of the staff. Thus, one should not, from the results of this one study, rush to the conclusion that infant day care will never be associated with increased incidence of illness. Obviously the data are from a high-quality program which strove for optimal conditions for the maintenance of health. They are in the least encouraging.

Effects on Parents

What are the effects of infant day care on parents? This is an extremely important question, but one for which no objective data can be offered at present. Although the main focus of infant day care obviously is on the child, all known programs have made some effort to have an impact on parents as well. Traditionally parent involvement in day care is hard to achieve, and infant day care is no different from day care for older children in this area. One reason is not hard to understand: working mothers by definition must combine home duties and work duties, and it is often difficult for them to find time to participate in day care activities.

Most infant day care programs have attempted at least an informal evaluation of the effects of the program on participating parents, and such reactions usually are positive. Infant care directors have reported that although parents complain about opening and closing hours, behavior of a particular staff member, fees, and other essentially administrative details, they are usually enthusiastic about how the program is helping their children.

It may well be that infant day care will have important tangential effects on parents which, in turn, can only further benefit the children. That is, most parents interact positively with their children when the children please them. And parents are invariably pleased by watching their children develop well. If infant day care helps children develop their abilities to their full potential and evolve healthy patterns of social and emotional functioning, then parents are going to enjoy their interaction with the children and offer them more social reinforcement.

A hint of this pattern can be found in the already described study

from the Syracuse project that suggested the mothers of more developmentally advanced infants were more attached to their infants. Thus,
if infant day care can foster developmental advance, it can indirectly
foster more positive maternal attachment. According to everything we
now know about how infants develop, such a process can benefit both
the child and the mother—and eventually the total society.

Experience Abroad

A number of recent studies have reported on the experiences in
Europe, the Soviet Union, and Israel concerning day care for infants.
Currently, Marsden and Mary Wagner are making an intensive study
of the day care programs in Denmark, which has had a long and successful experience with group care of infants.

That country has found that it is better to locate day care centers
near the children's residence rather than the place of work for the
mother. Small neighborhood centers are preferable to large centralized
ones and all care services should be provided in the center, including
health and social services. Children up to the age of 3 are divided into
three care groups—3 to 10 months, 10 to 18 months, and 18 to 36
months. The staff ratio varies from 1 to 2 to 1 to 4 for the younger
infants and increases to 1 to 8 for the older children.

The infant care worker is a trained secondary school graduate who has
had a 1-year specialized course followed by a year's internship.

Price Tag

The cost of infant day care, of course, is extremely important. Unfortunately, at this time we do not have any firm figure for quality infant
care. In all of the Children's Bureau research and demonstration projects
care has been expensive—ranging from $2,400 to $8,000 per child per
year. These figures can be misleading, however, because a major portion of cost in every one of these programs is the research and evaluation component. In addition to the salary of all persons whose assignment is to conduct research and the cost of all research-related equipment and supplies, there are usually a large number of free personnel
who contribute to the program in one way or another—students who
work directly with the children, faculty members who offer free supervision, visitors with special competencies, and volunteers who like to
work in high-visibility programs.

Of course, one major difficulty in computing the cost of quality infant
day care is the difficulty in defining quality infant day care operationally.

Today in the field of evaluation the key word is "accountability"—the operators of programs must specify precise behavioral objectives and demonstrate that the programs do indeed accomplish these objectives. In the data of infant day care, we are trying to create settings in which little children can develop well and happily. We know that we do not wish to equate such a diffuse goal with so many points on a developmental test.

So what can we use instead? Those who are interested in spreading the potential benefits of infant day care to a wider group must be willing to come to grips with this unpleasant but essential question. Until such time as our society has adequate resources to meet every social need, every service must justify its claim on the public resources. At this juncture it appears that infant day care will be able to do that. A necessary first step is the accumulation of much more objective information about the effects of such an experience on all aspects of infant and family functioning.

REFERENCES

1. HUNT, J. McV.: *Intelligence and Experience*. New York: Ronald Press, 1961.
2. BRUNER, J. S.: *The Process of Education*. Cambridge, Mass.: Harvard University Press, 1960.
3. BLOOM, B. S.: *Stability and Change in Human Characteristics*. New York, N. Y.: John Wiley and Sons, 1964.
4. CALDWELL, B. M.: "Impact of Interest in Early Cognitive Stimulation." In H. E. Rie (Ed.): *Perspectives in Child Psychopathology*. New York, N. Y.: Aldine-Atherton, 1971.
5. KEISTER, M. E.: *"The Good Life" for Infants and Toddlers*. Washington, D. C.: National Association for the Education of Young Children, 1970.
6. CALDWELL, B. M., WRIGHT, C. M., HONIG, A. S., & TANNENBAUM, J.: "Infant Day Care and Attachment." *American Journal of Orthopsychiatry*, April 1970.
7. AINSWORTH, MARY: "Object Relations, Dependency, and Attachment: A Theoretical Review of the Infant-Mother Relationship." *Child Development*, December 1969.
8. SCHAFFER, H. R. & EMERSON, P. E.: "The Development of Social Attachments in Infancy." *Monograph of the Society for Research in Child Development*, 1954.
9. GLEZEN, W. P., LODA, F. A., CLYDE, W. A., JR., SENIOR, R. J., SCHEAFFER, C. I., CONLEY, W. G., & DENNY, F. W.: "Epidemiologic Patterns of Acute Lower Respiratory Diseases of Children in a Pediatric Group Practice." *Journal of Pediatrics*, March 1971

PART III: PARENT-CHILD SEPARATION

16

CHARACTERISTICS OF THE EMO-
TIONAL PATHOLOGY OF THE
KIBBUTZ CHILD

Mordecai Kaffman, M.D.

Medical Director, Kibbutz Child and Family Clinic,
Tel Aviv, Israel

Over the past twenty years, the author has had the oppor-
tunity to study the developmental patterns as well as the
incidence and nature of emotional disorders exhibited by
the kibbutz child population. Kibbutz children and youth
do not reveal any specific personality type, developmental
deviations, or distinctive psychiatric syndromes. The author
has not found a single case of non-organic early childhood
psychosis among 3,000 kibbutz emotionally disturbed chil-
dren referred to the kibbutz clinics.

To the casual observer, the kibbutz might seem the ideal milieu for
establishing stereotyped patterns of normal and abnormal behavior and
definite similarities in the personality structure of children. The basic
conditions appear to be so homogeneous and stable that one may be led
to believe there is a reasonable chance of discovering a distinctive, collective prototype of child and adolescent kibbutz personality, as well as a
uniform type of child psychopathology.

Reprinted from the AMERICAN JOURNAL OF ORTHOPSYCHIATRY, 42 (4), July 1972, pp.
692-709. Copyright © 1972, the American Orthopsychiatric Association, Inc. Reproduced by permission.

241

KIBBUTZ PERSONALITY TYPES

In our modern Western society, it is difficult to find an example of egalitarian and homogeneous cultural and environmental conditions parallel to those of the kibbutz. Kibbutz children grow up and develop in a cultural and economic framework rooted in the principles of cooperation and equality. Each child enjoys a common standard of accommodation, food, clothing, education, and cultural facilities. The kibbutz knows no slums, economic insecurity, or disadvantaged families of low socio-economic status. The children are brought up in a group in which there are no significant variations in child-rearing aims, methods and practices; in the standards of its schools, in the content and form of its educational program; in its pedagogic systems; and in the quality of its teachers. Kibbutz children are exposed to similar kinds of cultural, entertainment, and mass media influences. The amount of time that children spend with their parents is also allocated on a standard basis. By general agreement, rules are laid down to determine the division of responsibility among the various parties with whom the child has contact in the process of its social development—parents, teachers, the children's group and, the kibbutz as a whole. Thus, this type of society apparently embodies ideal conditions for transforming the literary fiction of *Brave New World* into an everyday reality.

In fact, this is not the case. Some authors (4, 15, 18) have indeed attempted to define the specific characteristics of the kibbutz *sabra,* and to isolate the modal personality prototype of this kibbutz child and adolescent, but their conclusions are confusing and contradictory. There are almost as many definitions of the personality of the sabra as there are researchers who have dealt with the subject, mostly through unsystematic observation, interviews, questionnaires, and psychological tests performed on small samples of kibbutz adolescents.

According to some of these definitions, the "typical" kibbutz adolescent appears to be decidedly introvert, emotionally insecure, inhibited, and shy with strangers or with members of the kibbutz outside of his own age group; at the other extreme, such adolescents have been described as emotionally stable and extroverted youngsters, capable of adapting themselves to any social environment. On the one hand, they have been described as emotionally and intellectually depleted, with uniform interests, narrow horizons, and little originality (4); on the other hand, as more intellectually gifted than other youth groups in Israeli society, able to perform non-routine tasks, and rich in emotional expression and creative ability in numerous fields of activity. The same kibbutz adolescent is sometimes described as a dependent personality incapable of individual initiative outside the framework of the kibbutz; at other times as the opposite—an independent personality, and capable of outstanding achievement in social activities, at work, in the management of diverse branches of the kibbutz, as an army officer, or as a university student.

It is no wonder that these reports, portraying a hypothetical, homogenized type of kibbutz *sabra,* have emanated mainly from authors whose representations of the adolescent personality structure were drawn up following a brief visit to a kibbutz frequently without knowledge of the language, and mainly on the basis of casual observations, anecdotal data, and psychometric responses of an unrepresentative sample of adolescents in the absence of adequate control studies. We should not, therefore, be too surprised that, in many cases, the "typical" personality structure of kibbutz youth, portrayed as characteristic of an entire generation of adolescents, is almost identical with the preconceived theoretical viewpoint of a particular author, as regards the emotional significance and potential effect of the form of upbringing practiced in the kibbutz on the development of the child's personality.

It follows that the child-parent relationship in the kibbutz can be described and analyzed from opposing standpoints and contradictory theoretical approaches. On the one hand, the kibbutz system of education can be defined as "intermittent multiple mothering" (15) or as "parental role rejection," implying some degree of maternal deprivation and diffusion of the mother-image, leading to excessive frustration, and impaired capacity on the part of the child to develop significant relationships in later life, due to "repression of affection and emotional flatness" (4). On the other hand, the same kibbutz system of education can be shown to produce a different type of child personality pattern when it is regarded as a "collaborative child-rearing program in which parents and other adults co-ordinate their child-rearing tasks on behalf of the child from infancy on" (11). In this case, the author probably assumes that the additional positive emotional centers and the dilution of the tight ties of dependency present in monomatric families should lead to increased personality autonomy along with "more subtle and more complex personality characteristics, presumably because of more varied identification figures" (20).

Despite all this, we do not contend that the various types of kibbutz *sabra* personality that we find portrayed in professional literature represent self-confirming conclusions that fit preconceived theoretical views on the psychological significance of kibbutz education. It stands to reason that the above-mentioned descriptions all contain elements of truth and untruth; in other words, that in reality there is no such things as an archetype of kibbutz *sabra,* but a wide spectrum of diverse personality patterns that make it very simple to find confirmation for the theoretical hypothesis one happens to believe in.

Consequently, it is much easier for the foreign investigator who spends only a short time in the kibbutz to discover an assumed homogeneous type of kibbutz adolescent than it is for the Israeli clinical workers who have spent twenty years or more in close contact with such youngsters, but have not yet succeeded in isolating a distinctive and singular kibbutz personality prototype.

THE INTERACTION OF PSYCHO-SOCIAL CONDITIONS

Naturally there are certain traits that distinguish the generation that founded the kibbutz from the following generation, born, reared and educated in the kibbutz. But these differences do not indicate the formation of a stereotyped personality in either generation. Generally, the first generation was, and is, more concerned than the succeeding generation with the ideological basis of their activities. It must be remembered that we are speaking of a highly selective group of people, most of whom left their countries of origin of their own free will, for idealistic reasons. In establishing the kibbutzim, they continued to seek an ideological *raison d'être* for the revolutionary step they had taken, and, in their new-found identity, to justify the change that had taken place in their lives. The kibbutz presented a many-sided challenge, a new form of enterprise that embraced all aspects of social life, work, culture, politics, education, and defense—each of them without blueprints or precedent. Ideology was essential for members of the founding generation. They were a select handful of people linked by common values that distinguished them from the majority in their immediate surroundings, who, though Jews of similar background, did not find their way to the kibbutz.

The second and third generations had no need for ideology to justify the special way of life of the kibbutz. Those born in the kibbutz grew up within an established socio-economic framework and a well-defined ideological program. The choice confronting the second generation was to conform to existing conditions, to preserve and develop them according to the tenets they had inherited, or to become a revolutionary generation by destroying the very framework of the kibbutz. Since conditions prevailing in Israel today are not conducive to radical change in the structure of the society as a whole, and of the kibbutz in particular, it is not surprising that the kibbutz-born generation is not concerned to the same degree as its parents' with the ideology underlying the meaning of the kibbutz. That the second generation exhibits some common peer-group values and judgments in regard to more immediate ideological and social problems is not sufficient to enable us to speak of the emergence of a uniform personality among kibbutz members, just as it cannot be deduced from the fact that a large number of soldiers fighting on the same front and identifying themselves with a common military objective have uniform personality characteristics.

Thus, even in a setting such as that of the kibbutz, where all children are exposed to similar external influences, the specific and divergent conditions under which each individual child grows up outbalance and supersede the common factors.

Marcus et al. (14), whose observations of a group of kibbutz children included an analysis of 201 behavior items embracing nine categories of temperament, confirmed what all parents and educators in the kibbutzim take for granted—that each child has his own individual psychology, his own particular pattern of development, and his own predominant temperamental traits, despite the relative similarity of environmental factors. (Though even in the kibbutz, environmental conditions and the various factors influencing the individual child are far from being stable and uniform; in fact, the list of distinctive variants with regard to each child is so lengthy that it would be impossible to deal with them all in a single paper.)

EMOTIONAL PROBLEMS

The specific influences surrounding the individual child manifest themselves first and foremost in the enormous diversity of psycho-social functioning patterns within the family and, secondly, in the wide degree of diversity in the personality of his educators and the composition of the child's group, as well as in peculiarities and variations in child rearing practices among different kibbutzim, and sometimes even within the same kibbutz.

Thus the interaction of *individualized* constitutional, temperamental, and environmental factors explains why we have failed to find a clear-cut common denominator in the personality structure of the second generation in the kibbutz. Apparently for the same reason, kibbutz children attending the Kibbutz Child Guidance Clinics do not reveal any psychiatric syndrome peculiar to the kibbutz nor any particular cluster of symptoms typical of, or prevalent in, kibbutz children. We do, however, find a large variety of psychiatric diagnostic entities that are generally analogous to the clinical syndromes described by other clinics dealing with children from private families.

The severity of emotional problems, the distribution of diagnostic groups, and the symptomatic manifestations may differ when one compares samples of kibbutz and non-kibbutz emotionally disturbed children (13). Yet, to the best of my knowledge, there are no psychiatric diagnostic categories detected among Western private families that cannot also be found among kibbutz children. To illustrate the point, we may mention that cases exist among kibbutz adolescents of anti-social personality, juvenile delinquency, drug addiction, and sexual deviation, even though their incidence is quite minimal and exceptional.

In regard to the frequency of emotional problems among kibbutz children, our figures do not reveal any fundamental differences between this group and other social groups of Western cultural origin. However, we cannot draw any definite conclusion in view of the paucity and inaccuracy of comparative epidemiological data regarding the frequency of emotional disorders in representative samples of children of different age-levels. Actually, it is hardly possible to compare respective statistical findings because of the variations in definitions, diagnostic criteria, and methods used by different professional people to identify patterns of emotional pathology.

It has been estimated by the U.S. Commission on the Mental Health of Children (17) that about ten percent of the children in the United States are in need of psychiatric help. This appears to be a rather conservative estimate reflecting the prevalent views expressed by various professional workers dealing with the subject (16). Other studies suggest a higher incidence of emotional disturbance in childhood. Chess et al. (8), in their longitudinal study of the behavioral development of 136 children who were observed from early infancy, reported an incidence of 21% of behavioral disturbances in children up to the age of seven years. These children were submitted for psychiatric observation as a result of persistent concern over their deviant behavior on the part of their parents, their teachers, or both. A screening survey of school children in a regular rural school in Minnesota (19) revealed that 22% of the children in the 10-12 year age group displayed evidence of moderate to serious emotional impairment. Actually, different epidemiological studies produce quite conflicting figures as to the "average" proportion of children in need of professional advice and care due to emotional problems, the figures ranging from 1% to 40% (6).

For the time being, we have no way of overcoming this embarrassing statistical situation, which results from lack of uniformity in research methods of detecting psychiatric disorders in children. On the other hand, the kibbutz would appear to be able to provide suitable conditions for obtaining more accurate and reliable figures on the frequency of psychopathological disorders in kibbutz children. One must, of course, be circumspect when making comparisons with other groups because of the different criteria adopted by the kibbutz in determining a child's need for treatment. Most kibbutzim possess not only the basic conditions and the practical tools for early diagnosis and treatment of children with psychological problems, but also a generally positive attitude towards mental problems, which encourages parents and teachers to seek professional advice in any case of behavior problems or maladjustment in the child (12). This is also made easier by the existence of centralized diagnostic therapeutic services provided by educational specialists in the kibbutzim and by the professional workers of the Kibbutz Children's Clinic, to which each individual kibbutz is attached.

Over the past twenty years, the author has had a unique opportunity to observe the incidence and nature of emotional disorders exhibited by the child population of one particular kibbutz settlement. The kibbutz in question may be regarded as typical from every point of view. It was founded 23 years ago and has a population of 500, including 200 children and adolescents under the age of eighteen. Each of these children has been under regular psychiatric observation, with the close cooperation of his parents and teachers, by means of systematic follow-up of the child within his group, within his family, and, if necessary, through individual psychiatric interviews. The psychiatrist meets regularly with each of the teachers of the various age groups in order to obtain an up-to-date report on the development, achievements, and problems of each child. For the past twenty years, the author has devoted an average of ten hours a week to this longitudinal study, being assisted by two special educators who work full-time in the kibbutz helping children who have emotional difficulties. Clearly this kibbutz is exceptional in having advanced facilities for the detection, diagnosis, therapy, and follow-up of the various types of psychological, developmental, and organic disturbances of the child. Indeed, it would be hard to find any other place in the world in which it would have been possible to carry out such intensive psychiatric observations over such an extended period of time on the emotional development of its entire child population.

It is not the purpose of this paper to give a detailed description of the findings of this longitudinal study. It will suffice to point out that

Table I

PSYCHIATRIC DIAGNOSTIC DISTRIBUTION OF
196 EMOTIONALLY DISTURBED KIBBUTZ
CHILDREN (EXCLUDING ORGANIC
CASES AND MENTAL DEFICIENCY)
AGED 3–18 YEARS

PSYCHIATRIC DIAGNOSIS	N	%
REACTIVE BEHAVIOR DISORDERS (ALL TYPES)	150	76
Overanxious (Neurotic Traits)	48	24
Unsocial-Aggressive	42	21
Infantile-Immature	39	20
Withdrawing	13	6
Hyperkinetic	8	4
PSYCHONEUROTIC DISORDERS (ALL TYPES)	26	13
Mixed or Undifferentiated Neurosis	12	6
Anxiety Neurosis	7	3
Obsessive-Compulsive Neurosis	4	2
Phobic Neurosis	2	1
Conversional Neurosis	1	.5
PERSONALITY DISORDERS (ALL TYPES)	10	5
Inadequate-Immature	5	2
Passive-Aggressive	2	1
Antisocial (Psychopathic)	2	1
Explosive-Epileptoid	1	.5
BORDERLINE PSYCHOSIS	2	1
SCHIZOPHRENIC PSYCHOSIS	2	1
OTHER DIAGNOSTIC CATEGORIES	6	3

in this kibbutz, which undoubtedly has ideal conditions for an accurate determination of the incidence of emotional disorders in children, we have found a strikingly constant annual proportion of children in need of help due to psychological difficulties, the rate being 12%-15% of the total sample. Out of a sample of 124 children ranging in age from 5-18, sixteen of them (13%) have been under psychiatric treatment for a year or more, the vast majority because of reactive behavior disorders, and only a small minority due to more internalized neurotic problems. The above-mentioned proportion of children needing systematic psychological treatment, at least once a week, relates to all the children in this kibbutz with moderate to serious psychiatric disturbances who have received psychotherapy in the course of the past five years. Boys were referred for psychological help in a consistently higher ratio than girls, especially during the primary school years. Altogether, three times more boys than girls were in need of prolonged forms of psychotherapy. Since, in this sample, both boys and girls lived in the same social environment, had the same educators as referral sources, and were screened by a single psychiatrist using uniform diagnostic criteria, the unequal sex distribution of emotional deviation during school years indicates that boys display more overt impressive types of clinical symptomatology, which increases the chances of earlier detection and/or of an open conflict with their surroundings.

In addition to the group of 13% of children receiving psychotherapy, there are other children with psychological problems who display only mild developmental or reactive disturbances, which did not necessitate regular therapy. When all types of non-organic behavioral disturbances, including children with relatively mild symptomatic clinical pictures, are combined together, we reach an impressive figure of 42% for kibbutz children aged 5-18 who have been referred to a psychiatrist at least once on account of psychological symptoms of varying severity.

Although we have no documentary evidence, it is our firm belief that, taken as a whole, this group of 200 kibbutz children whom we have followed for twenty years does not exhibit exceptional features in the incidence of pathology. On the contrary, it is our impression that, on the whole, they have fewer serious problems than children from comparable non-kibbutz settings. If our assumption is correct, we would then have proof that there is, after all, no serious danger inherent in a close, long-term relationship with a psychiatrist.

PSYCHOPATHOLOGY OF THE KIBBUTZ CHILD:
PREVALENT PSYCHIATRIC CATEGORIES

With a view to demonstrating the basic features that characterize the psychopathology of the kibbutz child, we will now present an analysis of our findings with respect to a group of 196 children and adolescents aged between three and eighteen who were referred to the Kibbutz Child and Family Clinic during the years 1966-1969, because of all types of emotional disorders (Table 1).

This group includes only children born in the kibbutz for whom a comprehensive diagnostic evaluation has been completed, including psychiatric and psychological assessment. A second group of 57 children showing clinical signs of neurological impairment (mainly cases of "minimal brain damage" and/or mental deficiency) are not included in this survey, which covers purely psychogenically determined disturbances.

Of the 196 children in the psychogenic group, three-quarters were under the age of twelve, most of them being in the 6-12 age group. A lower proportion of children in the 12-18 age group were referred to the Clinic, but this fact should not be used as a basis for conclusions as to the real frequency of emotional disturbances in the preadolescent and adolescent years, since these age groups show an increasing reluctance to agree to attend consultations or treatment. It must be borne in mind that at adolescence there is less close contact between the youth and his educators and also less possibility for close observation of his problems in contrast to the lower age groups, when the kibbutz child is in a small group and subject to much more concentrated educational supervision.

There exists a distinct and understandable difference in the nature and severity of psychiatric problems exhibited by kibbutz children before and after puberty. Up to the age of twelve, the most prevalent diagnosis is that of "Behavior Disorders of Childhood." Out of the total number of children in the 3-12 age range who were referred to the Clinic, 96% fell into this category. The frequency of "Reactive Behavior Disorders" in the complete sample of 196 children through age eighteen amounted to 76%. Needless to say, this common diagnostic label relates to a heterogeneous group of out-turning patterns of deviant behavior, which have developed as a symptomatic reaction to an unfavorable environment or to traumatic occurrences in the absence of a crystallized neurotic conflict or chronic personality disorder. In the 12-15 age group, the relative frequency of reactive disorders among kibbutz children decreases, while there is a steady increase as the age curve rises in the frequency of neurotic and personality disorders, which are the most usual diagnostic categories in the 12-18 age group. The severity of emotional pathology becomes increasingly intensified after the age of 12—a phenomenon readily understood in consequence of the rise in the proportion of diagnostic categories related to internalized psychoneurotic conflicts and well-structured personality disorders after the age of puberty.

In the 12-18 age range, a sample of 50 youngsters referred to our Clinic revealed the following psychiatric diagnostic distribution: psychoneurosis, all types, 46%; personality disorders, all types, 20%; behavior disorders, 20%; borderline patients, 4%; schizophrenic process, 4%; other diagnostic categories, 6%.

Table 2

DIAGNOSTIC DISTRIBUTION OF 150 KIBBUITZ CHILDREN WITH REACTIVE BEHAVIOR DISORDERS, BY AGE

TYPE OF BEHAVIOR DISORDER	AGE 3-6		AGE 6-9		AGE 9-12		AGE 12-18		AGE 3-18	
	N	%	N	%	N	%	N	%	N	%
Overanxious (Neurotic Traits)	6	27	19	33	18	30	5	45	48	32
Unsocial-Aggress've	10	45	19	33	11	18	2	18	42	28
Infantile-Immature ("Spoiled")	3	14	13	23	21	35	2	18	39	26
Withdrawing	0	0	2	3	9	15	2	18	13	9
Hyperkinetic	3	14	4	7	1	2	—	—	8	5

The integrated evaluation of the family therapist and the psychiatrist, as the degree of severity of the emotional disorders, rated 26% of the cases in the 12-18 age group as severe pathology, as compared with about half this proportion (14%) among children under twelve.

BEHAVIOR DISORDERS OF CHILDHOOD

We have attempted to classify the kibbutz children belonging to the primary or reactive behavior disorder group into seven major categories in accordance with the directives and definitions proposed in the Second Edition of the Diagnostic and Statistical Manual of Mental Disorders published by the American Psychiatric Association (10). We found that the great majority of those kibbutz children diagnosed as "Behavior Problems" fit into three diagnostic subcategories, each of which encompassed a fairly similar proportion of the children with behavior problems, namely 26-32% (see Table 2).

The three subgroups of behavior problems that appear to reflect the most prevalent and characteristic representation of the psychopathology of pre-adolescent kibbutz children are:

1) The familiar picture of the immature "spoiled" child, who retains an exaggerated feeling of omnipotence and is confident of his power to control his surroundings mainly through nagging demand or antagonistic behavior. The child's frustration tolerance is low; he expects immediate gratification of his desires. His behavior is childish and unbefitting to his age, and he exhibits excessive dependence, immaturity, and inadequate achievement in diverse areas of socialization and training. However, overtly aggressive actions do not play a central role in the symptomatic reactions present in this type of behavior disorder.

2) The unsocial aggressive type of reaction: this group includes kibbutz children with a recurring behavioral pattern of physical and verbal hyperaggressiveness. They do not get along well with their group peers and their siblings, and often become involved in quarrels and fights. They maintain a belligerent attitude of hostile disobedience in their relationships with parents and educators. They may react to frustrating situations with explosive outbursts of anger, destructiveness, and loss of control. Sometimes these children show antisocial responses such as repeated lying, truancy, and pilfering. However, we do not include in this group children who show a consistent pattern of delinquent actions and ego-syntonic antisocial behavior, since the latter are classified in the psychiatric category of psychopathic personality disorders.

In both of the above-mentioned groups, we often come across two widespread symptomatic manifestations at school age, namely, manifold types of scholastic problems and persistent enuresis.

3) The third group includes children evidencing overanxious reaction types of behavior disorders. This diagnosis is actually a semantic variation of what we generally term "neurotic traits" (1). The predominant elements in their clinical make-up are excessive anxiety, with symptomatic behavior such as general inhibition and apprehension, lack of self-confidence, fear in facing new situations, oversensitivity, shyness, passivity, sleep difficulties, exaggerated fears, and so on. The over-anxious type of behavior disorder constitutes a more flexible and changeable in-turning pattern than do psychoneurotic cases characterized by rigidly internalized and repetitive symptomatic patterns.

It goes without saying that, in practice, one rarely finds sharply delineated, self-contained symptomatic clusters, and the symptoms of two or more subcategories often appear concurrently. For instance, one may find a combination of marked emotional immaturity together with hyperaggressiveness, or the concomitant presence of inadequate control of hostile impulses, overanxiety, and fear. However, in most cases, it is possible to identify the central core of the prevalent symptomatology for the purpose of determining the appropriate subcategory in classifying the behavioral problems.

Our sample of 150 kibbutz children with behavior disorders showed a significantly higher proportion of boys than girls (96 as against 54), equivalent to a male-female ratio of 1.8 to 1. This ratio is comparable to the sex ratio revealed in the overall sample of 196 psychogenic children referred to our clinic. Here, too, we found a clear preponderance of males (1.7 boys to 1 girl).

There is a significant difference in the respective prevalence of the various types of behavior disorders as between boys and girls. The frequency of the unsocial-aggressive types of reaction is considerably higher in boys than in girls. For each girl diagnosed in this sub-category of behavioral disorder, we found 3.2 boys in whom excessive aggressiveness constituted the central clinical manifestation. Out of 96 boys with behavior disturbances, 32 of them (33%) were classified as having unsocial-aggressive types of reactions, as compared with only 10 girls out of 54 (18%).

Since environmental and educational conditions are very similar for both sexes among kibbutz children, it would appear reasonable to conclude that the difference is determined primarily by constitutional factors. Our observations are in accord with the common finding outside the kibbutz that preschool boys tend to show a higher frequency of aggressive behavior in reacting to frustrating situations and environmental inadequacies than do preschool girls.

In contrast to the preponderance of boys with aggressive behavior disorders, when we turn to the emotionally immature, "spoiled" type of child, we find a relatively higher frequency among girls. Out of the group of 54 girls with diverse behavior disorders, 33% fell into this category of arrested emotional development, as compared with 22% of the boys. The overanxious type of behavior disorder showed much the same incidence in boys (31%) as in girls (33%).

Thus we can discern two dominant, though apparently contradictory, clinical pictures among kibbutz boys under the age of 12: 1) exaggerated out-turning aggressive reactions and impulsive overactivity, and 2) overanxiety, fears, and general inhibition. The latter pattern also appears frequently among girls with behavior disorders (one-third of the sample), but in another third of the girls we find the symptomatic cluster of infantile omnipotence and underdeveloped emotional maturity instead of the reactive behavior pattern of uninhibited aggressiveness typical of the male sex. We believe it important to draw attention to the fact that the breakdown of the various symptomatic clusters of behavioral disorders differs from one age group to another. The incidence of aggressive types of behavioral disorders declines noticeably as the children get older. After the age of nine, kibbutz children show a distinct tendency to discontinue or modify aggressive patterns of reaction in response to emotional frustration or deprivation.

It would appear that the specific structure of the kibbutz (a closed cohesive society sharply critical of any dissident conduct, particularly with regard to violence, which might threaten the stability or the very existence of the group) does not foster the occurrence or maintenance of aggressive behavior. The group dynamics of children brought up together in an atmosphere that stresses the values of co-operation and mutual assistance, acts as an important restraining factor and as a positive model of identification, which neutralizes or channels away individual anti-social responses. Perhaps the early and progressive inclusion of work assignments and other responsibilities in the daily schedule of the kib-butz child (from the first grade in primary school) also contributes towards mitigating symptoms of aggressive conduct and diverting them into more socially acceptable patterns of behavior.

It is not the intention of this paper to analyze the significance of our findings in respect of the relative prevalence of the referral symptoms in the psychogenic group included in our study. For the present, we will simply draw attention to the fact that the most frequent symptom from age six onwards was learning difficulties, accompanied by scholastic under-achievement. In the kibbutz school we meet with a wide span of learn-ing problems that do not differ symptomatically from those learning disorders observed elsewhere.

Enuresis is a frequent symptom under the age of twelve (appearing in one-third of our cases), but becomes very rare among kibbutz pre-adolescents and adolescents (only 4% of our cases in the 12-plus group). Antisocial behavior such as truancy, lying, stealing, and other delinquent actions are very unusual referral symptoms.

PSYCHONEUROSIS AMONG KIBBUTZ ADOLESCENTS

The diagnosis of psychoneurosis was made in 26 children (13%) of the group of 196 included in our study. We are unable to point to any particularly characteristic symptoms or signs of neurosis in kibbutz children. The vast majority of cases diagnosed as childhood neurosis were adolescents. Below the age of nine we found no clear-cut fixated neurotic patterns, but only transient or reactive types of phobic and anxiety symptoms, including animal phobias, sleep disturbances, and diverse fears. These younger children with transitory unstructured types of anxiety reaction were included in the "overanxious" category of be-havior disorders (10), which appears to be a semantic innovation re-placing the former diagnostic categories of "neurotic traits" (1) and "neurotic behavior disorders" (7).

Psychoneurosis is the most frequently met emotional disturbance among kibbutz children over the age of 12 (46% of the children be-longing to the psychogenic group in the 12-18 age range).

In conformity with our findings in a previous study (9), the present group of 26 neurotic kibbutz adolescents also shows a clear-cut tendency of higher frequency of neurotic conditions in girls parallel to increase in age. The current survey shows a male-female sex ratio of 1.6 to 1 in the occurrence of psychoneurosis under the age of fifteen, while in the 15-18 age group, we find an equal number of boys and girls with neurotic problems, although even at this age a larger number of boys than girls were referred to the Clinic.

This progressive trend in the frequency of neurotic disorders in girls continues even more strikingly after the age of eighteen. Of the kibbutz-born young men and women in the 20-30 age group who have been referred to our Clinic because of neurotic disturbances, there are twice as many women as men.

We will not attempt here to analyze the possible reasons for the gradual change in the relative incidence of each of the various diagnostic categories in relation to age and sex. But it is clearly evident that, up to the age of adolescence, far more boys are referred for treatment as a consequence of externalized conflicts taking the form of behavior disorders. Later on, in the teens, the proportion of girls with internalized neurotic conflicts increases considerably, until it equals and gradually exceeds the proportion of males with neurotic disturbances. It is by no means certain that this particular feature is characteristic only of kibbutz children and adolescents; indeed, it is our impression that a parallel picture prevails outside the kibbutz, apparently for similar reasons.

As to the characteristics of the symptoms and clinical features observed in the group of 26 neurotic kibbutz children and adolescents, we found that in a high proportion of cases we were dealing with a mixed type of neurosis. Anxiety constitutes the most outstanding primary feature and is associated with several other neurotic manifestations, such as general inhibition, fear of some bodily, intellectual, or psychic abnormality, feelings of inferiority, preoccupation with health problems, diverse phobic fears, etc. Approximately two-thirds of our cases of neurosis were diagnosed as anxiety neurosis or mixed-undifferentiated types of neurosis. The remaining third is divided according to the central cluster of symptoms between obsessive-compulsive neurosis, phobic neurosis, and conversional neurosis.

PERSONALITY DISORDERS

The diagnosis of personality disorders involving a deep-seated characterologic constellation of maladaptive patterns of behavior was established as a principal or sole diagnostic category in ten children aged

12-18 (5% of the whole psychogenic group). This diagnosis did not appear at all in children below the age of twelve.

The following subcategories of personality disorders were found among 10 out of 50 kibbutz adolescents aged 12-18 who were referred to our Clinic because of emotional difficulties: five cases of Inadequate-Immature Personality (10% of the group); two cases of Passive-Aggressive Personality (4%); two cases of Antisocial Personality (4%); and one Explosive-Epileptoid Personality (2%).

We think it important to stress that the incidence of antisocial types of personality disorder (psychopathic or sociopathic personality) was extremely low, constituting only one percent of our total simple of 196 kibbutz children. In the light of twenty years of clinical experience in diagnosing and treating kibbutz children with emotional problems, we believe that this very low percentage of sociopathic children is a characteristic of the psychopathology of the kibbutz child. In this matter, there is a clear and substantial difference in the diagnostic distribution of the children referred to the Kibbutz Clinic, as compared with a parallel group of non-kibbutz children referred to an urban Child Guidance Clinic. In working with urban children referred to the Kupat Holim (Sick Fund) Mental Health Clinic in Haifa, we found that seven percent were diagnosed as sociopathic adolescents (13)—in other words, that there were seven times the number of cases of structured antisocial personality than in kibbutz children of the same age. We have already drawn attention to the fact that, among the unsocial type of reactive behavior disorders, a gradual decline occurs in the frequency and intensity of aggressive symptoms as age increases. The very rare appearance of fixed antisocial or sociopathic personality disorders would appear to be further evidence of the same process, indicating that the kibbutz system of education provides adequate means for socializing and positive models of identification, so as to modify and attenuate both reactive and structured patterns of antisocial behavior.

A combination of several factors may explain the apparently low incidence of hostile social responses. It should be borne in mind that, from many points of view, kibbutz methods of upbringing and education embody some of the essential conditions for moderating excessive aggressive responses on the part of the child. Generally speaking, kibbutz child-rearing practices are characterized, both in the parents' home and in the children's quarters, by a considerable tolerance for "normal" expression of aggressive behavior in young children, through limited use of punitive, frustrating, or restrictive forms of control, and through ample availability of motor outlets, social activity, and group interaction from an early age. Incidentally, the kibbutz peer group can exercise considerable pressure against dissident aggressive behavior. The peers tend to replace parents and educators as interpreters and enforcers of their moral code.

The kibbutz peer group constitutes a very influential socializing agent, and acceptance or rejection by one's peers becomes an important source of positive or negative self-evaluation, especially over the age of eight. There would appear to be a direct connection between the degree of cohesiveness within the group from this age onwards and its influence as a restraining factor in cases of antisocial behavior. Naturally, the hundreds of children's groups in the many kibbutzim differ one from another in their degree of unity according to variables such as the number of children in the group, whether they are of the same or mixed ages, the personalities and stability of their educators, the general social structure of the kibbutz, etc. We also believe that the inclusion of work assignments in the child's daily routine represents an additional factor in socializing aggressiveness. As has been pointed out, work, in the sense of regular assignments and responsibilities for service chores in the children's quarters, starts as early as the first school grade. These work assignments are increased gradually as the child grows older and play an increasingly important part in his activities. From the age of 15-16, successful work performance in the various branches of the kibbutz can be an important factor in social adaptation, in identifying the adolescent with the values of adult society, and in raising his self-esteem in cases of emotional conflict.

Devotion to duty, a volunteer spirit, and significant achievements in the sphere of work are basic requisites for winning the appreciation of kibbutz members and the peer group. Our experience shows that the early introduction of productive work that encourages young people to take over responsible adult jobs in the kibbutz economy is an important factor in the rehabilitation of emotionally maladjusted kibbutz adolescents and in reducing the incidence of anti-social manifestations at this age.

Of course, in the kibbutz, there is less likelihood of finding antisocial acting-out models to identify with, than in other non-kibbutz social environments. In recent years, however, there have been substantive changes in the composition and size of the kibbutz population, accompanied by a pronounced modification in the original image of the kibbutz as an intimate, closed, well-knit, and united group in its values and way of life. Among other things, the kibbutzim have opened their gates to temporary groups of young volunteers, mainly students from various overseas countries, who come to stay for a few months as a supplement to the labor force and to gain first hand knowledge of the kibbutz way of life. These temporary residents undoubtedly include all types of socially maladjusted people with neurotic and personality disorders. They are liable to introduce into the kibbutz their own ecological model of rebellion against the norms of their own society, including delinquent behavior, drug addiction, and asocial or antisocial "new" moral codes and values. A steadily increasing percentage of marijuana, LSD, and other drug users, who have infiltrated into the kibbutzim from overseas "developed" countries, now constitute an integral part of the surroundings of the kibbutz-born youth. Until now, we have found only rare instances of kibbutz youth using drugs, and even in these isolated cases most of the subjects were not kibbutz-born youth but adolescents who had joined the kibbutz from outside. However the real test as to whether kibbutz youth is or is not immune to drug addiction or other manifestations of digressive social behavior has still to be met. The change in the ecological climate of the kibbutz in terms of enhanced contact with people whose values conflict sharply with accepted kibbutz norms, is a feature mainly of the last four years, following the Six Day War. It is still too early to make a reliable assessment as to the manner and degree in which the kibbutz has been influenced by contact with people coming from different cultures and introducing unconventional customs and ways of life. In the meantime, we have not discerned any disturbing indications among kibbutz youth of an increased appearance of unusual antisocial behavior. The kibbutz child and adolescent continues to be bound both socially and in his standards of values to his peer group, which in turn still faithfully reflects the essential norms of social behavior and moral values of the kibbutz adult model.

PSYCHOTIC DISORDERS: THE ABSENCE OF PSYCHOGENIC EARLY CHILDHOOD AUTISM

Over the past ten years, we have had the opportunity of studying eight kibbutz children (five boys and three girls) with a typical clinical picture of early childhood psychosis. Their psychotic condition was diagnosed during the preschool years, mostly before the age of three. The group includes four children referred to the Tel Aviv Kibbutz Clinic and four children examined by us at the Oranim Kibbutz Clinic. They have been followed up for three to ten years.

All of these eight children completely met the diagnostic criteria put forward by the British working group, under the Chairmanship of

Creak (9). These children presented typical severe patterns of autistic, atypical and withdrawn behavior, failure to develop adequate person-to-person relationships, uneven development, abnormalities in verbal communication, dereistic thinking and activity, disturbed expression of feelings, ritualistic and stereotyped mannerisms, sustained resistance to change, poor body image, etc. All of them showed evidence of total or scattered areas of mental subnormality of varying degrees of severity.

Due to the small number of children involved in our study, no definite conclusions can be drawn; however, it seems to us worth emphasizing that, without exception, in all of our eight cases of early childhood autism the psychotic condition was invariably associated with some kind of organic CNS disturbance. All eight children displayed "soft" signs of neurologic impairment similar to the features regularly found in cases labeled as "minimal brain damage" or "cerebral dysfunction" (5). Our findings included motor disturbances (e.g., hyperkinesis, abnormal gait, poor motor coordination, difficulties in executing fine motor movements, choreiform movements); diverse perceptual and cognitive defects; expressive types of dysphasia and aphasia; as well as other objective signs of structural pathology of the CNS. In two cases, epileptic seizures developed in the course of the follow-up. A history of complications in pregnancy, which may have caused injury to the fetus or other perinatal or postnatal pathological conditions, was recorded in almost every case. Four of our psychotic cases were premature babies.

The fact that until now we have not revealed a single case of non-organic autistic or symbiotic type of early childhood psychosis does not seem to us to be related—in contrast to Bettelheim's (4) hypothesis—to existing differences in the child-rearing practices of kibbutz and private families. Bettelheim assumes that the kibbutz infant's lessened dependence on its mother, as a result of the transfer of several important infant care functions to the kibbutz *metapelet,* would eliminate the danger that "autism might develop as a response to extreme negative feelings shown by the mother to the specific child."

We do not share this view because, in the kibbutz, too, the child's contact with his parents, and especially with his mother, is sufficiently close and intense during infancy and early childhood. Actually, a baby in a Kibbutz Infant's Home reacts exactly as any non-kibbutz baby would in displaying symptoms of restlessness, excessive crying, vomiting, eating and sleep disturbances, in response to inappropriate maternal handling and attitudes.

All types of child psychological disorders described in psychiatric textbooks, as deriving from a disturbed parent-child relationship, can and do develop within the specific framework of the kibbutz from infancy onwards. It is therefore strange that, of all the possible diagnostic categories, psychogenically determined early childhood psychosis is absent while the organic type of psychosis appears in its place. We believe that there is another and simpler explanation than that advanced by Bettelheim, who assumes emotional separation between mother and child.

The medical, psychological, and educational services provided for kibbutz children enable us to assemble and reliably trace pathogenic organic factors that may have brought about the neurological damage to the child, as well as to arrive at early exposure of deviant development and detection of objective findings of innate or postnatal CNS pathology. The child is observed daily throughout the years in a small group, in everyday life situations, by experienced nurses. This allows them and the parents to make a continuous evaluation of the child as compared with others in his peer-group. Any deviation from "normal standards" can usually be detected sooner and more easily in the kibbutz setting than in the rather closed setting of a private family. Furthermore, the accurate evaluation of the pathology of psychotic kibbutz children is made easier by the centralization of diagnostic, management, and follow-up procedures in the Kibbutz Clinics from early childhood through adolescence.

Once again, we would emphasize that out of 3,000 emotionally disturbed children referred to two Kibbutz Child Clinics in the course of approximately fifteen years, we have so far failed to reveal a single case of "pure" psychogenic psychosis prior to the age of twelve. Our cases of non-organic psychosis relate exclusively to adolescents over twelve, and especially over the age of fifteen. In this age range, overtly psychotic kibbutz adolescents seem to present a clinical picture similar to non-kibbutz adolescents in the context of an acute schizophrenic episode or a chronic schizophrenic pattern, both types of psychosis fitting into the symptomatic model of adult schizophrenia.

In the light of our experience, we cannot but agree with the view (5) that neurological damage related to so-called "minimal brain damage" or "cerebral dysfunction" may result in multiplicity of disorders and in clinical pictures ranging from diverse kinds of deviant developmental patterns to childhood psychosis, including the typical syndrome of early autistic psychosis.

It is true that the vast majority of kibbutz and non-kibbutz children diagnosed as brain damaged are not psychotic or autistic; and we should seek an explanation as to why a minority does become psychotic. But the fact remains that the kibbutz children examined by us and diagnosed as cases of early childhood psychosis, all present what seem to be unmistakable signs of organic neurologic pathology. Of course, even the symptomatic picture of children with organic psychosis includes and reflects the participation of psychogenic influences related to the interplay between the child and his family and social environment. However, in these eight cases, which we diagnosed as organic types of childhood psychosis, we found that the superimposed psychological elements played only a subsidiary role in producing the symptoms.

The clinical evidence of an irreversible CNS abnormality in all our cases may explain the unfavorable course and poor prognosis of the disease in each of these psychotic children. Despite the systematic use of diverse eclectic types of therapy and intensive and continuous teaching and training programs carried out by individual educators in the kibbutz setting, or at residential therapy centers, we did not encounter a single instance of psychological independence and adequate adjustment to regular school and group life. In this respect, kibbutz children with an unequivocal diagnosis of early childhood psychosis share the same unfortunate fate as the group of 150 New York schizophrenic children who, when followed up twenty years or more after the onset of the disease, revealed a continuation of their childhood illness into adulthood in nearly every case. It would appear to be true that "schizophrenia evidenced any time in childhood, leads to a life course of schizophrenia" (3).

CONCLUSIONS

Undoubtedly there are several factors that contribute to reducing the severity of clinical types of emotional pathology among kibbutz children. They include the special child-rearing practices of the kibbutz, the fact that it is a selective society from the point of view of its ideals, aspirations, and culture, as well as its extensive facilities and services for diagnosis and early treatment of cases of pathological abnormality. Naturally, the unique system of child rearing in the kibbutz framework also produced definite dissimilarities in the symptomatic characteristics and distribution of the various psychiatric categories.

Our main conclusion as a result of more than twenty years' work with "normal" and disturbed kibbutz children may be summed up in two central facts:

1) We have failed to uncover any clinical entity recognizable as a specific or prevalent emotional disturbance of kibbutz children. In fact, the usual psychiatric syndromes observed in children and adolescents raised in the traditional Western family may also be observed among

kibbutz youngsters. It should be noted, however, that out of 3,000 emotionally disturbed children referred to the Kibbutz Clinics, we have so far failed to reveal a single case of psychogenically determined early childhood psychosis.

2) On the other hand, the kibbutz system of upbringing permits the rearing of normal children showing an ample diversity of personality patterns, all of which are certainly covered by the wide concept of "normalcy."

REFERENCES

1. ACKERMAN, N. (1958): *The Psychodynamics of Family Life.* New York: Basic Books.
2. AMIR, Y. (1967): Adjustment and promotion of soldiers from kibbutzim. (In Hebrew) *Megamot,* 15:250-258.
3. BENDER, L. & FARETRA, G. (1969): *Psychiatric News* (July):25.
4. BETTELHEIM, B. (1969): *The Children of the Dream.* New York: Macmillan.
5. BIRCH, H. ET AL. (1969): Neurological findings in minimal brain damage. *Amer. J. Orthopsychiat.,* 39:437-446.
6. BUCKLE, D. & LEBOVICI, S. (1960): *Child Guidance Centres.* World Health Organization, Monograph Series No. 40, Geneva.
7. CHESS, S. (1959): *An Introduction to Child Psychiatry.* New York: Grune and Stratton.
8. CHESS, S., ET AL. (1963): Interaction of temperament and environment in the production of behavioral disturbances in children. *Amer. J. Psychiat.,* 120:142-147.
9. CREAK, M. (Chairman) (1961): Schizophrenic syndrome in childhood: British Working Party. *Brit. Med. J.,* 2:889-890.
10. *Diagnostic and Statistical Manual of Mental Disorders (DSM-II)* (1968): American Psychiatric Association, Washington, D. C.
11. EISENBERG, L. & NEUBAUER, P. (1965): Mental health issues in Israeli collectives. *J. Amer. Acad. Child Psychiat.,* 4:426-442.
12. KAFFMAN, M. (1967): Survey of opinions and attitudes of kibbutz members toward mental illness. *Israel Annals Psychiat. and Related Disciplines,* 5:17-31.
13. KAFFMAN, M. (1965): A comparison of psychopathology: Israeli children from kibbutz and from urban surroundings. *Amer. J. Orthopsychiat.,* 35:509-520.
14. MARCUS, J., THOMAS, A., & CHESS, S. (1969): Behavioral individuality in kibbutz children. *Israel Annals Psychiat. and Related Disciplines,* 7:43-54.
15. RABIN, A. (1965): *Growing in the Kibbutz.* New York: Springer Publishing Co.
16. REXFORD, E. (1966): Discussion of Dr. Solnit's paper. *J. Amer. Acad. Child Psychiat.,* 5:26.
17. SOWDER, B. (1969): Report of the Joint Commission on the Mental Health of Children. *Psychiatric News* (May).
18. SPIRO, M. (1958): *Children of the Kibbutz.* Cambridge, Mass.: Harvard University Press.
19. STENNETT, R. (1966): Emotional handicap in the elementary years: Phase or disease? *Amer. J. Orthopsychiat.,* 36:444-449.
20. YARROW, L. (1964): Separation from parents during early childhood. In M. Hoffman and W. Hoffman (Eds.), *Child Development Research.* New York: Russell Sage Foundation (vol. 1:89).

Part IV

LANGUAGE AND LEARNING

Linguistic deviation is a central issue in the psychiatric diagnosis of children. It is often a key to a youngster's thinking processes and intellectual level. Yet those not working in the field of linguistics often find discussions in this area difficult to follow. In the papers in this section, Macnamara considers the cognitive basis of language learning clearly and critically in an easily comprehensible fashion. The report by Marwit and his colleagues shows that the language of black, non-middle-class children has consistent rules and is a legitimate and logical grammar intelligently applied. Their study adds further weight to the thesis that the linguistic usage of lower socioeconomic class black children is not simply a substandard form of English.

Kline and Lee, in an unusual study, compare bilingual Chinese children in terms of their competence in reading English and Chinese. A challenging fact that only 6% of the children had difficulty in both languages raises new questions about the nature of learning.

Birch supplies a comprehensive and analytic review of the relationship of malnutrition, learning and intelligence. Questions about degree of malnutrition, its timing and duration are examined. The interaction of social and cultural factors is given consideration.

17

COGNITIVE BASIS OF LANGUAGE LEARNING IN INFANTS

John Macnamara, Ph.D.

Department of Psychology, McGill University

The main point of the paper is that infants learn their language by first determining, independent of language, the meaning which a speaker intends to convey to them, and by then working out the relationship between the meaning and the expression they heard. The assumptions on which the thesis rests are discussed, the main one being that a speaker's linguistic system and his intentions are distinguishable. Evidence in support of the thesis itself is adduced at three levels: lexicon, syntax, and phonology. An attempt is made to describe the strategies, nonlinguistic as well as linguistic, by which children use meaning to decipher language.

The thesis of this paper is that infants learn their language by first determining, independent of language, the meaning which a speaker intends to convey to them, and by then working out the relationship between the meaning and the language. To put it another way, the infant uses meaning as a clue to language, rather than language as a clue to

Reprinted from PSYCHOLOGICAL REVIEW, Vol. 79, No. 1, January 1972: pp. 1-13. Copyright © 1972 by the American Psychological Association and reproduced by permission.

Many of the ideas in this paper come from discussion with Nancy Katz of the McGill psychology department whose doctoral work is in this area. I am particularly grateful to her. I also owe much to Dick Tucker, Rose-Marie Weber, Charles Taylor, Roy Wright, Harry Bracken, Michael Corballis, all of whom either were or are my colleagues at McGill, and to Gillian and David Sankoff of the University of Montreal.

meaning. This thesis is a strong form of the theory that meaning plays an important part in language learning. Its most respectable antecedent is Brown's (1958) "original word game." I would like, however, to make use of recent developments in linguistics and psycholinguists in developing the theory and I would also like to present a theory which, unlike earlier ones, integrates vocabulary, syntax, and phonology.

The theory relates mainly to the beginning of language learning. Obviously once he has made some progress in language a child can use language to develop his thinking. I am not, therefore, casting doubt on the belief that our thinking is enriched or brought into focus by language. Further, I am prescinding from the more general question of the extent to which our thinking is conditioned by the linguistic environment in which we live, and from problems relating to advanced levels of language, in particular certain aspects of poetic expression.

The approach to language learning which I am proposing had for some time been neglected in linguistics and in psycholinguistics. Part of the reason for this was the uneasiness with which behaviorism handled semantics. Even more important, however, was the impact of structuralism in linguistics which, following a suggestion of Bloomfield's (1933), sought to settle all grammatical questions without appeal to meaning. The advent of transformational grammar, in many respects so critical of linguistic structuralism, did nothing to change this situation. Indeed, in *Syntactic Structures*, Chomsky (1957, Ch. 9) went a little further than Bloomfield and seriously questioned the view that meaning could be an aid to the discovery of grammar. The paucity of references to meaning in the literature on child language during the 10 years that follow the appearance of *Syntactic Structures* is scarcely a coincidence (for overviews see McNeill, 1966a, 1966b). In the late 1960s, however, grammarians came to rely more on semantics than before. Chomsky (1968) uses semantics to counter several arguments against the grammar which he had proposed; the arguments against him came from a group of transformational grammarians, such as Lakoff (1968), Lakoff and Ross (1967), Fillmore (1968), and McCawley (1968), who largely abolished the distinction between grammar and syntax. This turn of events, whatever the ultimate fate of the contending grammars with which it is associated, has engendered a readiness to seek a basis for language learning in infants among nonlinguistic cognitive principles. Perhaps the earliest and so far the most important study of child language in the new key is Bloom (1970). (A general swing in this direction can be seen in several books and articles, e.g., Brown, 1970; Ervin-Tripp, 1970; Kernan, 1969; McNeill, 1970; Slobin, 1971.)

While most of what has appeared on child language has focused on the production of speech, I would like to focus on the comprehension of speech. Some recent papers have indeed studied comprehension (Clark, 1971; Chomsky, 1969; Donaldson & Balfour, 1968). These, however, deal with children well beyond the initial stages of language learning. I know of only a very few papers which deal with the ability of two-year-old infants to comprehend speech (Shipley, Smith, & Gleitman, 1969; Smith, 1970). I would like to get behind these fine studies and to draw attention to the cognitive strategies which an infant brings to the task of comprehending speech. Apart from some very general remarks on such strategies (see, e.g., Chomsky, 1965, pp. 31 ff.; Fodor, 1966), the topic has been quite neglected. It is, however, a topic which is basic to the whole examination of language learning and, moreover, one which, as I hope to show, permits us several possibilities for empirical research. But first, some remarks on meaning.

I will use *meaning* to refer to those intentions which a speaker wishes to express in language, and following the lead of Frege (1952), I will regard sentences as names for the intentions which they express. Meanings can be assertions, negations, commands, and questions; they may include a reference to the speaker's physical environment, to his feelings (of pain, pleasure, uneasiness, etc.), and to his ideas or concepts. They may also include his attitudes of belief or doubt toward his assertions. In other words, meaning refers to all that a person can express or designate by means of a linguistic code. The code on the other hand consists of a set of formatives and syntactic devices whose main function is to relate meaning to the phonological system of the language.

I prefer to leave the problem of meaning at that, simply because I do not believe that we are able to define it more precisely without losing it. Perhaps the clearest attempts of behaviorists to treat meanings as mediating responses are those of Osgood (1963) and Mowrer (1960). With Fodor (1965), however, I regard all such attempts as unfortunate and misguided. Equally unfortunate and misguided, in my opinion, are the attempts of positivists such as Carnap (1956) and Quine (1960, 1961) to eliminate as far as possible talk about meaning and to replace it with talk of things present to the senses. All such attempts seem to me to purchase clarity by impoverishing human intelligence and by ignoring the dynamism of the act of understanding. Further than this, there is no need to go for the purposes of the present paper.

In stressing the distinction of meaning and linguistic code, I do not wish to imply a functional separation of thought and language. This would end up in what Quine (1960, p. 206) calls the "fallacy of subtraction," that is, the fallacy that meaning is what is left over when language has been filtered out. The fallacy can be avoided if with Saussure (1959, pp. 111 ff.) we regard an utterance as the embodiment of thought in language. Saussure points out that without thought, language is useless, and he also claims that thought without language is nebulous. While not going so far as to say that without language all thought is nebulous, I find Saussure's general thesis reasonable. Meaning and the linguistic code are best treated as though they were elements of a compound, much in the way that oxygen and hydrogen are the separate elements which combine to form molecules of water. That is, the two are not usually experienced separately, though they are distinguishable.

The thesis that infants use meaning as a clue to the linguistic code rests on the assumption that in the period when infants begin to learn language, their thought is more developed than their language. Support for this assumption is to be found in the work of Vygotsky (1962), Piaget (1963), and Sinclair-de-Zwart (1969), who adduce evidence that the development of thought is at first independent of language. They emphasize that at about the age of one, when an infant begins to understand language, he has already made many observations on the world about him, on himself, and on his own activities: he has succeeded in classifying many things and has seen the relationship between, for example, his own activities and the movement of various objects.

The thesis also has the support of the findings on cognition and affect in the deaf (for an overview see Vernon, 1971). Though there are difficulties in the interpretation of this work, it seems reasonably clear that persons who are severely retarded in language development nevertheless reveal all the essentials of human thought processes and human affect. It follows that thought and affect are distinguishable from language and that they can develop without benefit of language. It also follows that initially they can develop, independent of language, and outpace the growth of language in normal children.

Evidence from Vocabulary

At first sight it might appear that to learn the vocabulary of his language is the simplest linguistic task which confronts the infant. It might appear that all he has to do is to relate objects to the external world with their names. However, this illusion of simplicity soon disappears when we reflect on the vocabulary itself. Not only are there numerous names and descriptive terms which can be applied to a single object, but it soon transpires that descriptive terms refer to objects only through the speaker's complicated network of concepts (see Odgen & Richards, 1938). But how is the infant to match words and concepts?

In *Word and Object,* Quine (1960) argues convincingly, it seems to me, that no empirical test or set of tests could ever convince a reasonable but skeptical linguist that what appeared to be equivalent terms in two languages were in fact equivalent in meaning. The example he gives is of a linguist in a strange country who hears what seems to be the word for a rabbit. How is he to know whether the word might not mean "fur" or "head" or "animal" or "rabbitlike shape" or indefinitely many other things? Since, however, linguists make such decisions all the time and since it would be obtuse to deny that they are highly successful, it follows that they do not behave like Quine's skeptical linguist. They must rely on cognitive strategies which they bring with them to the task of describing a language.

Quine's arguments can be applied (though my use of them would not have his support) with few changes to the infant in the process of learning vocabulary. Like the adult linguist, the child's success depends on a set of cognitive strategies which function as shortcuts in the task of relating symbols to a speaker's intentions. That there must be such a set is evident from the fact that neither in the linguistic code nor in the physical environment are there sufficient constraints to explain how an infant could have even the most superficial success. For example, children do not form bizarre concepts to include foot and floor and exclude all else. There are quite marked constraints on what will be grouped together in a concept. Unfortunately the study of these cognitive constraints, which at the perceptual level interested the Gestalt psychologists, has been largely neglected, so most of what can be said about them is of a very tentative nature.*

It is obvious that an infant has the capacity to distinguish from the rest of the physical environment an object which his mother draws to his attention and names. It seems clear too that in such circumstances he adopts the strategy of taking the word he hears as a name for the object as a whole rather than as a subset of its properties, or for its position, or weight, or worth, or anything else. The same strategy would serve equally well in the numerous cases where something happens which

---

* In addition to the gestalt work on perception, which is surely related to concept formation, there is the extensive work of the ethologists on innate release mechanisms in lower animals and the part played in such mechanisms by selective attention to certain aspects or events of the environment (see Miller, Galanter, & Pribram, 1960, Ch. 5). The impact of the ethological work is to increase the credibility of a theory which incorporates restraints on perceptual attention and on concept formation in humans.

draws an infant's and other people's attention to a particular object and they use the occasion to mention the object's name. Indeed the literature records several errors which, on the reasonable assumption that adults are good at guessing what children mean, show that the child is using just such a strategy (e.g., Blount, 1969, p. 62). An example is to be found in Hoffman (1968) who recounts that at the age of 17 months, one infant whom she was studying used to refer to the kitchen stove as *hot*. The likely explanation is that her mother told the infant not to touch the stove saying *"it's hot,"* and the infant took *hot* to be the object's name. The theory thus exemplified fits in with some facts. Children learn names for colors, shapes, and sizes only after they have learned names for many objects. That is, names for entities are learned before names for certain attributes.

However, names for at least some of the various states, conditions, and activities of entities come very early. *Daddy* can be *gone, sitting down,* or *clipping the hedge.* A *toy* can be *broken.* One can *open* a *book* or *close* it. It is not that a state like *sitting down* is more clearly delineated than a color like *red;* the referents for each category show enormous variability. But the categories differ in at least one important and highly relevant respect. States and activities such as those just mentioned are not permanent attributes of entities, whereas colors and shapes usually are. If there is a differential set in small children to attend to varying states and activities rather than unvarying attributes, we need look no further for an explanation for the order in which the corresponding terms are learned.

A further hypothesis is that the child will not learn the name for states or activities until he has firmly grasped the name for at least some entities which exemplify such states and activities. Thus the order of learning would be as follows: names for entities, names for their variable states and actions, and names for more permanent attributes such as color. Perhaps the best research strategy would be first to test this hypothesis on clear-cut examples of each class. If the results are favorable, an argument based on construct validity would subsequently enable us to determine whether a particular doubtful term referred to a variable state or to a permanent quality in the child's world. The age at which the child learns the term would be the clue.

Some of the earliest words an infant learns to understand are proper names which single out the named object's individuality, for example, the names of his brothers and sisters and the name of the family dog. Other names are shared by many objects and connote what these objects hold in common. There are syntactic consequences attached to the distinction; one cannot speak of *a Fido,* but one can speak of *a dog.* Yet it seems unlikely that the young infant can use such evidence to distinguish between the two types of names. On the other hand, it is not at all improbable that he should assume that certain objects such as spoons have only common names, while other objects such as dogs and people should have proper names.* He may at first treat common and proper names when referring to the same objects—*Fido is a dog*—as optional proper names. If so, he will learn to differentiate when he discovers that only the family dog is called *Fido,* whereas all dogs are called *dog.*

Initial investigation suggests that infants treat higher order common names as collective nouns.** For example a two-year-old child will treat "toys" as a collective noun which refers to a group of objects. Thus, while allowing that a particular object is a *truck* or a *train,* he will deny that it is a *toy.* On the other hand, he knows well what is meant by his *toys.* Moreover his response—that the *truck* is not a *toy*—does not seem to depend on what the surrounding objects are. It is the same whether or not the truck is surrounded by other toys or by objects which are clearly not toys, like spoons and cups. Thus it seems as if, for the child, *toy* is not a hierarchical term which contains *trucks* as a subcategory. It remains to be seen how children get themselves out of this situation, but presumably it is by a process similar to that which enables them to distinguish between proper and common nouns.

The pronouns, too, might appear impossibly difficult if we did not presuppose on the child's part in the ability to guess their semantic force. How else could he learn to say *I* when he is addressed as *you?* Indeed autistic children usually fail to make this reversal.

So far we have dealt with some of the aspects of learning words which have referents in the concrete world of the environment, but there are also words which seem to refer primarily to cognitive operators and only secondarily to physical objects. Some such words, for example, *and, or,* and *true,* are acquired very early. Slobin and Welsh (in press) record a 27-month-old child's correct and spontaneous use of *and.* Brown, Fraser, and Bellugi (1964) record *all* and *more* as well as *some* for a 24-month-old boy. Even if some of the instances when such words are used are of doubtful validity, others seem genuine enough. It is inconceivable that the hearing of a logical term should generate for the first time the appropriate logical operator in a child's mind. Indeed the

---

* Indeed some preliminary observations made by Nancy Katz of small babies support the idea that they do make this discrimination.

** The work referred to in this paragraph is being done by Nancy Katz.

only possibility of his learning such a word would seem to be if he experienced the need for it in his own thinking and looked for it in the linguistic usage about him.

Evidence from Syntax

One might imagine that an infant who addresses himself to the task of learning syntax would to begin with adopt a simple hypothesis. He might, for example, suppose that a single semantic relationship would always be expressed by means of a single syntactic device or structure. Conversely, he might adopt the hypothesis that any change in syntactic structure signalled a change in semantic structure. However, such strategies would probably be less of a help than a hindrance. Consider 1 and 2 in each of which the same message is expressed by two different surface structures:

> 1. a. Give the book to me.
>   b. Give me the book.
>
> 2. a. My hair is black.
>   b. I have black hair.

Consider, too, 3 in which there is even a change in the syntactic category to which *kiss* belongs without any change in meaning:

> 3. a. Give me a kiss.
>   b. Kiss me.

On the other hand, 4 shows that a single syntactic device can signal several different semantic structures:

> 4. a. In a minute (time "when").
>   b. In a minute (time "how long").
>   c. In a box.
>   d. In a temper.

The task of the child is to detect the structures of syntax and relate them to semantic structures. The preceding examples show that the two are related in a rather flexible manner. The consistencies and regularities of syntax are to some extent independent of those of semantics. How, then, does the infant manage to relate the two? In keeping with the main lines of this paper, my answer will be that he uses independently attained meaning to discover at least certain syntactic structures that are of basic importance.

While I imagine that this position has the intuitive support of many students of child language, it runs counter to the assumption once wide-spread among linguists that syntax can be, even must be, described without recourse to meaning. Though few linguists would subscribe to this assumption today, the matter is so basic to the present discussion that it merits more than a cursory dismissal. Consider 5:

> 5. a. The boy struck the girl.
>   b. The girl struck the boy.

How is the infant to know that these two sentences are not stylistic variants like 1a and 1b, or like 2a and 2b? There is in fact no way to decide the matter unless one has independent access to the meaning, probably through observing what is happening at the time sentences such as 5a and 5b are uttered. This is to say that without recourse to meaning, one could not discover so basic a syntactic device as the use of word order in English to express the subject-predicate relationship. The decision to treat 1a and 1b as stylistic variants must depend on the child's appreciation that while books can be given to people, people cannot be given to books. Thus the child must use his nonlinguistic knowledge to arrive at the notions of direct and indirect object and at the alternative ways of signaling them in English.

Before going on to speculate about how a child might use meaning to unravel syntactic puzzles, there are two qualifications to be made. First, not all syntactic puzzles must be or can be solved by semantic means. For example, gender in Indo-European languages does not correlate with any nonlinguistic classification of objects. Further, the rule that determines the number of the verb in English on the basis of the number of the surface subject is surely a purely syntactic one. Thus, though 6a and 6b mean roughly the same thing, the number of the verb is different in the two sentences:

> 6. a. The boys strike the girl.
>   b. The girl is struck by the boys.

It is quite apparent then, that the child must have great skill in detecting the syntactic regularities of his language whether or not they can be tied in some way to meaning. Something of the French child's skill in relating word endings to gender can be seen in Tucker (1967).

The second qualification relates to the difference between *discovering* the syntactic devices of a language and stating them. A syntactic device which could not have been discovered without the aid of meaning might nevertheless be stated without any reference to meaning. To illustrate, a person who was intent on distinguishing Fords from Chevrolets might begin by reading the trade names which appear somewhere on every car. After a time, however, he might come to rely on the shapes of fenders, rear windows, etc. There would even be a certain advantage in switching from trade name to distinctive features, since the latter can be recognized at a greater distance. Similarly in the realm of language. For example, it is altogether improbable that a child could discover the difference between transitive and intransitive active verbs without the aid of meaning. The presence or absence of following noun phrases is not an adequate criterion, as the examples of 7 show:

> 7. a. John drove.
>   b. John drove a car.
>   c. John drove home.
>   d. I walked.
>   e. I walked home.

The child must appreciate at some cognitive level that the action of driving has an effect on "car" but not on "home," and that the action of walking does not have an effect on "home."

The grammarian, on the other hand, might distinguish the two sorts of verbs by whether or not they have passives. Actually, this test is inadequate (see Lyons, 1968, Ch. 8), but it will serve as an illustration. Let us now suppose that a list of verbs which have no passive forms has somehow been formed. It follows that one can tell whether or not a verb is intransitive by whether or not it appears on the list. There is no need to refer to meaning. The fact, then, that children need meaning to establish the two classes of verbs and to decide which class a particular verb belongs to does not preclude the possibility or usefulness of formal tests which make no reference to meaning.

But to return to the main line of the discussion, how does the infant use meaning as a clue to certain syntactic devices? The most likely avenue to explore here is the prior learning of vocabulary, principally nouns, verbs, and adjectives. It seems natural to suggest that children initially take the main lexical items in the sentences they hear, determine referents for these items, and then use their knowledge of the referents to decide what the semantic structures intended by the speaker must be. This is in fact the strategy implicit in my treatment of examples 1 to 7. Once the children have determined the semantic structures, their final task is to note the syntactic devices, such as word order, prepositions, number affixes, etc., which correlate with the semantic structures. Such a strategy will yield most of the main syntactic devices in the language.

It is important to note, however, that the establishment of different semantic relationships among the formatives of a sentence does not immediately establish different syntactic relationships. For example, the relationship between *boy* and *ball* in 8a is quite different from the relationship between them in 8b:

> 8. a. The boy kicked the ball.
>   b. The boy liked the ball.

Yet in each, *ball* can be taken as the grammatical object of the verb. On the other hand, the relationship between *I* and *home* in 9a is different both syntactically and semantically from the relationship between them in 9b:

> 9. a. I like home.
>   b. I walk home.

The fact that *home* is not the direct object of *walk* in 9b is indicated by the fact that most nouns which follow *walk* are preceded by *to* or *toward*: one *walks to town, to the table, toward the door.* Perhaps the child notes this fact and combines it with the semantic information to arrive at the conclusion that syntax of sentences such as 9b is different from that of sentences like 9a. This is of course highly speculative, but two general conclusions seem warranted: (a) the child cannot discover many syntactic structures without the aid of meaning, and (b) the child is prodigiously skilled at noting the regularities in the language which he hears.

The hypothesis that prior knowledge of vocabulary items and their referents is basic to the learning of syntax suggests that we return for a moment to some of the ideas discussed in the section on vocabulary. There it was noted that children at one stage take a word like *toys* as a collective noun rather than as a higher order noun with subcategories, *truck* and *doll*. It follows that *toys* should always be plural for the child at that stage, and that while he will understand 10a he will either not understand 10b or treat it as equivalent to 10a:

> 10. a. Those are your toys.
>   b. That is your toy.
>   c. A truck is a toy.

It follows further that he will not understand sentences like 10c in which the same referent is placed in two classes at once. Some of these matters are testable, but to go further at the present time would be to court disaster.

So far in this section, we have been concerned with declarative sentences, but there are of course many other forms of speech act such as questions and commands. How the child learns to categorize speech acts correctly is almost a complete mystery, except that his doing so also presupposes an ability to determine the nature of the act independent of its syntactic form. In this connection, two observations will have to suffice. Lieberman (1967, pp. 44ff.) cites evidence for the existence of an innate tendency in babies to react positively to friendly tones of voice and negatively to angry ones. Perhaps repeated commands tend to assume an angry tone, and so an angry tone might come to be taken by the child as an indication that he is either to do something or stop doing it. Later in the same book (p. 132), Lieberman examines 14 languages and finds that in 12 of them, questions can be signaled by means of rising pitch. While rising pitch is not then a universal marker of questions, it seems to have very wide currency as such. Could it be that children tend naturally to take rising pitch as a marker that a question is being asked?

But apart from such suprasegmentals, it seems clear that there must be a set of universal signs, of face, physical gesture, and bodily movement which the child interprets correctly and thus among other things comes to distinguish among speech acts. The evidence for such a set is growing (see Vernon, 1971), but as yet little is understood about how they relate to the learning of language. This is surely an important area of research. In the meantime we will have to content ourselves with the observation that the different forms of speech act probably correspond to deeply rooted mental attitudes of asserting, seeking for information, wishing to have others perform certain acts, etc. Indeed, such attitudes must be either innate or develop almost without benefit of learning. Endowed with such a set of attitudes, the child will be on the lookout for means of expressing them, nonverbal as well as verbal, and in this way come to discriminate the forms of different speech acts.

These suggestions of how an infant might use independently attained meaning to discover syntax are of course tentative. Yet they have the general support of several of the findings about the *production* of speech. For example, the suggestion that prior knowledge of vocabulary is vital to the learning of syntax fits well with the initial stages of speech production. First come single words that, as Bloom (1970), McNeill (1970), and several others have pointed out, infants employ to express a variety of semantic structures. Thus the single word milk can express: "This is milk," "Is this milk?" "I want milk," "I want more milk," etc. This indicates a heavy reliance on vocabulary items without supporting syntax. Moreover, when the child comes to combine words into two-word sentences, he continues to omit many of the syntactic features which adults include, such as plural and possessive markers, tense markers, auxiliaries, articles, etc. Yet Bloom (1970) has argued very forcibly that he does so for lack of syntactic processing space rather than for lack of semantic sophistication, and she has the support of many scholars in the area (see, e.g., Brown, 1970; McNeill, 1970; Schlesinger, 1971).

The point is equally clear when we consider children's attempts to repeat adult sentences. Brown and Bellugi (1964) and Brown and Fraser (1964), for example, pointed out that when required to repeat sentences, small children fasten onto meaning, drop the function words such as prepositions, and convey the substance of the message by means of the principal words. Slobin (1971) examines the data from several studies of child language in many countries and many different languages, and claims that such "telegraphese" is one of the universals of language learning.

In this connection it is also interesting to note the several suggestions in the literature that parents pay little attention to their small children's grammar, and only correct them on points of fact and discipline (see Bellugi-Klima, cited in Cazden, 1969). This observation, which is repeated in Gleason (1967), in Brown, Cazden, and Bellugi (1961), and in Brown and Hanlon (1970), implies that children learn grammar incidentally while parents attempt to put their thoughts and behavior right. However, too much must not be made of this point since children can learn from their parents' remarks only if they can understand them, which probably implies, after the very earliest stages, some knowledge of adult syntax. Indeed Shipley et al. (1969) found that small children made good use of adult syntactic devices in understanding adult sentences even if the children did not employ such devices in their own speech.

There is one further support in the literature for the thesis that in language learning the thrust to learn syntax comes mainly from meaning. It is the observation that children acquire first those grammatical devices which have a clear semantic force, such as numerous uses of tense and number markers, and only later acquired those which, like gender, have not (see Slobin, 1966). Indeed Slobin (1971) erects this into a tentative universal:

> Rules related to semantically defined classes take precedence over rules relating to formally defined classes.

I only know of one argument against the general thesis of this section. In an otherwise stimulating paper, Bever (1970, pp. 305-306) argued against the primacy of semantics in language learning. He presented sentences such as 11a and 11b to small children of varying ages:

> 11. a. The mother pats the dog.
>   b. The dog pats the mother.

He required them to act out the meanings of the sentences with toys and found that relative to their performance on sentences like 11a, two-year-olds performed better than older children on sentences like 11b. That is, the two-year-olds seemed to be less upset by the improbability of the second type of sentence. Bever argues:

> The implication of this is to invalidate any theory of early language development that assumes that the young child depends on con-textual knowledge of the world to tell him what sentences mean independent of their structure [p. 306].

This is a perplexing interpretation, seeing that in fact the younger children had interpreted the improbable sentences correctly more often than one might have expected. After all they were doing just what they were told. Besides, in absolute terms, the older children gave more correct responses to the improbable sentences. Indeed all sorts of explanations for the results other than the one given by the author come readily to mind.

Evidence from Phonology

The relationship between speech sounds and meaning is quite as loose as that between syntactic structures and meaning. A single speech sound either on its own or in combination with others frequently signals many different meanings, while just as frequently a variety of speech sounds signal a single meaning. Examples of the first sort of complexity are well known and beloved by punsters. There is *meat* and *meet,* or *watch* in the sense of "look at" and *watch* in the sense of "time piece." The other type of complexity is less well known and is worth spending some time on.

Phonological theory distinguishes between two major sorts of variation in the speech sounds of a language, one which is accompanied by varia-tion in meaning and one which is not. Languages vary considerably, however, in their rules for assigning a particular variation to one cate-gory rather than another, and so the infant has to *learn* which is which. Examples of variation in sounds which are not accompanied by variation in meaning are many of the regional variations in the pronunciation of English or even the peculiarities of individual speakers. An example of the variation in sound which in English conveys a difference in meaning is that between *ship* and *sheep*. The interest of this example is that Spanish speakers have great difficulty in noticing the change because in Spanish it is of no importance.

I will give one further example to underscore the complexities in phonology which an infant may encounter and the need for access to meaning in order to master them. In modern Irish, the initial consonant of the word *bád* (boat) is modified after the definite article as indicated in 12:

12. Case	Normal script	First consonant
Nom.	*An bád*	[b]
Gen.	*An bháid*	[v]
Dat.	*An mbád*	[m]

What is noteworthy is that elsewhere in Irish, initial [m] and [b], for example, are contrasted as can be seen from the pair, *moladh* (praise) and *boladh* (smell). However, after the article in the dative case the initial [b] of *boladh* is replaced by [m] so that it sounds identical with *moladh*. We have, then a variation in sound which is sometimes accompanied by a variation in meaning and sometimes not.

In all, we have discussed three types of phonological variation, one accompanied by change of meaning, one not accompanied by change of meaning, and one which is sometimes accompanied by change in meaning and sometimes not. We began this section with changes in meaning without any change in sound. How is the infant to find his way through this many-branched puzzle?

The answer must be that the infant is able to relate sound and meaning because he is able to tell what the speaker is speaking about independent of the speaker's language. This follows naturally from the evidence presented. The infant cannot use the sound system of a language to get at the meaning until he has learned the system. There seems to be little in the sound system itself which could direct the child in the choice of which sound differences to attend to and which to ignore. However, if he can determine the meaning and has sufficiently acute powers of auditory discrimination to begin with,* the infant can use meaning as the key to the sound system and thus arrive at the most elementary building blocks of his language.

---

* There is now some evidence that infants are born with very fine powers of discrimination for speech sounds, and that learning for them consists mainly in ignoring differences in sound. The relevant material is well reviewed in Kaplan and Kaplan (in press).

Roger Brown (1958, pp. 213 ff.) describes a highly relevant experiment in his chapter on the original word game. He showed chips of different colors to native English speakers; each color was "named" with a nonsense syllable. Certain syllables differed only in vowel length which is not phonemic in English. The subjects were asked to group the chips in accordance with their names. Brown found that length of vowel was ignored if the corresponding chips differed little in color, but if the difference in color was marked, then different groups of chips were formed to correspond to the long and short vowels. In other words, subjects used the physical properties of the objects named as clues to the phonological units employed in naming them. Though his subjects were adults, the conclusion can be extended to infants without undue hesitation.

The claim that the infant uses meaning as the key to phonology needs to be filled out with details of how he does so, but unfortunately we know very little of the process. My remarks here are intended mainly as suggestions for further investigation. Let us begin by returning to the Irish example. Clearly the infant must use the fact that the referent is constant to arrive at the appreciation that [bád], [váid], and [mád] are all different realizations of the same phonological entity. In other words there are three different surface realizations of the same underlying morphophonemic form. Similarly, he must use the fact that *moladh* and *boladh* refer to different things (at least in equivalent environments) to avoid the mistake of treating these two words as different realizations of the same morphological entity. But while such a strategy works well for the examples I gave, how is the infant to avoid applying the constancy-of-referent strategy indiscriminately with disastrous phonological consequences? For example, *Fido* and *dog* might well be used to refer to a single animal, but to treat them as different surface realizations of the same phonological deep structure would be fatal. *Little* and *small* have more or less the same meaning, but they are phonologically quite distinct. The solution is that the various realizations of the Irish word *bád* are instances of a very general and simple phonological regularity. The rule for the dative (somewhat simplified), for example, is to voice the initial consonant if it is unvoiced and if it is voiced to replace it with the homorganic nasal (i.e., the nasal most closely related from an articulatory point of view). Part of the child's capacity to learn a language is his ability to detect such phonological regularities. Meaning alone cannot reveal them, though it probably directs the child to look for them. There are no phonological regularities relating *Fido* and *dog* or *little* and *small*. In the absence of such regularities the infant does not attempt to relate them phonologically despite the correspondences in meaning.

To learn a language involves relating a system of intentions to a phonological system. To know the one is not *ipso facto* to know the other. Indeed the two are often related only through a complex system of syntax. I have had to have recourse to the syntactic system more than once in the foregoing discussion. For example, the phonological modifications of initial consonants in Irish are a function of syntactic rules which presumably must be learned together with the phonological modifications themselves. The combination of phonology and syntax are also presumably involved in the explanation of how the infant manages to distinguish such homonyms as *meat* and *meet,* and such nonhomonyms as *moladh* and *boladh.* This is hardly surprising in view of the fact that phonology and syntax are theoretical distinctions which are employed in the description of what is experientially a unit, the speech act. To explain the learning of phonology by means of syntax is not, however, to abandon the main thesis of this paper. In the previous section I argued that the learning of most basic syntactic relationships is possible only with the aid of meaning.

CONCLUDING REMARKS

I have treated of the learning of vocabulary, syntax, and phonology in separate sections, but the three could not be kept apart. It was necessary to base the learning of syntax in large part on knowledge of vocabulary, and it was necessary to base the learning of phonology in some part on knowledge of syntax. At this point it might be as well to correct the impression that infants use meaning to learn vocabulary, vocabulary to learn syntax, and syntax to learn phonology. It was not my intention to propose anything so neat. It is evident that some syntactic learning cannot be based on a knowledge of the referents of the lexical items employed. Similarly, phonology cannot be entirely dependent on prior knowledge of syntax. To argue that it was would be to argue in a circle, because without some independent grasp of phonology one could not perceive either words or syntactic devices. One cannot at once make the perception of vocabulary and syntax dependent on knowledge of phonology and make knowledge of phonology dependent on knowledge of vocabulary and syntax. The way out of this circle is to recognize that the interdependencies are only partial, though it is important to appreciate that at present they are quite obscure.

I have continually insisted on the child's possessing nonlinguistic cognitive processes before he learns their linguistic signal. By this I do not intend to endow the infant at birth with a complete ready-made set of cognitive structures. I accept Piaget's thesis that children gradually develop many of the cognitive structures, which they employ in association with language. Neither do I suggest that the child has a complete set of cognitive structures at the moment when he begins to learn language. All that is needed for my position is that the development of those basic cognitive structures to which I referred should precede the development of the corresponding linguistic structures. Since the acquisition of linguistic structures is spread over a long period, there is no reason that the acquisition of the corresponding nonlinguistic ones should not also extend well into the period of language learning.

I have repeatedly compared the infant to a linguist engaged in describing a language which to him is new. This seems a fair comparison provided the limp is recognized. Clearly, the infant does not produce explicit rules whereas the linguist does. The linguist aims to make explicit the native speaker's latent knowledge. Otherwise the tasks of infant and linguist are similar. Hockett (1961) points out that in fact no linguist has ever succeeded in deciphering a language without making use of meaning. He instances the Rosetta Stone which carried the same message in three languages, Greek, Demotic, and Hieroglyphic Egyptian. Because they knew Greek, Young and Champollion succeeded in deciphering the other two languages which no one at the time was able to read or understand. Similarly, Old Irish was deciphered by a Bavarian scholar named Johanne Kasper Zeuss. He worked on seven Latin manuscripts which carried glosses in Old Irish explaining the text. His great work, *Grammatica Celtica,* appeared in Latin in 1853, the first grammar of Old Irish.

It is not too fanciful to think of the infant as treating the sentences he hears as glosses on the events that occur about him. The grammar he writes is not in Latin or in any other language, but in some neurological code of which as yet not a single letter has been deciphered.

REFERENCES

BEVER, T. G.: The cognitive basis for linguistic structures. In J. R. Hayes (Ed.), *Cognition and Language Learning.* New York: Wiley, 1970.

BLOOM, L.: *Language Development: Form and Function in Emerging Grammars.* Boston: M.I.T. Press, 1970.

BLOOMFIELD, L.: *Language.* New York: Holt, Rinehart & Winston, 1933.

BLOUNT, B. G.: *Acquisition of Language by Luo Children.* Berkeley: Language Behavior Research Laboratory, University of California, 1969.

BROWN, R.: *Words and Things.* New York: Free Press, 1958.

BROWN, R.: *Stage 1. Semantic and Grammatical Relations.* Cambridge, Mass.: Harvard University, Department of Psychology, 1970. (Mimeo)

BROWN, R., & BELLUGI, U.: Three processes in the child's acquisition of syntax. *Harvard Educational Review,* 1964, 34, 133-151.

BROWN, R., CAZDEN, C. B., & BELLUGI, U.: The child's grammar from I to III. In J. P. Hill (Ed.), *1967 Minnesota Symposium on Child Psychology. Minneapoliss* University of Minnesota Press, 1969.

BROWN, R., & FRASER, C.: The acquisition of syntax. In U. Bellugi & R. Brown (Eds.), The acquisition of language. *Monographs of the Society for Research in Child Development,* 1964, 29, 43-79.

BROWN, R. & HANLON, C.: Derivational complexity and order of acquisition in child speech. In J. R. Hayes (Ed.), *Cognition and the Development of Language.* New York: Wiley, 1970.

CARNAP, R.: *Meaning and Necessity.* (2nd ed.) Chicago: University of Chicago Press, 1956.

CAZDEN, C. B.: The psychology of language. In L. E. Travis (Ed.), *Handbook of Speech, Hearing and Language Disorders.* (Rev. ed.) New York: Appleton-Century-Crofts, 1969.

CHOMSKY, C.: *The Acquisition of Syntax in Children 5 to 10.* (Res. Mono. No. 57) Cambridge, Mass.: M.I.T. Press, 1969.

CHOMSKY, N.: *Syntactic Structures.* The Hague: Moulton, 1957.

CHOMSKY, N.: *Aspects of the Theory of Syntax.* Cambridge, Mass.: M.I.T. Press, 1965.

CHOMSKY, N.: *Deep Structure, Surface Structure, and Semantic Interpretation.* Bloomington: Indiana University, Linguistics Circle, 1968. (Mimeo)

CLARK, E. V.: On the acquisition of the meaning of *before* and *after. Journal of Verbal Learning and Verbal Behavior,* 1971, 10, 266-275.

CROMER, R. F.: "Children are nice to understand": Surface structure, clues for the recovery of a deep structure. *British Journal of Psychology,* 1970, 61, 397-408.

DONALDSON, H., & BALFOUR, G.: Less is more: A study of language comprehension in children. *British Journal of Psychology,* 1968, 59, 461-471.

ERVIN-TRIPP, S.: Structure and process in language acquisition. In, *Report of the Twenty-first Annual Round Table Meeting on Linguistics and Language Studies.* Washington, D. C.: Georgetown University Press, 1970.

FILLMORE, C. J.: The case for case. In E. Bach & R. T. Harms (Eds.), *Universals in Linguistic Theory.* New York: Holt, Rinehart & Winston, 1968.

FODOR, J. A.: Could meaning be an r_m? *Journal of Verbal Learning and Verbal Behavior,* 1965, 4, 73-81.

FODOR, J. A.: How to learn to talk: Some simple ways. In F. Smith & G. A. Miller (Eds.), *The Genesis of Language.* Cambridge, Mass.: M.I.T. Press, 1966.

FREGE, G.: *Philosophical Writings.* (Ed. by Peter Geech & Max Black) Oxford: Basil Blackwell, 1952.

GLEASON, J. B.: Do children imitate? Paper presented at the international conference on oral education of the deaf, Lexington School for the Deaf. New York, June 1967.

HOCKETT, C. F.: Linguistic elements and their relations. *Language,* 1961, 37, 29-53.

HOFFMAN, M.: Child language. Unpublished master's thesis, McGill University, Department of Psychology, 1968.

KAPLAN, E. L., & KAPLAN, G. A.: Is there any such thing as a pre-linguistic child? In J. E. Lot (Ed.), *Human Development and Cognitive Processes.* New York: Holt, Rinehart & Winston, in press.

KERNAN, K. T.: The acquisition of language by Samoan children. Unpublished doctoral dissertation, University of California, Berkeley, Department of Anthropology, 1969.

LAKOFF, G.: Instrumental adverbs and the concept of deep structure. *Foundations of Language,* 1968, 4, 4-29.

LAKOFF, G. & ROSS, J. R.: *Is Deep Structure Necessary?* Cambridge, Mass.: Author, 1967.

LIEBERMAN, P.: *Intonation, Perception and Language.* Boston: M.I.T. Press, 1967.

LYONS, J.: *Introduction to Theoretical Linguistics.* Cambridge: Cambridge University Press, 1968.

MCCAWLEY, J. D.: The role of semantics in a grammar. In E. Bach & R. T. Harms (Eds.), *Universals in Linguistic Theory.* New York: Holt, Rinehart & Winston, 1968.

MCNEILL, D.: Developmental psycholinguistics. In F. Smith & G. A. Miller (Eds.), *The Genesis of Language.* Cambridge, Mass.: M.I.T. Press, 1966. (a)

MCNEILL, D.: The creation of language by children. In J. Lyons & R. J. Wales (Eds.), *Psycholinguistics Papers: Proceedings of the 1966 Edinburgh Conference.* Edinburgh: Edinburgh University Press, 1966 (b)

MCNEILL, D.: *The Acquisition of Language: The Study of Developmental Psycholinguistics.* New York: Harper & Row, 1970.

MILLER, G. A., GALANTER, E., & PRIBRAM, K. H.: *Plans and the Structure of Behavior.* New York: Holt, Rinehart & Winston, 1960.

MOWRER, O. H.: *Learning Theory and the Symbolic Process.* New York: Wiley, 1960.

OGDEN, C. K. & RICHARDS, I. A.: *The Meaning of Meaning.* New York: Harcourt, Brace & World, 1938.

OSGOOD, C. E.: *Psycholinguistics.* In S. Koch (Ed.), *Psychology: A Study of a Science.* Vol. 6. New York: McGraw-Hill, 1963.

PIAGET, J.: Le langage et les opérations intellectuelles. In *Problèmes de psycholinguistique.* (Symposium de l'association de psychologie scientifique de langue française.) Paris: Presses Universitaires de France, 1963, 51-72.

QUINE, W. V.: *Word and Object.* New York: Wiley, 1960.

QUINE, W. V.: *From a Logical Point of View.* Cambridge, Mass.: Harvard University Press, 1961.

SAUSSURE, F. DE: *Course in General Linguistics.* New York: McGraw-Hill, 1959.

SCHLESINGER, I. M.: Production of utterances and language acquisition. In D. Slobin (Ed.), *The Ontogenesis of Grammar.* New York: Academic Press, 1971.

SHIPLEY, E. F., SMITH, C. S., & GLEITMAN, L. R.: A study of the acquisition of language: Free responses to commands. *Language,* 1969, 45, 322-342.

SINCLAIR-DE-ZWART, H.: Developmental psycholinguistics. In D. Elkind & J. H. Flavell (Eds.), *Studies in Cognitive Development: Essays in Honor of Jean Piaget.* New York: Oxford University Press, 1969.

SLOBIN, D. I.: Acquisition of Russian as a native language. In F. Smith & G. A. Miller (Eds.), *The Genesis of Language.* Cambridge, Mass.: M.I.T. Press, 1960.

SLOBIN, D. I.: Universals of grammatical development in children. In G. B. Flores d'Arcais & W. J. M. Levelt (Eds.), *Advances in Psycholinguistics.* Amsterdam: North Holland, 1971.

SLOBIN, D. I. & WELSH, C. A.: Elicited imitation as a research tool in developmental psycholinguistics. In C. A. Ferguson & D. J. Slobin (Eds.), *Readings on Child Language Acquisition.* New York: Holt, Rinehart & Winston, in press.

SMITH, C.: An experimental approach to children's linguistic competence. In J. R. Hayes (Ed.), *Cognition and the Development of Language.* New York: Wiley, 1970.

TUCKER, G. R.: French speaker's skill with grammatical gender. Unpublished doctoral dissertation, McGill University, Department of Psychology, 1967.

VERNON, M.: Language development's relationship to cognition, affectivity and intelligence. Paper presented at the meeting of the Canadian Psychological Institute, St. John's Newfoundland, June 1971.

VYGOTSKY, L. S.: *Thought and Language.* Cambridge, Mass.: M.I.T. Press, 1962.

18

NEGRO CHILDREN'S USE OF NONSTANDARD GRAMMAR

Samuel J. Marwit, Karen L. Marwit and

John J. Boswell

University of Missouri at St. Louis

Two Negro and two white examiners presented 93 Negro and 108 white second graders with a task requiring them to derive the present, plural, possessive, and time extension forms of nonsense syllables. The hypothesis that white subjects would supply more standard English forms and Negro subjects more nonstandard English forms was supported. The hypothesized characteristics of nonstandard English were upheld in all but one category. The possibility of Negro nonstandard English being a distinct "quasi-foreign" language system and its implications were discussed.

It has been noted for a long time (Klineberg, 1935; Pasamanick & Knobloch, 1955) that Negro children, primarily those of lower socioeconomic status, appear deficient in language functioning. Many of these linguistic "deficiencies" are similar to those noted among white children of low socioeconomic status (Bernstein, 1961; Templin, 1957); others appear specifically related to race (Deutsch, 1965). Most of the litera-

Reprinted from JOURNAL OF EDUCATIONAL PSYCHOLOGY, 1972, Vol. 63, No. 3, pp. 218-224.

This research was supported by United States Department of Health, Education, and Welfare, Office of Education Grant No. OEG-6-70-0041 (509) and by funds supplied by Office of Research Administration, University of Missouri-St. Louis. The opinions expressed herein do not necessarily reflect the position or policy of the United States Office of Education and no official endorsement by them should be inferred.

ture to date has been focused either on the relationship of these deficits to specific cognitive impairments (Deutsch, 1965; John, 1963; John & Goldstein, 1964; Klineberg, 1935) or to those social conditions that might be responsible for the manifestation of such problems (Gray & Klaus, 1963; McCarthy, 1969; Milner, 1951; Nisbet, 1961). Regardless, the traditional view of Negro children's language is that it represents a "substandard" language relative to white middle-class norms and expectations (S. Baratz, 1968).

Recently, however, some linguists and educators (Bailey, 1968; J. Baratz, 1969; S. Baratz, 1968; Labov, 1967; Stewart, 1967, 1968; Vetter, 1969) have come to regard "black language" as a uniquely different linguistic system from that of standard American English. Instead of considering it *sub*standard American English, they have come to view it as *non*standard American English. They point out that black language follows a consistent and predictable set of phonological and grammatical rules that are highly elaborated and sophisticated, and different from those governing the standard English used by most white Americans. If this is the case, Negro children are approaching the traditional school situation with the overwhelming disadvantage of speaking a "quasi-foreign language" (Stewart, 1968) which is neither fully recognized nor openly accepted. The problems this poses in holding one's own in reading, writing, communication, and concept formation have been clearly illustrated by Bailey (1968) and Vetter (1969). These problems, according to Deutsch (1965), are "cumulative" and therefore increase over the child's academic career.

Using standard English as a reference point, the major distinguishing syntactical features of Negro nonstandard English are (a) the zero copula (absence of the verb "is" in the present tense); (b) singularization of plural objects; (c) the zero possessive (lack of a morphological possessive); and (d) the use of "be" to represent time extension. Examples of each of these, respectively, are, "He go," "There are two hat," "The man hat," and "He be going."

Unfortunately, most of the literature pertaining to these nonstandard patterns has been descriptive and observational. Few attempts, if any, have been made to study them empirically. If Negro nonstandard English is, in fact, a well-ordered, highly structured, highly developed language system, we must assume, as does J. Baratz (1969), that by the time the Negro child is 5, he has learned the rules of *his* linguistic environment. The present study investigates this by employing a design similar to that used by Berko (1958) in studying white children's acquisition of the rules of standard English. Negro and white second graders were required to transform nonsense syllables in ways designed to represent each of the above four distinguishing grammatical features. Nonsense syllables were used to insure that the child was responding in terms of internalized rules and not in terms of familiarity with preexisting vocabulary. It was hypothesized that for each category, white children would supply significantly more standard English forms and Negro children significantly more nonstandard English forms of the variety described above.

METHOD

Subjects

A total of 229 second graders from 10 classrooms of four elementary schools in a St. Louis County public school system were tested by two Negro and two white examiners. Nineteen of these subjects were discarded because of an examiner's failure to present standard instructions, 8 because information relevant to socioeconomic status could not be obtained, and 1 because of oriental origin. The remaining sample consisted of 93 Negro subjects, 38 of whom were tested by Negro examiners, 55 by white examiners; and 108 white subjects, 49 tested by Negro examiners, 59 by white examiners. Subjects were further subdivided into high, middle, and low socioeconomic status by applying Hollingshead's (1958) Occupational scale from his Two Factor Index of Social Position to subjects' parents' occupation. High, middle, and low were arbitrarily represented by Categories 1-3, 4, and 5-7, respectively. Unfortunately, parental occupation was the only demographic datum provided by the schools. The absence of supportive educational and/or income information necessarily reduces the validity of the scale (Light & Smith, 1969) and any effects due to socioeconomic status must be interpreted with this in mind.

Apparatus

Each subject was administered a test consisting of 24 ambiguous drawings each accompanied by sentences read by the examiner describing the drawing as either an object or a person engaged in some action. In all cases, the object or action was labeled by a nonsense syllable and presented to the subject in such a way that he was required to derive the present, plural, possessive, or time extension form of the nonsense syllable. The first four items were sample items offered to (a) familiarize the subject with the task and (b) to assure the examiner that his subject understood and was able to perform it. These were followed by 20 test items arranged sequentially such that each of the 5 items assessing present tense was followed by one testing the formation of plural objects, followed by possessive, followed by time extension. This order was chosen to minimize the generalization of a set established on one item to any of the four related items. Examples of each test item and the order of presentation are given below:

(1) Present tense. Stick figure reclining with legs crossed and head on hand. "This is a man who knows how to pid. What is he doing now? Now he ————."

(2) Pluralization. One, then two figures resembling musical notes. "This is a lun. No there is another one. There are two of them. There are two ————."

(3) Possessive. Cup, lun holding cup. "This is a cup that belongs to the lun. Whose cup is it? It is the ————."

(4) Time extension. Stick figure positioned for throwing. "This is a man who knows how to mork. He does this *all the time. All the time, he* ————."

The 18 nonsense syllables employed for the total 24 items (12 used only once as in 1 and 4 above, 6 duplicated as in 2 and 3 above) were selected from a total of 25 nonsense syllables on the basis of association values obtained from an independent sample of 60 Negro and 22 white second graders from a school system other than the one under study (J. J. Boswell, K. L. Marwit, & S. J. Marwit, unpublished data, 1970). Those 15 syllables which had the lowest association value and the highest frequency of independent responses were employed as test stimuli. The next three highest in "nonsensibility" were employed as sample items. The remaining six were discarded from study.

All sessions were recorded on Ampex 641-¼-1800 tape using a Wollensak 1500 tape recorder at 3¾ inches per second.

Testing Procedure

Prior to testing, examiners attended four 2-hour training sessions, half of each being devoted to the practice testing of children (four per examiner) from schools other than those used in the study, and half devoted to a discussion of problems in test administration and to practice in the verbatim recording of subjects' responses. Examiners were told that they were participating in a study of language development but never informed of the hypothesis being tested. They were instructed to accept all subject responses as being "inherently correct for that particular child at his particular stage of linguistic development." Posttest interviews confirmed each examiner's ignorance of the purpose of the research.

Testing for data collection was performed in rooms set aside by each school for the express purpose of conducting this study. Each subject was tested individually. Each was seated at a table opposite the examiner and told that he was "about to play a little word game using a tape recorder" and that he was to speak directly into the microphone placed before him. The task was then introduced to the child as follows:

> We are going to play a silly word game with a bunch of silly words that somebody made up. I think you will find this a lot of fun. What I am going to do is this. I am going to say some sentences but I will leave off the last part. What you are to do is finish the last part for me. OK? (Answer any questions that might arise). Now let's practice.

The examiner then administered the four sample items which could be repeated for the child, if necessary. Examiners were not permitted, however, to repeat anything more than the sentence stem. Most children comprehended the task by Item 2, all by Item 3. Practice was followed by the examiner's presentation of the 20 test items, for which no repetition was permitted. Each subjects' responses were recorded verbatim in a test booklet which also provided space for his name, sex, age, race, and "comments."

Rating Procedure

All tapes of all sessions were given to two student speech clinicians who independently recorded all subjects' responses verbatim in test booklets identical to those used by examiners. It was felt that "trained ears" whose sole task was to listen and record would provide an accurate assessment of each subject's responses as well as a reliability check on the examiners' ability to record these responses. Responses recorded by examiners and speech clinicians were then rated by the three principal investigators blind to subjects' identifying information. The rating scale provided categories for standard English, nonstandard English as hypothesized, and nonstandard English other than hypothesized. This scale and examples utilizing sentence stems from the sample items above are included in Table 1.

A kappa coefficient (k) of agreement for nominal scale data (Fleiss, Cohen, & Everitt, 1969) was used to test interrecorder reliability. All ks were highly significant $(p < .001)$. Tests of significance between ks

TABLE 1

RATING SCALE AND EXAMPLES OF STANDARD ENGLISH, NONSTANDARD ENGLISH AS HYPOTHESIZED, AND
NONSTANDARD ENGLISH OTHER THAN HYPOTHESIZED

Task and category	Rating	Example
Present tense		Now he_____.
SE	1	is pidding, pids
NSE as hypothesized	2	pid
NSE other than hypothesized	3	is pid
NSE other than hypothesized	4	pidding
No response	5	
Pluralization		There are two ____.
SE	1	luns
NSE as hypothesized	2	lun
No response	5	
Possessive		It is the _____.
SE	1	lun's
NSE as hypothesized	2	lun
No response	5	
Time extension		All the time, he _____.
SE	1	is morking, morks
NSE as hypothesized	2	be morking
NSE other than hypothesized	3	mork
NSE other than hypothesized	4	morking
No response	5	

Note.—Abbreviations: SE = standard English, NSE = nonstandard English.

were nonsignificant. While the vast majority of test items showed triple agreement, those that did not showed at least double agreement. Thus, the "test two out of three" was defined as the criterion for obtaining scores for the final data analyses.

RESULTS

Individual Differences between Examiners

It was decided, *a priori,* to initially test for differences between examiners. Univariate analyses of variance comparing all examiners for each rating category for each of the four tasks revealed only one significant main effect. That was for the number of standard English forms elicited on the present tense task $(F = 2.86, df = 3/197, p < .05)$. A Duncan multiple-range test (Winer, 1962) showed this to be the result of differences between Negro and white examiners and not between examiners of the same race. On this basis, both Negro examiners' scores were combined as were both white examiners' scores. All ensuing analyses of variance, therefore, employed two levels of examiner race in addition to the two levels of subject race and three levels of subject socioeconomic status.

TABLE 2
ANALYSIS OF VARIANCE OF NUMBER OF STANDARD
AMERICAN ENGLISH FORMS SUPPLIED BY
NEGRO AND WHITE SUBJECTS ON
FOUR TASKS

Source	df	MS	F
Between			
Examiner race (A)	1	6.22	.55
Subject race (B)	1	140.07	12.45**
Subject socioeconomic status (C)	2	34.96	3.11
A × B	1	1.48	.13
A × C	2	3.40	.30
B × C	2	12.08	1.07
A × B × C	2	3.47	.31
Error	189	11.25	
Within			
Task (D)	3	62.84	64.58***
A × D	3	1.76	1.80
B × D	3	5.17	5.31**
C × D	6	1.37	1.41
A × B × D	3	2.73	2.80*
A × C × D	6	.73	.75
B × C × D	6	2.97	3.05*
A × B × C × D	6	.59	.60
Error	378	.97	

* $p < .05$.
** $p < .01$.
*** $p < .001$.

Standard English

The multivariate analysis of variance used to test the hypothesis that white subjects supply significantly more standard English forms than Negro subjects on all four tasks is presented in Table 2. The mean number of standard English endings supplied by both races on all tasks can be obtained from Table 3. While all four mean comparisons are in the hypothesized direction and a strongly significant effect of subject race was obtained, a Subject Race × Task interaction was also obtained indicating significant race effects on certain tasks only. Univariate analyses of variance analyzing each task separately indicate significant effects of subject race on the plural ($F = 7.78$, $df = 1/189$, $p < .005$), possessive ($F = 12.11$, $df = 1/189$, $p < .0001$), and time extension ($F = 20.03$, $df = 1/189$, $p < .0001$) dimensions but not on the present tense task.

Two significant triple interactions were obtained. Observation of the relevant means indicates that the Examiner Race × Subject Race × Task interaction is the result of Negro examiners eliciting more standard English from Negro subjects on all but the time extension task and from white subjects on all but the plural task. Whether this is primarily an examiner effect with Negro examiners facilitating or white examiners suppressing the occurrence of standard English regardless of subject race, or an interactive effect dependent upon particular examiner—subject combinations cannot be ascertained from the present design, nor can the reason for the reversal of these effects in one of four cases. The Subject Race × Subject Socioeconomic Status × Task interaction was analyzed by applying Scheffé's (1953) test to all pairs of mean differences in the amount of standard English endings supplied by each race on each task at each socioeconomic level ($k = 24$). In all comparisons, white subjects supplied more standard English than Negro subjects. Neither Negro nor white subjects of high socioeconomic status nor Negro and white subjects of middle socioeconomic status differed in their relative rates of supplying standard English endings to each of the four tasks. In other words, the functions depicting both races' performances across the four tasks at these socioeconomic levels were essentially parallel. On the other hand, a significant difference was obtained when comparing Negro and white subjects of low socioeconomic status in their relative rates of responding to the present and time extension tasks as vs. the plural and possessive tasks ($F = 53.27$, F' $(_{.01}) = 43.31$). Plotting the means for these groups across tasks indicates nonparallel functions and suggests that the major contributing factor in the triple interaction is the differential rate of responding on the time extension task. Whether white subjects are overproducing or Negro subjects underproducing standard English forms on this task relative to their performance on the other three tasks cannot be determined, nor can the reason for this discrepancy occurring among subjects of one socioeconomic level only.

Nonstandard English

Inherent in the white subject's significantly greater productivity of standard English is the implication that Negro subjects respond significantly more with either one or a number of nonstandard English forms. To determine whether these are of the variety hypothesized, a multivariate analysis of variance, similar in structure to that found in Table 2, was run for the total number of hypothesized nonstandard English

TABLE 3

MEAN NUMBER OF STANDARD AMERICAN ENGLISH AND NONSTANDARD AMERICAN ENGLISH AS HYPOTHESIZED FORMS SUPPLIED BY NEGRO AND WHITE SUBJECTS ON PRESENT, PLURAL, POSSESSIVE, AND TIME EXTENSION TASKS

Form	Race	n	Task							
			Present		Plural		Possessive		Time extension	
			M	SD	M	SD	M	SD	M	SD
Standard	White	108	2.65	1.94	3.91	1.81	3.93	1.75	4.00	1.78
	Negro	93	1.80	1.80	2.89	2.01	2.73	1.93	2.45	2.11
Nonstandard	White	108	1.15	1.83	1.06	1.78	1.04	1.71	.90[a]	1.71
	Negro	93	1.75	1.92	2.04	1.99	2.25	1.95	2.43[a]	2.14

[a] No nonstandard English as hypothesized, rated 2, was obtained for time extension. Scores entered represent the mean number of 3 ratings obtained.

forms obtained from subjects of both races on the present, plural, and possessive tasks. Time extension was omitted from analysis because no nonstandard English as hypothesized was obtained. In other words, no subject responded to the sentence stem "All the time, he ———" by supplying "be" followed by the gerund form of the nonsense syllable.

As can be seen in Table 3, all means for the three comparisons are in the predicted direction. The analysis of variance displayed a significant effect of subject race ($F = 8.80$, $df = 1/189$, $p < .01$) and a significant Subject Race $\times$ Task interaction ($F = 3.18$, $df = 2/378$, $p < .05$) which complements results obtained in the analysis of standard English forms described above. Univariate analyses of variance analyzing each task separately again showed significant effects of subject race for the plural ($F = 8.10$, $df = 1/189$, $p < .005$) and possessive ($F = 12.92$, $df = 1/189$, $p < .0005$) tasks and again failed to reach significance for the present tense variable. Regarding time extension, while no hypothesized nonstandard English forms were obtained, Negro subjects did consistently offer a nonhypothesized nonstandard English form. Significantly more Negro than white subjects responded to the time extension stem by supplying the stimulus syllable, without modification ($F = 20.07$, $df = 1/189$, $p < .0001$) thereby obtaining a rating of 3 (see Table 1).

DISCUSSION

In general, the results support the hypothesis that white children supply more standard English endings to response syllables designed to represent the plural and possessive of nouns and the present and time extension forms of verbs, and that Negro subjects, consequently, supply more nonstandard English forms. Significant syntactical differences due to subject race were obtained on all but the present tense task. The hypothesized characteristics of Negro nonstandard English were supported for all but the time extension dimension.

The failure to obtain significant subject race differences on the present tense task was a particularly unexpected finding. While it is possible that, in actuality, no differences exist, it is unlikely since it is this category, more than any other, that is referred to in the literature when documenting racial differences in language functions. A second possibility is that differences do exist but that the grammatical rules involved are particularly difficult to learn and are not incorporated by the time children reach second grade. However, this too is unlikely since it is hard to see what is more difficult about learning these rules than those governing the other three tasks for which significant differences were obtained. More likely, the failure to obtain significance resulted from the investigators' poor assignment of nonsense stimuli to this task. Of the five words used to test present tense, one was ris, another zub. To the first, subjects could respond with ris which would be rated nonstandard English as hypothesized or risses, rated standard English. The final s on the stimulus syllable makes the auditory discrimination of these forms difficult, especially if the response is slurred or spoken rapidly. Similarly, with zub, subjects could respond with either, "Now he's zubbing," a standard English form, or "Now he zubbing," a nonstandard English form. Research now in progress has substituted more easily discernible stimuli; that is, nonsense syllables not containing sibilants in the initial or final position, and should help determine whether or not the hypothesized differences exist.

Regarding the preponderance of nonstandard English given by Negro subjects, the hypothesized form was given to a significant degree on the plural and possessive tasks. A noteworthy but nonsignificant trend in this direction was also obtained for the present tense task. The failure to reach significance in this latter case is probably the complementary result of the poor choice of present tense nonsense syllables discussed above. The complete failure of the time extension task to elicit any nonstandard English as hypothesized was surprising. Either the hypothesized form was incorrect or the sentence stem was improperly structured to elicit it. According to J. Baratz (1969) and others, "be" followed by the "ing" form of the verb in and of itself denotes time extension for the Negro child. It is therefore possible that the authors' use of the stem "all the time" obviated the Negro subjects' need to supply "be-ing." To do so would have simply been redundant and poor grammatical form in any man's language. Just what stimulus, if any, is required to elicit the hypothesized nonstandard form of time extension must remain a question for future investigation. More important for the present hypothesis, however, is recognition of the fact that even though Negro subjects failed to respond with the hypothesized nonstandard form, they did supply an alternate nonstandard form with significant regularity.

The consistent use of nonstandard English forms by Negro subjects is probably the most remarkable finding of this study. It lends empirical support to those who have claimed that "black language" is a separate, highly consistent language with fixed grammatical rules that differ in particular ways from the rules governing the language used by most white Americans. If black language were nothing more than a substandard form of standard English, a sloppy array of nonstandard forms should have emerged. Instead, well-defined nonstandard forms differing in set ways from standard English were elicited for the most part by each sentence stem. The problems inherent in a culture supporting languages differing in grammar yet sharing the same vocabulary are too immense to be elaborated upon here. Yet, it seems imperative to note, in conclusion, that unless the distinguishing features of one language are recognized and accepted by speakers of the other, no one stands to gain.

REFERENCES

BAILEY, B. L.: Some aspects of the impact of linguistics on language teaching in disadvantaged communities. Elementary Education, 1968, 45, 570-579.

BARATZ, J. C.: Language and cognitive assessment of Negro children: Assumptions and research needs. Asha, 1969, 11, 87-91.

BARATZ, S. S.: Social science strategies for research on the Afro-American. Paper presented at the meeting of the American Psychological Association, San Francisco, September, 1968.

BERKO, J.: The child's learning of English morphology. Word, 1958, 14, 150-177.

BERNSTEIN, B.: Social structure, language, and learning. Educational Research, 1961, 3, 163-176.

DEUTSCH, M.: The role of social class in language development and cognition. American Journal of Orthopsychiatry, 1965, 35, 78-88.

FLEISS, J. L., COHEN, J., & EVERITT, B. S.: Large sample standard errors of kappa and weighted kappa. Psychological Bulletin, 1969, 72, 323-327.

GRAY, S. W. & KLAUS, R.: Early Training Project: Interim report. Murfreesboro, Tenn.: The City Schools and Peabody College for Teachers, November, 1963. (Mimeo)

HOLLINGSHEAD, A. B. & REDLICH, F. C.: Social Class and Mental Illness. New York: Wiley, 1958.

JOHN, V. P.: The intellectual development of slum children: Some preliminary findings. American Journal of Orthopsychiatry, 1963, 33, 813-822.

JOHN, V. P. & GOLDSTEIN, L. S.: The social context of language acquisition. Merrill-Palmer Quarterly, 1964, 10, 265-276.

KLINEBERG, O. A.: Negro Intelligence and Selective Migration. New York: Columbia University Press, 1935.

LABOV, W.: Some suggestions for teaching standard English to speakers of nonstandard urban dialects. In *New Directions in Elementary English.* Champaign, Ill.: National Council of Teachers of English, 1967.

LIGHT, R. J. & SMITH, P. V.: Social allocation models of intelligence: A methodological inquiry. *Harvard Educational Review,* 1969, 39, 484-510.

McCARTHY, D. A.: Affective aspects of language learning. (Presidential address, Division of Developmental Psychology, American Psychological Association, September, 1961.) *APA Newsletter,* Division of Developmental Psychology, Fall, 1961, 1-11.

MILNER, E.: A study of the relationship between reading readiness in grade one school children and patterns of parent-child interaction. *Child Development,* 1951, 22, 95-112.

NISBIT, J. P.: Family environment and intelligence. In A. H. Halsey, J. Floud, & C. A. Anderson (Eds.): *Education, Economy, and Society.* New York: Free Press of Glencoe, 1961.

PASAMANICK, B. & KNOBLOCH, H.: Early language behavior in Negro children and the testing of intelligence. *Journal of Abnormal and Social Psychology,* 1955, 50, 401-402.

SCHEFFÉ, H.: A method for judging all contrasts in the analysis of variance. *Biometrika,* 1953, 40, 87-104.

STEWART, W. A.: Sociolinguistic factors in the history of American Negro dialects. *The Florida FL Reporter,* 1967, 5 (No. 2, 1-4).

STEWART, W. A.: Continuity and change in American Negro dialects. *The Florida FL Reporter,* Spring, 1968.

TEMPLIN, N. C.: *Certain Language Skills in Children.* Minneapolis: University of Minnesota Press, 1957.

VETTER, H. J.: *Language Behavior and Communication.* Itasca, Ill.: Peacock Publishing Company, 1969.

WINER, B. J.: *Statistical Principles in Experimental Design.* New York: McGraw-Hill, 1962.

19

A TRANSCULTURAL STUDY OF DYS-LEXIA: ANALYSIS OF LANGUAGE DISABILITIES IN 277 CHINESE CHIL-DREN SIMULTANEOUSLY LEARNING TO READ AND WRITE IN ENGLISH AND IN CHINESE

Carl L. Kline, M.D., C.R.C.P.(C)

Clinical Associate Professor

and

Norma Lee, B.A.

University of British Columbia

A unique opportunity to study some important aspects of language disability was afforded by the large group of Chinese children in Vancouver, British Columbia, who were simultaneously learning to read and write in English and Chinese. English is largely phonetic, and Chinese is completely pictorial—a difference that enabled us to conduct parallel studies on learning to read and write two entirely different language systems.

Reprinted from THE JOURNAL OF SPECIAL EDUCATION, Vol. 6, No. 1, 1972. Pp. 9-26. This study was made under a grant from the Educational Research Institute of Vancouver, British Columbia. Paper presented at the Annual Meeting of the American Orthopsychiatric Association, San Francisco, March 1970.

The term "dyslexia" as used here refers to a specific reading disability occurring in a child who has adequate intelligence, vision, and hearing and is without brain damage or primary significant emotional disability. Reading disability is viewed as a continuum, and therefore no dvision into primary and secondary groups was attempted (Rabinovitch, Drew, DeJong, Ingram, & Withey, 1954).

PURPOSE OF THE STUDY

Written Chinese is ideographic, nonphonetic, and virtually without mnemonic-device possibilities. Although the written language is essentially the same throughout China, numerous dialects are spoken that bear little or no resemblance to each other. For example, Cantonese dialect is not understood by those speaking Mandarin, now the official language of China. Spoken Chinese is tonal, so that the same basic word has different meanings depending upon the inflection. "Mai" pronounced with a falling tone means "sell," but with a rising tone it means "buy," an obviously crucial difference. Because of these characteristics of Chinese, reading and writing can be mastered only by rote memory. In order to read the newspaper, 3,000 characters must be memorized. In contrast, English is about 86% phonetic and is best learned as a sound-sight association system, which also lends itself to mnemonic devices as aides in mastering many of the irregular words. Kinesthetic reinforcement is helpful in learning either Chinese or English.

If certain theoretical premises about factors in learning to read, spell, and write English are valid, then certain expectations follow in regard to learning Chinese by the same children. The authors could find no published study on learning disabilities in Chinese children. There is one important recent study on the incidence of reading disabilities in Japanese children (Makita, 1968).

The present study attempts to answer the following questions:

1. What is the incidence of dyslexia in Chinese children learning to read and write Chinese?

2. What is the incidence of dyslexia in these same children studying to read and write English?

3. How many of the children studied have a significant disability in both languages?

4. Will analysis of the results support assumptions of diagnostic specificity, utilizing a group of tests to which diagnostic specificity is often assumed in literature?

5. Do the present findings support the following assumptions: (a)

Table 1

Number of Chinese Children and Number Studying Chinese in Grades 1-3,
Strathcona Public School, Vancouver, B.C.

Grade	Total no. of children	No. of Chinese children	% Chinese children	No. Chinese children study-ing Chinese	% Chinese children study-ing Chinese
1	116	102	88	28	27
2	125	103	82	50	48
3	121	107	88	58	54
Total	362	312	86	136	43

Table 2

Number of Children Tested in Mon Keang Chinese
Language School

Grade	No. of children
1	37
2	27
3	29
4	25
5	23
Total	141

that more boys than girls (4 to 1) are affected by dyslexia; (b) that reading disability is closely tied to intelligence; (c) that dyslexic children have lower verbal than performance scores on the WISC; (d) that problems in the home are a major factor in reading disability.

6. Do the findings provide leads to effective methodology in teaching reading or remedial techniques?

METHODOLOGY

Vancouver has the second largest Chinese community outside of the Orient. Of the pupils at Strathcona Public School, 96% were Chinese at the time of the study; but of the 362 children in grades 1, 2, and 3, just 86% were Chinese, as indicated in Table 1. After a full day in public school, 43% of these Chinese children attended one of the three private Chinese language schools for 2 hours daily, where they were taught to read and write Chinese and learn something about Chinese culture and history.

Many of the teachers in the Mon Keang school, whose children we also studied, spoke only Chinese. Some of the children were recent immigrants from Hong Kong or China who spoke and understood very little English. Therefore the ability of Norma Lee, research assistant in this study, to speak, read, and write fluent Cantonese was essential.

The following plan was followed, except that the children in first grade were not tested until March and were not given the Ayers Spelling Test (Monroe, 1932): We surveyed 312 Chinese children attending the Strathcona Public School in Chinatown in grades 1, 2, and 3. Of these, 136 were attending a Chinese language school for 2 hours each afternoon after regular school.

An additional 141 Chinese children were studied in the Mon Keongt Chinese Language School; all of these children attended public schools other than Strathcona. Tables 1 and 2 show the distribution of the totals studied from the two schools. All 277 children were learning to read and write in both English and Chinese simultaneously.

All children in the study were given the Iota Oral Reading Test as an indicator of reading disability (Monroe, 1932). In order to have a comparable test in Chinese, the Chinese Iota Test was devised, standardized, and validated (see Figure 1). From scores on the Iota (English), the Dyslexia Quotient (Kline, Kline, Ashbrenner, & Calkins, 1968) was calculated and used as an index of the presence of a reading problem in English. (The Dyslexia Quotient is obtained by subtracting the child's score on the Iota from his school placement, stated in years and months; the remainder is then divided by the minuend and the result multiplied by 100. When the child's reading performance is below grade level, the result is a negative number. Normal scores are to —15). The children were also asked to read from a standard basic reader (McCracken & Walcutt, 1963) for comparison with the Iota scores. Disability in reading Chinese was determined by scores on the Chinese Iota Test together with assessment by the Chinese language teachers. These teachers were interviewed in Chinese by Norma Lee, who also asked them to complete questionnaires on each child found to have a problem in reading Chinese.

When the above procedures indicated the presence of a problem in *either* language, the following tests were administered: Ayers Spelling Test (Silver, 1961), Monroe Auditory Discrimination Test (Monroe, 1932), Monroe Auditory-Visual Learning Test (Monroe, 1932), Bender-Gestalt (Koppitz, 1964), Draw-a-Person Test (Goodenough, 1926), the Wechsler Intelligence Scale for Children (WISC), and tests for cerebral dominance (Monroe, 1932). The WISC and Bender-Gestalt tests were given by a qualified psychologist; the others were administered by Miss Lee. The parents of all Strathcona school children who were also attending Chinese language school were asked to complete a questionnaire written in Chinese (Figure 2). A low return ratio had been predicted,

爸 媽 哥
弟 姊 妹
好 說 孩
來 手 也
走 做 拍

CHINESE IOTA TEST: English Meanings

CARD 1

father	mother	(elder)brother
(younger) brother	(elder)sister	(younger)sister
good	talk	child
come	hand	also
run	make	clap

車 張 紙 六
角 蝶 蜜 時
常 事 物 怕
小 古 高 深
便 該 應 習

CHINESE IOTA TEST: English Meanings

CARD II

car	piece	paper	six
horn	butterfly	honey	time
always	matter	thing	fear
little	ancient	high	deep
convenient	ought.	respond	custom

我 跳 面
唱 歌 狗
歡 初 迎
過 四 幾
大 教 五

CHINESE IOTA TEST: English Meanings
CARD III

I	jump	face
sing	song	dog
joy	original	receive
pass	four	several
big	teach	five

Figure 1
Chinese Iota Test

but 88% were returned without the need for follow-up letters or phone calls.

This study covers pupils enrolled in the first 5 years at the Mon Keang Chinese Language School because age distribution there varies from that in public school classes. Children often start in Chinese language school at age 5, but some older children start as beginners. Some who had just moved to Vancouver did not previously have the opportunity to attend, while others were delayed in starting because of the expense or parental ambivalence.

Chinese children without reading problems, attending Strathcona school, served as controls. They were given the same battery of tests as those with reading disabilities.

SOCIOECONOMIC BACKGROUND

The Chinatown population in Vancouver characteristically maintains Chinese customs and standards, although Westernization is increasingly in evidence. Among the parents of the children studied, 92% were born in China or Hong Kong. Chinese is spoken almost exclusively in the homes of 92% of the children, and most of the time in the other 8%. All of the children studied are bilingual. Teachers in the Strathcona

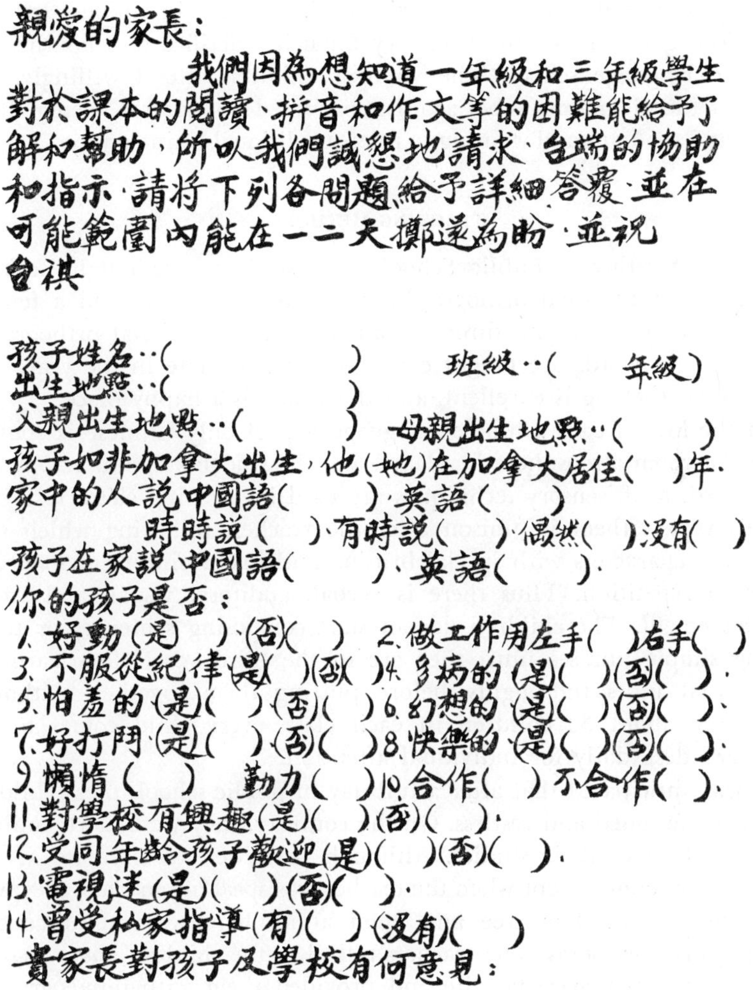

親愛的家長：

我們因為想知道一年級和三年級學生對於課本的閱讀、拼音和作文等的困難能給予了解和幫助，所以我們誠懇地請求 台端的協助和指示 請將下列各問題給予詳細答覆 並在可能範圍內能在一二天擲還為盼 並祝

台祺

孩子姓名‥(　　　　) 班級‥(　年級)
出生地點‥(　　　　)
父親出生地點‥(　　　) 母親出生地點‥(　　　)
孩子如非加拿大出生，他(她)在加拿大居住( )年.
家中的人說中國語( )、英語( )
　　　　　時時說( )、有時說( )、偶然( )沒有( )
孩子在家說 中國語( )、英語( ).
你的孩子是否：
1. 好動 (是)( )、(否)( ) 2. 做工作用左手( )右手( )
3. 不服從紀律(是)( )(否)( )4. 多病的(是)( )(否)( ).
5. 怕羞的 (是)( )(否)( )6. 幻想的 (是)( )(否)( ).
7. 好打鬥 (是)( )(否)( )8. 快樂的 (是)( )(否)( ).
9. 懶惰( ) 勤力( )10. 合作( )不合作( ).
11. 對學校有興趣(是)( )(否)( ).
12. 受同年齡孩子歡迎(是)( )(否)( ).
13. 電視迷(是)( )(否)( ).
14. 曾受私家指導(有)( )(沒有)( )
貴家長對孩子及學校有何意見：

Figure 2

Questionnaire Sent to Parents of All Strathcona School Children Who Were Studying Chinese

school commented on the rapidity with which most of the recent Chinese immigrant children learned to read English.

The families of the children are at essentially the same socioeconomic level. They are hardworking, thrifty, honest, steeped in Confucian principles, and patriarchal. In regard to discipline, the fathers are not harsh or authoritarian, depending instead on the traditional Chinese respect for elders. Parents anxious for their children to retain Chinese cultural traditions gladly make the necessary financial sacrifice to send them to Chinese language school. The younger children attend willingly, but some of the older ones rebel against continued attendance, seeing them-selves as Canadians and wanting to reject traditional Chinese ways.

TEACHING METHODS

In the Strathcona Public School most students are taught to read English by traditional orthography, many by "look-say," and a few by ITA, color phonics, and direct phonics. In the traditional orthography groups, sight words are taught early, and phonics late in the year. The quality of teaching is excellent, and the school is a happy place.

In the Mon Keang Chinese Language School only Chinese is spoken. The classroom atmosphere is relaxed and the students appear happy and interested. Multisensory techniques are used in teaching characters. The pupils repeat them in unison after the teacher, following which they draw the characters with special brushes and ink. Reinforcement occurs through repetition. Thus there is verbal, auditory, visual, and tactile reinforcement. The children do not start composing sentences or trans-lating simple phrases until they are in the third year; they learn the individual units thoroughly before putting them together. Although there are about 30 children in each class, every child comes to the teacher's desk daily for individual attention.

It was anticipated that after a full day in public school, these children might be fatigued and restless. On the contrary, they were alert, smiling, and involved in their studies. Although permitted to circulate at will around the room, except when the teacher was speaking in class, they were well disciplined. The free and open atmosphere was reminiscent of Montessori classrooms. The teachers talked to the children about matters relevant to their everyday life and provided them with mimeographed material featuring appropriate Chinese characters.

RESULTS OF THE STUDY

A preliminary report of this study was published in the Bulletin of the Orton Society (Kline & Lee, 1969). This more extensive and intensive analysis of the data alters some of the findings reported there. Tables 3, 4, and 5 reveal the incidence of significant reading disability in Eng-lish, Chinese, and languages as found in each school. These findings are shown by grade level and then combined to show the incidence in

Table 3
Incidence of Language Problems in Mon Keang Chinese Language School

Chinese grade level	No. of children in grade	Children with problems in English only		Children with problems in Chinese only		Children with problems in both languages	
		No.	% of total no. in grade	No.	% of total no. in grade	No.	% of total no. in grade
1	37	4	11	4	11	2	5
2	27	0	0	3	11	0	0
3	29	3	10	6	20	2	7
4	25	1	4	4	16	0	0
5	23	0	0	1	4	0	0
Total	141	8	5.6	18	13	4	3

Table 4
Incidence of Language Problems in Strathcona Public School

Grade	No. of children in grade[a]	Children with problems in English only		Children with problems in Chinese only		Children with problems in both languages		Children with problems in English only and in both languages (total)		Children with problems in Chinese only and in both languages (total)	
		No.	% of total in grade	No.	% of total in grade	No.	% of total in grade	No.	% of total in grade	No.	% of total in grade
1	28	7	25	6	21	9	32	16	57	15	53
2	50	9	18	9	18	4	8	13	26	13	26
3	58	2	3	3	5	1	2	3	5	4	7
Total	136	18	13	18	13	14	10	32	23	32	23

[a] Includes only those children enrolled in Chinese Language School.

Table 5
Incidence of Language Problems in both Strathcona and Mon Keang Schools

School	No. of children tested	Children with problems in English only		Children with problems in Chinese only		Children with problems in both languages		Children with problems in English only and in both languages (total)		Children with problems in Chinese only and in both languages (total)	
		No.	% of total no. in school	No.	% of total no. in school	No.	% of total no. in school	No.	% of total no. in school	No.	% of total no. in school
Strathcona	136	18	13.0	18	13.0	14	10	32	23	32	23
Mon Keang	141	8	5.6	18	12.0	4	3	12	8	22	15
Total	277	26	9.0	36	13.0	18	6	44	16	54	19

each school; finally, the figures from the two schools are combined to show the total incidence of disability.

Examination of the data in these tables reveals the following:

1. The incidence of difficulty in each language dropped significantly over a 3-year period. The Strathcona school figures are especially interesting because the children there were in the traditional age-grade groupings, which was not true at the Mon Keang school. Note the nearly identical dropping off of incidence of difficulty in each of the three categories over the 3-year period. These figures are strikingly similar to Makita's figures in his study of reading disabilities in Japanese children (1968). Why did this large sample of children have such a low incidence of reading disability at the end of grade 3? I would like to speculate here that this may well be due to the multisensory training received in Chinese language school.

2. The children tested at the Mon Keang school were having significantly fewer difficulties in all areas than those at the Strathcona school. In view of the fact that the same tests were given by the same research assistant in both schools, there is no discernible explanation for this discrepancy.

3. Of the children studying both languages, 28% were having a problem in one or both (Table 5).

4. In this same group, 16% were having difficulty with English (Table 5). This figure is close to the incidence figure (15%) arrived at by the HEW National Advisory Committee on Dyslexia and Related Reading Disorders (*Reading Disorders in the United States,* 1969).

5. Despite the fact that Chinese is a more difficult language to read than English, only 19% were having difficulty in Chinese (Table 5).

6. Just 6% were having a problem in both languages, a significant finding which will be commented on below (Table 5).

SEX DISTRIBUTION

In the total sample of 277 children, 152 were boys (54%) and 125 were girls (46%). Of those with a language problem, males comprised 19% and females 6%, giving a ratio of 3 males to 1 female. Table 6 provides the details of sex distribution in this study.

Durrell's study in 1940 showed that among 1,130 children aged 11-13, 20% of the boys and 10% of the girls were backward in reading. Alden, Sullivan, & Durrell (1941) reported on 6,000 children aged 7-11, in which 18.6% of the boys were dyslexic compared with 9.8% of the girls. Monroe (1932) reported 86% males among her cases of reading disability.

A recent nationwide study (Pringle, Butler, & Davie, 1966), of 11,000 7-year-old children found that 11.2% of boys and 5.9% of girls had not progressed beyond their first reading book after 2 years of elementary school instruction.

In this study only 1% of the girls had trouble in *both* languages compared with 10% of the boys; whereas the sex differences in English alone and in Chinese alone were essentially in keeping with other figures reported.

AUDITORY DISCRIMINATION

The Monroe Auditory Discrimination Test (Monroe, 1932) was given to all children with a language problem and to 35 children in a control group of Chinese children. Difficulty in auditory discrimination is indicated if three or more errors are made. Table 7 reveals the results of the testing. In the Chinese language, auditory discrimination is important only in regard to the tonal qualities in the spoken language. In English, which is basically phonetic, the letters and letter combinations represent specific sounds, and auditory discrimination of these sounds is essential. Although Chinese children are especially tone conscious because of the tonal quality of the spoken Chinese language, they still had difficulty in this test in about the same ratio as English speaking children with reading disabilities. This fact alone tends to minimize the importance of auditory discrimination as a prominent *cause* of reading disability.

It should also be noted that the controls had a higher percentage of errors than did either Group 1 or 2. Group 3 had significantly more errors than the control group, suggesting that difficulty in auditory discrimination may be one factor in children with very severe language problems. However, the findings are inconclusive and do not indicate that problems in auditory discrimination play a key etiological role in reading disabilities.

MONROE'S AUDITORY-VISUAL LEARNING TESTS

Visual-auditory association pathways are essential in transmodal learning and are basic to the process of learning to read. Regardless of the method by which reading is taught, associations between visual and auditory stimuli must be made. Children with difficulty in this area require (a) simplification of the stimuli (code approach rather than whole-word approach); (b) considerable reinforcement via auditory, visual, and kinesthetic combinations; and (c) repetition. (The Orton-Gillingham method [Gillingham & Stillman, 1960] is especially helpful to children with problems in transmodal learning.)

Table 6
Sex Distribution among Chinese Children with Language Problems

Language problem	Males (N=152)		Females (N=125)	
	Number	%	Number	%
English only	33	21	7	5
Chinese only	37	24	13	10
Both languages	16	10	2	1
Total	54	35	18	14

Table 7
Results of Monroe Auditory Discrimination Test in Chinese Children with Language Problems

Groups of children	No. of children tested	No. of children making errors				% children making errors
		3 errors	4 errors	5 errors	Total	
(1) Difficulty in Chinese	50	5	3		8	16
(2) Difficulty in English	40	4	1	1	6	15
(3) Difficulty in both	18	5	2		7	39
(4) Controls	35	6	0	2	8	23

Table 8
Results of Monroe Auditory-Visual Learning Test
in Chinese Children with Language Problems

Groups of children	No. of children tested	No. of abnormal scores	% abnormal scores
Problem both languages	18	3	16
Problem English only	40	4	10
Problem Chinese only	50	1	2
Controls	30	2	6

The Auditory-Visual Learning Test (Monroe, 1932) consists of five nonsense symbols, similar in appearance to Oriental characters, printed on individual white cards. Each symbol has a name: ree, sōō, ma, fō, and kī. The child is shown the cards one at a time, told the name of the symbol, and then allowed to study it for 5 seconds. After having been shown all five cards in this manner, the child is shown the cards again and asked to give the names of those he can remember. This procedure is followed three times. On a fourth turn the cards are shown in random order to eliminate the possibility of the child having learned them on the basis of auditory recall. Scores are obtained by adding the correct answers in the first three trials. Scores of 2-5 indicate difficulty, and scores below 2, severe difficulty. Table 8 presents the results obtained in this study.

The process of memorizing these symbols is very similar to the process involved in learning Chinese characters, except that tonal factors are absent and there is no kinesthetic reinforcement. Surprisingly few children had difficulty with this test, in contrast with the usual clinical experience in testing English-speaking children with language disabilities, in whom a high incidence of abnormal tests occurs. Perhaps their practice in learning Chinese characters accounts for this phenomenon.

Fildes (1921) concluded that slowness in visual perception is not an important factor in reading difficulties. Instead the failure is due partly to an inability to retain the visual impressions and partly to slowness of association processes, which hinder finding the appropriate name. The Monroe Auditory-Visual Learning Test appears to be specific for this process.

Vernon (1957) too could not find in her cases evidence of any general disorder of the visual perception of shapes. She indicated that a deficiency in the accurate discrimination of detail or in spatial orientation, related possibly to a general lack of maturation in analysis and visual memory, may be present; but that these are more likely the result rather than the cause of reading disability.

Finally, Benton (1962) points out that when visuopsychic defects were demonstrable in dyslexics, they only occurred in the younger subjects. He concluded that deficiency in visual perception is not an important correlate of developmental dyslexia.

The results reported here on the Monroe Auditory-Visual Learning Test appear to support these ideas of Fildes (1921), Vernon (1957), and Benton (1962). The findings also raise further serious questions about the validity of the whole concept of visual perception as a meaningful factor in learning to read. Certainly if these children had a defect in so-called "visual perception," those with difficulty in learning Chinese characters would be expected to show this defect. Yet only 2% had such a problem.

CEREBRAL DOMINANCE

In recognition of the work of Orton (1937), Silver & Hagin (1960), and others, 108 children with language problems and 30 controls were tested for handedness, footedness, and eyedness. The testing was carried out according to the criteria established by Silver (1960). Results are detailed in Table 9.

Table 9

Cerebral Dominance among 108 Children with Language Problems

Hand, foot, and eye preference	Percentage of preference					
	Control group (30)	Total tested (108)	Children with problems in both languages	Children with problems in English only	Children with problems in Chinese only	Total children with language problems
Right hand, right foot, right eye	68%	55%	50%	70%	50%	50%
Right hand, right foot, left eye	32	34	50	26	38	40
Right hand, left foot, right eye	0	3.7	0	4	6	4
Left hand, right foot, right eye	0	2	0	0	3	2.
Right hand, left foot, left eye	0	4	0	0	0	2
Left hand, right foot, left eye	0	0	0	0	3	2

Table 10

Monroe Hand-Eye Relationships[a]

Hand-eye preference	Percentage of preference	
	Control group (101)	Reading-disability (215)
Right hand, right eye	59%	47%
Right hand, left eye	21	35
Left hand, right eye	6	3
Left hand, left eye	5	8

[a] Based on data presented in M. Monroe, Children who cannot read, Chicago: University of Chicago Press, 1932.

Table 11

WISC Scores on 72 Children with Language Problems

Test	MS	Range
Verbal	105.7	68-134
Performance	111.2	83-154
Full scale	105.0	74-147

Monroe (1932) analyzed hand-eye preferences of the children in the reading-defect groups and in the control group of 101 school children, and found that the reading-disability cases and the controls had about the same percentage of right- and left-handedness. Her results on hand-eye relationships are reproduced in Table 10 for comparison. Other authors have reported similar findings, indicating that left-eyedness is apparently not a significant factor in reading disability. The findings in the present study suggest the problems in cerebral dominance may not be a significant factor in reading disabilities.

WECHSLER INTELLIGENCE SCALE FOR CHILDREN

The Wechsler Intelligence Scale for Children (WISC) was administered to 110 children (72 with language problems, 38 controls); the results were analyzed in terms of distribution of verbal, performance, and full-scale scores. The data are reproduced in Tables 11 and 12. Peters & Ellis (1970) analyzed the WISC data from this study and found that:

> The WISC does not show any differences between those children who have reading problems with Chinese only and those who do not have any reading difficulties. It seems therefore that for this group the WISC provides no information that distinguishes between the two groups [and] . . . may have no predictive value in identifying those children who will have no difficulty learning to read in English but have difficulty learning to read Chinese.
>
> Secondly, when learning to read in English is a problem, the WISC *does* indicate some specific weaknesses. When learning to read in English was the only problem, Chinese children tended to be lower than the control group in Information, Vocabulary, Digit Span and Verbal I.Q. When the children had problems reading in both languages, they were significantly low in these areas and were also significantly lower than the control group in the Arithmetic. Similarities and Picture Arrangement subtests and on the Full Scale I.Q. score [p. 8].

As in most of the studies of dyslexia, our subjects tended to be weak on the arithmetic and digit-span tests. However, the study does not indicate that Chinese children with reading disabilities do more poorly on coding subtests, as is the case for children studied by some other researchers (Altus, 1956; Shedd, 1967).

It is of interest here to refer briefly to significant studies reported in the literature. Fildes (1921) studied 25 children of low intelligence (IQ 50-82) and found no close relationship between intellectual level and reading ability. Wall (1946) and others have shown that children with IQs below 70 can learn to read. After reviewing the available material on the subject, Vernon (1957) concluded: "Learning to read depends more on mental age, that is to say, level of maturation, than upon intelligence as such; and specific reading disability cannot be directly attributed to subnormality of intelligence."

An important study of WISC scores in dyslexic children is that of

Table 12

Relationships between WISC Performance and Verbal Scales for 72 Children with Language Problems and 38 Controls

Subtest relationship	Children with problems in Chinese	Children with problems in English	Children with problems in both languages	Control group	Total
Performance > verbal	29	21	14	34	98
Verbal > performance	3	1	3	3	10
Performance = verbal	0	0	1	1	2

Table 13

WISC Verbal, Performance, and Full-Scale Mean
Scores in 72 Children with Language Problems
and 38 Controls

Groups of children	Mean scores		
	Verbal	Performance	Full-Scale
Problem in Chinese only	100.4	113.1	107.0
Problem in English only	92.2	110.4	101.4
Problem in both languages	86.4	105.1	94.8
Controls	101.0	112.9	107.3

Wolf (1967): From a group of 250 dyslexic boys, 32 were selected, on the basis of carefully determined criteria, who showed clear-cut developmental dyslexia. A matched group of 23 served as controls. The author states that some, but not all, clinical studies suggest that dyslexic individuals produce a low verbal-scale IQ in comparison with the performance scale IQ. The study found that the experimental group of 32 scored a group mean on the WISC verbal scale of 108.53; whereas the mean for the control group was 115.13 ($p = .0190$). The experimental group also performed less well on digit span, mazes, and vocabulary.

In our study, the verbal, performance, and full-scale WISC scores were compared for the three groups ($N = 72$) and a control group ($N = 38$). The control was a group of Chinese children, also studying both languages, but without any reading disability. Results are indicated in Table 13.

The differences between verbal and performance scores in all groups are significant. It is of interest to note how closely the scores of those with trouble only in Chinese resemble the mean scores of the control group. Those having a problem in both languages showed significantly lower scores than did the controls of the other group. Those having trouble in English scored somewhat below the mean of the control group.

Table 14

Abnormal Bender-Gestalt and Draw-a-Person Tests

Students tested	Number tested	Abnormal Bender[a]		Abnormal DAP[a]		Both Bender and DAP abnormal		Total with abnormal tests	
		Number	% of those tested	Number	% of those tested	Number	% of those tested	Number	% of those tested
Students with difficulties in Chinese only	36	12	33	14	38	8	22	18	50
Students with difficulties in English only	18	10	55	9	50	7	38	12	66
Students with difficulty in both English and Chinese	18	15	83	14	77	13	72	16	88
Controls	38	8	21	9	24	5	13	12	31

[a] Includes students with both Bender and DAP abnormal.

THE BENDER-GESTALT AND DRAW-A-PERSON TESTS

All children presenting a language disability were given both of these tests (Goodenough, 1926; Koppitz, 1964). In addition, the tests were administered to 38 Chinese children who were not having difficulty in either language, and these served as controls. The results are presented in Table 14.

A high percentage of abnormal tests occurred in all categories, including controls. Those children having difficulty only with Chinese had the lowest percentage of abnormal Benders, with a markedly increased level of abnormality in those having difficulty in English. Children having difficulty in both languages had an 83% incidence of abnormal Benders. The controls had a 21% incidence of abnormal Bender-Gestalts.

Draw-a-Person Test

Here again, the same distribution of abnormal scores prevailed. The controls had a 24% incidence of abnormal tests, while those with difficulty in Chinese had a 38% incidence. Although the figures are somewhat lower than those for the abnormal Bender-Gestalts, 50% of children having difficulty with English had abnormal Bender-Gestalts; 50% of children having difficulty with English had abnormal DAPs; while 77% of the children having a problem in both languages produced abnormal DAP tests.

Bender-Gestalt and DAP Both Abnormal

Among the controls, 13% produced abnormal Benders and DAPs. The same distribution of abnormal scores occurred in the other three categories as with the Benders and DAPs. Again, those having trouble in both languages had a very high error score (72%). Finally, in examining the totals for those with any combination of abnormal tests, the same distribution of percentage of errors prevails.

What do these tests actually indicate regarding disturbances in function among children with language problems? Both tests rely on eye-hand coordination; both rely on ability to revisualize; obviously cognitive processes are involved in both tests. Attitudes towards the testing and towards the examiner are important, as is the child's ability to perceive the directions accurately. A child with a problem in receptive language, auditory recall, or sequencing might have special problems performing on these tests. It is of interest that only 30% of the children drew Oriental persons, despite the fact that they are Chinese and live in a predominately Chinese culture. Silver's (1961) criteria were used in evaluating these tests.

The fact that a high percentage of the controls showed abnormal findings in all categories indicates the lack of specificity of these tests. At the same time, the much higher incidence of abnormal tests in all three categories in children with problems in *both* languages suggests some kind of significant relationship factor.

Why should the children with problems only in English have more difficulty with these tests than the children having a problem only in Chinese? Empirically the possibility suggests itself that the children doing well in Chinese are successful in the rote memorization of the Chinese characters through the process of auditory-visual association with multisensory reinforcement. Perhaps the drill entailed in attaining such success also enables them to function better in the revisualizing required in both of these tests. Skill in forming the Chinese characters also demands good eye-hand coordination.

The results on the Draw-a-Person Test do not in any way indicate that so-called "body image" is a factor in learning to read. If it were, there should be nearly an identical percentage of abnormality in those having trouble reading in each language; but this is not the case. Also, the 24% of control cases with abnormal DAPs should be having difficulty with reading if poor body image, as reflected in the DAP, is a factor in reading disability.

It has often been suggested that abnormal Benders and abnormal

Table 15

Compiled Results of Questionnaire Sent to Parents of
Strathcona School Children[a]

Characteristic of Child	Parent response			
	Yes	No	Does not know	Left blank
Restless	84	26	9	2
Left-handed	3	117	0	1
Hard to discipline	19	82	17	3
Sick a lot	4	114	1	2
Shy or bashful	42	64	13	2
A daydreamer	16	70	33	2
A fighter	20	83	17	1
Unhappy	8	104	5	4
Lazy	37	70	10	4
Uncooperative	29	69	17	6
Hard worker	58	42	16	5
Interested in school	99	5	13	4
Liked by his peers	107	2	9	3
Watches too much TV	62	55	1	3
Ever tutored	18	94	4	5

[a]See Figure 2 for original in Chinese.

DAPs indicate physiological or emotional immaturity, and that these are important factors in reading disability. It is also suggested that abnormality on these tests indicates organicity. While any of these three possibilities may well be true in selected cases, in this series the children were singularly free of clinical evidence of organic brain disease and emotional immaturity.

The findings in this study suggest that the appearance in a child of an abnormal Bender-Gestalt, DAP, or both may or may not be correlated with reading disability. There is no evidence to suggest that these tests are diagnostic. In my opinion, it is unlikely that they have predictive value unless included in a battery of other predictive tests (de Hirsch, 1966). Factors that might account for the prevailing tendency to misinterpret these tests and to misconstrue their significance in reading disabilities are poor standardization, lack of skill in administering and interpreting the tests, and erroneous theoretical premises.

PARENT AND TEACHER QUESTIONNAIRES

Questionnaires written in Chinese (Figure 2) were sent to all parents of Strathcona school children who were studying Chinese. The results compiled from the 121 questionnaires returned (out of 136) appear in Table 15. A large number of Chinese parents reported their children as shy or bashful. This was also a frequent comment by teachers about these youngsters. The word "lazy" is overworked in our Western culture and, unfortunately, also seems to be popular with the Chinese. Chinese parents also feel that their children watch too much television.

A cultural difference is reflected in the variation of ways in which Chinese and Caucasian teachers viewed the concept of disciplinary problems. In the Chinese language school, the teachers indicated that 3 girls and 13 boys were disciplinary problems (out of 141 children). At Strathcona school, out of 136 children, teachers saw only 5 boys as presenting discipline problems. Mr. Wark, the principal at Strathcona, confirms the low incidence of behavior problems in the school. It seems possible that the Chinese teachers had somewhat higher expectations of their students relative to classroom behavior; however, the reported difference could also be due to poor motivation of some students in the Chinese language school or increased fatigue and irritability at the end of a long day.

SUMMARY AND CONCLUSIONS

1. Bilingual Chinese children in grades 1-3 learning to read and write both in English and Chinese were studied for evidence of reading disabilities. The following incidence of disabilities was found: (a) in Chinese only, 13%; (b) in English only, 9%; (c) in both languages, 6%. Combining the figures, the total having trouble in English was 15%, and the total having difficulty with Chinese 19%. These differences are not felt to be significant, considering the possibilities for scientific error in the studies. The incidence of reading disability reported in the recent Health, Education, and Welfare study was 14.7%.

If *specific* etiological factors are operating in a child to produce a reading disability in one language, it seems likely that the child would also have a problem in learning to read another language. Yet only 6% of the children in this study had difficulty in both languages. Interestingly, the dropping off of incidence of disability in each language from grade 1 to 3 parallels the same phenomenon reported in Japan by Makita. In contrast, most studies done with English-speaking students do not show this pattern of rapid decrease in disabilities as the child ascends the grade-level ladder. At the end of grade 3, the children in our study had only a 3% incidence of difficulty in English, 5% in Chinese, and 2% in both languages. It is possible that these few residual cases represented the "hard-core" developmental dyslexics (Critchley, 1971).

2. The sex distribution in this sample is similar to that reported in

most other studies, except for the wide disparity between boys and girls (10-1) for those having trouble in both languages. If a familial or genetic factor is operating to account for the higher incidence in boys, it should operate equally for both languages in the *same sample* of children. The fact that the ratio of boys to girls differed in the three categories raises a question about the validity of the genetic factor in reading disability. Perhaps the familial factor is only important in specific developmental dyslexia (Critchley, 1971).

3. The findings in this study suggest that problems in auditory discrimination are not a major cause of reading disability. Although no tests for auditory discrimination were conducted in the Japanese study by Makita (1968), the low incidence of reading disabilities reported indicates either that Japanese children are singularly free of problems in auditory discrimination or that it is not a significant factor in learning to read. To the often-quoted comment from Hermann (1959) that "not the eye but the brain learns to read," we add that it is not the ear either. In my experience, when a problem in auditory discrimination is present, remedial therapy with a phonetic approach usually alleviates it.

4. The relatively low incidence of difficulty in transmodal learning in those with reading problems in Chinese, as reflected by the Monroe Auditory-Visual Learning Test, suggests either that difficulties in visual-auditory association were rare or had been overcome by the teaching methods in the Chinese language school. Also, if the Japanese children in Makita's study (1968) ever had problems in transmodal learning, they apparently overcame them in the process of learning to read in Japanese schools. I have found, in testing hundreds of Caucasian children, that most of those with developmental dyslexia have an abnormal Monroe Auditory-Visual Learning Test; in contrast, those without specific reading disabilities nearly always have normal tests. After remediation of the reading disability, the Monroe test becomes normal. This underlines the basic importance of teaching methodology. Teaching to read with a code approach (synthetic-analytic) utilizing multisensory reinforcement actually develops visual-auditory association, a process essential to learning to read. Incidentally, the fact that Japanese is largely a phonetic language may account for the low incidence of reading disability reported by Makita.

5. This study suggests that the WISC has no predictive value in identifying children who will have difficulty in learning to read. However, children who develop reading problems tend to have significantly lower verbal than performance scores. When learning to read English is a

problem, below-normal scores tend to occur in the following WISC subtests: information, vocabulary, digit span, and verbal IQ. Children with difficulty in both languages scored significantly lower in these same areas and also in arithmetic, similarities, and picture arrangement. Obviously intelligence is important in comprehension and, in older children, in abstract thinking; but it does not appear to be a factor in *learning* to read.

6. The data in this study do not support the idea that crossed cerebral dominance correlated in a significant manner with reading disabilities.

7. The distribution of abnormal findings on the Bender-Gestalt and Draw-a-Person tests in this sample suggests that these tests do not serve as reliable indicators of etiological factors in reading disability.

Together with our data on the Monroe Auditory-Visual Learning Test these findings indicate that Mann (1970) is correct in his recent criticism of the role attributed to perceptual problems in reading disability.

8. Questions are often raised as to whether parents who speak in their native tongue should expose their children to that language as well as to English. Sometimes fear is expressed that speaking two languages might confuse the child and create problems in learning to read. This study appears to discredit such fears. All of these children spoke both languages; many spoke Chinese more fluently than English. Yet their incidence of reading disability at the end of grade 3 was much lower than the reported national average. The children at Strathcona school, which is almost completely Chinese in population, consistently have the highest scholastic average in the Vancouver public school system. This paper lends support to the cognitive psychologists' recommendation that a second language should ideally be taught in the preschool years.

9. The findings here raise the question of the necessity for extensive testing procedures in the diagnosis of reading disability. For example, if such factors as "perceptual disorders" are not basic causes of reading problems, then tests for these problems are irrelevant. Other recent studies (Falik, 1969; Klim, 1970; McGrady & Olsen, 1970; Olson & Johnson, 1970) have questioned the validity of the Frostig test and remedial program. In fact, the whole concept of "visual perception" seems open to serious doubt. The present findings support other authorities who are raising serious questions about the mystique of testing in relationship to reading disabilities. Expensive, time-consuming diagnostic testing programs often leave the child exhausted and the parents bewildered and confused. Educators can be misled into embarking upon ill-conceived, often expensive remedial programs—programs that often fail to meet the basic problem.

In this study, all of the testing did not provide essential diagnostic information that was not provided by the Iota Oral Reading Test. (Probably the best basic test for the identification of reading and spelling disabilities is the Jastak because of its wide age-grade range and its correlation with achievement potential as related to intelligence percentiles [Jastak & Jastak, 1965]. We have found that the Iota correlates well with the reading section of the Jastak, and the Iota was used here because of the young age group involved and the ease of administration.)

On the basis of the findings reported here, together with other data recently reported in the literature, it is suggested that children with reading disabilities are being subjected to unnecessary testing. Furthermore, certain tests are being used with the assumption that they have a specificity that they do not possess. The resulting prescriptions are then erroneous, often failing to effectively remediate the child's problem. In fact, the child's disability may get worse and become so fixed that later efforts to help may be too late.

10. Teaching methodology appears to be of key importance in terms of prevention of learning disabilities. Early identification of children with reading problems through use of a simple test battery, followed by intensive remedial therapy utilizing techniques such as those of Anna Gillingham (Gillingham & Stillman, 1960), should meet the needs of nearly all children who are developing reading disabilities.

REFERENCES

ALDEN, C. L., SULLIVAN, H. B., & DURRELL, D. D.: *Education*, 1941, 62, 32.

ALTUS, G. T.: A WISC profile for retarded readers. *Journal of Consulting Psychologists*, 1956, 20, 155-156.

BENTON, A. L.: Dyslexia in relation to form perception and directional sense. In J. Money (Ed.): *Reading Disability, Progress and Research Needs in Dyslexia*. Baltimore: Johns Hopkins Press, 1962.

CRITCHLEY, M.: *The Dyslexic Child*. Springfield, Ill.: Charles C Thomas, 1971.

DE HIRSCH, K., JANSIER, J. J., & LANGFORD, W. S.: *Predicting Reading Failure*. New York: Harper, 1966.

DURRELL, D. D.: The improvement of basic reading abilities. *Journal of Education*, February, 1958.

FALIK, L. H.: The effects of special perceptual-motor training in kindergarten on reading readiness and on second grade reading performance. *Journal of Learning Disabilities*, 1969, 2, 10-16.

FILDES, L. G.: A psychological inquiry into the nature of the condition known as congenital word blindness. *Brain*, 1921, 44, 286-307.

GILLINGHAM, A., & STILLMAN, B. W.: *Remedial Training for Children with Specific Disability in Reading, Spelling, and Penmanship*. (7th ed.) Cambridge, Mass.: Educators Publishing Service, 1960.

GOODENOUGH, F.: *Measurement of Intelligence by Drawings*. Yonkers, N. Y.: World Book Company, 1926.

HERMANN, K.: *Reading Disability*. Springfield, Ill.: Charles C Thomas, 1959.

JASTAK, J. F., & JASTAK, S. R.: The wide range achievement test: Manual and instructions. Wilmington: Guidance Associates, 1965.

KLIM, R. P.: Visual-motor training, readiness, and intelligence of kindergarten children. *Journal of Learning Disabilities*, 1970, 3, 5.

KLINE, CARL L., KLINE, CAROLYN L,, ASHBRENNER, M., & CALKINS, S.: The treatment of specific dyslexia in a community mental health center. *Journal of Learning Disabilities*, 1968, 1, 457-466.

KLINE, C. L. & LEE, N.: A transcultural study of dyslexia: Analysis of reading disabilities in 425 Chinese children simultaneously learning to read and write in English and Chinese. A preliminary report. *Bulletin of the Orton Society*, 1969, 19, 67-81.

KOPPITZ, E.: *The Bender-Gestalt Test for Young Children*. New York: Grune & Stratton, 1964.

MAKITA, K.: The rarity of reading disabilities in Japanese children. *American Journal of Orthopsychiatry*, 1968, 38, 599-613.

MANN, L.: Perceptual training: Misdirection and redirection. *American Journal of Orthopsychiatry*, 1970, 40, 1.

McCRACKEN, G. & WALCUTT, C. C. *Basic Reading*. Philadelphia: Lippincott, 1963.

McGRADY, H. J., & OLSEN, D. A.: Visual and auditory learning processes in normal children and children with specific learning disabilities. *Exceptional Children*, April, 1970, 581-589.

MONROE, M.: *Children Who Cannot Read*. Chicago: University of Chicago Press, 1932.

OLSON, A. V. & JOHNSON, C.: Structure and predictive validity of the Frostig developmental test of visual perception in grades one and three. *Journal of Special Education*, 1970, 4, 49-52.

ORTON, S. T.: *Reading, Writing and Speech Problems in Children*. New York: Norton, 1937.

PETERS, L. & ELLIS, E. N.: An analysis of WISC profiles of Chinese-Canadian children with specific reading disabilities in Chinese, English or both languages. Unpublished manuscript. Vancouver, B.C.: Vancouver School Board, June 1970.

PRINGLE, K., BUTLER, N. R., & DAVIE, R.: 11,000 seven-year-olds: Studies in child development. London: Longmans, 1966.

RABINOVITCH, R., DREW, A. C., DE JONG, R. N., INGRAM, W., WITHEY, L.: *Approach to Reading Retardation: Proceedings of the Association for Research in Nervous and Mental Disease*. Baltimore: Williams & Wilkins, 1956.

RAWSON, M. B.: *Developmental Language Disability: Adult Accomplishments of Dyslexic Boys*. Baltimore: John Hopkins Press, 1968.

Reading Disorders in the United States. Report of the Secretary's National Advisory Committee on Dyslexia and Related Reading Disorders. Washington, D. C.: U.S. Department of Health, Education, and Welfare, 1969.

SHEDD, C. L.: Some characteristics of a specific perceptual-motor disability dyslexia. *Journal of the Medical Association of Alabama*, 1967, 37, 150-162.

SILVER, A. A.: Diagnostic considerations in children with reading disabilities. *Bulletin of the Orton Society*, 1961, 11, 5-12.

SILVER, A. A. & HAGIN, R.: Specific reading disability: Delineation of the syndrome and relationship to cerebral dominance. *Comprehensive Psychiatry*, 1960, 1, 126-134.

VERNON, M. D. *Backwardness in Reading: A Study of Its Nature and Origin*. Cambridge University Press, 1957.

WALL, W. D.: Article in *British Journal Education Psychology*, 1946, 16, 133.

WOLF, C. W.: An experimental investigation of specific language disability (dyslexia). *Bulletin of the Orton Society*, 1967, 17, 32-39.

20

MALNUTRITION, LEARNING, AND INTELLIGENCE

Herbert G. Birch, M.D., Ph.D.

INTRODUCTION

Research on the relation of nutrition factors to intelligence and learning has burgeoned over the past decade. Its resurgence after a period of nearly thirty years of quiescence which followed Patterson's (1930) review of studies conducted in the first three decades of the century reflects a number of social and historical currents. Newly emerging nations as well as aspiring underprivileged segments of the population in more developed parts of the world have increasingly come to be concerned by the association of social, cultural and economic disadvantage with depressed levels of intellect and elevated rates of school failure. Attention has variously been directed at different components of the combined syndromes of disadvantage and poverty in an effort to define the causes for such an association. Sociologists, psychologists and educators have advanced reasons for intellectual backwardness and school failure relevant to their particular concerns. They have pointed to particular patterns of child care, cultural atmosphere, styles of play,

Reprinted from AMERICAN JOURNAL OF PUBLIC HEALTH, Vol. 62, No. 6, June 1972, pp. 773-784.

Dr. Birch (deceased) was Professor of Pediatrics, Yeshiva University, Albert Einstein College of Medicine, New York. The research for this study was supported in part by the National Institutes of Health, National Institute of Child Health and Human Development (HD 00719), and by the Association for the Aid of Crippled Children. This paper was presented before the Food and Nutrition, Maternal and Child Health, and Mental Health Sections of the American Public Health Association at the Ninety-Ninth Annual Meeting in Minneapolis, Minnesota on October 13, 1971.

depressed motivation, particular value systems, and deficient educational settings and instruction as factors which contribute to lowered intellectual level and poor academic performance in disadvantaged children. The importance of such variables cannot be disputed and studies and findings relevant to them expand our understanding of some of the ways in which poor achievement levels are induced. However, it would be most unfortunate if by recognizing the importance of these situational, psychological and experimental components of the syndrome of disadvantage we were to conclude that they represented the whole of the picture or even its most decisive components. Any analysis of the content of poverty and disadvantage rapidly brings to our notice the fact that these negative features of the behavioral and educational environment take place within the pervasive context of low income, poor housing, poor health and, in general, defective circumstances for the development of the individual as a biologic organism who interacts with the social, cultural and educational circumstances.

Such considerations inevitably cause us to expand the range of our concern to include a fuller range of factors contributing to lowered intellect and school failure. In this larger perspective the health of the child and, in particular, his nutritional opportunities must assume a position of importance. It has long been recognized that the nutrition of the individual is perhaps the most ubiquitous factor affecting growth, health and development. Inadequate nutrition results in stunting, reduced resistance to infectious disease, apathy and general behavioral unresponsiveness. In a fundamental sense it occupies a central position in the multitude of factors affecting the child's development and functional capacity. It is therefore entirely understandable that in a period dedicated to the improvement of man and his capacities that renewed attention has come to be directed to the relation of nutrition to intelligence and learning ability.

As is almost always the case in new areas of inquiry, clarity of thought and concept has not kept pace with zeal. Confusion has resulted from extravagant claims as to the unique contribution of malnutrition to brain impairment and intellectual deficit. Further confusion has been contributed by those who have with equal zeal sought to minimize the importance of nutritional factors and to argue for the primacy of social, genetic, cultural, or familial variables in the production of deficit. Little that is useful emerges from such sterile controversy. It is a truism that malnutrition occurs most frequently in those segments of the population who are economically, socially and culturally disadvantaged. When lowered intellect is demonstrated in malnourished children coming from such groups, it is not difficult to ignore a consideration of the possible contribution of nutritional and health factors by pointing to the possibility that the children affected are dull because they are the offspring of dull parents; or that the general impoverishment of their environments has resulted in experiential deprivations sufficient to account for reduced intellectual function. Such an argument implies that the children are malnourished because their parents are dull and that their functional backwardness stems from the same cause as their malnutrition. On logical grounds one could of course argue the very opposite from the same bodies of data. However, to do so would not be to consider the issue seriously, but to engage in a debater's trick. The serious task is to disentangle, from the complex mesh of negative influences which characterize the world of disadvantaged children, the particular and interactive contributions which different factors make to the development of depressed functional outcomes. A responsible analysis of the problem, therefore, seeks to define the particular role which may be played by nutritional factors in the development of malfunction, and the interaction of this influence with other circumstances affecting the child.

Before considering the ways in which available research permit us to achieve this objective, it is of importance to clarify the term malnutrition. Characteristically, we in the United States tend to react to the word in terms of a crisis model. When we think of malnutrition our imaginations conjure up images of the Apocalypse. We have visions of famines in India, of victims of typhoons, and of young Biafrans starved by war. These images reflect only a highly visible tip of an iceberg. Intermittent and marginal incomes as well as a technology which is inadequate to support a population result less often in the symptoms characteristic of starvation than in subclinical malnutrition or what Brock (1961) has called "dietary subnutrition . . . defined as any impairment of functional efficiency of body systems which can be corrected by better feeding." Such subnutrition when present in populations is reflected in stunting, disproportions in growth, and a variety of anatomic, physiologic, and behavioral abnormalities (Birch and Gussow, 1970). Our principal concern in this country is with these chronic or intermittent aspects of nutritional inadequacy.

In less highly developed regions of the world, and indeed in the United States as well, chronic subnutrition is not infrequently accompanied by dramatic manifestations of acute, severe and, if untreated, lethal malnutrition, particularly in infants and young children. These illnesses variously reflected in the syndromes of marasmus, kwashiorkor, and marasmic-kwashiorkor are conditions deriving from acute exacerbations of chronic subnutrition which in different degrees reflect caloric deficiency, inadequacy of protein in the diet, or a combination of both states of affairs. Studies of children who recover from such disorders provide significant information on the effects of profound nutrition inadequacy on behavioral development.

In addition to the already mentioned conditions, malnutrition has classically been manifested as a consequence of the inadequate ingestion of certain essential food substances. The diseases of vitamin lack, such as scurvy, rickets, pellagra, and beri-beri, as well as the iron deficiency anemias are representative of this class of disorders.

None of the foregoing should be confused with the term hunger, which has often indiscriminately been used as a synonym for malnutrition. Hunger is a subjective state and should not be used as the equivalent of malnutrition, which is an objective condition of physical and physiologic suboptimum. Clearly, malnourished children may be hungry, but equally, hungry children may be well-nourished.

With these introductory considerations in mind we can now approach a series of questions. We shall be concerned with two issues: First, what is the state of sound knowledge of the relation of malnutrition in its various forms to intellect and learning and what is the significance of the evidence for psychology and education. And second, what are the implications of the evidence for improved functioning.

THE EVIDENCE

A number of model systems have been used to explore the relationship of malnutrition to behavior. At the human level these have consisted of a) comparative studies of well- and poorly-grown segments of children in populations at risk of malnutrition in infancy; b) of retrospective follow-up studies of the antecedent nutritional experiences of well-functioning children in such populations; c) of intervention studies in which children in the poor-risk population were selectively supplemented or unsupplemented during infancy and a comparative evaluation made of functioning in the supplemented and unsupplemented groups; d) follow-up studies of clinical cases hospitalized for severe malnutrition in early childhood; and e) intergenerational studies seeking to relate the degree to which conditions for risk of malnutrition in the present generation of children derived from the malnutrition or subnutrition experienced by their mothers when these latter were themselves children. Studies of human populations have been supplemented by a variety of animal models. These animal studies have been: a) direct comparative follow-up investigations of the effects of nutritional difficulties in early life on subsequent behavioral competence; and b) the study of the cumulative effects of malnutrition when successive generations of animals have been exposed to conditions of nutritional stress. The available evidence will be considered in relation to these investigative models.

In two of our reports (Cravioto, DeLicardie and Birch, 1966; Birch, 1970) we have reviewed many of the earlier studies which have sought to explore the association between malnutrition and the development of intellect and learning. Perhaps the most complete study of the relation of growth achievement to neurointegrative competence in children living in environments in which severe malnutrition and chronic subnutrition are endemic is our study of Guatemalan rural Indian children. The children lived in a village having a significant prevalence level of both severe acute malnutrition and prolonged subnutrition during infancy and the preschool years. At school age, relatively well-nourished children were identified as the better grown, and children with the highest antecedent risk of exposure to malnutrition identified as those with the lowest growth achievements for age. On the basis of this reasoning, two groups of children were selected from all village children in the age range 6 to 11 years. These groups encompassed the tallest and shortest quartiles of height distribution at each age for the total population of village children. In order to avoid problems associated with the use of intelligence tests as measures of functioning in pre-industrial communities, levels of development in the tall and short groups were compared by means of evaluating intersensory integrative competence by a method developed by Birch and Lefford (1963). In this method of evaluation children are required to judge whether geometric forms presented in different sensory modalities are the same or different. Competence in making such judgments follows a clearly defined developmental course in normal children in the age range studied.

At all ages taller children exhibited higher levels of neurointegrative competence than did the shorter group. Overall, the shorter children lagged by two years behind their taller agemates in the competence which they exhibited in processing information across sensory systems.

In order to control for the possibility that height differences were reflecting differences in antecedent nutritional status rather than familial differences in stature, the child's height was correlated with that of the parents. The resulting correlation was extremely low and insignificant. This stands in marked contrast to the finding in the same ethnic group living in more adequate nutritional circumstances. Under these latter conditions the height of children correlates significantly with that of their parents.

Secondly, it was possible that the shorter children were, in the community at risk as well as in communities not at risk of malnutrition, merely exhibiting generalized developmental lag both for stature and for neurointegrative competence attached to differences in stature in the children not exposed to endemic malnutrition.

And finally, it was possible that the shorter children came from home environments significantly lower in socioeconomic status, housing and parental education, and that both the malnutrition and the reduced neurointegrative competence stemmed independently from these environmental deficits. When differences in these factors were controlled they did not erase the differences in intersensory integrative competence between children of different growth achievements for age in the community at nutritional risk.

Over the past several years replications of this study have been conducted in Mexico by Cravioto and DeLicardie (1968), and in India by Champakam et al. (1968). In addition, Cravioto, Espinoza and Birch (1967) have examined another aspect of neurointegrative competence and auditory-visual integration, in Mexican children of school age. Once again in children in communities at risk of malnutrition differences in growth achievement at school age were reflected in differences in auditory-visual integration favoring the taller children. These latter findings are of particular importance because of the demonstrated association between such competence and the ability to acquire primary reading skill (Birch and Belmont, 1964, 1965; Kahn and Birch, 1968).

A major consideration in interpreting the findings of all these studies is the fact that antecedent malnutrition is being inferred from differences in height rather than by direct observation of dietary intakes during the growing years. However, a multitude of data from earlier studies beginning with those of Boas (1910) on growth differences in successive generations of children of Jewish immigrants, of Greulich (1958) on the height of Japanese immigrants, of Boyd-Orr (1936) on secular trends in the height of British children, of Mitchell (1962, 1964) on the relation of nutrition to stature, of Boutourline-Young (1962) on Italian children, as well as the recent study of heights of 12-year-old Puerto Rican boys in New York City by Abramowicz (1969) all support the validity of such an inference.

It should be noted too that findings similar to those obtained in the Guatemalan and Mexican studies have been reported by Pek Hien Liang et al. (1967) from Indonesia, and Stoch and Smythe (1963, 1968) from

South Africa. In the Indonesian study 107 children between 5 and 12 years of age all deriving from lower socioeconomic groups were studied. Forty-six of these children had been classified as malnourished during a previous investigation into nutritional status in the area carried out some years earlier. All children were tested on the WISC and Goodenough tests with scores showing a clear advantage for the better-grown and currently better-nourished children. Moreover, the data indicated that the shortest children were markedly overrepresented in the group that had been found to be malnourished in the earlier survey, with the largest deficits in IQ found to be associated with the poorest prior nutritional status.

Stoch and Smythe have carried out a semi-longitudinal study of two groups of South African Negro children, one judged in early childhood to be grossly underweight due to malnutrition, and the other considered adequately nourished. At school age, the malnourished children as a group had a mean IQ which was 22.6 points lower than that of the comparison group. Moreover, these relative differences were sustained through adolescence. Unfortunately, the interpretation of the findings in this study is made difficult because the better-nourished children came from better families and had a variety of nursery and school experiences unshared by the poorly grown children.

Comparative studies of differential cognitive achievement in better and less well-nourished groups in communities at high levels of subnutrition have been supplemented by a relatively large number of follow-up evaluations of children who had been hospitalized for serious nutritional illness (marasmus or kwashiorkor) in infancy. As will be recalled from our earlier remarks, marasmus is a disorder produced by an insufficient intake of proteins and calories and tends to be most common in the first year of life. Kwashiorkor—a syndrome produced by inadequate protein intake accompanied by a relatively adequate caloric level, or in its marasmic form associated with reduced calories as well—is more common in the post-weaning between 9 months and 2 years of age.

As early as 1960 Waterlow, Cravioto and Stephen (1960) reported that children who suffered from such severe nutritional illnesses exhibited delays in language acquisition. In Yugoslavia, Cabak and Najdanvic (1965) compared the IQ levels of children hospitalized for malnutrition at less than 12 months of age with that of healthy children of the same social stratum and reported a reduced IQ in the previously hospitalized group. Of perhaps greater interest was their report of a significant correlation between the severity of the child's illness on admission as estimated in his deficit of expected weight for age with depression of IQ in school years. Indian workers (Champakam, et al. 1968) studied many variables in a group of 19 children who between 18 and 36 months of age had been hospitalized and treated for kwashiorkor. When compared at school age with a well-matched control group, significantly depressed IQ was found in the children previously severely malnourished.

In order to control more fully for differences in the child's genetic antecedents microenvironment, which may still exist even when more genetical controls for social, class and general circumstances are used in the selection of a comparison group, we in two studies (Birch, Cravioto et al., in press, 1971) and Hertzig, Birch, Tizard and Richardson, in preparation, 1971) have compared children previously malnourished in infancy with their siblings as well as with children of similar social background. In the first of these studies intelligence at school age was compared in 37 previously malnourished Mexican children and their siblings. The malnourished children had all been hospitalized for kwashiorkor between the ages of 6 and 30 months. The siblings had never experienced a bout of severe malnutrition requiring hospitalization. Sibling controls were all within 3 years of age of the index cases. Full scale WISC IQ of the index cases was 13 points lower than that of the sibling controls. Verbal and Performance differences were of similar magnitude and in the same direction. All differences were significant at less than the 0.01 per cent level of confidence. These findings are in agreement with those of the Yugoslav and Indian workers and the use of sibling controls removes a potential contaminant for interpretation.

In the second study, Tertzig, et al. (in preparation, 1971), a large sample of 74 Jamaican children, all males, who had been hospitalized for severe malnutrition before they were two years of age were compared with their brothers nearest in age, and with their classmates whose birthdate was closest to their own. All children were between 6 and 11 years of age at follow-up. On examination, neurologic status, intersensory competence, intellectual level, and a variety of language and perceptual and motor abilities were evaluated. Intellectual level was significantly lower in the index cases than in either the siblings or the classmate comparison groups. As was to be expected, the order of competence placed the classmate comparison group at the highest level, the index cases at the lowest, and the sibs at an intermediate level. The depressed level of the siblings in relation to classmates suggests one disadvantage in sibling studies. Clearly, the presence of a child hospitalized for severe malnutrition identifies a family in which all children are at a high level of risk for significant undernutrition on a chronic basis, the index child merely representing an instance of acute exacerbation of this chronic marginal state. Therefore, the index cases and sibs are similar in that they share a common chronic exposure to subnutrition and differ only in that the index cases have experienced a superimposed episode of acute nutritional illness as well. Thus, the use of sibling controls, in fact, does not compare malnourished with the non-malnourished children. Rather, it determines whether siblings who differ in their degree of exposure to nutritional risk differ in intellectual outcomes and supports the view that graded degrees of malnutrition result in graded levels of intellectual sequelae.

Other follow-up studies of acutely malnourished children such as those of Cravioto and Robles (1965) in Mexico, Pollitt and Granoff (1967) in Peru, Botha-Antoun, Babayan and Harfouche (1968) in Lebanon, and Chase and Martin (1970) in Denver, have all been shorter-term follow-ups of younger children. Cravioto and Robles (1965) studied the developmental course of returning competence in children hospitalized for malnutrition during the period of their treatment and recovery while in hospital. Their findings indicated that behavioral recovery was less complete in the youngest children (hospitalized before 6 months of age) than in older children. They posed the possibility that this earliest period of infancy was the one most critical for insult to the developing brain and thus to eventual intellectual outcome. However, the study of Jamaican children (in preparation, 1971) does not have findings which supported this possibility. In that study approximately equal numbers of children having experienced an acute episode of malnutrition in each of the four semesters of the first two years of life were examined. Equivalent depression of IQ was found to characterize each of the groups when these were separated by age at hospitalization.

In the Lebanese (1968), Peruvian (1967) and Venezuelan (1963) short-term follow-up studies depression in intellectual level tended to be found in the index cases. In the American study (1970) and in a Chilean study (Monckeberg, 1968) the findings have shown depression in intellectual function in the preschool years in children hospitalized for malnutrition during the first year of life. The American investigators working in Colorado found that 20 children who had been hospitalized for malnutrition before the age of one year had a mean development quotient on the Yale Revised Developmental Examination which was 17 points lower than that achieved by a matched control group of children who had not been malnourished. All of these studies suggest strongly that malnutrition of severe degree in early life tends to depress the intellectual functioning at later ages.

In summary, the follow-up studies of children who have been exposed to hospitalization for a bout of severe acute malnutrition in infancy indicate an association of significant degree between such exposure and reduced intellectual level at school age. The studies, involving careful social class controls and sibship comparisons, suggest that it is not general environmental deprivation but rather factors which are uniquely related to the occurrence of severe malnutrition that are contributing to a depression in intellectual outcome. However, there is some indication that different degrees of recovery may be associated with different post-illness conditions. Thus, urban and rural differences in intellectual outcomes are reported in the sibship comparison studies of Jamaican children earlier referred to (in preparation, 1971).

The fact of such an association provides strongly suggestive but by no means definitive evidence that malnutrition directly affects intellectual competence. As Cravioto, DeLicardie and Birch (1966) have pointed out, at least three possibilities must be considered in the effort to define a causal linkage. The simplest hypothesis would be that malnutrition directly affects intellect by producing central nervous system damage. However, it may also contribute to intellectual inadequacies as a consequence of the child's loss in learning time when ill, of the influences of hospitalization, and of prolonged reduced responsiveness after recovery. Moreover, it is possible that particular exposures to malnutrition at particular ages may in fact interfere with development at critical points in the child's growth course and so provide either abnormalities in the sequential emergence of competence or a redirection of developmental course in undesired directions. Although certain of these possibilities (such as hospitalization and post-illness opportunities for recovery) can be explored in children, others for moral and ethical reasons cannot. Thus, it is impermissible to establish appropriate experimental models either for interfering with development at critical periods, or for inducing brain damage. The approach to these problems requires either detailed analyses of naturally occurring clinical models or the development of appropriate animal investigations.

Animal models of the effects of malnutrition on brain and behavior have been used to study the issue with a degree of control that is quite impossible in human investigation. In a series of pioneering investigations (Widdowson, 1966, Dobbing, 1964, Davison and Dobbing, 1966) have demonstrated that both severe and modest degrees of nutritional deprivation experienced by the animal at a time when its nervous system was developing most rapidly results in reduced brain size and in deficient myelination. These deficits are not made up in later life even when the animal has been placed on an excellent diet subsequent to the period of nutritional deprivation.

More recent studies (Zamenhof, 1968) as well as by Winick (1968) have demonstrated that the deprivation is also accompanied by a reduction in brain cell number. This latter effect has been demonstrated too in human brain in infants who have died of severe early malnutrition (Winick and Rosso, 1969).

Enzymatic maturation and development in brain is also affected, and Chase et al. (1967, 1970), have demonstrated defective enzyme organization in the brains of malnourished organisms.

In all of these studies the evidence indicates that the effects of malnutrition vary in accordance with the time in the organism's life at which it is experienced. In some organisms the effects are most severe if the nutritional insult occurs in the prenatal period, in others during early postnatal life.

Some confusion in the interpretation of evidence has occurred because of the use of different species, since in different organisms the so-called critical periods occur at different points in the developmental course. Thus, in pigs' brain, growth and differentiation are occurring most rapidly in the period prior to birth, whereas in the rat the most rapid growth occurs when the animal is nursing. In human beings the period for rapid growth is relatively extended and extends from mid-gestation through the first six through nine months of postnatal life. In man, the brain is adding weight at the rate of one to two mg/minute at birth and goes from 25 per cent of its adult weight at birth to 70 per cent of its adult weight at one year of age. After this age, growth continues more slowly until final size is achieved. Differentiation as well as growth occurs rapidly during the critical periods, with myelination and cellular differentiation tending to parallel changes in size.

Since brain growth in different species is occurring at different points in the life course it is apparent that deprivations that are experienced at the same chronologic ages and life stages will have different effects in different species. Thus deprivation during early postnatal life will have little or no effect upon brain size and structure in an organism whose brain growth has largely been completed during gestation. Conversely, intrauterine malnutrition is likely to have only trivial effects on the growth of the brain in species in which the most rapid period for brain development has occurred postnatally. When these factors are taken into account the data leave no doubt that the coincidence of malnutrition with rapid brain growth results in decreased brain size and in altered brain composition.

It would be unfortunate if brain growth in terms of cell number were to be viewed as the only definers of rapid change and thus of critical periodicity. In the human infant, neuronal cell number is most probably fully defined before the end of intrauterine life. Thereafter, through the first 9 months of postnatal life, cell replication is that of glial cells, a process which terminates at the end of the first year. However, myelination continues for many years thereafter as does the proliferation of dendrite branchings and other features of brain organization. It is most probable, therefore, that in man the period of vulnerability extends well beyond the first year of life and into the preschool period. Such a position is supported by the findings of Champakam et al. (1968). These workers, it will be recalled, found significant effects on intellect in their group of malnourished children who had experienced severe malnutrition when they were between 18 and 36 months of age.

Other workers who have used animal models have sought to study the effects of malnutrition on behavioral outcomes, rather than on brain structure and biochemical organization. The typical designs of these studies are investigations in which animals have been raised upon diets which were inadequate with respect to certain food substances, or in which general caloric intake has been reduced without an alteration in the quality of the nutriments. Such animals have been compared with normally nourished members of the species with respect to maze learning, avoidance conditioning, and open field behavior. Unfortunately, most of the investigations have suffered from one or another defects in design which make it difficult to interpret the findings. Though in general the nutritionally deprived organisms have tended to be disadvantaged learners, it is not at all clear whether this is the result of their food lacks at critical points in development or whether the differences observed stem from the different handling, caging, and litter experiences to which the well- and poorly-nourished animals were exposed. Moreover, in a considerable number of studies food or avoidance motivation have been used as the reinforcers of learning. There is abundant evidence (Mandler, 1958; Elliott and King, 1960; Barnes, et al. 1968; Levitsky and Barnes, 1969) that nutritional deficiency in early life affects later feeding behavior. Consequently, it is difficult to know whether the early deprivation has affected food motivation or whether it has affected learning capacity. The use of learning situations which do not involve food, but are based upon aversive reinforcement, do not remove difficulties for interpretation, since early malnutrition modifies sensitivity to such negative stimuli (Levitsky and Barnes, 1970).

One must therefore recognize that at present, although the animal evidence suggests that early malnutrition may influence later learning and behavior, it is by no means conclusive. Moreover, when learning has been deleteriously affected the mechanisms through which this effect has been mediated is by no means clear. What is required is a systematic series of experiments in which behavioral effects are more clearly defined, and in which the use of proper experimental designs accompanied by appropriate controls permits the nature of the mechanisms affected to be better delineated.

Thus far both in our consideration of the human and animal evidence we have been considering the direct effects of nutritional deprivation on the developing organism. Clearly, this is too limited a consideration of the problem. It has long been known (Boyd-Orr, 1936) that nutritional influences may be intergenerational and that the growth and functional capacity of an individual may be affected by the growth experiences and nutrition of his mother. In particular the nutritional history of the mother and its effect upon her growth may significantly affect her competence as a reproducer. In its turn, this reproductive inadequacy may affect the intrauterine and birth experiences of the offspring.

Bernard (1952) working in Scotland has clearly demonstrated the association between a woman's nutritional history and her pelvic type. He compared one group of stunted women in Aberdeen with well-grown women and found that 34 per cent of the shorter women had abnormal pelvic shapes conducive to disordered pregnancy and delivery as compared with 7 per cent of the well-grown women with whom they were compared. Greulich, Thoms and Twaddle (1939) still earlier had reported that the rounded or long oval pelvis which appears to be functionally superior for childbearing was much more common in well-off, well-grown women than in economically less-privileged clinic patients. They further noted, as had Bernard, that these pelvic abnormalities were strongly associated with shortness.

Sir Dugald Baird and his colleagues in the City of Aberdeen, Scotland, have from 1947 onward conducted a continuing series of studies on the total population of births in this city of 200,000 in an effort to define the patterns of biologic and social interactions which contribute to a woman's growth attainments and to her functional competence in childbearing. More than 20 years ago Baird (1947) noted that short stature, which was five times as common among lower-class women than in upper-class women, was associated with reproductive complications. He pointed out (1949), on the basis of analyzing the reproductive performances of more than 13,000 first deliveries, that fetal mortality rates were more than twice as high in women who were under five feet one inch in height than in women whose height was five feet four inches or more. Baird and Illsley (1953) demonstrated that premature births were almost twice as common in the shorter than in the taller group. Thomson (1959a) extended these observations by analyzing the relation between maternal physique and reproductive complications for the more than 26,000 births which had occurred in Aberdeen over a 10-year period and found that short stature in the mother was strongly associated with high rates of prematurity, delivery complications and perinatal deaths at each parity and age level. He concluded that "it is evident that whatever the nature of the delivery the fetus of the short woman has less vitality and is less likely to be well-grown and to survive than that of a tall woman."

It was of course possible that these findings simply reflected differences in social class composition of short and tall women and were based upon differences in "genetic pool" rather than in stunting as such. To test this hypothesis the Aberdeen workers (Baird, 1964) re-examined their data for perinatal mortality and prematurity rates by height within each of the social classes for all Aberdeen births occurring in the 10-year period from 1948 to 1957. They found that shortness in every social class was associated with an elevated rate of both prematurity and perinatal deaths. Concerned that the findings in Aberdeen might not be representative they also analyzed the data from the all-Britain perinatal mortality survey of 1958 and confirmed their findings. Moreover, Thompson and Billewicz (1963) in Hong Kong, and Baird (1964) have substantiated the Aberdeen findings for Chinese and West African women respectively. Other findings on a similar vein from this series have been summarized by Illsley (1967).

The available data therefore suggest that women who are not well-grown have characteristics which negatively affect them as childbearers. In particular, short stature is associated with pregnancy and delivery complications and with prematurity. Since growth achievement within ethnic groups is a function of health history and in particular nutrition, it is clear that the mother's antecedent nutritional history when she herself was a child can and does significantly influence the intrauterine growth, development and vitality of her child. Moreover, an inadequate nutritional background in the mother places this child at elevated risk for damage at delivery.

It is instructive to consider the consequences for mental development and learning failure that attach to the most frequently occurring consequence of poor maternal growth—prematurity. Concern with the consequences of this condition is hardly new, with Shakespeare indicting it as one element in the peculiarities of Richard III, and Little (1862) linking it with the disorder we now call cerebral palsy. Benton (1940) reviewed the literature up to that time and found that though most students of the problem maintained that prematurity was a risk to later mental development, others could find no negative consequence attaching to it. At that time no resolution of disagreement could be made because most of the early studies had been carried out with serious deficiencies in design and in techniques of behavioral evaluation. Groups who were of low birth weights or early in gestational age were often compared with full-term infants who differed from them in social circumstances as well as in perinatal status. Estimates of intellectual level were made with poor instruments and often dependent on "clinical impression" or testimony from parents or teachers.

Serious and detailed consideration of the consequences of low birth for later behavioral consequences can properly be said to have begun by Pasamanick, Knobloch, and their colleagues shortly after World War II. These workers were guided by a concept which they referred to as a "continuum of reproductive casualty." They argued that there was a set of pregnancy and delivery complications which resulted in death by damaging the brain and hypothesized that in infants who survived exposure to these risks "there must remain a fraction so injured who do not die, but depending on the degree and location of trauma, go on to develop a series of disorders extending from cerebral palsy, epilepsy and mental deficiency, through all types of behavioral and learning disabilities, resulting from lesser degrees of damage sufficient to disorganize behavioral development and lower thresholds to stress" (Pasamanick and Knoblock, 1960). In a series of retrospective studies prematurity and low birth weight were identified by them as being among the conditions most frequently associated with defective behavioral outcomes. They therefore, in association with Rider and Harper (1956), undertook a prospective study of a balanced sample of 500 premature infants born in Baltimore in 1952 and compared them with full-term control infants born in the same hospitals who were matched with the prematures for race, maternal age, parity, season of birth and socioeconomic status. Four hundred pairs of cases and controls were still available for study when the children were between six and seven years of age, and examination of the sample indicated that at this age the prematures and full-term children continued to be matched for maternal and social attributes (Wiener, et al. 1965). Findings at various ages persistently showed the prematures to be less intellectually competent than the controls. At ages three to five the prematures were relatively retarded intellectually and physically and had a higher frequency of definable neurologic abnormalities (Knobloch, et al. 1959; Harper, et al. 1959). At ages six through seven, IQ scores on the Stanford-Binet test were obtained and at ages eight to nine, WISC IQs are available. At both age levels, lower birth weights were associated with lower IQs (Wiener, et al. 1965, 1968).

Although certain British studies such as that of McDonald (1964) and of Douglas (1956, 1960) appear to be somewhat discrepant with these findings, reanalysis of their findings (Birch and Gussow, 1970) indicates a similar trend. More dramatic differences between prematures and full-term infants have been reported by Drillien (1964, 1965) but interpretation of her data is made difficult by complexities in the selection of the sample studied.

A number of analyses suggest that the effects of prematurity are not the same in different social classes, with children from the lowest social classes appearing to have subsequent IQ and school performances more significantly depressed by low birth weight than in the case for infants in superior social circumstances. This has been reported for Aberdeen births (Illsley, 1966; Richardson, 1968), and for Hawaiian children in the Kauai pregnancy study of Werner (1967). There appears to be an interaction between birth-weight and family social condition in affecting intellectual outcome, but the precise mechanisms involved in this interaction are as yet unclear.

If the risk of deficient intellectual outcome in prematurity is greatest for those children who are otherwise socially disadvantaged as well, our concern in the United States with the phenomenon of prematurity must be increased. In 1962 more than 19 per cent of non-white babies born in New York City had a gestational age of less than 36 weeks as compared with 9.5 per cent of white babies, and in Baltimore this comparison was 25.3 per cent in non-white infants as compared with 10.3 per cent in whites (National Center for Health Statistics, 1964). In 1967 (National Center for Health Statistics, 1967) nationally, 13.6 per cent of non-white infants weighed less than 2,500 grams as compared with 7.1 percent of white infants. Other relevant and more detailed analyses of the social distribution of low birth weight and gestational age on both national and regional bases, together with an analysis of their secular trends, provides additional support for these relationships (Birch and Gussow, 1970). Thus, prematurity is most frequent in the very groups in which its depressing effects on intelligence are greatest.

On the basis of the evidence so far set forth it may be argued with considerable justification that one can reasonably construct a chain of consequences starting from the malnutrition of the mother when she was a child, to her stunting, to her reduced efficiency as a reproducer, to intrauterine and perinatal risk to the child, and to his subsequent reduction in functional adaptive capacity. Animal models have been constructed to test the hypotheses implied in this chain of associations, most particularly by Chow and his colleagues (1968; Hsueh, 1967), as well as by (Cowley and Griesel, 1963, 1966). The findings from these studies indicate that second and later generation animals who derive from mothers who were nutritionally disadvantaged when young are themselves less well-grown and behaviorally less competent than animals of the same strain deriving from normal mothers. Moreover, the condition of the offspring is worsened if nutritional insult in its own life is superimposed on early maternal malnutrition.

A variety of factors would lead us to focus upon the last month of intrauterine life as one of the "critical" periods for the growth and development of the central nervous system. Both brain and body growth together with differentiation are occurring at a particular rapid rate at this time. It has been argued, therefore, that whereas marginal maternal nutrition resources may be sufficient, adequately to sustain life and growth, during the earlier periods of pregnancy, the needs of the rapidly growing infant in the last trimester of intrauterine existence may outstrip maternal supplies. The work of Gruenwald et al. (1963), among others, would suggest that maternal conditions during this period of the infant's development are probably the ones which contribute most influentially to low birth weight and prematurity. Such concerns have led to inquiries into the relation of the mother's nutritional status in pregnancy to the growth and development of her child. In considering this question it is well to recognize that as yet we have no definitive answer to the question of the degree to which maternal nutrition during pregnancy contributes to pregnancy outcome. Clearly, whether or not nutritional lacks experienced by the mother during pregnancy will affect fetal growth is dependent upon the size and physical resources of the mother herself. Well-grown women are most likely to have tissue reserves which can be diverted to meet the nutritional needs of the fetus even when pregnancy is accompanied by significant degrees of contemporary undernutrition. Conversely, poorly grown women with minimal tissue reserves could not under the same set of circumstances be expected to be able to provide adequately for the growing infant.

Children coming from families in which the risks for exposure to malnutrition are high are unlikely to experience nutritional inadequacies only in early life. It is far more likely that earlier nutritional inadequacies are projected into the preschool and school years. Such a view receives support from numerous surveys as well as from recent testimony presented before the Senate Committee on Nutrition and Human Needs (1968-1970). Our knowledge of the degree to which children and families at risk continue to be exposed to nutritional inadequacies derives from a series of indirect and direct methods of inquiry. At an indirect level it can be argued that family diet in the main is very much dependent upon family income level. The report *Dietary Levels of Households in the United States* (1968) published by the United States Department of Agriculture underscores this proposition. According to a household survey conducted in the spring of 1965, only 9 per cent of families with incomes of $10,000 and over a year were judged as having "poor diets." However, the proportion of poor diets increased regularly with each reduction in income level, with 18 percent of the families earning under $3,000 a year reporting poor diets, that is, diets containing less than two-thirds of the recommended allowance of one or more essential nutrients. Conversely, the proportion of "good" diets went from 63 percent in the $10,000 and over category down to 37 per cent in the under $3,000 group. Of course, income alone is not an adequate indicator of socioeconomic status since in families with equal incomes more education appears to produce a better diet (Jeans, Smith & Sterns, 1952; Murphy & Wertz, 1954; Hendel, Burke & Lund, 1965). But, at the least, such figures suggest that we must be seriously concerned with just how badly nourished are our poor in what we often claim is the "best-fed nation in the world."

Reports of the survey type may be supplemented by inquiries in which mothers are asked what they feed their families and how much of what kinds of food they purchase. Similarly actual food intakes may be estimated by requests for the retrospective recall of all foods eaten over the last 24 hours. Owen and Dram (1969) studying nutritional status in Mississippi preschool children found not only that the poorer children were on the average smaller than more affluent children but that their diets were significantly low in calories, vitamin C, calcium and riboflavin. Dibble, et al. (1965) in Onondaga County, New York, found that among students drawn from a junior high school which was 94 per cent Negro and predominantly laboring class, 41 per cent had come to school without breakfast; but in two "overwhelmingly white" junior high schools, only 7 per cent in one school and 4 per cent in the other had skipped breakfast. In recent studies among teen-agers in Berkeley, California, Hampton et al. (1967) and Huenemann et al. (1968) have found intakes of all nutrients declining with socioeconomic status, with

Negro girls and boys having worse intakes than those in other ethnic groups. Huenemann also found that among junior and senior high school students studied over a two-year period, 90 per cent of the Negro teen-agers had irregular eating habits and many appeared to be "fending for themselves."

Christakis et al. (1968) who carried out the first dietary study of New York school children in 20 years found that in an economically depressed district the diets of 71 per cent of children examined were poor and less than 7 per cent had excellent diets. Moreover, his data demonstrated that if the child's family were on welfare the likelihood of his having a poor diet was much increased.

The situation is not markedly different in the Roxbury district of Boston. In this area Meyers et al. (1968) studied the diets and nutritional status of 4th, 5th and 6th graders, about two-thirds of whom were black. Meals were ranked as "satisfactory" or "unsatisfactory." Four satisfactory ratings for a given meal over the 4-day period produced a "satisfactory" rating for the meal. Fifty-five per cent of the children failed to get such a satisfactory rating for breakfast, 60 per cent of them did not have satisfactory lunches, and 42 per cent had less than four satisfactory evening meals in 4 days. "Satisfactory" scores declined with age for all meals, and Negroes generally had more unsatisfactory ratings than Caucasians. The school had no school-lunch programs, and lunches were the poorest meals, with 33 per cent of the children having two or more unsatisfactory lunch ratings in 4 days. During the 4-day period 64 per cent of the children had less than two glasses of milk a day, 132 children had *no* citrus fruit, and only 1 child had a green or yellow vegetable; 37 per cent of the Negro and 46 per cent of the Caucasian children had "unsatisfactory" intakes of the protein foods in the meat, fish, poultry, eggs, and legume group. "It is evident," the authors concluded, "that many of the children were eating poorly."

These data are illustrative and not atypical of the national picture. The preliminary reports deriving from the National Nutrition Survey serve to confirm these findings on a national scale. The evidence though scattered and of uneven quality indicates strongly that economically and ethnically disadvantaged children eat poorly in both the preschool and school age periods.

Direct clinical studies occurring largely within the Head Start Program serve to support the impression produced by the data of nutritional surveys. One way of examining possible sub-nutrition on an economical clinical basis is to define the prevalence of iron deficiency anemia. Hutcheson (1968), reporting on a very large sample of poor white and

Negro children in rural Tennessee, found the highest level of anemia among children around 1 year old. Of the whole group of 15,681 children up to 6 years of age, 20.9 per cent had hematocrits of 31 per cent, indicating a marginal status. Among the year-old children, however, the incidence of low hematocrits was even higher: 27.4 per cent of the whites and 40 per cent of the nonwhites had hematocrits of 31 per cent or less, and 10 per cent of the whites and one-quarter of the nonwhites had hematocrits of 30 per cent or under, indicating a more serious degree of anemia. Low hemoglobin level was also most common among the younger children in a group whom Gutelius (1969) examined at a child health center in Washington, D. C. Iron-deficient anemia, determined by hemoglobin level and corroborative red cell pathology, was found among 28.9 per cent of the whole group of 460 Negro preschoolers, but children in the age group 12-17 months had a rate of anemia of 65 per cent. Gutelius points out, moreover, that these were probably not the highest-risk children, since the poorest and most disorganized families did not come for well-baby care at all, and of those who did attend, the test group included only children who had not previously had a hemoglobin determination—that is, they were children judged to be "normal" by the clinic staff. Thus "many of the highest risk children had already been tested and were not included in this series."

Even in the summer 1966 Head Start program, in which the incidence of other disorders was surprisingly low (North, 1967), studies indicated that 20-40 per cent of the children were suffering from anemia, a proportion consistent with the findings of various studies summarized by Filer (1969) as well as with the level of anemia found in a random sample of predominantly lower-class children coming into the pediatric emergency room of the Los Angeles County Hospital (Wingert, 1968). Anemia rates as high as 80 per cent among preschool children have been reported from Alabama (Mermann, 1966) and Mississippi (Child Development Group of Mississippi, 1967).

It is clear from such evidence that some degree of malnutrition is relatively widespread among poor children; but we have already seen that the effects of inadequate nutrition on growth and mental development depend to a very large extent on the severity, the timing, and the duration of the nutritional deprivation. Inadequate as are our data on the true prevalence of malnutrition among children in this country, we are even less informed about its onset or about its severity and quality. The absence of such knowledge must not be taken to reflect the absence of the problem but rather the lack of attention which has been devoted to it.

IMPLICATIONS

The evidence we have surveyed indicates strongly that nutritional factors at a number of different levels contribute significantly to depressed intellectual level and learning failure. These effects may be produced directly as the consequences of irreparable alterations of the nervous system or indirectly as a result of ways in which the learning experiences of the developing organism may be significantly interfered with at critical points in the developmental course.

If one were to argue that a primary requirement for normal intellectual development and for formal learning is the ability to process sensory information and to integrate such information across sense systems the evidence indicates that both severe acute malnutrition in infancy as well as chronic sub-nutrition from birth into the school years results in defective information processing. Thus by inhibiting the development of a primary process essential for certain aspects of cognitive growth, malnutrition may interfere with the orderly development of experience and contribute to a suboptimal level of intellectual functioning.

Moreover, an adequate state of nutrition is essential for good attention and for appropriate and sensitive responsiveness to the environment. One of the most obvious clinical manifestations of serious malnutrition in infancy is a dramatic combination of apathy and irritability. The infant is grossly unresponsive to his surroundings and obviously unable to profit from the objective opportunities for experience present in his surroundings. This unresponsiveness characterizes his relation to people, as well as to objects. Behavioral regression is profound; and the organization of his functions is markedly infantilized. As Dean (1960) has put it, one of the first signs of recovery from the illness is an improvement in mood and in responsiveness to people—"the child who smiles is on the road to recovery."

In children who are subnourished one also notes a reduction in responsiveness and attentiveness. In addition the subnourished child is easily fatigued and unable to sustain either prolonged physical or mental effort. Improvement in nutritional status is accompanied by improvements in these behaviors as well as in physical state.

It should not be forgotten that nutritional inadequacy may influence the child's learning opportunities by yet another route, namely, illness. As we have demonstrated elsewhere (Birch & Cravioto, 1968; Birch & Gussow, 1970) nutritional inadequacy increases the risk of infection, interferes with immune mechanisms, and results in illness which is both more generalized and more severe. The combination of sub-nutrition and illness reduces time available for instruction and so by interfering with the opportunities for gaining experience disrupts the orderly acquisition of knowledge and the course of intellectual growth.

We have also pointed to intergenerational effects of nutrition upon mental development. The association between the mother's growth achievements and the risk to her infant is very strong. Poor nutrition and poor health in the mother when she was a girl result in a woman at maturity who has a significantly elevated level of reproductive risk. Her pregnancy is more frequently disturbed and her child more often of low birth weight. Such a child is at increased risk of neurointegrative abnormality and of deficient IQ and school achievement.

Despite the strength of the argument that we have developed, it would be tragic if one were now to seek to replace all the other variables —social, cultural, educational, and psychological—which exert an influence on intellectual growth with nutrition. Malnutrition never occurs alone; it occurs in conjunction with low income, poor housing, familial disorganization, a climate of apathy, ignorance and despair. The simple act of improving the nutritional status of children and their families will not and cannot of itself fully solve the problem of intellectual deficit and school failure. No single improvement in conditions will have this result. What must be recognized rather is that within our overall effort to improve the condition of disadvantaged children, nutritional considerations must occupy a prominent place, and together with improvements in all other facets of life including relevant and directed education, contribute to the improved intellectual growth and school achievement of disadvantaged children.

REFERENCES

ABRAMOWICZ, M.: Heights of 12-year-old Puerto Rican boys in New York City: Origins of differences. *Pediatrics,* 43, 3:427-429, 1969.

BAIRD, D.: Social class and foetal mortality. *Lancet,* 253:531-535, 1947.

BAIRD, D.: Social factors in obstetrics. *Lancet,* 1:1079-1083, 1949.

BAIRD, D. & ILLSEY, R.: Environment and childbearing. *Proc. Roy. Soc. Med.,* 46:53-59, 1953.

BAIRD, D.: The epidemiology of prematurity. *J. Pediat.,* 65:909-924, 1964.

BARNES, R. H., NEELY, C. S., KWONG, E., IABADAN, B. A., & FRANKOVA, S.: Postnatal nutritional deprivations as determinants of adult behavior toward food, its consumption and utilization. *J. Nutr.,* 96:467-476, 1968.

BARRERA-MONCADA, G.: *Estudios sobre alteraciones del crecimiento y del desarrollo psicologico del sindrome pluricarencial (kwashiorkor).* Caracas, Editora Grafos, 1963.

BENTON, A. L.: Mental development of prematurely born children: A critical review of the literature. *Amer. J. Orthopsychiat.,* 10:719-746, 1940.

BERNARD, R. M.: The shape and size of the female pelvis. Transactions of the Edinburgh Obstetrical Society. *Edin. Med. J.*, 59, 2:1-16, 1952 (Transactions bound at end).

BEVAN, W. & FREEMAN, O. I. Some effects of an amino acid deficiency upon the performance of albino rats in a simple maze. *J. Genet. Psychol.*, 80:75-82, 1952.

BIRCH, H. G. & LEFFORD, A.: Intersensory Development in Children. Monographs. *The Society for Research in Child Development*, 28:1-48, 1963.

BIRCH, H. G. & BELMONT, L. Auditory-visual integration in normal and retarded readers. *Amer. J. Orthopsychiatry*, 44, 5:852-861, 1964.

BIRCH, H. G. & BELMONT, L.: Auditory-visual integration, intelligence and reading ability in school children. *Percept. Mot. Skills*, 20:295-305, 1965.

BIRCH, H. G. & CRAVIOTO, J.: Infection, nutrition and environment in mental development. In H. F. Eichenwald (Ed.): *The Prevention of Mental Retardation Through the Control of Infectious Disease*. Public Health Service Publication, 1962. Washington, D. C.: U.S. Govt. Printing Office, 1968.

BIRCH, H. G. & GUSSOW, J. D.: *Disadvantaged Children: Health, Nutrition and School Failure*. New York: Harcourt Brace and World, and Grune and Stratton, Inc., 1970, pp. 322.

BIRCH, H. G.: Malnutrition and early development. In E. Grotberg (Ed.): *Day Care: Resources for Decisions*. Office of Economic Opportunity: Office of Planning, Research and Evaluation: Experimental Research Division, 349-372, 1971.

BIRCH, H. G., PINEIRO, C., ALCALDE,, E., TOCA, T., & CRAVIOTO, J. Kwashiorkor in early childhood and intelligence at school age. *Pediat. Res.*, 5:579-585, 1971.

BOAS, F.: *Changes in the Bodily Form of Descendants of Immigrants*. Immigration Commission Document No. 208. Washington, D. C.: U.S. Govt. Printing Office, 1910.

BOTHA-ANTOUN, E., BABAYAN, S., & HARFOUCHE, J. J.: Intellectual development relating to nutritional status. *J. Trop. Pediat.*, 14:112-115, 1968.

BOUTOURLINE-YOUNG, H.: Epidemiology of dental caries: Results from a cross-cultural study in adolescents of Italian descent. *New Eng. J. Med.*, 267-843-849, 1962.

BROCK, J.: *Recent Advances in Human Nutrition*. London: J. & A. Churchill, 1961.

CABAK, V. & NAJDANVIC, R.: Effect of undernutrition in early life on physical and mental development. *Arch. Dis. Child.*, 40:532-534, 1965.

CHAMPAKAM, S., SRIKANTIA, S. G., & GOPALAN, C.: Kwashiorkor and mental development. *Amer. J. Clin. Nutr.*, 21:844-852, 1968.

CHASE, H. P., DORSEY, J., & MCKHANN, G. M.: The effect of malnutrition on the synthesis of a myelin lipid. *Pediatrics*, 40:551-559, 1967.

CHASE, H. P. & MARTIN, H. P.: Undernutrition and child development. *New Eng. J. Med.*, 282:933-976, 1970.

Child Development Group of Mississippi: Surveys of Family Meal Patterns. Nutrition Services Division. May 17, 1967, and July 11, 1967. Cited in *Hunger, USA*.

CHOW, B. F., BLACKWELL, B., HOU, T. Y., ANILANE, J. K., SHERWIN, R. W., & CHIR, B.: Maternal nutrition and metabolism of the offspring: Studies in rats and man. *A.J.P.H.*, 58:668-677, 1968.

CHRISTAKIS, G., MIRIDJANIAN, A., NATH, L., KHURANA, H. S., COWELL, C., ARCHER, M., FRANK, O., ZIFFER, H., BAKER, H., & JAMES, C.: A nutritional epidemiologic investigation of 642 New York City children. *Amer. J. Clin. Nutr.*, 21:107-126, 1968.

COWLEY, J. J. & GRIESEL, R. D.: The development of second generation low protein rats. *J. Genet. Psychol.*, 103:233-242, 1963.

COWLEY, J. J. & GRIESEL, R. D.: The effect on growth and behavior of rehabilitating first and second generation low protein rats. *Anim. Behav.*, 14:506-517, 1966.

CRAVIOTO, J. & ROBLES, B.: Evolution of adaptive and motor behavior during rehabilitation from kwashiorkor. *Amer. J. Orthopsychiat.*, 35:449-464, 1965.

CRAVIOTO, J., DELICARDIE, E. R., & BIRCH, H. G.: Nutrition, growth and neurointegrative development and experimental and ecologic study. *Pediatrics*, 38:2, Part II, Suppl. 319-372, 1966.

CRAVIOTO, J., ESPINOZA, C. G., & BIRCH, H. G.: Early malnutrition and auditory-visual integration in school age children. *J. Spec. Ed.*, 2:75-82, 1967.

CRAVIOTO, J. & DELICARDIE, E. R.: Intersensory development in school age children. In N. S. Scrimshaw and J. E. Gordon (Eds.): *Malnutrition, Learning, and Behavior.* Massachachusetts: MIT Press, 1968, pp. 252-269.

DAVISON, A. N. & DOBBING, J.: Myelination as a vulnerable period in brain development. *Brit. Med. Bull.*, 22, 1:40-44, 1966.

DEAN, R. F. A.: The effects of malnutrition on the growth of young children. *Mod. Probl. Pediat.*, 5:111-122, 1960.

DIBBLE, M., BRIN, M., MCMULLEN, E., PEEL, A., & CHEN, N.: Some preliminary biochemical findings in junior high school children in Syracuse and Onondaga County. New York: *Amer. J. Clin. Nutr.*, 17:218-239, 1965.

DOBBING, J.: The influence of early nutrition on the development and myelination of the brain. *Proc. Roy. Soc.*, 159:503-509, 1964.

DOUGLAS, J. W. B.: Mental ability and school achievement of premature children at 8 years of age. *Brit. Med. J.*, 1:1210-1214, 1956.

DOUGLAS, J. W. B.: "Premature" children at primary schools. *Brit. Med. J.*, 1, 2:1008-1013, 1960.

DRILLIEN, C. M.: *The Growth and Development of the Prematurely Born Infant.* Baltimore: Williams & Wilkins, 1964, p. 376.

DRILLIEN, C. M.: Prematures in school. *Pediatrics Digest*, September, 1965, pp. 75-77.

ELLIOTT, O. & KING, J. A.: Effect of early food deprivation upon later consumatory behavior in puppies. *Psychol. Rep.*, 6:391-400, 1960.

FILER, L. J., JR.: The United States today: Is it free of public health nutrition problems?—anemia. *A.J.P.H.*, 59:327-338, 1969.

GREULICH, W. W., THOMS, H., & TWADDLE, R. C.: A Study of pelvis type and its relationship to body build in white women. *J.A.M.A.*, 112:485-492, 1939.

GREULICH, W. W.: Growth of children of the same race under different environmental conditions. *Science*, 127:515-516, 1958.

GRUENWALD, P., DAWKINS, M., & HEPNER, R.: Chronic deprivation of the fetus. *Sinai Hosp. J.*, 11:51-80, 1963.

GUTELIUS, M. F.: The problem of iron-deficiency anemia in preschool Negro children. *A.J.P.H.*, 59:290-295, 1969.

HAMPTON, M. C., HUENEMANN, R. L., SHAPIRO, L. R., & MITCHELL, B. W.: Caloric and nutrient intakes of teenagers. *J. Amer. Diet. Ass.*, 50:385-396, 1967.

HARPER, P. A., FISCHER, L. K., & RIDER, R. V.: Neurological and intellectual status of prematures at three to five years of age. *J. Pediat.*, 55:679-690, 1959.

HENDEL, G. M., BURKE, M. C., & LUND, L. A.: Socioeconomic factors influence children's diets. *J. Home Econ.*, 57:205-208, 1965.

HERTZIG, M. E., BIRCH, H. G., TIZARD, J., & RICHARDSON, S. A.: *Growth Sequelae of Severe Infantile Malnutrition.* 1971 (in preparation).

HERTZIG M. E., TIZARD, J., BIRCH, H. G., & RICHARDSON, S. A.: *Mental Sequelae of Severe Infantile Malnutrition.* 1971 (in preparation).

HSUEH, A. M., AGUSTIN, C. E., & CHOW, B. F.: Growth of young rats after differential manipulation of maternal diet. *J. Nutr.*, 91:195-200, 1967.

HUENEMANN, R. L., SHAPIRO, L. R., HAMPTON, M. C., & MITCHELL, B. W.: Food and eating practices of teenagers. *J. Amer. Diet. Ass.*, 53:17-24, 1968.

HUTCHESON, H. A. & WRIGHT, N. H.: Georgia's family planning program. *Amer. J. Nurs.*, 68:332-335, 1968.

ILLSEY, R.: Early prediction of perinatal risk. *Proc. Roy. Soc. Med.*, 59:181-184, 1966.

ILLSLEY, R.: The sociological study of reproduction and its outcome. In S. A. Richardson and A. F. Guttmacher (Eds.): *Childbearing: Its Social and Psychological Aspects*. Baltimore: Williams & Wilkins, 1967, pp. 75-135.

JEANS, P. C., SMITH, M. B., & STEARNS, G.: Dietary habits of pregnant women of low income in a rural state. *J. Amer. Diet. Ass.*, 28:27-34, 1952.

KAHN, D. & BIRCH, H. G.: Development of auditory-visual integration and reading achievement. *Percept. Motor Skills*, 27:459-468, 1968.

KNOBLOCH, H., PASAMANICK, B., HARPER, P. A., & RIDER, R.: The effect of prematurity on health and growth. *A.J.P.H.*, 49:1164-1173, 1959.

LEVITSKY, D. A. & BARNES, R. H.: Effects of early protein calorie malnutrition on animal behavior. Paper read at meeting of American Association for Advancement of Science, Dec. 1969.

LEVITSKY, D. A. & BARNES, R. H.: Effect of early malnutrition on reaction of adult rats to aversive stimuli. *Nature*, 225:468-469, 1970.

LIANG, P. H., HIE, T. T., JAN, O. H., & GIOK, L. T.: Evaluation of mental development in relation to early malnutrition. *Amer. J. Clin. Nutr.*, 20:1290-1294, 1967.

LITTLE, W. J.: On the influence of abnormal parturition, difficult labour, premature birth, and asphyxia neonatorum on the mental and physical conditions of the child, especially in relation to deformities. *Trans. Obstet. Soc. London*, 3:293-344, 1962.

MANDLER, J. M.: Effects of early food deprivation on adult behavior in the rat. *J. Comp. Physiol. Psychol.*, 51:513-517, 1958.

McDONALD, A. D.: Intelligence in children of very low birth weight. *Brit. J. Prev. Soc. Med.*, 18:59-74, 1964.

MERMANN, A. C.: Lowndes County, Alabama, TICEP Health Survey, Summer 1966; and Statement Prepared for the U.S. Senate Sub-Committee on Employment. Manpower and Poverty. Washington, D. C.

MITCHELL, H. S.: Nutrition in relation to stature. *J. Amer. Diet. Ass.*, 40:521-524, 1962.

MITCHELL, H. S.: Stature changes in Japanese youth and nutritional implications. *Fed. Proc.*, 28:877, No. 27, 1964.

MONCKEBERG, F.: Effect of early marasmic malnutrition on subsequent physical and psychological development. Chap. In N. S. Scrimshaw, & J. E. Gordon (Eds.): *Malnutrition, Learning and Behavior*. Cambridge: MIT Press, 1968, pp. 269-277.

MURPHY, G. H. & WERTZ, A. W.: Diets of pregnant women: Influence of socioeconomic factors. *J. Amer. Diet. Ass.*, 30:34-48, 1954.

MYERS, M. L., O'BRIEN, S. C., MABEL, J. A., & STARE, F. J.: A nutrition study of school children in a depressed urban district. 1. Dietary findings. *J. Amer. Diet. Ass.*, 53:226-233, 1968.

National Center for Health Statistics. Vital Statistics of the United States, 1965. Washington, D. C., U.S. Govt. Printing Office, 1967.

National Center for Health Statistics: Natality Statistics Analysis, United States, 1962. Vital and Health Statistics, PHS Pub. No. 1000, Series 21, No. 1. Public Health Service. Washingon, D. C.: U.S. Govt. Printing Office, 1964.

NORTH, A. F.: Project Head Start and the pediatrician. *Clin. Pediat.*, 6:191-194, 1967.

ORR, J. B.: *Food, Health and Income*. London: Macmillan, 1936.

OWEN, G. M. & KRAM, K. M.: Nutritional status of preschool children in Mississippi: Food sources of nutrients in the diets. *J. Amer. Diet. Ass.*, 54:490-494, 1969.

PASAMANICK, B. & KNOBLOCH, H.: Brain damage and reproductive casualty. *Amer. J. Orthopsychiat.*, 30:298-305, 1960.

PATTERSON, D. G.: *Physique and Intellect*. New York: Appleton-Century-Crofts, 1930.

RICHARDSON, S. A.: The influence of social, environmental and nutritional factors on mental ability. In N. S. Scrimshaw and J. E. Gordon (Eds.): *Malnutrition, Learning and Behavior*. Cambridge: MIT Press, 346-360, 1968.

POLLITT, E. & GRANOFF, D.: Mental and motor development of Peruvian children treated for severe malnutrition. *Revista Interamericana de Psicologia,* 1: (2), 93-102, 1967.

Senate Committee on Nutrition and Human Needs. cf. parts 1 et seq. 1968-70.

STOCH, M. B. & SMYTHE, P. M.: Does undernutrition during infancy inhibit brain growth and subsequent intellectual development? *Arch. Dis. Child.,* 38:546-552, 1963.

STOCH, M. B. & SMYTHE, P. M.: Undernutrition during infancy, and subsequent brain growth and intellectual development. In N. S. Scrimshaw and J. E. Gordon (Eds.): *Malnutrition, Learning and Behavior.* Cambridge: MIT Press, 1968, pp. 278-289.

THOMSON, A. M.: Diet in pregnancy. III. Diet in relation to the course and outcome of pregnancy. *Brit. J. Nutr.,* 13:4:509-525, 1959a.

THOMSON, A. M. & BILLEWICZ, W. Z.: Nutritional status, physique and reproductive efficiency. *Proc. Nutr. Soc.,* 22:55-60, 1963.

WATERLOW, J. C., CRAVIOTO, J., & STEPHEN, J. K. L.: *Protein Malnutrition in Man. Advances in Protein Chemistry.* New York: Academic Press, Inc., 15:131-238, 1960.

WERNER, E.: Cumulative effect of perinatal complications and deprived environment on physical, intellectual and social development of preschool children. *Pediatrics,* 39:490-505, 1967.

WIDDOWSON, E. M.: Nutritional deprivation in psychobiological development: Studies in animals. In: *Deprivation in Psychobiological Development.* Pan American Health Organization Scientific Pub. No. 134. Washington, D. C., WHO, 1966, pp. 27-38.

WIENER, G., RIDER, R. V., OPPEL, W. C., FISCHER, L. K., & HARPER, P. A.: Correlates of low birth weight: Psychological status at 6-7 years of age. *Pediatrics,* 35:434-444, 1965.

WIENER, G., RIDER, R. V., OPPEL, W. C., & HARPER, P. A.: Correlates of low birth weight: Psychological status at eight to ten years of age. *Pediat. Res.,* 2:110-118, 1968.

WINGERT, W. A.: The demographical and ecological characteristics of a large urban pediatric outpatient population and implications for improving community pediatric care. *A.J.P.H.,* 58:859-876, 1968.

WINICK, M.: Nutrition and cell growth. *Nutr. Rev.,* 26:195-197, 1968.

WINICK, M. & ROSSO, P.: The effect of severe early malnutrition in cellular growth of human brain. *Pediat. Res.,* 3:181-184, 1969.

ZAMENHOF, S., VAN MARTHENS, E., & MARGOLIS, F. L.: DNA (cell number) and protein in neonatal brain: Alteration by maternal dietary protein restriction. *Science,* 160:322-323, 1968.

Part V

RACIAL IDENTIFICATION

While the papers in this section deal specifically with black children and their identification, the questions they examine are pertinent to other important issues as well: how do children develop self-esteem, what events will enhance this, how can we recognize subtle factors that undermine a child's opportunity to form a positive self-image?

Fish and Larr and Ward and Brown indicate a measurable rise in black children's willingness to identify themselves racially and to give black characteristics a positive connotation. These data offer an antidote to the "mark of oppression" thesis that the pathological effects of racism on blacks are permanent and crippling. Coates' paper is a reminder that when racism is institutionalized, attitudes may be transmitted subtly and covertly without the individual being conscious that he is so doing.

347

21

A DECADE OF CHANGE IN DRAWINGS BY BLACK CHILDREN

Jeanne E. Fish, Ph.D.

*Division of Child Psychiatry, University of Kansas
Medical Center (Kansas)*

and

Charlotte J. Larr, M.A.

Children's Mercy Hospital, Kansas City (Missouri)

Comparison of human figure drawings made by black children before 1960 with those made by black children after 1970 indicated that more black racial indicators are included in current drawings. These results suggest that black children are now more positively aware and accepting of their racial and ethnic background than was the case before 1960. The authors offer possible explanations.

Informal clinical observations of the human figure drawings that black children recently made suggested that there has been a considerable increase in the number of black racial characteristics included in such drawings compared with those collected several years ago as part of routine psychiatric evaluations.

Reprinted from the AMERICAN JOURNAL OF PSYCHIATRY, 129:4, October 1972, pp. 421-426. Copyright © 1972, the American Psychiatric Association.

Read at the 125th annual meeting of the American Psychiatric Association, Dallas, Tex., May 1-5, 1972. Collection of data for this investigation was made possible through a grant from the Department of Psychiatry, University of Kansas Medical Center.

Machover (1) has suggested that the figure drawn reflects the impulses, anxieties, conflicts, and compensations characteristic of the individual producing the drawing. Dennis (2) has stated that children include in their drawings those features they most admire and wish were characteristic of themselves. He cited art objects and children's drawings from other cultures (Hasidic, Japanese, pre-Columbian Indian, and pre-slavery African) to support his statement that the arts and crafts of a culture depict humans with physical characteristics similar to and valued by the culture.

One would expect the current emphasis on Black Power, Afro-American culture, black history, and the like to have had an effect on human figure drawings if these programs are succeeding in their efforts to influence the black value system and identification. There is some other evidence that this is so. Black college students included more identifiable black racial characteristics in their human figure drawings in 1967 than students from the same college did in 1957 (3). Casual observation of recent drawings suggested that relatively young and unsophisticated black children were drawing human figures that seemed to more closely resemble blacks than whites. Questions that arose in relation to these observations have been investigated.

1. Are human figure drawings currently being made by black children more easily identified as representing black people than are drawings made by black children ten or more years ago?

2. Is there an age progression in the ability to depict accurately the black racial characteristics of which one is aware?

3. If drawings by black children are now more easily identified, what details of the drawings convey the racial group membership?

4. Are black judges more accurate than white judges in judging whether a drawing is by a black person?

Method

The pre-1960 files of the division of child psychiatry at the University of Kansas Medical Center and at Children's Mercy Hospital, Kansas City, Mo., were searched, and 56 human figure drawings by black children were identified. In addition, drawings collected in 1958 from second-, fourth-, and sixth-grade children were searched, and ten more drawings by black children were located. This group of 66 drawings makes up the pre-1960 data. The age and sex distributions for these drawings are summarized in Table 1.

The current drawings were collected during the summer of 1970 at

TABLE 1
Distribution of Pre-1960 and 1970 Drawings
by Age and Sex of Child

AGE	BOYS	GIRLS
Pre-1960		
6	3	1
7	6	5
8	4	1
9	1	8
10	17	3
11	2	0
12	0	1
13	6	1
14	1	1
15	4	0
16	1	0
Total	45	21
1970		
5	11	9
6	3	8
7	12	8
8	12	11
9	12	14
10	24	19
11	9	21
12	16	20
13	22	14
14	15	10
15	2	4
Total	138	138

two general medical outpatient clinic facilities maintained by the department of pediatrics, University of Kansas Medical Center, and from the division of child psychiatry at Children's Mercy Hospital.[1] The distribution of the 276 drawings according to age and sex of the children is shown in Table 1.

In addition, 58 drawings by white children from the second, fourth, and sixth grades were added to the group of drawings by black children.

The drawings were randomly assembled and divided into two groups of 200 drawings each. The drawings were then shown by opaque projector to groups of judges. Each judge was asked to indicate whether each drawing, in his opinion, illustrated any identifiable black characteristics such as hair or facial features, skin coloring, style of dress, or other indications of racial group membership. The judges were not asked to specify such characteristics but only to make an overall judgment as to whether each drawing contained any such features.

---

[1] Standard instructions are: "Draw a picture of a person. Make all of it and do the best you can." After he completes the first drawing the child is instructed to make a drawing of a person of the opposite sex from that in the first drawing.

TABLE 2
Comparison of Sex Distribution of Accurately Identified Drawings

GROUP	PRE-1960		1970		VALUES OF x^2	SIGNIFICANCE
	NUMBER	CORRECT	NUMBER	CORRECT		
Girls	21	3	138	48	2.64	p = .05
Boys	45	2	138	49	14.60	p = .001
All subjects	66	5	276	97	18.67	p = .001˜

TABLE 3
Comparison of Age Distribution of Accurately Identified Drawings

AGE GROUP	PRE-1960		1970		VALUE OF x^2	SIGNIFICANCE
	NUMBER	CORRECT	NUMBER	CORRECT		
7 or younger	15	3	51	11		n.s.
8–9	14	1	49	15	2.05	p = .10
10–11	22	1	73	25	6.08	p = .005
12–13	8	0	72	29	3.46	p = .025
14–15	6	0	31	17	4.08	p = .025

All of the judges were mental health professionals, teachers, or graduate students in psychology or education. One group of 200 drawings was
judged by two black and four white judges; the other was judged by
three black and seven white judges.

Results

Each judge's impression of each drawing was tabulated, and the number of pre-1960 and 1970 drawings that most of the judges identified as
having been done by black children was compared with the number of
drawings in that group. Table 2 summarizes these data.

The data indicate that between 1960 and 1970 there has been a significant increase in the number of drawings that can be correctly identified as having been done by black children. These results are consistent
with the studies by Dennis (2, 3), as well as those by Spurlock (4) and
Wise (5).

When the data are examined by age levels, the significant differences
hold, beginning with children of ten years. Table 3 summarizes these
data.

One possible explanation for these results is that the drawing skills
of the youngest children are simply not refined or accurate enough for
them to depict the racial characteristics of which they may be perfectly
aware. Since none of the children was interviewed about his drawings
after he completed them, it is not possible to evaluate this possibility.
Furthermore, once a child begins to move into the community and away
from his close family circle, he becomes the target of all the educational
and social efforts of various civil rights and other groups to increase his

awareness, understanding, and acceptance of his racial identity. These educational efforts may well have influenced not only the inclusion of racial detail, but also the age at which such details are incorporated. Many of the children whose figure drawings are included in the 1970 group were active in an Afro-American cultural center maintained in the community center near their homes.

The foregoing data clearly indicate that black children's figure drawings have become more easily identified as drawings of black people. What is the source of the change? Sociological and psychological studies in the past have documented the reluctance of blacks to value their physical racial characteristics. In addition to the studies of Dennis (2, 3) cited earlier, Frisch and Handler (6) found that drawings collected from 122 black children and 103 white children were the same except for the emphasis on hair in the black children's drawings. The hair in these drawings was more elaborate and emphasized. Black children were then instructed to draw black figures. With such specific instructions, 88 percent of them made drawings that had distinctively black features.

Social scientists have also documented the extent to which blacks have rejected their own physical characteristics (7, 8). White skins have been preferred to dark skins, and a higher social status has been given to the lighter-skinned individual; children have preferred white-skinned, blue-eyed, and/or blond dolls and have even been known to insist that they, themselves, were blond, blue-eyed, and white-skinned. Dennis' recent study (3) of the drawings of college students suggests that this trend is beginning to change in favor of a higher value being placed on distinctly black features and characteristics.

What, then, were the graphic cues that led a majority of judges to score a particular drawing as being produced by a black child? Spontaneous comments suggested that hairstyle, earrings, and incomplete bodies all played their parts in conveying racial group membership to the individual judges. The investigators developed a scoring system that included positive scores for such details as hairstyle, facial features (full lips, wide nose), facial hair (mustaches, beards, and/or sideburns), indication of skin color, earrings, peace gestures or symbols, Afro-style costume, profile head, head only, and omission of arms, hands, legs, or feet.

All drawings in the 1970 group were scored, and the average scores for the drawings identified as black and for those not so identified were calculated. A t test for differences between means for each category's mean score and for the total mean scores resulted in significant differences in the scores received for feature details (hair, eyes, facial hair, profile

TABLE 4
Comparison of Racial Details Included in Identified and Nonidentified 1970 Drawings

CATEGORY	POSSIBLE POINTS	MEAN SCORES		VALUE OF T	SIGNIFICANCE
		IDENTIFIED	NONIDENTIFIED		
Features	7	2.826	1.084	2.051	p < .05
Body	8	1.734	1.067	.506	n.s.
Costume	7	.551	.134	1.176	p < .10
Total	22	5.112	2.320	2.330	:p = .02

head, lips, nose, or skin color) and total detail scores. Table 4 summarizes these data.

These data are not surprising when one considers that most people, after noting a person's sex, mostly notice his face. And the emphasis on facial detail is the only subgroup of details that, when included, was likely to be judged as indicating the black racial group. The idea that black children are more likely to draw incomplete human figures was of no help to the judges in assigning drawings to racial groups. Such omissions were likely to occur with drawings by black children not judged as black. Contrary to informal expectations, costume factors such as clothing with large designs indicated, dark glasses, peace symbols, cigarettes or pipes, and jewelry were of no significance in determining whether a drawing was judged as produced by a black child.

The decision to use both black and white judges was based on the often-voiced complaint of blacks that whites are outsiders who cannot really be empathetic with or appreciative of the special position of the black person in the community (8). However, when we examine the accuracy of the individual judge in assessing whether a particular drawing was drawn by a black child or by a white one, the opposite seems to be true. In judging pre-1960 drawings, 1970 drawings, or drawings by white children, the overall accuracy of the white judges was significantly better than that of the black judges. Because of the slight variation in the number of drawings from each population judged by individual judges, the percentage accuracy scores were used to evaluate differences in performance, using the Mann-Whitney U test. These data are summarized in Table 5.

When the opinions of individual judges were evaluated to determine whether significant differences existed in accuracy in judging pre-1960 and 1970 drawings, only four judges did not show significantly greater accuracy in judging the more recent drawings. Only one of these four judges were black. The comparison between accuracy of judgments for pre-1960 and 1970 drawings is summarized in Table 6.

These data indicate that the white judges were more accurate in their

TABLE 5
Comparison of Percentage Accuracy Scores
Between Black and White Judges

DRAWINGS	MANN-WHITNEY U VALUE	SIGNIFICANCE
Pre-1960	27	p = .001
1970	23	p = .001
White	9	p = .001

TABLE 6
Comparison of Accuracy for Each Judge

JUDGES	PERCENTAGE CORRECT		SIGNIFICANCE
	PRE-1960	1970	
1*	21.2	41.1	p = .025
2	45.4	67.3	p = .0125
3	6.0	29.7	p = .005
4	45.1	63.4	p = .05
5	19.3	53.9	p = .0025
6	9.0	40.0	p = .0025
7	6.0	37.0	p = .0025
8*	12.1	38.5	p = .005
9*	36.3	62.9	p = .005
10	15.1	51.7	p = .0025
11	30.3	45.3	n.s.
12	21.2	49.6	p = .001
13	18.1	30.4	n.s.
14*	18.1	42.5	p = .01
15	15.1	29.0	n.s.
16*	12.1	24.8	n.s.

*Black

judgments than were the black judges. Why? All the black judges were in their middle 20s or older and therefore had spent their early formative years in the time before civil rights and other positive black programs and groups were so active and effective. They grew up during the time when, sociologists suggest, the successful black was the one who most closely approximated white appearance and white values and who rejected black characteristics as not valuable. Perhaps these attitudes, ingrained early, served to prevent recognition of the sorts of ethnic details that white judges, with their background of white supremacy, were supersensitive to.

In addition, members of one racial group have often complained of difficulty in differentiating among members of another racial group, in spite of biologic and sociologic evidence to suggest there is greater variability within a group than there is between the extreme members of one group and the extreme members of another group. Perhaps "out-group" whites pay too much attention to common black racial physical characteristics, while "in-group" blacks are more aware of the individual distinguishing characteristics and overlook the more "racial" characteristics as of no significance.

Experience with other drawings of black children also may have been advantageous. Two judges, one a black teacher of black children and the second a white psychologist in a clinic that serves a predominantly black population, were highly successful in judging both the pre-1960 and 1970 drawings.

When judges were ranked for accuracy, the judges who were teachers or psychologists did better in judging the drawings than did social workers or psychiatrists, perhaps because psychologists and teachers are simply more familiar with children's drawings in general. Only two of the black judges were teachers (judges 1 and 8). Eight of the 11 white judges were psychologists. The failure to include more black judges familiar with children's drawings in general also may have contributed to the significant difference in accuracy between the white and black judges.

Conclusions

The findings in the current investigation of black children's drawings are consistent with results reported by Dennis (2, 3), Spurlock (4) and Wise (5), among others, that drawings by black children are becoming more clearly drawings of black people. Periodic collection of drawings to follow the trend is indicated, since the inclusion of racially identifiable details seems related to the values the group assigns to those attributes.

Many observers of the integration scene suggest that without a positive self-image that accepts and incorporates all the physical and psychological attributes of oneself, the individual cannot make a comfortable or appropriate adjustment to any community. Nor, if he does not value himself, will others accept him as valuable. The periodic collection of human figure drawings may be an effective and efficient, although gross, measure of the success of the various programs to upgrade and revalue the status of the black person in the group.

Unfortunately, the pre-1960 drawings in this study were taken almost entirely from files of psychiatric facilities, which means that all of them were by children whose behavior had brought them to the attention of school authorities, community authorities, or parents and then to psychiatric evaluation. In answer to this criticism, one can only cite Dennis' investigation of college students in 1957 and 1967, which indicated that in 1957 black college students did not produce racially identifiable figure drawings, either. Furthermore, of the ten pre-1960 drawings that were collected from a public school, only one drawing was identified as having been done by a black child.

Another avenue of investigation suggested but not explored by this study is to evaluate the effect on black identity and value systems of the many Afro-culture, Black Power, and other civil rights programs. The striking increase over the past ten years in the number of black children's drawings that can be identified as drawings of black people indicate such programs may have a positive effect. Collection of drawings from children who do not participate in such educational programs and from children who do not participate should give an objective indication of the effectiveness of such programs.

REFERENCES

1. MACHOVER, K.: *Personality Projection in the Drawings of the Human Figure.* Springfield, Ill.: Charles C Thomas, 1949.
2. DENNIS, W. (Ed.): *Readings in Child Psychology,* 2nd ed. Englewood Cliffs, N. J.: Prentice-Hall, 1963.
3. DENNIS, W.: Racial change in Negro drawings. *J. Psychol.,* 69:129-130, 1968.
4. SPURLOCK, J.: Problems of identification in young black children—static or changing? *J. Nat. Med. Ass.,* 61:504-507, 1969.
5. WISE, J. H.: Self-reports by Negro and white adolescents to the Draw-A-Person. *Percept. Motor Skills,* 28:193-194, 1969.
6. FRISCH, G. R. & HANDLER, L.: Differences in Negro and white drawings: A cultural interpretation. *Percept. Motor Skills,* 24:667-670, 1967.
7. MYRDAL, G.: *An American Dilemma,* 20th anniversary ed. New York, Harper & Row, 1962.
8. GULLATTEE, A. C.: The Negro psyche: Fact, fiction, and fantasy. *J. Nat. Med. Assn.,* 61:119-129, 1969.

22

SELF-ESTEEM AND RACIAL PREFERENCE IN BLACK CHILDREN

Susan Harris Ward, B.S., and John Braun, Ph.D.
University of Bridgeport

In the 1950s and early 1960s, studies of racial preference of children consistently showed black children choosing white models and rejecting dark models. The present study of black children growing up since 1963 indicates a reversal of this position. The authors interpret their findings as a reflection of a more accepting incorporation of racial identity and pride within the child's self-concept.

Three- to seven-year-old black children have a well developed knowledge of the concept of racial differences between *white* and *colored,* as this is indicated by the characteristic of skin color (6). Blacks living in the South as well as the North (5, 14, 19), and integrated as well as segregated children (8, 11, 19) consistently preferred the white color and rejected the dark color. However, it should be noted that the environment of today's black children is strikingly different from that of the children previously tested. Various social changes as well as social and political movements, have evolved. Possibly such changes or move-

Reprinted from the AMERICAN JOURNAL OF ORTHOPSYCHIATRY, 42 (4), July 1972, pp. 644-647. Copyright © 1972, the American Orthopsychiatric Association, Inc. Reproduced by permission.

Mrs. Ward is currently staff psychologist at Children's Hospital of Pittsburgh, Pittsburgh, Pa.; Dr. Braun is Chairman of the Psychology Department, University of Bridgeport, Bridgeport, Conn.

ments might contribute to increased feelings of competence, and encourage blacks to identify or adopt their own group as a social comparison model. It has been stated that at the same time that the child is learning to understand his social environment, he is developing a concept of himself. The group to which he belongs becomes a factor in his self-concept. "Self and group evaluation furnish forceful motivation for a variety of specific behavior" (16).

Butts (3) found that black children with impaired self-concepts, as measured by the California Test of Personality, perceived themselves less accurately in terms of skin color. Asher and Allen (1) reported that middle-class blacks show greater white preference than do lower-class blacks, and that black males are more outgroup oriented than are black females.

The present study investigated the interrelation of self-esteem and racial preferences in black children. Reasoning from the previous studies the following hypotheses were generated:

1. Subjects with impaired self-concepts will be more outgroup oriented than those with unimpaired self-concepts.

2. White preference will be greater among middle-class than among lower-class black children.

3. There will be a significant difference between boys and girls in their choice of the black or white puppet on each of the racial preference statements. Black males will show greater white preference than will black females.

METHOD

Ss were 60 black girls and boys between the ages of seven and eight. Thirty were from a middle-class interracial, suburban school (Media, Pa.) and the remaining 30 were from a lower-class interracial inner-city school (Chester, Pa.). All Ss were judged to be of at least normal intelligence.

Ss from the suburban school were selected from a second- and third-grade class list. Since the number of blacks enrolled in the school was very small, all of the black students in each of the six second- and third-grade classes were included in the sample. However, in the inner-city school, every fifth child who was black was selected from the class list of second and third graders.

The test instrument for self-esteem was the Piers-Harris (17) Children's Self-Concept Test. This 80-item "yes-no" questionnaire was read aloud to the children by the black female E. The test device for assessing racial preference was an adaptation from the Clark and Clark (5) dolls test. There were two pairs of puppets chosen to match as closely as possible the sex and ages of the subjects. Within each pair, the puppets were identical except for skin and hair color. The black puppet was of medium brown facial color with black hair, and the white puppet had light skin and light hair. The puppets were placed in prone position before each child, who was asked to make fixed alternative responses to each of the following directions:

1. Give me the puppet that you would like to play with.
2. Give me the puppet that is a nice puppet.
3. Give me the puppet that is a nice color.
4. Give me the puppet that looks bad.

Since research has consistently found no effects of race of the E upon performance in this situation (9, 11, 13), this factor was not varied in the present study. A black preference choice was defined as choosing the black puppet for the racial preference statements "play with," "nice puppet," and "nice color," but choosing the white puppet as the one that "looks bad."

RESULTS

The Mann-Whitney U Test indicated a significant relationship between self-esteem and racial preference. The median self-concept score for those subjects who made at least three of the four black preference choices (63.06 vs. 55.5; $p < .01$). Chi-square tests yielded no significant sex nor social class differences in racial preferences among black children. The majority of the black children preferred the black puppet. For example, 70% of the subjects chose the black puppet as the "nice puppet," and 82% chose the black puppet as the one that is a "nice color." A majority of these subjects (79%) chose the white puppet as the one that "looks bad." This finding of a preference by black children for black dolls confirms the recent results of Hraba and Grant (13) and Fox and Barnes (7). It is interesting to note that the median self-concept scores for the suburban (middle class) and the inner-city (lower class) children were at the 77th and 66th percentiles.

DISCUSSION

This study demonstrated a relationship between self-esteem and racial preference. The Mann-Whitney U Test indicated that those subjects who made *more* black color preferences had higher self-concept scores than those who made *fewer* black color preferences. It is possible that this relationship between self-esteem and racial preference may signify a new spirit of dignity in the lives of Afro-American children. This suggested that "Black is beautiful" and that black children have come to appreciate their uniqueness, beauty, and special value. Blacks who evidenced this feeling for their own group are experiencing, at some level of awareness, self-love. Personal pride is essentially the expression of group pride (4, 12, 15). Also, Chein (4) has stated that adequate self-perception and feelings of personal continuity are the major psychological functions of group identity for the person.

The results did not support the hypothesis that white preference will be greater among middle-class black children and black preference will be greater among lower-class black children. Perhaps the lack of a significant difference between middle- and lower-class black children suggests that middle-class black children are currently as ethnocentric as are lower-class black children. A second possibility may be that, regardless of socio-economic status, black children who attend schools with a heterogeneous social class and racial population, compete more and develop more self-esteem (2). Hraba and Grant (13) found that black children in an interracial setting are not necessarily white oriented.

Contrary to the views of Asher and Allen (1), and of Ausubel (2), this study did not find a significant sex difference. This lack of a significant difference between black males and females implied that black males are currently as racially aware as are black females. A second possibility may be that a black male maintains his self-respect as a unique and worthwhile human being apart from the position of inferior being that the racists insist he assume.

The results of the present study suggest questions for future research. First, there is a need to determine what effect an interracial vs. a uniracial situation has in shaping the black personality development. Does an interracial or a uniracial situation enhance or impede a black child's self-esteem? Second, there is a need to examine the effect on self of black peoples' participation in social and political movements. Exactly what effect has the black awareness movement or the new "Freedom" schools had on the self-esteem of young black children. Pouissant and Comer (18) have stated that drilling "Black is beautiful" in a rote memory fashion may have a reverse effect. It may give rise to the same doubts, self-hatred, and guilt a child experiences when his mother constantly insists that he be proud of being black. Are children who come from Freedom schools or other schools that use these slogans ("I'm an Afro-American" and "Black is beautiful") more likely to choose a black puppet? Finally, what is the relationship between racial preference and behavior. Are black children who express black preference more militant, more likely to succeed in school? Hraba and Grant (13) found that racial preference does not correspond with interpersonal behavior. Although black children may prefer a doll or puppet of their own race when race is the only cue, other criteria may be more important in establishing interpersonal relationships or in executing certain kinds of behavior. Nevertheless, the factor of racial preference, which can be conceptualized as an attitude and behavior, is worthy of scrutiny.

REFERENCES

1. ASHER, S. & ALLEN, V. (1969): Racial preference and social comparison processes. *J. Soc. Issues*, 25:157-166.
2. AUSUBEL, D. & AUSUBEL, P. (1963): Ego development among segregated Negro children. In A. Passow (Ed.), *Education in Depressed Areas*. New York: Bureau of Publications, Teachers College, Columbia University.
3. BUTTS, H. (1963): Skin color perception and self-esteem. *J. Negro Ed.*, 32:122-128.
4. CHEIN, I. (1948): Group membership and group belonging. American Jewish Congress, New York. (mimeo)
5. CLARK, K. & CLARK, M. (1947): Racial identification and preference in Negro children. In T. Neucomb and E. Hartley (Eds.), *Readings in Social Psychology*. New York: Holt.
6. CLARK, K. (1950): Emotional factors in racial identification and preference in Negro children. *J. Negro Ed.*, 19:341-350.
7. FOX, D. & BARNES, U. (1971): Racial preference and identification of black, Chinese, and white children. Paper presented at American Educational Research Association meetings, New York.
8. GOODMAN, M. (1952): *Race Awareness in Young Children*. Reading, Mass.: Addison-Wesley.
9. GREENWALD, H. & OPPENHEIM, D. (1968): Reported magniture of self-misidentification among Negro children—artifact? *J. Pers. Soc. Psychol.*, 8:49-52.
10. GREGOR, A. (1964): Integrated schools and Negro character development. *Psychiatry*, 24:69-72.
11. GREGOR, A. (1966): Racial attitudes among white and Negro children in a deep south metropolitan area. *J. Soc. Psychol.*, 68:95-190.
12. GROSSACK, M. (1966): Group belongingness among Negroes. *J. Soc. Psychol.*, 43: 167-180.
13. HRABA, J. & GRANT, J. (1970): Black is beautiful: A re-examination of racial preference and identification. *J. Pers. Soc. Psychol.*, 16 (3):398-402.
14. MORLAND, J. (1966): A comparison of race awareness in northern and southern children. *Amer. J. Orthopsychiat.*, 36:22-31.
15. NOEL, D. (1964): Group identification among Negroes: An empirical analysis. *J. Soc. Issues*, 20:71-84.
16. PETTIGREW, T. (1964): *A Profile of the Negro American*. Princeton, N. J.: Van Nostrand (pp. 6-11).
17. PIERS, E. & HARRIS, D. (1969): *The Piers-Harris Children's Self-Concept Scale*. Nashville, Tenn.: Counselor Recordings and Tapes.
18. POUISSANT, A. & COMER, P. (1971): The question every black parent asks: What shall I tell my child? *Redbook* (McCall Publishing Co.), 136:64.
19. STEVENSON, H. & STEWART, E. (1958): A developmental study of racial awareness in young children. *Child Development*, 29:399-409.

23

WHITE ADULT BEHAVIOR TOWARD BLACK AND WHITE CHILDREN

Brian Coates, Ph.D.

Assistant Professor, Department of Child and Family Studies
Washington State University

Twenty-four males and 24 female white adults used verbal statements to train 9-year-old black or white male children on a discrimination problem. Bogus information on the children's performance was given to the adults and the dependent variable was the adults' statements to the children. A sex of adult × race of child interaction was found. Males were more negative with black children than with white children whereas there was a nonsignificant difference between the two races for females. On trait ratings of the children following the training session, both males and females rated black children more negatively than white children.

Research on social interaction between adults and children has been dominated by a unidirectional model which assumes that the adult influences the child. In recent years, however, this model has been questioned by several writers (Bell 1968; Gewirtz 1961; Kessen 1963; Korner 1965; Rheingold 1969; Wenar & Wenar 1963), and the necessity of in-

Reprinted from CHILD DEVELOPMENT, 1972, 43, 143-154. © 1972 by the Society for Research in Child Development, Inc. All rights reserved.

This research was supported in part by a grant from the University Research Council, University of North Carolina. The author is grateful to Elizabeth H. Foster and Jane D. Furr for assistance in collecting the data and David Goldstein and G. Josh Haskett for help in its processing.

vestigating the effects of children on adults has become clear. Bell argues persuasively for a bidirectional model and suggests that an adequate understanding of the socialization process will be obtained only when the effects of children on adults are assessed independently of the effects of adults on children.

The major purpose of the present study was to assess the effects of race of the child on the behavior of adults toward children. Male and female adults participated in an experiment which they were told was designed to "facilitate children's learning." Each adult trained a 9-year-old male (black or white) on a discrimination problem by using positive, neutral, or negative statements following each trial of the problem. Although the children worked on the problem, their performance was not presented to the adults. Rather, bogus information was presented to the adults. With this method, the performance of each child was seen to be the same, and the effects of race of the child on the adults' statements to the children could be examined independently of performance differences between the two races.

It has been found consistently in research on interracial attitudes that white adults have negative attitudes toward Negro adults (e.g., Noel & Pinkney 1964; Sheatsley 1966). I reasoned that these attitudes would be generalized to children and would be expressed in the statements used by adults in training a black child on a learning problem. Thus, it was predicted that white adults would be more negative in their statements when training a black child than when training a white child. Predictions were not made for differences between male and female adults in their use of statements for the two races.

METHOD

Subjects.—The *S*s were 48 *adult* volunteers, 24 males and 24 females, from introductory psychology classes at the University of North Carolina who were meeting part of the course requirement for research participation. All *S*s were white and ranged in age from 18 to 23 years (*M*=18-9 years). The majority of the *S*s (77%) were residents of North Carolina; with two exceptions, the remaining *S*s were from the eastern United States, most of them from the southeastern United States.

Children.—The children (i.e., confederates) were two white and two black third-grade males, from a local elementary school. In order to provide comparability of the children in the two racial groups, each of the children was 9 years of age, which is 1 year older than the average child in the third grade, and scored below the fiftieth percentile on national norms for standard achievement tests. Thus, in terms of their progress in school and performance on achievement tests, the children were below average.

Experimental design.—A 2 (Sex of Adult) × 2 (Race of Child) design was employed. Each adult was randomly assigned to a black or white child with each of the four children performing the discrimination problem in the presence of six male and six female adults. It should be noted that the adult thought that he was testing the child.

Apparatus.—The stimulus materials for the discrimination problem were outlined on sheets of paper which were stacked on a table to the left of the adult. The discrimination problem was similar to one used by Stevenson, Hale, Klein, and Miller (1968). Briefly, four letter-like forms (Gibson 1963) appeared in a row at the bottom of a page, with one of the four cues (circle, diamond, rectangle, square) centered at the top of a page. The four correct answers for the problem were obtained by randomly pairing each of the cues with each of the letter-like forms. There were six sets of 16 pages, a total of 96 trials. The stick of pages was constructed so that no two successive pages were identical, the same cue did not appear on two successive pages, within each set of 16 pages no page occupied the same position, and each of the cues appeared once with each of the forms in each spatial position. Within these restrictions, the order of the pages was random.

The adult and the child sat at opposite ends of a table with a wooden screen (25 inches wide and 14½ inches high) between them. The screen enabled the adult to see the child's face and shoulders, but prevented any observation of the child's responses to the discrimination problem. On the adult's side of the screen was a panel containing four colored lights which indicated to the adult the nature of the child's responses on the problem. The lights were placed horizontally and were labeled, from left to right, A, B, C, and D. On the table in front of the adult was a list of the correct responses (labeled as A, B, C, or D) for the discrimination problem and a list of five statements, one of which the adult was to say to the child following each trial of the problem.

On the child's side of the screen was a response panel which contained four buttons. The buttons were placed horizontally, were not labeled in any way, and were used by the child to indicate his response on each trial. A cable connected the child's response panel with the adult's light panel. This cable was *not* connected to an electrical outlet; thus the child's responses were *not* recorded on the adult's light panel.

A second response panel, identical with the child's response panel, was located behind a one-way mirror. This panel was connected to the adult's light panel and to an electrical outlet, and enabled an observer to *systematically program* the child's responses on the discrimination problem.

Procedure.—A female white experimenter explained the general procedure of the experiment to each child prior to the first session for that child. She also encouraged the child to structure his behavior so that the adult thought the child was making every effort to learn the discrimination problem. Finally, the experimenter told the child he should not be concerned with the statements made by the adult, since the purpose of the study was to test the adult. Adverse effects on the children from their participation in the study were not detected. There appeared to be no systematic differences between the black and white children in either their desire or ability to serve as confederates, and the motivation of the children remained at a high level throughout the experiment.

The experimenter met the adult and escorted him to the experimental room. The experimenter then gave the following instructions:

"The purpose of this experiment is to facilitate children's learning. On each stimulus sheet you will see four nonsense forms and one standard shape. There are four standard shapes: circle, diamond, rectangle, and square. Each nonsense form has been paired with one of these standard shapes throughout the entire experiment. Your job is to teach the child which nonsense form goes with each standard shape."

Following instructions on the location of the experimenter, the adult, and the child in the experimental room, the experimenter then said:

"The stimulus sheets will be at your left. On each of the 96 trials, you will hand a sheet to me, I will announce the trial number, and will hand the sheet to the child. The child has four buttons in front of him, one for each of the nonsense forms. He will indicate his response by pressing one of the four buttons in front of him. The child's response will illuminate one of the colored lights on the light panel on your side of the table. You will compare his response with the correct response on the answer sheet in front of you. When you have determined whether the child was correct, you may make one of the five statements from another sheet which will also be in front of you. You must make one of these statements after each of the child's responses; do not vary the wording of the statements. It is important for you to understand that these statements are your only way of teaching the child the task. Except for the statements that you make, there should be no talking during the experiment. This task has been shown to be of moderate difficulty for a child of this age."

The experimenter then took the adult to another room and introduced him to the child. Following their return to the experimental room, the experimenter gave the child instructions for the discrimination problem. The experiment was then begun.

Child's performance.—As indicated above, the child's actual performance on the discrimination problem was neither seen by nor presented to the adult. Rather, the child's responses were determined by an observer behind a one-way mirror who followed a prepared schedule of correct and incorrect responses to be attributed to the child. The schedule was arranged so that the adult thought that the child made 32 correct responses and 64 incorrect responses over the 96 trials of the discrimination problem. The schedule of correct and incorrect responses was ordered so that the child gave the appearance of a slow "learning curve." The schedule was as follows, with the first number indicating the trial block (16 trials for each block) and the second number, the number correct during that block: 1,3; 2,4; 3,5; 4,6; 5,6; 6,8. The order of the correct and incorrect responses within each trial block was random with the restriction that the child make no more than three correct responses in a row.

Adult's statements.—The adult could make one of five statements following each of the child's responses on the discrimination problem. The five statements, which were designed to range from positive to negative, were chosen on the basis of a rank-ordering of 12 statements by 46 students in an introductory child psychology class at the University of North Carolina. The five statements were: "Great, you're really catching on"; "Hey, you're doing pretty good"; "Okay, let's go on to the next one"; "You should do better than that"; and "That's bad; you're not doing very well." The adult's statements were recorded by the observer.

Rating scales.—Following the training session, each adult was asked to complete a questionnaire in order "to obtain some additional information about the child that you saw." The questionnaire was designed to provide information on the adult's ratings of the personality traits of the child. The adult rated the child on a series of seven-point scales patterned after the semantic differential. Each scale consisted of a pair of adjectives (e.g., shy-bold) which was selected from the pair used by Stevenson, Hill, Hale, and Moeley (1966). The instructions indicated that the adult was "to place a check in the interval that you think best describes the child that you saw." The adult was told to check the extreme intervals if the adjective described the child "very well," the next two intervals if the adjective described the child "fairly well," and so on.

The serial position of each adjective pair and the right-left position of each adjective within each pair was random. The positioning of the adjectives was constant for all subjects.

An additional item asked the adult to rate the difficulty of the task for the child. The ends of this seven-point scale was labeled "high" and "low."

Scoring.—On each of the 96 trials of the discrimination problem, the most positive statement that the adult could make to the child arbitrarily received a score of 1, with successively more negative statements receiving scores 2-5. The scores were then summed within each of the six trial blocks for correct and incorrect responses which were attributed to the child. Since the child did not make the same number of correct and incorrect responses within each trial block, the scores were divided by the number of opportunities that the adult had to make a statement for each type of response. For example, if the child made three correct responses during a trial block, then the score for each adult for correct responses was divided by 3.

The trait-rating scales were scored on a seven-point scale. A check in the interval nearest the adjective on the left arbitrarily received a score of 1, with succeeding intervals receiving scores 2-7.

RESULTS

The differences between the adults' statement scores and the ratings of the two children within each of the racial groups were evaluated by t tests. These differences were not significant. Consequently, the scores for children within each racial group were combined in subsequent analyses.

The means of the adults' statement scores for each of the four experimental groups are presented in Table 1. The scores are presented separately for each of the six trial blocks and for the correct and incorrect responses which were attributed to the child. The major questions of interest are the effects of sex of adult and race of child on the adults' statements. Thus, a 2 × 2 analysis of variance was performed on the total scores for statements (correct + incorrect responses across trial blocks). The main effects for Sex of Adult and Race of Child were not significant, F's = 1.18 and .37. However, a significant Sex of Adult × Race of Child interaction was found, $F(1,44) = 5.38$, $p < .025$. Follow-up tests (Winer 1962) on this interaction revealed that the males were significantly more negative to the black children than to the white children, $F(1,44) = 4.26$, $p < .05$, whereas the difference between the two groups of children was not significant for the females, $F = 1.47$. In

TABLE 1

MEANS OF ADULT STATEMENT SCORES ACCORDING TO RACE OF CHILD, SEX OF ADULT, TYPE OF RESPONSE, AND TRIAL BLOCK

GROUP	CORRECT RESPONSE							INCORRECT RESPONSE						
	1	2	3	4	5	6	M	1	2	3	4	5	6	M
White:														
Male..........	1.37	1.77	1.62	1.58	1.67	1.59	1.60	3.44	3.36	3.48	3.55	3.53	3.64	3.50
Female	1.61	1.60	1.70	1.63	1.67	1.62	1.64	3.58	3.70	3.58	3.62	3.66	3.86	3.67
Negro:														
Male..........	1.36	1.88	1.88	1.86	1.97	1.70	1.78	3.76	3.80	3.78	3.83	3.90	3.79	3.81
Female	1.44	1.54	1.55	1.56	1.50	1.52	1.52	3.47	3.48	3.44	3.48	3.49	3.62	3.50

NOTE.—Higher score indicates more negative statements.

addition, the males were significantly more negative to the black children than were the females, $F(1,44) = 5.79$, $p < .025$. Each of the remaining four contrasts was not significant.

A series of subsidiary analyses of variance was performed to test the remaining effects in the four-factor design. The tests were the exact tests needed to eliminate the problem of unequal correlations among scores in a repeated measures design (Greenhouse & Geisser 1959; Lana & Lubin 1963).[1] The major findings were: (a) no significant effects for the interaction of Race of Child with Type of Response (correct and incorrect) and trials; (b) a highly significant effect for Type of Response—the adults were more negative when the child made an incorrect response than when he made a correct response, $F(1,42) = 673.46$, $p < .01$. Significant Type of Response × Trials, $F(2,40) = 3.73$, $p < .05$, and Sex of Adult × Trials, $F(1,42) = 7.31$, $p < .01$, interactions were also found. Inspection of Table 1 reveals that the Type of Response × Trials interaction is due to a gradual increase across trial blocks in the negativeness of the statements for an incorrect response, whereas for a correct response there was an increase from trial block 1 to trial block 2 and then a gradual decrease for the remaining trial blocks. The Sex of Adult × Trials interaction appears to be due to a gradual increase in the negativeness of the statements across trials for females, whereas for males there is a complex relation between trial blocks and the negativeness of the statements (see Table 1).

The mean scores for each of the four experimental groups for each of the 19 trait-rating scales are presented in Table 2. A 2 (Sex of Adult) × 2 (Race of Child) analysis of variance was performed for each of the scales. For each analysis, the main effect of Sex of Adult and the interaction between Sex of Adult and Race of Child was not significant. For 16 of the 19 scales, however, a significant main effect for Race of Child was found (see Table 2 for F values). From middle-class cultural standards, it appears that in each case black children were rated more negatively (e.g., dull, passive, unfriendly) than were white children (Table 2). An analysis of variance of the ratings for difficulty of the task for the child revealed no significant effects.

In view of the limited information on the stability of adult behavior toward children (e.g., Halverson & Waldrop 1970), it was of some interest to assess the stability of the adults' statements to the children across the six trial blocks. The total scores (correct + incorrect responses)

---

[1] The author thanks Elliot Cramer and John Draper of the Psychometric Laboratory, University of North Carolina, for advice on these analyses.

TABLE 2

MEAN TRAIT RATINGS ACCORDING TO RACE OF CHILD AND SEX OF ADULT

SCALES (1–7)	WHITE		NEGRO		F VALUE FOR
	Male	Female	Male	Female	RACE OF CHILD
Shy-bold	3.17	2.17	1.58	1.67	11.71**
Attractive-unattractive ...	3.42	3.00	2.92	2.50	3.58
Sociable-unsociable	3.50	3.42	4.92	4.50	10.88**
Colorful-colorless	3.58	3.92	4.75	4.67	9.55**
Unenthusiastic-enthusiastic	4.50	4.08	2.58	2.42	23.62**
Timid-forceful	3.33	2.58	2.08	1.67	9.81**
Pleasant-unpleasant	2.33	1.92	3.17	2.75	8.43**
Nonassertive-assertive	4.33	3.75	2.17	2.58	13.64**
Immature-mature	4.50	4.67	4.08	3.67	5.38*
Sober-jolly	4.50	3.58	2.17	2.00	23.12**
Uncertain-certain	3.67	4.17	2.75	3.25	4.68*
Agitated-calm	5.25	4.75	4.83	5.83	<1
Unfriendly-friendly	5.33	5.75	3.67	4.08	20.80**
Insensitive-sensitive	4.83	4.83	5.00	4.58	<1
Passive-active	4.17	4.00	2.75	3.00	12.06**
Bored-interested	4.08	4.08	3.17	2.67	6.41*
Bright-dull	3.08	3.08	4.00	4.92	17.59**
Unreliable-reliable	4.50	5.33	4.33	4.33	4.18*
Cold-warm	4.58	5.17	3.83	4.25	4.34*

* $p < .05.$
** $p < .01.$

for the adults were transformed to standard scores in order to remove the effects of the experimental conditions. Correlations were then computed among the scores for each trial block. As shown in Table 3, each of the correlations is of high magnitude and statistically significant. Thus, the data indicate that there were stable individual differences in the adults' statements to the children across the six trial blocks.

DISCUSSION

White male adults used more negative statements when training a black male child on a discrimination problem than when training a white male child. White female adults, in contrast, did not employ the statements differently for the two racial groups. In rating of personality traits, both males and females judged black children more negatively than white children.

This study was based on the assumption that the adults, in both their statements and ratings, were responding to the "race" and not to other characteristics of the child. An alternative possibility is that the adults were responding to differences in the behavior of the two races during the experiment. This assumption would be supported if the trait ratings were based on the personality characteristics of the children

TABLE 3

INTERCORRELATIONS AMONG TRIAL BLOCK SCORES
FOR ADULTS' STATEMENTS

Trial Block	1	2	3	4	5	6
1	...	.69	.62	.63	.58	.63
2	...	...	.70	.77	.54	.61
3	...	...	...	.80	.63	.73
4	...	...	...	...	.73	.81
5	...	...	...	...	...	.72
6	...	...	...	...	...	...

NOTE.—$N = 48$, $r = .37$, $p < .01$.

themselves. But the findings may only be a consequence of the stereo-typed attitudes that adults hold toward black and white children, and the same findings would have occurred even if only pictures of the children had been presented.

The procedures and findings of the present study provide evidence that the adults were not responding to behavioral differences in children of the two races. For example, steps were taken to minimize such differences. The perceived performance of the child on the discrimination problem was the same for each adult, and the children were told to structure their behavior so that the adults thought that they were making every effort to learn the task. Additional evidence against the assumption that the adults were responding to behavioral differences between the races is provided by the t tests on the adults' scores for statements and ratings for the children within each racial group. As mentioned previously, these tests revealed no significant differences. Such differences would have been evident if the adults were responding to the characteristics of each child and not to his "race." Next, if the assumption about behavioral differences is correct, then the males should not have used the statements differently for the two races on the initial trials of the discrimination problem. During these trials, they would have had little opportunity to observe the behavior of the child. Table 1, how-ever, shows that the males were more negative to the black children than to the white children on the initial trial blocks, as well as on later trial blocks. (The lack of a difference for correct responses during trial block 1 is probably due to the fact that there were only three correct responses by the children during this trial block.) Similar reasoning suggests that the differences between the two races should become more pronounced over trials as the males had a greater opportunity to observe the behavior of the black children. Again, Table 1 shows that such increasing differentiation between the two sets of children was not evi-dent. Also, in the analysis of variance of the adults' statements to the children, the interaction between Race of Child and Trials was not sig-nificant. For these reasons, then, the findings do not appear to have been caused by differences in the behavior of the black and white children.

Some caution must be exercised in interpreting the results for the training session. On the one hand, the results do indicate that males were significantly more negative to black children than to white chil-dren. On the other hand, the small mean difference between the two racial groups (Table 1) raises a number of questions. For example, what effect would the males' behavior have on the child's behavior?

Would the difference be larger or smaller with the other samples (e.g., teachers)? What would the difference be outside the laboratory situation? These questions must be considered in future research in order to further increase our knowledge of adult behavior toward black and white children.

It was found that the sex of the adult and race of the child influence the statements used by adults when training children on a discrimination problem and their subsequent trait ratings of the children. The study illustrates a method for investigating social interaction between adults and children which is independent of the child's performance on a task. Future research with this technique should increase our knowledge of the interaction between adults and children and between blacks and whites.

REFERENCES

BELL, R. Q.: A reinterpretation of the direction of effects in studies of socialization. *Psychological Review*, 1968, 75, 81-95.

GEWIRTH, J. L.: A learning analysis of the effects of normal stimulation, privation and deprivation on the acquisition of social motivation and attachment. In B. M. Foss (Ed.): *Determinants of Infant Behavior*. New York: Wiley, 1961. Pp. 219-299.

GIBSON, E. J.: Development of perception: Discrimination of depth compared with discrimination of abstract forms. In J. C. Wright & J. Kagan (Eds.): Basic cognitive processes in children. *Monographs of the Society for Research in Child Development*, 1963, 28 (2, Serial No. 86).

GREENHOUSE, S. W., & GEISSER, S.: On methods in the analysis of profile data. *Psychometrika*, 1959, 24, 95-112.

HALVERSON, C. F., JR. & WALDROP, M. F.: Maternal behavior toward own and other preschool children: The problem of "ownness." *Child Development*, 1970, 41, 839-845.

KESSEN, W.: Research in the psychological development of infants: An overview. *Merrill-Palmer Quarterly*, 1963, 9, 83-94.

KORNER, A. F.: Mother-child interaction: One- or two-way street? *Social Work*, 1965, 10, 47-51.

LANA, R. E. & LUBIN, A.: The effect of correlation on the repeated measures design. *Educational and Psychological Measurement*, 1963, 23, 729-739.

NOEL, D. L., & PINKNEY, A.: Correlates of prejudice: Some racial differences and similarities. *American Journal of Sociology*, 1964, 69, 609-622.

RHEINGOLD, H. L.: The social and socializing infant. In D. H. Goslin (Ed.): *Handbook of Socialization Theory and Research*. Chicago: Rand McNally, 1969. Pp. 779-790.

SHEATSLEY, P. B.: White attitudes toward the Negro. In T. Parsons & K. B. Clark (Eds.): *The Negro American*. Boston: Houghton Mifflin, 1966. Pp. 303-324.

STEVENSON, H. W., HALE, G. A., KLEIN, R. E., & MILLER, L. K.: Interrelations and correlates in children's learning and problem solving. *Monographs of the Society for Research in Child Development*, 1968, 33 (7, Serial No. 123).

STEVENSON, H. W., HILL, K. T., HALE, G. A., & MOELEY, B. E.: Adult ratings of children's behavior. *Child Development*, 1966, 37, 929-941.

WENAR, C. & WENAR, S. C.: The short-term prospective model, the illusion of time, and the tabula rasa child. *Child Development*, 1963, 34, 697-708.

WINER, B. J.: *Statistical Principles in Experimental Design*. New York: McGraw-Hill, 1962.

Part VI

CLASSIFICATION AND DIAGNOSIS

The importance of classification and diagnosis is still all too frequently minimized by many mental health professionals. The papers included in this section reemphasize the contribution that careful clinical studies in this area can make to improving patient care and to enlarging our understanding of the nature of psychopathological syndromes.

In their review article, Anders and Weinstein relate sleep disturbances to stages of sleep. This provides a rational basis for therapeutic intervention by facilitating a distinction between those disturbances which represent developmental deviations and those which are psychologically initiated.

Lesser and Easser's clinical review describes the special stresses of the deaf and the coping and defensive strategies they develop to deal with these stresses. The authors emphasize the danger of inaccurate diagnosis if these special issues are not properly evaluated.

Chess investigates the relationship between neurological dysfunction and childhood behavioral pathology in a series of 88 patients and compares the findings in this group with those in a control sample. She pays special attention to the frequency of those symptoms which have traditionally been considered typical of the brain-damaged child.

Cytryn and McKnew reflect the growing interest in depressive symptomatology in childhood. It is now recognized that this occurs more frequently than had previously been thought, and these authors contribute a classification system for such reactions that points toward specific strategies of intervention.

24

SLEEP AND ITS DISORDERS IN INFANTS AND CHILDREN: A REVIEW

Thomas F. Anders, M.D.,

and

Pearl Weinstein, M.S.

From the Infant Development Laboratory, Department of Psychiatry, Montefiore Hospital and Medical Center, and The Rose F. Kennedy Center for Research in Mental Retardation and Human Development, Albert Einstein College of Medicine

ABSTRACT. Recently the polygraphic study of sleep has provided techniques for the assessment of central nervous system (CNS) functioning in newborn infants and the diagnosis of sleep disorders in children. First, in this review, the normal developmental course of the "active" and the "quiet" sleep states from birth through childhood is described. Then, within the context of these recent electrophysiologic findings, the abnormalities of sleep state organization during the neonatal period, the physiologic disorders of sleep in older children, and finally, the physiological disturbances manifested through sleep are reviewed.

Reprinted with permission from THE JOURNAL OF PEDIATRICS, Vol. 50, No. 2, August, 1972, pp. 311-324. Copyright © by The C. V. Mosby Co., St. Louis, Mo.

This work was supported by National Institute of Mental Health Research Development Award K1-MH-43340 (T.F.A.) and by the W. T. Grant Foundation, Inc. Drs. M. Cohen, L. Finberg, M. Gersch, and H. Gordon graciously reviewed earlier versions of this report.

Abbreviations: CNS: Central nervous system; EEG: Electroencephalogram; NREM: Nonrapid eye movement; REM: Rapid eye movement; REMs: Rapid eye movements; SWS: Slow wave sleep.

In 1955 Aserinsky and Kleitman (1), observing sleeping infants, described a "rest-activity" cycle characterized by *quiet* periods of no body movements and no eye movements and *active* periods of body movements and rapid eye movements (REMs) under closed lids. Dement and Kleitman (2) first confirmed these observations by electrophysiologic recording from sleeping adults in 1957. More than 15 years later, after a virtual explosion of investigative interest into the functions and mechanisms of sleep in man and other animals, it is well recognized that sleep is not a unitary physiologic state of restitution, but rather two cycling states of differing physiologic activity. Several texts indicate the scope of this work (3-5), and sleep studies during infancy have recently been reviewed by Lenard (6).

Although the sleep of infants and adults differs in minor details, the basic alternation of an "aroused" state with an "inhibited" one is similar. An initial description of the *adult* sleep cycle provides the background for the understanding of developing sleep patterns and sleep stages sequencing in the infant and young child. Dement and Kleitman (2) described four stages of electroencephalogram (EEG) activity during adult sleep: Stage 1 is typified by low voltage, fast activity; Stage 2 by the presence of sleep spindles and K-complexes against a low voltage background; and Stages 3/4 by varying degrees of slow, high voltage activity. Stages 3/4 have been called slow wave sleep (SWS). Rapid eye movement (REM) sleep is defined by the occurrence of a Stage I EEG, binocularly synchronous rapid eye movements, the suppression of muscle tone as recorded from chin muscles, and accelerated, irregular respiratory and heart rates. The nonrapid eye movement (NREM) stages (1 to 4) of sleep lack REMs and are accompanied by the presence of muscle tone, and slowed, regular cardiac and respiratory rates. The alternating REM and NREM states, occurring during sleep, define two distinct states of neurophysiologic activity. The REM state is highly activated; the NREM state is basal and highly regulated. They follow each other in a periodic fashion and together they comprise the sleep cycle.

A typical adult sleep cycle starts (as does sleep onset) with "descending" NREM sleep stage shifts, moving from Stage I to 4, then "emergent" shifts through Stages 3 and 2 to a REM period after which the cycle is repeated. The typical night's sleep involves 4 to 6 REM/NREM cycles.

The REM phase of the cycle is associated with what typically has been defined as dreaming though some mental activity does occur during Stages 1 and 2 of NREM sleep (7, 8).

The present paper considers sleep and its disorders in infants and children with respect to recent findings emanating from polygraphic studies of sleep. The psychological disturbances of sleep, not associated with abnormal polygraphic findings, are differentiated from the physiologic disorders. Three broad areas are reviewed: (1) the development of normal and abnormal sleep patterns in infancy, (2) physiologic disorders of sleep and arousal in children, and (3) psychological stresses manifested by disturbances of sleep. Although these areas differ slightly in their subject matter, the role of sleep is central and the polygraphic recording of sleep parameters is relevant to both development and physiologic studies. For the sake of completeness they are included in this single review. It is hoped that continuing investigation will provide the links, if any, between early developmental deviations and the later disorders of sleep and arousal. For the present, it is possible only to review the three areas independently.

THE DEVELOPMENT OF SLEEP PATTERNS IN INFANCY

The changing electrophysiologic and organizational characteristics of infant sleep, as maturation progresses, provide new indices for early developmental assessment. Several of the differences between infant and adult sleep patterns and sleep cycles are worthy of note:

Organization

All of the sleep occurring during the adult's night sleep can readily be classified as either REM or NREM sleep and staged accordingly. During the newborn period, in contrast, the physiologic and behavioral activities routinely recorded during a sleep period are not as readily classified into two distinct sleep states. In a recent attempt at standardization of terms and techniques, an infant scoring manual has been published which defines three sleep states: . . . *active-REM* sleep, *quiet* sleep and *indeterminate* sleep (9). Whereas active-REM sleep and quiet sleep may be precursors of adult REM and NREM sleep respectively and seem, even in infancy, to share the "activated" and "basal" characteristics of the two adult sleep states, indeterminate sleep represents an "immature" state of poorly organized sleep, predominant in premature infants but also present in young, term infants and some abnormal infants. For more precise definitions of these sleep states the reader is referred to the infant scoring manual (9).

Proportions

Sleep state proportions change with age. Indeterminate sleep, predominant in the premature infant of 34 weeks, diminishes and most often disappears by 3 months of age. At term, active-REM sleep occupies 45 to 50% of total sleep time, indeterminate sleep occupies 10 to 15%, and quiet sleep occupies 35 to 45%. With increasing age, the proportion of quiet sleep increases and active-REM sleep decreases until late childhood when young adult normative amounts are achieved (20% REM sleep; 80% NREM sleep) (10-12). Furthermore, by 3 months of age, quiet sleep EEG patterns can begin to be subclassified into NREM sleep stages (13).

The predominance of an activated state of sleep during the early months of life has led Roffwarg, et al. (14) to put forward the ontogenetic hypothesis which, restated, suggests, "the REM sleep mechanisms of the brainstem constitute a CNS auto-stimulating system particularly important during uterine development and early post-natal life when the young organism is relatively cut off from external stimulation. Since growth and maintenance of neural tissue are enhanced by stimulation, according to this view, the cyclic excitatory activation provided to much of the brain by REM sleep serves to augment differentiation of neuronal structures and lay down the rudiments of neurophysiological discharge patterns in the developing organism" (15).

Periodicity and Sequencing

The length of the sleep cycle (active-REM/quiet sleep) changes with age. The cycle of normal infants at term has a periodicity of 45 to 50 minutes. More immature infants have shorter cycles and premature infants of less than 34 weeks' conceptual age do not demonstrate sleep cycling (16). The sleep cycle of adolescents and adults approximates 90 to 100 minutes.

The temporal patterning of individual sleep states within a sleep period also changes with age. Whereas adults enter sleep with an initial sustained NREM period and have most of their REM sleep during the last third of the night, newborn infants enter sleep initially through active-REM sleep and cycle, at regular intervals, with quiet sleep. Thus there is as much active-REM sleep in the first half of the newborn's sleep period as in the second half.

Day-Night Shifts

Diurnal patterning of sleep and wakefulness develops with maturation. In adults, wakefulness and sleep are associated most commonly with light and dark respectively. In newborn infants, daytime wakefulness and night time sleep is evident by 3 months of age, though indications of the diurnal rhythm have been reported as early as the first 10 days of life (17, 18). These day-night shifts occur while the overall 24-hour amounts of sleep and wakefulness change only minimally. Initial brief, individual sleep and wake periods coalesce into longer periods as the diurnal pattern develops. By 8 months of age a sustained period of daytime wakefulness, interrupted by two brief naps, and an uninterrupted period of night time sleep are characteristic (19). This process of "settling" or sleeping through the night is discussed further in the section on psychological disturbances of sleep. It is unclear what, if any, environmental influences retard or enhance the progression of these developmental changes. On the one hand, early adequate mother-infant regulation including appropriate feeding procedures, diet, absence of excessive anxiety, sufficient handling, and so forth have been implicated; on the other hand, maturation of the CNS alone has been felt to be sufficient. Most likely, the combination of a sensitive, responsive environment and normal maturation is optimal.

Miscellaneous

Several minor differences between adult sleep and infant sleep have also been noted. It is possible to deprive adult sleepers of a single sleep state, such as REM sleep, for a period of time and demonstrate a selective "rebound" of that state during subsequent uninterrupted recovery sleep (20). Neither deprivation nor recovery of sleep states is as clearcut in the newborn period. Rather, the infant demonstrates a "tenacity" for his ongoing sleep state, returning to it immediately following disturbance (15). Finally, hormones such as human growth hormone and cortisol have been associated with particular sleep stages in adults (21, 22). These relationships do not seem to exist during the first 3 months of life for the human infant (23, 24).

The assessment of sleep state organization, proportions and rhythmicity, by the polygraph has resulted in a new tool—the sleep polygram —useful in the diagnosis of a wide variety of developmental abnormalities. The areas of clinical applicability can be enumerated briefly:

Dreyfus-Brisac and Monod (25) have reported a complete lack of cycling in the sleep of severely brain-damaged newborn infants and unusually frequent and irregular sleep state shifts in infants with lesser degrees of neurological impairment. Infants with mild degrees of birth trauma (26), infants born to diabetic mothers (27) and to toxemic mothers (28), and infants born to heroin-addicted mothers (29) have all demonstrated abnormalities in their quiet sleep state organization and/ or in the maturation of various EEG wave forms. Abnormalities of active-REM sleep have been reported in a variety of pathological conditions including chromosomal abnormalities (30), infantile autism (31), and nonspecific mental retardation (32). The reversal of sleep EEG abnormalities associated with thyroid deficiency closely parallels clinical improvement (33).

More experience with the sleep polygram during early development will provide the basis for a much needed sensitive early indicator of neurological integrity, especially in the early detection and prognostic determination of children with minimal brain damage. The efficacy of various therapeutic regimens may prove to be another area in which sleep studies will provide clinically useful information.

DISORDERS OF SLEEP AND AROUSAL IN CHILDREN

In children older than 2 years, although sleep stage proportions have not achieved adult ratios, the characteristics of the physiologic measures recorded during sleep have by and large assumed adult forms. Therefore, as in the adult, it is possible to define a state of REM sleep alternating with a state of NREM sleep which can be subdivided further into Stages 1 to 4 according to previously described EEG criteria (2).

Nocturnal enuresis, somnambulism, somniloquy, pavor nocturnus (night horrors) and narcolepsy are generally considered to be the most common physiologic childhood disorders of sleep. In the past they have been classified in a variety of ways depending on their motor, autonomic, or psychophysiologic components (34). Through the use of the sleep polygraph, the widely held belief that these disorders were associated with seizure activity has not been confirmed (35-40). Rarely, temporal lobe seizures may mimic these disorders, but adequate study in the sleep laboratory readily differentiates epileptic disorders from sleep disorders. Currently a helpful classification has been with respect to their relationship to the REM/NREM sleep cycle. After a prolonged initial period of Stage 3/4 NREM sleep, the ascending or "emergent" shifts to Stages 2, 1, and REM sleep represent the "lightening" of sleep in the direction of arousal. Accordingly bed wetting, sleep walking, sleep talking, and night terrors are all associated with emergence from Stage 3/4 NREM sleep and consequently are defined as disorders of *arousal*. Narcolepsy, on the other hand, is associated with the abnormal occurrence of REM sleep and is thus regarded as a disorder of *sleep* (41-43). It is becoming increasingly evident that the disorders of arousal are most often associated with signs of neurological immaturity especially upon their initial occurrence in younger children.

The various disorders of arousal often appear in the same person at different times and often with a family history of the disorders (44-46). They are further linked by common aspects of their symptomatology: They are paroxysmal in nature and are characterized by nonresponsiveness to the environment, automatic appearance to actions, and retrograde amnesia for the episode. Prior to their study by sleep polygraphy, these disorders were commonly regarded as dream equivalents or "acting out" of dreams (47, 48). Dissociating these disorders from REM or "dreaming" sleep, however, are: (1) episodes occur during REM periods in less than 10% of polygraphic recordings; (2) REM sleep is most abundant during the last third of the night, whereas these disorders occur mainly during the first 3 hours of sleep; (3) dream recall is present after awakening from REM sleep while there is total amnesia following arousal from these episodes, and (4) children suffering from these disorders have normal REM sleep patterns and proportions (36, 40).

Still poorly understood is the reason that specific disorders occur in particular individuals and in those individuals only at certain times. There is evidence that the susceptibility to particular sleep disorders is related to individual physiologic differences and possible genetic factors (40, 49). Psychological anxiety and environmental stress are also frequently recognized, particularly where symptoms persist in late childhood and early adulthood, suggesting multiple interacting etiologies.

Nocturnal Enuresis

Bed wetting past the age of 3 is the most prevalent childhood sleep disorder. Rarely an organic etiology such as genitourinary pathology, epilepsy, or diabetes may be associated with enuresis but more often it is considered to be functional or idiopathic. In the pediatric literature childhood enuresis has been classified in various ways: Primary enuresis refers to the enuresis of children who have never developed bladder control, whereas secondary enuresis refers to children who have developed bladder control and then lost it. This secondary loss of control is often attributed to psychological stresses or intervening organic pathology. Night time enuresis has also been differentiated from daytime enuresis. In studies relating enuresis to sleep stage patterns, these distinctions have not been maintained and the results suggest that all categories of enuresis share varying proportions of a common physiological imbalance, at least when the symptoms first occur. Ritvo, et al. (50) have suggested that the initial psychophysiologic substrate for enuresis may provide a basis for perpetuation of the condition through later neurotic conflicts especially where enuresis occurs during Stages 1 and 2 NREM sleep in older children and adolescents.

Depending on the definition of enuresis and the methods of sampling, 5 to 17% of children between 3 and 15 years of age exhibit the disorder. The condition, more common in males, usually diminishes with maturation, rarely persisting into adulthood (44, 51, 52).

Broughton and Gastaut (53), by polygraphic monitoring, have defined an "enuretic episode" which generally occurs 1 to 3 hours after falling asleep, as the child is arousing from NREM Stage 3 or 4 sleep prior to entering his first REM period. The sleep stage change is often associated with body movements and increased muscle tone followed by tachycardia, tachypnea, erection in males, and decreased skin resistance. Micturition occurs ½ to 4 minutes after the start of the spisode in a moment of relative quiet. Immediately following micturition, children are difficult to awaken and when aroused indicate that they have not dreamed (47). There is total amnesia for the event. Adolescents and young adults are more likely to be enuretic when arousing from NREM Stages 1 or 2 (40, 54).

Broughton (40) has suggested that the arousal from slow wave sleep provides the appropriate dissociative state in which enuresis may occur. Evidence has been obtained that enuretics have higher intra-vesical pressure, especially in Stage 4 NREM sleep, than controls, have more frequent and intense spontaneous bladder contractions, and have more secondary contractions in response to naturally and artificially occurring increases in pressure (55, 56).

Treatment has taken many forms including drugs, conditioning techniques, and psychotherapy. Presently the drug of choice for severe enuresis is imipramine which reportedly increases Stage 2 NREM Sleep and decreases Stage 4 NREM sleep and REM sleep. It is unclear whether the effects of imipramine are due primarily to its anticholinergic properties effecting bladder control or to its stimulant effect. A flexible dosage and slow withdrawal schedule are recommended (57, 58). Ritvo, et al. (50) noted that imipramine was most effective for enuretic episodes that occurred during Stages 3 and 4 NREM sleep transitions.

Attempts to control enuresis through conditioning techniques or psychotherapy have met with mixed results (52, 59-63). Bakwin (63) noted the lack of evidence for clear-cut behavioral differences between enuretic and normal subjects, but stressed the psychological value of the physician's supportive role. When viewed as disorders of developmental immaturity, most cases (Stage 3/4 enuresis) subside spontaneously; intractable cases (Stage 1/2 enuresis) require more vigorous intervention.

Somnambulism and Somniloquy

Perhaps 15% of all children between the ages of 5 and 12 have walked in their sleep at least once (36). Occurring in 1 to 6% of the population, somnambulism or persistent walking is a fairly common disorder afflicting more males than females, more children than adults, and often associated with nocturnal enuresis (36, 46, 49). Of enuretic naval recruits, 34% reported a positive past history, and 25% a family history of sleepwalking (45). Monozygotic twins are concordant for the disorder six times as often as dizygotic twins (49). A typical somnambulistic episode consists of the following behavioral sequence: A body movement is followed by the subject abruptly sitting upright in bed. The eyes are open, glassy, and appear "unseeing." The subject may or may not actually get up and leave the bed. Doors and drawers may be opened, furniture skirted. The movements are clumsy but collisions and actual physical injury are generally avoided. Efforts to communicate with the sleepwalker may elicit mumbled and slurred speech with monosyllabic answers that are poorly related to the question. Occasionally spontaneous somniloquy is observed. The total duration of the episode may range from 15 to 30 seconds when sitting in bed, to 5 to 30 minutes, or more, when actual walking occurs. Walking generally ends with the child returning to his bed to sleep. There is amnesia for the event upon awakening. Severe sleepwalkers may have episodes 1 to 4 times weekly.

The majority of the somnambulistic episodes occur in the 1 to 3 hours immediately following sleep onset. They appear, as do enuretic episodes, to be associated with transitions from Stages 3/4 NREM sleep to lighter stages, prior to the first REM period. Kales, et al. (64), recording polygraphically during somnambulistic episodes, never found sleepwalking to arise during REM sleep. In this same report, sleepwalking could be induced in 7 of 38 sleepwalkers by standing them up during Stage 3 or 4 NREM sleep but not in REM sleep. Normal controls could not be induced to walk during any stage of sleep. When restricted from walking, somnambulists, compared to controls, tend to make many movements of a complex nature during slow wave sleep (34). They also exhibit longer than normal confusional episodes following forced awakenings from these stages (40).

The sleep EEG of somnambulists reveal the presence of rhythmic, paroxysmal, high voltage, slow frequency delta bursts (1-3 Hz) preceding each event (65). These paroxysmal bursts also occur in somnambulists at times unassociated with the event. Gibbs and Gibbs (66) have described these bursts as present in 85% of normal 6- to 11-month-old infants, decreasing to 3% in 7- to 9-year-olds. Their continued presence in somnambulists has suggested to Kales, et al. (65) an organic index of CNS immaturity in such patients.

Administration of a wide variety of psychological and personality tests has shown no single constellation of traits characteristic of somnambulists. A wide range of personality traits, emotional responsiveness and heterogeneous psychopathology marks these patients (67). Somnambulists in the military, on the other hand, exhibit greater psychopathology than controls (46). Sleepwalking incidents, despite their distinctive physiological signs and lack of specific psychological symptoms, are not divorced from psychological and environmental factors. Investigators report less sleepwalking in the laboratory than in the home (40, 65). Individuals who have had long periods without sleepwalking may revert under stress (67).

Sleep-talking is often observed during somnambulistic episodes. When it occurs alone it is most often associated with emergent stage transitions during NREM sleep. In these instances, speech content is related to immediately preceding experience (68).

As with enuresis, the therapy of somnambulism has included drugs, situational manipulation, and psychotherapy. The drug of choice for intractable, frequent occurrences is diazepam (Valium) which significantly reduces Stage 4 NREM sleep and also may reduce the number and intensity of emergent sleep stage shifts (69). As CNS maturation progresses, somnambulistic episodes usually diminish and disappear spontaneously.

Pavor Nocturnus

Attacks of childhood night terror must be differentiated from the more common nightmare or anxiety dream. In pavor nocturnus, the child suddenly sits upright in bed and screams. He appears to be staring at an imaginary object, breathes heavily, often perspires, and is in obvious distress. He is usually inconsolable for 10 minutes or more, then finally relaxes and returns to sleep. Immediate dream recall is fragmentary, if present at all, and in the morning there is amnesia for the attack. Though seen in older children and adults, night terrors are most common in the preschool age group.

Gastaut and Broughton (34) polygraphically recorded seven episodes of night terror in seven children. In all cases, the attack occurred during intense and sudden arousal from slow wave sleep. It was further noted that these children had relative tachycardia during slow wave sleep and hyperactive heart rates during arousal episodes. Fisher et al. (69) have confirmed these electrophysiologic findings in young adults.

For severe cases, the drug of choice, as in somnambulism, is diazepam. Most episodes in children occur so infrequently, however, that no medication is indicated.

Nightmares and anxiety dreams, which will be discussed more fully in the next section, are not considered disorders of arousal. Rather, they occur during REM sleep, are associated with vivid recollections, and often make the child fearful of going to bed.

Narcolepsy

Narcolepsy, in contrast to disorders of arousal, has been defined as a disorder of sleep. The characteristic symptom is recurrent daytime episodes of irresistible drowsiness and sleep. These sleep attacks may or may not be associated with the three auxiliary symptoms of cataplexy, sleep paralysis, and hypnagogic hallucinations to form the "narcoleptic tetrad" (39, 70). Cataplexy is the sudden loss of muscle tone resulting in falling to the ground while consciousness is maintained. Sleep paralysis is the sudden awareness, while falling asleep or during sleep, that one can not move or cry out. Hypnagogic hallucinations consist of vivid visual or auditory imagery occurring at sleep onset. Sleep attacks are associated with cataplexy about 75% of the time and with sleep paralysis and hypnagogic hallucinations 20 to 30% of the time. The full blown narcoleptic tetrad occurs about 10% of the time (70). A genetic factor is suggested by the higher familial incidence of the disorder (70, 71).

While most sufferers are brought to a physician in their teens or early adult years, it is probable that childhood symptoms of recurrent drowsiness are present but not considered remarkable. The interval between the first sleep attack and the occurrence of the other symptoms may vary from hours to years (39). The symptoms, themselves, also may vary between attacks and do not always occur together. Partial remissions have been reported, but complete remission is doubtful.

Electrophysiologic studies of the narcoleptic tetrad confirm its relationship to REM sleep (41-43, 72). In patients with a history of cataplexy or other auxillary narcoleptic symptoms, sleep attacks during the daytime are episodes of REM sleep intruding upon wakefulness. Cataplectic attacks during the day and sleep paralysis at sleep onset represent the loss of peripheral muscle tone, a normal physiologic correlate of REM sleep. The vivid imagery of the hypnagogic hallucinations resembles dreams recounted after REM sleep awakenings. In contrast to normal adults who enter sleep through a prolonged NREM period, sufferers of cataplexy, sleep paralysis and hypnagogic hallucinations exhibit a prolonged initial REM period, both in daytime attacks and in nocturnal sleep, reminiscent of newborn sleep.

Individuals who have only sleep attacks without a history of any auxiliary symptoms may not demonstrate this unusual transition to REM sleep, but rather the normal descending pattern from wakefulness to NREM sleep in both daytime attacks and, nocturnal sleep (42, 43, 72). That is, all daytime sleep attacks are not episodes of REM sleep. This has led Dement, et al. (42) to propose a compelling argument to limit the definition of narcolepsy to those disorders characterized by attacks of REM sleep and relegate other episodes of involuntary sleep to another diagnostic category.

The etiology of the disorder remains obscure but emotional experience and increases in tension and anxiety are known to precipitate attacks. Treatment with analeptic drugs has proved effective. The amphetamines, which reduce REM sleep while minimally interfering with other sleep stages are most commonly used (39, 42). Methylphenidate hydrochloride (Ritalin) has also been tried (73). Although numerous investigators have confirmed the nonepileptic form of narcolepsy, the anticonvulsant phenacemide (Phenurone) has achieved some success (74). Most recently the use of the REM suppressing MAO inhibitors have had marked success (75).

Hypersomnia refers to an excessive amount of sleep. It generally starts during adolescence. Though often confused with narcolepsy, it is not a disorder of REM sleep. Hypersomniacs fall into three categories: Daytime hypersomnia refers to excessive sleepiness during daylight hours when wakefulness is desired; nocturnal hypersomnia is characterized by excessively long nocturnal sleep periods with difficulty in arousal; and post-dormital hypersomnia refers to extreme confusion and drowsiness, lasting for 1 to 2 hours, upon awakening (76). The nocturnal sleep of hypersomniacs exhibits normal REM/NREM sleep cycles and patterns. The hypersomniac episodes generally represent periods of Stages 1 and 2 NREM sleep. The incidence, etiology, and management of this disturbance remains unclear, but it is generally felt to be largely associated with psychological conflicts.

PSYCHOLOGICAL DISTURBANCES OF SLEEP

"A sleepless baby is a reproach to his guardians" wrote Sundell (77) in 1922 suggesting that the full responsibility for sleep disturbance belonged to parents. Anna Freud (78), on the other hand, suggesting cultural sources of sleep disturbances, has pointed out that the human infant is perhaps the only creature among mammals who sleeps without the direct contact and warmth of another's skin. Regardless of their source, virtually all parents anticipate some sleep disturbances in their children.

Prior to sleep polygraphy, many of the previously described disorders were considered psychological in etiology. Indeed, many of them are associated with or induced by psychological conflicts or situations of heightened anxiety. All are a source of psychological suffering. The disorders to be described in this section, however, are those characterized by normal sleep polygrams. They are more common, often are reflections of normal phases of development, and have been loosely labeled by parents and pediatricians as "insomnia" and "nightmares." By far the majority are transient and, though a source of irritation, are inconsequential. Sometimes when bizarre or fixed, however, they may be indicators of more serious psychopathology. Medication, by and large, is not indicated though the *short*-term use of chloral hydrate has been advocated to promote peace and quiet in the family and prevent the sleep disturbance from becoming ingrained by "positive" reinforcement. Understanding the source of the child's anxiety, the parental concerns, and the current family situation are most often sufficient to enable the pediatrician to provide supportive guidance until the disturbance subsides.

Sleep disturbances may occur from the imminent approach of bedtime to the time of awakening. Nagera (79) has extensively reviewed these disturbances and classified them according to the most common age of appearance. This system of classification affords optimal understanding of the disturbance within the context of the child's developmental stage.

The First Year of Life

Two major concerns of the infant's family during the first year of life are sleeping through the night ("settling") and night awakenings. Settling, most comprehensively studied by Moore and Ucko (80), refers to sleeping from around midnight to early morning. These authors report that 70% of babies settle by 3 months, and another 13% have settled by 6 months. Ten percent never sleep uninterruptedly during the first year. The factors which promote settling are unknown though it is generally felt that it is related to the process of CNS maturation. Infants who have suffered some perinatal insult, such as anoxia, settle later (81). Sex, birth weight, and weight at 6 months do not seem related. Environmental conditions such as feeding schedule, sleeping arrange-ment, minor illness, and so forth, also do not seem related though high levels of maternal anxiety, reflected by inconsistent handling or insuffi-cient nonfeeding play, does seem to delay settling. Interestingly, 3 months of age (the age at which most infants are settling) is the time when infants' sleep polygrams assume more adult characteristics. At that time infants enter sleep via a sustained NREM period and the NREM EEG begins to be differentiated into NREM sleep stages (13). A study of the relationship between the age of settling and the maturity of the sleep polygram would be of interest.

Once the process of settling has occurred, waking normally recurs in 50% of infants between 5 and 9 months. During the second half of the first year environmental factors such as changed sleeping arrangements, separations, minor trauma, and new family members have been reported to be associated with wakenings. These disruptions are usually transient, though severe trauma may result in more prolonged disturbances. After 6 months of age parental concern and anger over poor sleeping habits may frequently compound the existing difficulty (82). Thus during the first year, if the babies' physiological needs are met adequately, empa-thetic understanding and guidance from the pediatrician to allay ex-cessive parental anxiety should lead to a rapid resolution of the sleep disturbance.

The Second Year of Life

During the second year of life, sleep disturbances often reflect infantile anxiety stemming from either developmental immaturity or neurotic conflict. At this age, psychological and cognitive components are added to the physiological requirements of sleep. With the strengthening of the child's ties to significant people and to the happenings of the external world, he clings all the more tenaciously to wakefulness (78). A preva-lent disturbance of this age, therefore, is reluctance to go to sleep (83). During the first half of the second year, the child's ego is still immature and can offer little comfort during times of separation. Since the child lacks the capacity to differentiate between absence and total disappear-ance of an object, he attempts to hold onto his important ties to avoid the fear of loss. Substitute objects, such as teddy bear or blankets, often tide him over these difficult times. By the end of the second year, with the acquisition of language and the development of a sense of object permanence, these difficulties often disappear.

Children in this age group are also easily overexcited by parents or upset by frightening daytime experiences. The resulting increased tension may lead to a second common disturbance: "bad" dreams or nightmares. Polygraphic studies have confirmed the presence of dream reports following REM sleep awakenings in 2-year-olds (84). Most often these elicited dream reports are re-enactments of daytime experiences, though the characters are frequently animals or monsters. Since the child, at this age, cannot distinguish between dreams and reality, fear of going to sleep because of bad dreams may develop. With an increase in ego development and the establishment of a clear-cut distinction between dreams and reality, this type of disturbance disappears.

To allay the anxiety associated with going to sleep, presleep habits or rituals develop during the second year. These include repetitive bedtime stories, last goodnights, and so forth. In a minority of cases, the rituals seem to stem from additional conflicts and become excessive, representing early precursors of more serious psychopathology. These instances are most often associated with overzealous attempts at early discipline (e.g. toilet training, limit setting, and so forth). It has been hypothesized that the anger generated by these parent-child power struggles is reduced by the child's presleep rituals. The youngster who repeatedly needs to kiss his parents goodnight, and so forth, indicates his love for them and in turn verifies their love for him.

The Third to Fifth Years of Life

It is rare to find a child in the 3- to 5-year age group who is not experiencing some difficulty over sleep, whether it be tardiness in falling asleep, night wakening, nightmares, projective fears of ghosts and wild animals, inability to sleep alone or in the dark, or ritualistic presleep behavior. Most of these disturbances are transient and responsive to minimal environmental manipulation. If refractive, the sleep disturbance most often represents only one symptom of a more profound conflict. Such conflicts in this age group most commonly are attributable to parental disturbances or reflect the child's inability to enter into the wider world of social relationships. Enlightened family counselling or psychotherapy for the child and family may be indicated.

Latency

During latency there usually is amelioration of most sleep disturbances. Reading before going to sleep often replaces other presleep rituals.

This avoids engaging in fantasies, mostly erotic, and the resulting secondary conflicts over masturbation. On occasion, however, the previous sleep disturbance may carry over, or even arise *de novo*. It may then persist through adolescence into adulthood.

SUMMARY

Recent electrophysiologic techniques have added considerably to the understanding of sleep and its disorders. Persistent nocturnal enuresis, somnambulism, somniloquy, and night terrors have been associated with emergent sleep stage transitions from Stage 4 to Stage 1 NREM sleep and have thus been classified as disorders of arousal. Narcolepsy, on the other hand, has been associated with the abnormal transition from wakefulness directly into REM sleep and has been termed a disorder of sleep. Though these disorders may be associated with psychological factors, psychophysiological factors have been demonstrated and specific pharmacologic agents have proved most effective in treatment.

The stresses and conflicts of growth and normal development may be expressed, from time to time, in various manifestations of disturbed sleep. Many complaints of "insomnia" and nightmares fall into this category and are misunderstood in terms of the developmental problem that the child and family face. Most often patience, support, and guidance are sufficient to alleviate the symptoms. Rarer, pathological disturbances must be differentiated from the more common developmental manifestations.

REFERENCES

1. ASERINSKY, E. & KLEITMAN, N.: A motility cycle in sleeping infants as manifested by ocular and gross bodily activity. *J. Appl. Physiol.*, 8:11, 1955.
2. DEMENT, W. & KLEITMAN, N.: Cyclic variation in EEG during sleep and their relationship to eye movements, body motility and dreaming. *Electroenceph. Clin. Neurophysiol.*, 9:673, 1957.
3. LUCE, G. & SEGAL, J.: *Sleep.* New York: Coward McCann, 1966.
4. KALES, A. (Ed): *Sleep—Physiology and Pathology, A Symposium.* Philadelphia: J. B. Lippincott, 1969.
5. HARTMANN, E. (Ed.): *Sleep and Dreaming.* Boston: Little, Brown, *Intl. Psychiat. Clin.*, 7: 1970.
6. LENARD, H.: Sleep studies in infancy—facts, concepts and significance. *Acta Paediat. Scand.*, 59:572, 1970.
7. DEMENT, W.: An essay on dreams. The role of physiology in understanding their nature. In F. Barron (Ed.), *New Directions in Psychology*, vol. 2. F. Barron. New York: Holt, Rinehart and Winston, p. 135, 1965.
8. FOULKES, D.: Nonrapid eye movement mentation. *Exp. Neurol.* (Suppl.), 4:28, 1967.

9. ANDERS, T., EMDE, R., & PARMELEE, JR., A. (Ed.): A manual of standardized terminology, techniques and criteria for scoring states of sleep and wakefulness in newborn infants. Los Angeles: UCLA Brain Information Service, NINDS, Neurological Information Network, 1971.

10. DREYFUS-BRISAC, C. & MONOD, N.: Sleep of premature and fullterm neonates—a polygraphic study. Proc. Roy. Soc. Med., 58:6, 1965.

11. PETRE-QUADENS, O.: Ontogenesis of paradoxical sleep in the human newborn. J. Neurol. Sci., 4:153, 1967.

12. FEINBERG, I. & CARLSON, V.: Sleep variables as a function of age in man. Arch. Gen. Psychiat., 18:239, 1968.

13. METCALF, D.: EEG sleep spindle ontogenesis. Neuropaediatrie, 1:428, 1970.

14. ROFFWARG, H., MUZIO, J., & DEMENT, W.: Ontogenetic development of the human sleep-dream cycle. Science, 152:604, 1966.

15. ANDERS, T. & ROFFWARG, H.: The effects of selective interruption and total sleep deprivation in the human newborn. Develop. Psychobiol., in press, 1972.

16. DREYFUS-BRISAC, C.: Ontogenesis of sleep in human prematures after 32 weeks of conception age. Develop. Psychobiol., 3:91, 1970.

17. PARMELEE, JR., A., SCHULTZ, M., & DISBROW, M.: Sleep patterns of the newborn. J. Pediat., 58:241, 1961.

18. SANDER, L., JULIA, H., STECHLER, G., & BURNS, P.: Continuous 24-hour interactional monitoring in infants reared in two different caretaking environments. Psychosom. Med., in press.

19. PARMELEE, JR., A.: Sleep patterns in infancy: A study of one infant from birth to eight months of age. Acta Paediat. Scand., 50:160, 1961.

20. DEMENT, W.: The effect of dream deprivation. Science, 131:1705, 1960.

21. SASSIN, J., PARKER, D., MACE, J., GOTLIN, R., JOHNSON, L., & ROSSMAN, L.: Human growth hormone release—relation to slow wave sleep and sleep-waking cycles. Science, 165:513, 1969.

22. WEITZMAN, E., SCHAUMBURG, H., & FISHBEIN, W.: Plasma 17-hydroxy-corticosteroid levels during sleep in man. J. Clin. Endocr., 26:121, 1966.

23. ANDERS, T., SACHAR, E., KREAM, J., ROFFWARG, H., & HELLMAN, L.: Behavioral state and plasma cortisol response in the human newborn. Pediatrics, 46:532, 1970.

24. FINKELSTEIN, J., ANDERS, T., SACHAR, E., ROFFWARG, H., & HELLMAN, L.: Secretion of growth hormone and behavioral state in the human infant. J. Clin. Endocr., 32:368, 1971.

25. DREYFUS-BRISAC, C. & MONOD, N.: Sleeping behavior in abnormal newborn infants. Neuropaediatrie, 3:354, 1970.

26. PRECHTL, H., WEINMANN, H., & AKIYAMA, Y.: Organization of physiological parameters in normal and abnormal infants. Neuropaediatrie, 1:101, 1969.

27. SCHULTE, F., LASSON, U., PARL, U., NOLTE, R., & JURGENS, U.: Brain and behavioral maturation in newborn infants of diabetic mothers, II. Sleep cycles. Neuropaediatrie, 1:36, 1969.

28. SCHULTE, F., HINZE, C., & SCHREMPF, G.: Maternal toxemia, fetal malnutrition and bioelectric brain activity of the newborn. Neuropaediatrie, 2:439, 1971.

29. SCHULMAN, C.: Alterations of the sleep cycle in heroin addicted and "suspect" newborns. Neuropaediatrie, 1:89- 1969.

30. PETRE-QUADENS, O. & JOUVET, M.: Sleep in the mentally retarded. J. Neurol. Sci., 4:354, 1967.

31. ORNITZ, E., RITVO, E., BROWN, M., LAFRANCHI, S., PARMELEE, JR., A., & WALTER, R.: The EEG and rapid eye movements during REM sleep in normal and autistic children. Electroenceph. Clin. Neurophysiol., 26:167, 1969.

32. FEINBERG, I.: Eye movement activity during sleep and intellectual function in mental retardation. Science, 159:1256, 1968.

33. Schultz, M., Schulte, F., Akiyama, Y., & Parmelee, Jr., A.: Development of electroencephalographic sleep phenomena in hypothyroid infants. *Electroenceph. Clin. Neurophysiol.*, 25:351, 1968.

34. Gastaut, H. & Broughton, R.: A clinical and polygraphic study of episodic phenomena during sleep. In J. Wortis (Ed.), *Recent Advances in Biological Psychiatry*. New York: Plenum, 7:197, 1965.

35. Gastaut, H., Broughton, R., Tassinari, C., & Rudkowska, A.: Polygraphic tests of paroxysmal phenomena occurring in night sleep. *Electroenceph. Clin. Neurophysiol.*, 18713, 1965.

36. Kales, J., Jacobson, A., & Kales, A.: Sleep disorders in children. *Prog. Clin. Pathol.*, 8:63, 1968.

37. Poussaint, A., Koegler, R., & Riehl, J.: Enuresis, epilepsy and the EEG. *Amer. J. Psychiat.*, 123:1294, 1967.

38. St. Laurent, J., Batini, C., Broughton, R., & Gastaut, H.: A polygraphic study of nocturnal enuresis in the epileptic child. *Electroenceph. Clin. Neurophysiol.*, 15:904, 1963.

39. Yoss, R., & Daly, D.: Narcolepsy in children. *Pediatrics*, 25:1025, 1960.

40. Broughton, R.: Sleep disorders: Disorders of arousal? *Science*, 159:1070, 1968.

41. Hishikawa, Y., & Kaneko, Z.: Electroencephalographic study on narcolepsy. *Electroenceph. Clin. Neurophysiol.*, 18:249, 1965.

42. Dement, W., Rechtschaffen, A., & Gulevitch, G.: A polygraphic study of the narcoleptic sleep attack. *Neurology*, 16:18, 1966.

43. Roth, B., Bruchova, S., & Lehovsky, M.: REM sleep and NREM sleep in narcolepsy and hypersomnia. *Electroenceph. Clin. Neurophysiol.*, 26:176, 1969.

44. Martin, C.: *A New Approach to Nocturnal Enuresis*. London: H. K. Lewis & Co. Ltd., 1966.

45. Pierce, C., Lipcon, H., McClary, J., & Noble, H.: Enuresis: Clinical, laboratory and electroencephalogcaphic studies. *U.S. Armed Forces Med. J.*, 7:208, 1956.

46. Pierce, C. & Lipcon, H.: Somnambulism: Electroencephalographic studies and related findings. *U.S. Armed Forces Med. J.*, 7:1419, 1956.

47. Pierce, C., Whitman, R., Maas, J., & Gay, M.: Enuresis and dreaming. *Arch. Gen. Psychiat.*, 4:166, 1961.

48. Sours, J., Frumkin, P., & Indetmill, R.: Somnambulism. *Arch. Gen. Psychiat.*, 9:400, 1963.

49. Bakwin, H.: Sleep walking in twins. *Lancet*, 2:446, 1970.

50. Ritvo, E., Ornitz, E., Gottlieb, F., Poussaint, A., Maron, B., Dittman, K., & Blinn, K.: Arousal and nonarousal enuretic events. *Amer. J. Psychiat.* 126:77, 1969.

51. Tapia, F., Jekel, J., & Domke, H.: Enuresis: An emotional symptom? *J. Nerv. Ment. Dis.*, 130:61, 1960.

52. Lovibond, S.: *Conditioning and Enuresis*. New York: Macmillan Co., 1964.

53. Broughton, R. & Gastaut, H.: Polygraphic sleep studies of enuresis nocturna. *Electroenceph. Clin. Neurophysiol.*, 16:625, 1964.

54. Ditman, K. & Blinn, K.: Sleep levels in enuresis. *Amer. J. Psychiat.*, 111:913, 1955.

55. Broughton, R. & Gastaut, H.: Further polygraphic sleep studies of enuresis nocturna (Intravesicular pressures.) *Electroenceph. Clin. Neurophysiol.*, 16:626, 1964.

56. Gastaut, H. & Broughton, R.: Conclusions concerning the mechanisms of enuresis nocturna. *Electroenceph. Clin. Neurophysiol.*, 16:625, 1964.

57. Poussaint, A. & Ditman, K.: A controlled study of Imipramine (Tofranil) in the treatment of childhood enuresis. *J. Pediat.*, 67:283, 1965.

58. Miller, P., Champelli, J., & Dinello, F.: Imipramine in the treatment of enuretic school children. *Amer. J. Dis. Child.*, 115:17, 1968.

59. DE ATAIDE, S.: Contributions to the study of enuresis in children. *Psychol. Abstr.*, 23: #4499, 1949.
60. HAMILL, R.: Enuresis. *J.A.M.A.*, 93:254, 1929.
61. KRIEGMAN, E. & WRIGHT, H.: Brief psychotherapy with enuretics in the army. *Amer. J. Psychiat.*, 104:254, 1947.
62. ZUFALL, R.: Adult male enuresis: A study of 200 cases. *J. Urol.*, 70:894, 1953.
63. BAKWIN, H.: Enuresis in childhood. *J. Pediat.*, 58:806, 1961.
64. KALES, A., JACOBSON, A., KUN, T., KLEIN, J., HEUSER, G., & PAULSON, M.: Somnambulism: Further all-night EEG studies. *Electroenceph. Clin. Neurophysiol.*, 21:410, 1966.
65. KALES, A., JACOBSON, A., PAULSON, M., KALES, J., & WALTER, R.: Somnambulism: Psychophysiological correlates. I. *Arch. Gen. Psychiat.*, 14:586, 1966.
66. GIBBS, F. & GIBBS, E.: *Atlas of Electroencephalography*, Vol. 1. Cambridge, Massachusetts: Addison Wesley Press Inc., 1950.
67. KALES, A., PAULSON, M., JACOBSON, A., & KALES, J.: Somnambulism: Psychophysiological correlates, II. *Arch. Gen. Psychiat.*, 14595, 1966.
68. RECHTSCHAFFEN, A., GOODENOUGH, D., & SHAPIRO, A.: Patterns of sleep talking. *Arch. Gen. Psychiat.*, 7:418, 1962.
69. FISHER, C., KAHN, E., EDWARDS, A., & DAVIS, D.: Effects of Valium on NREM night terrors. Psychophysiology, *Abstr. Assoc. Psychophysiol. Study of Sleep.* In press.
70. YOSS, R. & DALY, D.: Criteria for the diagnosis of the narcoleptic syndrome. *Proc. Staff Mtgs. of the Mayo Clinic*, 32:320, 1957.
71. DALY, D. & YOSS, R. A family with narcolepsy. *Proc. Staff Mtgs. of the Mayo Clinic*, 34:313, 1959.
72. HISHIKAWA, Y., NAN'NO, H., TACHIBANA, M., FURUYA, E., KOIDA, H., & KNEKO, Z.: The nature of sleep attack and other symptoms of narcolepsy. *Electroenceph. Clin. Neurophysiol.*, 24:1, 1968.
73. YOSS, R. & DALY, D.: Treatment of narcolepsy with Ritalin. *Neurology*, 9:17, 1957.
74. AIRD, R., GORDON, N., & GREGG, H.: Use of Phenacemide (Phenurone) in treatment of narcolepsy and cataplexy. *Arch. Neurol. Psychiat.*, 70:510, 1953.
75. WYATT, R., FRAM, D., BUCHBINDER, R., & SNYDER, F.: Treatment of intractable narcolepsy with a monoamine oxidase inhibitor. *New Eng. J. Med.*, 285:987, 1971.
76. RECHTSCHAFFEN, A. & ROTH, B.: Nocturnal sleep of hypersomniacs. *Activitas nervosa Superior*, 11:229, 1969.
77. SUNDELL, C.: Sleeplessness in infants. *Practitioner*, 109:89, 1922.
78. FREUD, A.: *Normality and Pathology in Childhood*. New York: International University Press, 1965.
79. NAGERA, H.: Sleep and its disturbances approached developmentally. *The Psychodynamic Study of the Child*. New York: International Universities Press, 21:393, 1966.
80. MOORE, T. & UCKO, L.: Night waking in early infancy: Part I. *Arch. Dis. Child.*, 32:333, 1957.
81. PRESTON, M.: Late behavioral aspects found in cases of prenatal, natal and postnatal anoxia. *J. Pediat.*, 26:353, 1945.
82. HIRSCHBERG, J.: Parental anxieties accompanying sleep disturbance in young children. *Bull. Menninger Clinic*, 21:129, 1957.
83. RAGINS, N., & SCHACTER, J.: A study of sleep behavior in two-year old children. *J. Amer. Acad. Child Psychiat.*, 10:464, 1971.
84. KOHLER, W., CODDINGTON, R., & AGNEW, H.: Sleep patterns in 2-year old children. *J. Pediat.*, 72:228, 1968.

25

PERSONALITY DIFFERENCES IN THE PERCEPTUALLY HANDICAPPED

Stanley R. Lesser, M.D.

Associate Professor of Psychiatry

and

B. Ruth Easser, M.D.

Associate Professor of Psychiatry
University of Toronto, Canada

Systems of personality development subsume a maturational and developmental ground plan. Within these ground plans there is the tacit assumption which Hartmann et al. (1946, 1949) have characterized as "an average expectable environment." From the findings of our own work we postulate that there is also the assumption of an "average constitutional endowment." We question whether one can assume either "an average expectable environment" or an "average constitutional endowment" in those individuals who have suffered from very early life a severe perceptual handicap such as a profound deafness. The limitations of the more established developmental theories have clearly been challenged when applied to those individuals reared in very different social environments. The need to adhere to pre-existing theoretical frameworks has led to evaluating the deviants from the usual maturational course in terms of this expected or so-called normal. This tendency has

---

Reprinted from THE JOURNAL OF THE AMERICAN ACADEMY OF CHILD PSYCHIATRY, Vol. 11, No. 3, pp. 458-466, July, 1972.

led to a set, so that the deviant has not been studied in his own right but rather has been understood by means of some distortion of the original theory.

Our thesis is that one cannot adequately evaluate or classify congenitally deaf persons unless one includes the knowledge of the very different developmental and experiential tracks over which these children have advanced. Furthermore, our broader assumption is that a study of the role of the sensory organs in such integrative psychological systems as that of self, identity, and the organization of the affective responses will shed new light on our understanding of personality development, particularly as it affects the emotive and defensive systems of the ego.

Although it is almost impossible for the investigator in a field in which a major perceptual faculty such as hearing has been eliminated or severely impaired to place himself in the shoes of the developing infant and child, it is valuable at least to start with the premises that such a child will in fact be a different organism from the child with no such impairment; he will be subjected to gross differences in mothering; in being confined to living within the shell of an incomplete perceptual environment. He will be dependent upon more concrete concepts for the control of his environment, and he also will be affected by his attitudes to other persons, their attitudes toward him, and finally in the integration of his own identity.

We would like to concentrate on some of our own findings and those of others which might cast a different evaluative light on certain accepted psychopathological syndromes and character traits and indicate our own evaluation of some of the factors in the developmental etiology of these disorders. We will limit ourselves, in the main, to a discussion of the congenitally deaf child and use the blind child only for contrast and emphasis.

Many deaf people have the following personality characteristics (Rainer and Altshuler, 1967): egocentricity, rigidity, impulsivity without accompaniment of anxiety or guilt, a paucity of empathy, and a lack of realization of the effect of their behavior on others. If we translate these findings into psychoanalytic terms, one might say that the deaf show a relative lack of the subtleties in their self-observing ego; a conscience formation different from that usually expected; a difficulty in the use of abstract symbols to test the environment and the self; and poor tension tolerance, which may be a reflection of the continued primacy of the pleasure principle over the reality principle. On the cognitive side, the major difficulty is the acquisition of words, symbolization, and abstraction, leading to a delay in the development of the sway of secondary process thinking over primary process thinking and the ease of regression to primary process thinking.

More specifically regarding the psychopathological syndromes, Rainer and Altshuler (1967) have observed that the incidence of schizophrenia in the deaf appears no different from that of the general population; however, retarded depressions, especially those characterized by guilt and delusions of personal culpability, are almost nonexistent. The agitated, hyperactive forms of depression are frequent (Wright, 1969) and the paranoid trends are at least as frequent, but not as systematized.

The incidence of psychoneurosis in the deaf has been little studied, but neuroticisms are taken for granted. No one has troubled to differentiate or characterize them. In our own survey we have found that sex would appear to be a taboo subject despite the prominence of the role that sexual development has been given in the understanding of development and in the psychoneuroses. Sexual difficulties were not even mentioned. We discussed this finding with the personnel of the Kinsey Institute, who reported that they had not considered doing such a sexual survey. The educators of residential training institutes for the deaf were bewildered and shocked by inquiry into such matters as childhood masturbation, sexual curiosity, and sexual play.

To return to the psychoneuroses, should the factor of deafness not be considered, many of the deaf could, using customary nosology, be placed under the rubric of obsessional-compulsive neurosis or obsessive-compulsive character disorders. Narcissistic character traits are prevalent (Kohut, 1968). Conversely, there are few instances of the dramatic, histrionic, hysterical personality and, in the more usual form, of the neurotic depressions. This finding is in marked contrast to that reported for the blind, who show a predominance of depressive, hypochondriacal, and hysterical modes.[1] All of the above is within the framework of those nosologies derived from the study of the perceptually intact.

Behavior disorders in childhood are almost ubiquitous. The behavior disorders often coexist with the aforementioned compulsive-like traits. The behavior disorders are often misdiagnosed as evidence of brain damage or, should they be accompanied by the not uncommon emotional withdrawal of the deaf, as autism or mental retardation (Minski, 1957). These behavior characteristics often show a dramatic reversal if the hearing loss can be corrected, e.g., when adequate hearing aids are provided, or after the child has developed good modes of communication, such as speech or sign language.

---

[1] Personal communication from V. Michaels.

Despite the common belief that other sensory modalities are hypertrophied to compensate for the absence of the lost modality, such as hearing, the fact is that the other modalities during infancy and early childhood are less developed in these handicapped children than in the children who possess the full range of perceptual faculties (Burlingham, 1964). The deaf child's increased ability to use touch or sight does not develop until other schemata have been organized. The integration of the relationship between touch and sight must occur before either can be used to compensate for the defect in the hearing. More generally, ego integration must have taken place before other channels can replace the deficient one (Piaget, 1923; Flavell, 1963). There can be no precept without concept. Thus, the ego organization of the deaf child, not only in areas close to his deficit, but in areas seemingly distant, such as emotional expression, is developed later than in his intact counterpart (Greenberg, 1970). The timing of these integrations imparts a different coloration to such matters as conscience formation, motor control, imitation, and identification.

A rather startling observation of ours has been the deaf child's high threshold of response to a painful stimulus. This is dramatically illustrated by Paul West (1970), the British poet, who wrote an accurate and lyrical description of his deaf child, *Words for a Deaf Daughter*. This child and others whom we have observed do not cry when they are subjected to inoculation but respond impassively to this and other injuries. Alternately, these same children will howl if their desires are not immediately comprehended and gratified. This impassiveness is rapidly reversed with language acquisition or other communicative devices. In fact, once this communicative capacity is established, these children often appear hypersensitive to pain and for the first time curious, overconcerned, and attuned to their own bodily sensations. This impassivity is closely related to their proneness to hypermotility. The motor restlessness is in itself worthy of discussion if only because it is often misdiagnosed as secondary to brain damage.

Unlike the brain-damaged youngster, these children alternate between periods of diffuse motor restlessness and periods of immobility. Should hearing aids permit the scanning of sound in the environment, this motor restlessness abruptly diminishes. The observer is struck by the immediate transformation in their facial expressiveness. A facies, emotionally blank except for the alertness of the eyes, attains the full panoply of emotional expression. These early characteristics of hyperactivity, diminished stimuli responsiveness, and blank faces have often been adjudged indicative of the autistic, retarded, or brain-damaged child. Fewer of these errors would be made if deafness were considered, if the alert ever-scanning eyes were noted, and if the nature of the child's object relations were carefully studied. (We have seen similar transformations when severe impairment was corrected.)

Myklebust (1960) has suggested that hearing gives us our background, vision our foreground. Hearing permits the diffuse scanning of our environment, vision the ability to focus on the particular or central object. The absence of hearing saddles vision with both tasks. Thus, the deaf child is not free to take for granted his consistent environmental background in order to concentrate on the stimulus at hand. This interferes with his ability both to sustain focused attention and to feel secure within his environment. In those people who suffer deafness at a later age a paranoid cast is often apparent. Analogies in these matters are open to question, but this dynamic may be one of the sources of the later suspiciousness and projective tendencies of the congenitally deaf. It also may partially explain the seeming withdrawal and aloofness of the deaf. This aloofness is by no means present when they themselves are talking or communicating through sign language, i.e., when they are active participants. Thus, the aloofness of the deaf in a speaking society is more apparent than real.

The impulsivity of the deaf child is closely connected with his lack of adequate communicative modalities to express his needs and feelings. Delay and detour depend at least in part on the capacity to understand one's needs and feelings. In this regard, the deaf child is greatly handicapped by lack of the verbal symbols with which to formulate. In the deaf child this is further restricted by the relative lack of the corrective reciprocal feedback which the child learns from an understanding of his effect upon others (Goldfarb, 1961).

The deaf child is not given a hearing, nor does he, nor can he, listen. We believe that impulsivity is directly related to the organization of emotions for the self and the understanding, the naming, if one likes, of the emotions by the self. This is analogous to Piaget's (1923) observations that a major part of the 3-year-old's speech is not directly communicative but serves the purpose of the child's organization of his "action self" (later schemata). Once an affect can be named, it can come under the sway of ego control and ego use. Our concept in this regard might be termed the self as an "emotional being."

This delay in organizing the "emotional self" is clearly related to the deaf child's difficulty with empathic responses. Emotions are used to feel out the other person and to adjust oneself quickly to the feelings noted in the other. This difficulty with the use of emotions creates a seeming bluntness in the deaf's social relationships. It delays and stunts the feelings of sorrow or shame. This may be one source of the deaf person's proneness to agitated responses rather than to guilty depressions.

With regard to depression, other facets must be noted. Putting aside the question of constitutional endowment, the major dynamics of depressive illness are: an inconsistency in the early child-mother relationship, with the mother's behavior alternating between hypersensitivity to her child's needs and gross maternal distraction, both emotional and physical; and identification with the emotional and physical suffering of the closest love objects, often mediated through the mother's demand that the child fill her void and reduce her suffering. As a result the child is overwhelmed and becomes ashamed of his inability to produce this response, or the child is frustrated and enraged at his parents and deflects this rage from his parents in reality to their representations within himself. Both dynamics may alternate or appear in various combinations.

Psychoanalytic studies of the handicapped have stressed the role of the mother's depressive response to her defective child and the subsequent affective deprivation in the child (Burlingham, 1964; Fraiberg and Freedman, 1964). In the deaf, unlike the blind and other handicapped children, the emotional communication of these depressive affects from the mother to her child is partially barred. Moreover, the mother of the deaf child, because of the communicative and other difficulties, does not tend to expect much solicitude from her child. These factors, while they create many other difficulties for deaf, partially immunize him from the guilt of having created his mother's suffering and from his not having satisfied her by living up to her ideals. This relative emotional obtuseness of the deaf leaves him prone to develop the more agitated, hyperactive forms of mental illness rather than the guilty and self-recriminatory forms.

Another prevalent characteristic of the deaf is the admixture of doubt and uncertainty which coexists with a rigidity and an obstinacy. These traits, combined with the deaf person's relatively dampened emotional display and with his characteristic ability at rote tasks, reproduce the picture of an obsessive-compulsive personality disorder. The major underlying dynamics of the obsessive-compulsive are generally ascribed to unconscious conflicts around aggression and sex. The obstinacy of the obsessive is related to his battle with authority; his doubts stem from the rapid swings between rage and fear; his ambivalences are due to his fluctuations from love to hate. The doubt in the deaf has quite another source. Doubt stems, in the deaf, from insecurity about what he perceives and what others perceive, and extends to a doubt about what he feels, what others feel, and particularly what others feel about him (Lipton, 1970). To restate, he is uncertain that his perceptions, comprehensions, and affects are commensurate or consensual with those of others. This would seem obvious until one considers that these doubts extend to all psychological areas and outlast the time when his perceptions are in fact accurate, sometimes more accurate than those of the persons upon whom he is relying to monitor him. This doubting characteristic does not lead to his becoming a "doubting Thomas," i.e., skeptical of the world and of others, but rather it is directed toward his own capacities. Moreover, the deaf are not overdependent, as are the blind. This doubt is much more specifically related to his uncertainty about his own capacity to organize his perceptions into more general and abstract concepts, whether these concepts concern the meaning of the perception itself (the cognitive), the emotional significance of his responses, or the accuracy of his motivations within the perceptual field. One might say he relies on a "seeing ear" for validation of the challenges of this environment.

For example, it has been noted that the deaf pupil will "cheat" on an examination without guilt or fear because to him looking at another's paper is an integral part of his checking on his environment and has not, as with the normal child, been equated with "stealing."

Later on, though usually not before his 7th or 8th year, pride and shame do assume inhibitory roles. The fear of making an error, of being mocked, the sensitivity about mishearing or misunderstanding, and the apprehension about making a fool of himself then become a strong regulating force. Once he has latched on to a mode that has given him a measure of internal and social security, he is loath to relinquish it. Rigidity and obstinacy allow him some degree of security and individuation.

These obsessivelike traits are reinforced by the usual rearing and educational practices met by the deaf (Furth, 1966). Both the parents and the teachers find little time to promote creativity and joy in learning when they feel overwhelmed by the task of training and teaching the rote and the habitual. Furthermore, fear of impulsivity and aggression tends to provoke a rigid and imaginative discipline. Although the deaf often simulate the obsessive-compulsive, careful scrutiny of the major modes of defense reveals essential differences. The deaf do not, in general, isolate affect from thought; are not particularly characterized by reaction formations; do not indulge in doing and undoing; and are not usually fearful of emotional outbursts. On the contrary, they often show an undue lack of concern if they lose control of their emotions. The deaf will plunge into activity without forethought, whereas in the obsessive-compulsive infrequent impulsivity follows a long period of ruminative thinking and doubting paralysis. The deaf person's actions may be accompanied by doubt, but rarely by anxiety; the obsessive-compulsive's activity is always accompanied by doubt and severe anxiety.

In summary, our thesis is that the usual psychopathological categories are poorly applicable to children whose development from birth must follow other pathways than those with which we are familiar. While all human beings are more alike than unlike, when we evaluate, diagnose, and treat, we must be aware of our own underlying sets and biases in order not to fall into the trap of too easily reaching conclusions which preclude our fuller understanding of both the usual and the deviant. That which looks alike is not always the same.

Further, we hope we have been able to convey that some psychic characteristics usually considered primary, such as organization of emotions, are in fact, subject to further analysis both genetically and organizationally. This may enable us both to delve further into their roots and to be more sensitive to their derivatives. There is a rich vein of knowledge to be mined in the study of the perceptually handicapped which we believe will enhance and possibly shift our understanding and our theoretical framework about such fundamental psychological characteristics as cognition, organization of emotions, defense organizations, identifications, ego organization, and the plasticity of men's adaptation.

REFERENCES

BENDER, R. E. (1960): *The Conquest of Deafness*. Cleveland: Press of Western Reserve University.

BURLINGHAM, D. (1964): Hearing and its role in the development of the blind. *The Psychoanalytic Study of the Child*, 19-95-112. New York: International Universities Press.

FLAVELL, J. H. (1963): *The Developmental Psychology of Jean Piaget*. Princeton, N. J.: Van Nostrand.

FRAIBERG, S. & FREEDMAN, D. A. (1964): Studies in the ego development of the congenitally blind child. *The Psychoanalytic Study of the Child*, 19:113-169. New York: International Universities Press.

FURTH, H. G. (1966): *Thinking Without Language*. New York: Free Press.

GOLDFARB, W. (1961): *Childhood Schizophrenia*. Cambridge, Mass.: Harvard University Press for the Commonwealth Fund.

GREENBERG, J. (1970): *In This Sign*. New York: Holt, Rinehart & Winston.

HARTMANN, H., KRIS, E., & LOEWENSTEIN, R. M. (1946): Comments on the formation of psychic structure. *The Psychoanalytic Study of the Child*, 2:11-38. New York: International Universities Press.

HARTMANN, H., KRIS, E., & LOEWENSTEIN, R. M. (1949): Notes on the theory of aggression. *The Psychoanalytic Study of the Child,* 3/4:9-36. New York: International Universities Press.

KOHUT, H. (1968): The psychoanalytic treatment of narcissistic personality disorders. *The Psychoanalytic Study of the Child,* 23:86-113. New York: International Universities Press.

LIPTON, E. L. (1970): A study of the psychological effects of strabismus. *The Psychoanalytic Study of the Child,* 25:146-174. New York: International Universities Press.

MINSKI, L. (1957): *Deafness, Mutism and Mental Deficiency in Children.* London: Heinemann.

MYKLEBUST, H. R. (1960): *The Psychology of Deafness.* New York: Grune & Stratton, 2nd ed., 1964.

PIAGET, J. (1923): *The Language and Thought of the Child.* London: Routledge & Kegan Paul, 1932.

PIAGET, J. (1936): *The Origins of Intelligence in Children.* New York: International Universities Press, 1952.

PIAGET, J. (1937): *The Construction of Reality in the Child.* New York: Basic Books, 1954.

RAINER, J. D. & ALTSHULER, K. Z., Eds. (1967): *Psychiatry and the Deaf.* Washington: Department of Health, Education and Welfare.

WEST, P. (1970): *Words for a Deaf Daughter.* New York: Harper & Row.

WRIGHT, D. (1969): *Deafness.* New York: Stein & Day.

26

NEUROLOGICAL DYSFUNCTION AND CHILDHOOD BEHAVIORAL PATHOLOGY

Stella Chess, M.D.

Professor of Child Psychiatry, New York University Medical Center

The relationship between neurological dysfunction and childhood behavioral pathology was examined in the case material of a 19-year child psychiatry consultation practice involving 1,400 patients, 838 boys and 562 girls, ranging in age from 13 weeks to 19 years at the time of initial consultation. Eighty-eight neurologically damaged children, 60 boys and 28 girls, and matched controls were compared for presenting complaints, psychiatric diagnoses, and the special group of symptoms commonly thought to be associated with brain damage: hyperactivity, short attention span, distractibility, mood oscillation, high impulsivity and perseveration. Perseveration was the sole symptom statistically more characteristic of the neurologically damaged children. Clustering of 3 or more of the special symptoms was significantly related to neurological damage; other than perseveration the presence of 1 or 2 of the special symptoms failed to distinguish the groups, while absence of all special symptoms characterized the neurologically intact controls. Clinical implications of the findings are discussed.

Reprinted from JOURNAL OF AUTISM AND CHILDHOOD SCHIZOPHRENIA, 1972, 2, 3, 299-311. Copyright © 1972 by Scripta Publishing Company. Requests for reprints should be sent to Dr. Stella Chess, Department of Psychiatry, New York University Medical Center, 550 First Avenue, New York, New York 10016.

The relationship between brain damage and behavioral deviation has long been a subject of debate in child psychiatry. At issue are two basic questions: (1) Do children with demonstrated cerebral pathology display an identifiable pattern of aberrant behaviors? and (2) Can a diagnosis of brain dysfunction, in the absence of specific neurological signs, be based solely on behavioral findings?

Confusion about these questions reigns in current discussion of such vaguely defined syndromes as "minimal brain dysfunction" and "mild brain damage" (Clements, 1966; Wender, 1971). These terms are too often used as all-inclusive labels for heterogeneous groupings of children whose deviant behavior may or may not have an organic basis. In many cases that offer no direct evidence of central nervous system pathology, the presence of brain disorders is inferred from the child's behavior.

This may open the door to inexact and overbold diagnosis, especially in the readiness to equate "hyperactivity" with "minimal brain dysfunction" (Birch, 1964). It is widely assumed that a hyperkinetic syndrome of distractibility, impulsiveness, and emotional lability must have an organic origin. The evidence is too scanty to justify confidence in such a diagnosis (Chess, 1969; Eisenberg, 1964). Moreover, many children who do have organic brain damage, verified by anatomic or neurologic examination, do not exhibit the patterns of behavior presumed to be characteristic of "brain damage." In my own extensive work with motorically handicapped children, many of whom had spastic diplegias and other disorders categorized under cerebral palsy, I have seen a large number who had no behavioral deviations. And of those children who did have behavioral problems, not all exhibited the same set of symptoms (Chess, 1968).

In some cases, of course, a causal relationship between cerebral dysfunction and behavioral aberrations is readily recognized. When a child has a degenerative disease of the brain, his loss of interest in his surroundings and his lowered intellectual functioning may be understood as direct symptoms of the organic changes. In the epileptic child, irritability in personality makeup may be a direct result of brain irritation. But in other cases, the ambiguities of the findings complicate the diagnostic problem. It then becomes hazardous to postulate a relationship between behavior and organic pathology.

In an effort to clarify this issue, I have reviewed the case records of 1,400 children who were brought to me for psychiatric evaluation from 1945 to 1964. The records include both behavioral and neurological findings. These were examined to determine if there are specific behaviors that seem to distinguish the child with neurological dysfunction

TABLE 1

ETIOLOGY OF NEUROLOGICAL DAMAGE IN 88 INDEX CHILDREN

Etiology	Male	Female	Total*
Intracranial infection	6	3	9
Brain trauma	5	2	7
Circulatory disturbance	2	1	3
Disturbance of growth, nutrition, metabolism	3	2	5
Intracranial neoplasm	0	1	1
Degenerative disease of CNS	0	0	0
Unspecified	28	7	35
Congenital cerebral palsy	6	4	10
Congenital hydrocephalus	2	1	3
Birth trauma	5	5	10
Epilepsy	12	7	20

* The total is higher than the number of children, since in some instances more than one category was implicated in the diagnosis.

from his peers who also present psychiatric problems but without any evidence of organic damage.

The findings should be of special interest because the study was based on an unusually large sample.

SAMPLE AND METHOD

In a 19-year period of private practice as a child psychiatrist, the author examined 1,400 youngsters brought for diagnosis because of behavior found troublesome by parents, teachers, playground supervisors, and others. The group comprised 838 boys and 562 girls, ranging in age from 13 weeks to 19 years at the time of initial consultation. Most of the children came from middle-class families.

A review of the case records identified 88 youngsters (60 boys and 28 girls) as having definite indications of central nervous system pathology. The neurological status of these index cases was based on hospital records, the examiner's own observations, and neurologists' reports.[1] To meet the criterion of neurological damage, a child had to manifest at least one hard or two soft signs. Hard signs are those which point to an anatomical locus, such as spasticity, anesthesias following nerve distribution, positive Babinski, definite ataxia. Soft neurological signs include mild hyperreflexia, mild adiodokokinesis, spooning of out-

---

[1] In all cases where the first suspicion of neurological damage had been raised in the psychiatric consultation, a neurologist was called in to confirm or rule out this possibility.

stretched hands, and clumsiness to a degree that interferes with ordinary levels of competence.

We classified the etiology of neurological damage according to the categories employed by the Diagnostic and Statistical Manual of Mental Disorders (DSM-II). Table 1 presents the distribution of etiologic categories in the 88 index children.

Each of the 88 index children was matched with a child whose records contained no indication of neurological damage (neither specific signs nor a history of neurological disease). The matching child had to be of the same sex and age as the index child, and the two children must have been brought for psychiatric consultation within a year of each other.

Eliminated from both the index and control groups were any equivocal cases. Historical data such as prematurity or anoxia at birth were viewed as risk factors, but not as evidence of existing pathology. To assure that no unequal variable was introduced in comparing the two groups, we had to determine whether they were equivalent in terms of general health or whether the neurologically damaged children had additional handicaps not noted in the matching youngsters. We therefore tabulated all complaints such as club feet, congenital dislocation of hip, celiac disease, eczema, hydrocele, and fractures. The incidence and severity of such complaints were similar in the two groups.

The 88 index cases represent 6.7% of the total of 1,400 children seen in private practice. Boys account for 59.9% of the total group and 58.2% of the index cases. This slight increase in boy-girl ratio is not statistically significant.

PRESENTING COMPLAINTS

Parental complaints about a child's behavior were classified according to 11 specific areas: sleep, eating, elimination, mood, discipline, habits, motor activity, somatic manifestations, speech, peer and social relationships, and learning. An additional category for "other" complaints include such behaviors as fears, desire to be of the opposite sex (with cross-dressing), frequent talking to oneself or to imaginary playmates, expressions of self-hate and the wish to die. Figure 1 illustrates the frequency of parental complaints in these specific areas comparing the neurological with matched cases.

As Table 2 shows, there were no significant differences in the presenting symptoms of index and matched cases in a number of categories. This equivalence is especially noteworthy in the categories of peer rela-

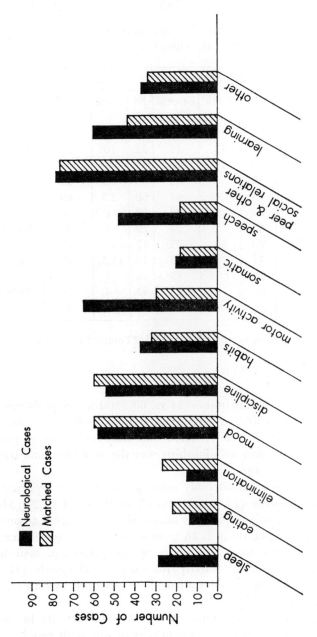

FIG. 1. Frequency of presenting symptoms.

Table 2

Frequency of Presenting Symptoms in Neurological and
Matched Cases

Category	Neurological			Matched			χ^2	p
	N*	Rank	Percent	N†	Rank	Percent		
Sleep	29	9	33	23	9	26		NS
Eating	13	12	15	22	10	25	2.314	NS
Elimination	14	11	16	27	8	31	4.122	< .05
Mood	58	4	66	60	2.5	68		NS
Discipline	54	5	61	60	2.5	68		NS
Habits	37	7	42	32	6	36		NS
Motor activity	65	2	74	29	7	33	13.788	< .01
Somatic	20	10	23	17	11.5	19		NS
Speech	47	6	53	17	11.5	19	14.062	< .01
Peer relationships	78	1	89	76	1	86		NS
Learning	60	3	68	43	4	49	2.806	NS
Other	36	8	41	33	5	38		NS

Note.—N = number of symptoms per child. *Total = 511, mean = 5.8. †Total = 439, mean = 5.0.

tionships (78 vs. 76), discipline (54 vs. 60), and mood problems (58 vs. 60). While there is little difference in frequency of these symptoms in our two groups, it should be noted that they rank high as presenting problems—in fact, peer relationships was the problem most frequently reported in both groups.

In two categories, considerably more problems were reported in the matched cases—eating (13 vs. 22), and elimination (14 vs. 27). However, the significance of this disparity is minor, since these areas accounted for relatively few complaints in both groups. In two categories, complaints were reported much more frequently by the parents of neurologically damaged children—motor activity (65 vs. 29) and speech (47 vs. 17). A less marked disparity not statistically significant was also noted in learning (60 vs. 43).

The preponderance of complaints about motor activity in the index children (ranking second in frequency) is in line with general expectations. This high frequency emphasizes that symptom complaints in this category should be taken most seriously as a possible indicator of neurological dysfunction. The fact that there were more than twice as many complaints about the index children than the matching group indicates a relationship that is more than casual. At the same time, the fact that 29 of 88 children without neurological damage presented symptoms in motor activity should put us on guard against automatically equating motor complaints with neurological damage in children who come to psychiatric notice.

The disparity in speech complaints is also in the direction of expected findings. What is striking, however, is the relatively low incidence of this presenting symptom in the matching cases. Its presence should alert one to investigate a child's neurological integrity.

The socioeconomic group represented in this study tends to focus on school problems. Indeed, the category of learning ranked third in frequency in the index cases and fourth in the controls. What seems significant is the relatively high ranking of this complaint in both groups, rather than the fact that there were about one-third as many more complaints in the neurologically damaged children. In itself, a learning complaint is not pathognomic of neurological damage. The presence of learning complaints, while a significant concomitant of neurological damage, does not significantly distinguish the organically damaged child from others who come to psychiatric attention.

SPECIAL SYMPTOMS

We were especially interested in determining whether children with neurological dysfunction show a disproportionate number of behavioral symptoms often reported to be associated with brain damage—hyperactivity, short attention span, distractibility, mood oscillation, high impulsivity, and perseveration. To explore this question we compared the frequency of such behaviors in the index and matched cases.

In categorizing these behaviors we required concrete descriptive data, with each area of judgment backed up by illustrations of the child's behavior. The following are some examples of the criteria for inclusion in the various categories:

(1) *Hyperactivity:* The child is characteristically described as "never sitting still," "always in motion," "restless," or several sources independently characterize him as "hyperactive" or "hyperkinetic."

(2) *Short attention span:* The data include objective descriptions supporting a general statement about brevity of attention—for example, a specific circumstance in which "attention was less than a minute."

Table 3

Frequency of Occurrence of Special Symptoms

Symptom	Neurological			Matched			χ^2 Total
	Male	Female	Total	Male	Female	Total	
Hyperactivity	23	5	28	16	9	25	
Short-attention span	15	2	17	6	3	9	
Distractibility	7	2	9	5	1	6	
Mood oscillation	16	11	27	11	5	16	
High impulsivity	22	10	32	22	7	29	
Perseveration	17	7	24	8	1	9	6.818*
Total	100	37	137	68	26	94	

*Significant beyond the .01 level of confidence.

(3) *Distractibility:* The child is described in such terms as "didn't pay attention—was listening to some other event," "mind wanders," "gets distracted easily," with illustrations.

(4) *Mood oscillation:* Descriptions may include situations in which the child "shows violent rage after a period of depression," "has crying spells," or "goes off in a huff and later apologizes."

(5) *Impulsivity:* The data include such observations as "when he loses his temper he breaks whatever he has in his hands," "bites and spits," "goes for children's eyes," "punches children without provocation." Impulsivity must be distinguished from mood oscillation, in which the mood itself is the issue. Here the sudden action is the crucial quality to be identified.

(6) *Perseveration:* Typical descriptions are "Repeats the same things over and over again," "repetitive questions," or "keeps a paper with the date on it always."

As Table 3 indicates, each of these special symptoms appeared more frequently in the index cases than in the controls. The degree of this discrepancy varies considerably with the category.

The number one special symptom in both groups was high impulsivity. This complaint was presented in 32 of the neurologically damaged children and 29 of the matched cases. Second highest complaint for both groups was hyperactivity (28 and 25). Mood oscillation was noted in 27 index cases as compared with 16 matched cases, but this differential

Table 4

Clusters of Special Symptoms

Number	Neurological			Matched			χ^2 Total
	Male	Female	Total	Male	Female	Total	
0 symptoms	14	6	20	24	11	35	4.090*
1 symptoms	15	12	27	14	10	24	
2 symptoms	15	6	21	15	5	20	
3 symptoms or more	16	4	20	7	2	9	4.172*
Total	60	28	88	60	28	88	

*Significant beyond the .05 level of confidence.

is short of statistical significance. Perseveration appeared in 24 of the index children as against only 9 of the controls, and this contrast is significant beyond the .01 level of confidence. Short attention span characterized 17 of the index group and 9 matched cases, another differential without statistical significance. The complaint of distractibility was presented in 9 index and 6 matched youngsters.

In sum, when the special symptoms are considered individually, perseveration alone appears so much more frequently among the neurological cases as to be statistically significant. This suggests that perseveration, while not pathognomic of an organic base, is sufficiently probable to signal the need for investigation. The other special symptoms also appear more often in the children with independently indicated neurological damage, but the greater frequency does not have statistical significance. While such symptoms should alert one to the possibility of neurological involvement, they cannot be a decisive argument for its probability.

In addition to considering the special symptoms individually, we wanted to ascertain whether these symptoms typically appear in clusters in children with neurological damage. We therefore examined the data to discover how many individual children in each group had 0, 1, 2, or 3 or more of the special symptoms. As Table 4 shows, the two categories that have statistical significance are 0 and 3 or more. The features that most clearly distinguish between the groups are: (1) The matched group has a significantly larger number of children without any of the special symptoms, and (2) the neurological cases have a significantly

TABLE 5

PSYCHIATRIC DIAGNOSES IN INDEX AND MATCHED CASES*

Diagnosis	Neurologically Damaged	Matched Cases
No behavior disorder	1	16
Developmental lag	0	5
Chronic brain syndrome	52	0
Reactive behavior disorder	16	23
Neurotic behavior disorder	18	20
Neurotic character disorder	0	3
Neurosis (anxiety; obsessive-compulsive)	1	6
Depression	0	1
Childhood schizophrenia	6	5
Childhood autism	0	1
Psychopathic personality	0	1
Mental Retardation	27	2
Hyperactive syndrome	0	5
No diagnosis reached	2	7

* Since multiple diagnoses are used, the total is greater than the 88 children represented in each column.

larger number of children who present a cluster of 3 or more special symptoms.

An individual child with none of the special symptoms may, of course, have both neurological dysfunction and behavioral symptoms, even though this is unlikely from a statistical point of view. At the other extreme, a child with 3 or more of these special symptoms may not have neurological dysfunction, but this possibility is strong enough to warrant a neurological investigation as an essential part of any workup.

PSYCHIATRIC DIAGNOSIS

Diagnoses were made in accordance with the categories defined by the author elsewhere (Chess, 1969). To make comparisons more meaningful for this study, the list was expanded to include "hyperactive syndrome" and "developmental lag." The following diagnoses were used: no behavioral disorder, developmental lag, chronic brain syndrome, behavior disorders due to cerebral dysfunction, reactive behavior disorder, neurotic behavior disorder, neurotic character disorder, neurosis, childhood schizophenia, autism, sociopathic personality, mental retardation, and hyperactive syndrome.

Several children fit into more than one diagnostic category, as shown in Table 5. Individual diagnoses of the index cases are detailed in Table 6.

TABLE 6
PSYCHIATRIC DIAGNOSES OF INDIVIDUAL NEUROLOGICALLY DAMAGED CHILDREN

Diagnosis	Number
No behavior disorder	1
Chronic brain syndrome (alone)	23
Chronic brain syndrome + reactive behavior disorder	6
Chronic brain syndrome + neurotic brain disorder	9
Chronic brain syndrome + retardation	7
Chronic brain syndrome + schizophrenia	3
Chronic brain syndrome + reactive behavior disorder + retardation	2
Chronic brain syndrome + neurotic behavior disorder + retardation	2
Reactive behavior disorder	7
Reactive behavior disorder + retardation	1
Neurotic behavior disorder	7
Neurosis (obsessive-compulsive; non-organic in nature)	1
Childhood schizophrenia	2
Childhood schizophrenia + retardation	1
Mental retardation	14
No diagnosis reached	2
	—
Total	88

First, we will consider the data on the neurologically damaged children. The majority of these children—52 of the 88—had chronic brain syndrome. This was the sole psychiatric finding in 23 youngsters. The next largest diagnostic category was mental retardation: 14 of the 27 retarded children had this as their only psychiatric diagnosis and the remaining 13 had additional problems. Of the 16 children with reactive behavior disorders, this was the sole problem for 7, while 8 others also had chronic brain syndrome. Finally, of the 18 youngsters with neurotic behavior disorders, 7 had this diagnosis alone. Only one of the neurologically damaged children in this group had no behavior disorder.[2]

In the 88 matched cases, 16 were behaviorally normal. Twenty-three had reactive behavior disorders and 20 had neurotic behavior disorders. Only two children in the control group were mentally retarded, while five had developmental lags. The remaining children were distributed among various other diagnostic categories.

One question that immediately occurs is: How can one account for the striking discrepancy between the number of behaviorally normal children in the index cases (N = 1) and the matched cases (N = 16)?

---

[2] It should be kept in mind that this is a sample drawn from psychiatric practice.

When behaviorally normal children are brought to a psychiatrist for consultation, it is usually because parents either find their behavior inconvenient or do not realize the great range of normal variability. One may surmise that parents of neurologically damaged children require a much greater degree of behavioral deviance before seeking a psychiatric consultation. In our sample, moreover, many of the neurologically damaged youngsters were under regular medical care for the neurological problem and their parents were therefore probably receiving some guidance on behavioral issues. In some cases it was a neurologist who referred the child. In other cases, school problems had made it necessary to obtain a comprehensive behavioral overview or an evaluation of possible retardation.

These factors probably also account for the greater number of neurologically normal children with the relatively mild diagnosis of *reactive behavior disorder*. In the neurologically damaged children it is likely that prenatal vigilance combined with the interpretation of a pediatrician or neurologist has defined the reactive issues, hence these may be less likely to come to psychiatric consultation.

The diagnostic categories of neurotic behavior disorder, neurotic character disorder, and neurosis were found in greater numbers among the matched cases. The virtual absence of neurotic diagnoses in the index cases reflects the fact that neurotic elements, when present in neurologically damaged children, are likely to be so overshadowed by behavioral elements reflecting the cerebral dysfunction that they are difficult to distinguish. The single neurologically damaged child with obsessive compulsive neurosis had spastic monoplegia. He had no behavior disorder until in early adolescence he was suddenly cut off from peer group by new socialization patterns in which he could not compete. His obsessive symptoms appeared soon after a leg operation which first immobilized him and then required him to learn new motor patterns.

Childhood schizophrenia appears for both groups well out of proportion to its general prevalence, but the ratio is in keeping with the author's consultation experience. Many children are brought to her for review of this diagnosis.

Developmental lag was diagnosed in 5 of the matched cases, but in none of the neurologically damaged children. A delay in development was not considered benign in a neurologically damaged youngster with a lag in language function, particularly if other competencies such as perceptual acuity were also delayed. In such cases the lag was attributed to the effect of the brain damage. But in the neurologically normal children, the delayed development of a single function, such as language, had to be seen in a different context. If such a child demonstrated a normal cognitive level in his nonverbal behavior, exhibited normal affective relatedness, and presented no history of a central nervous system disease, we identified a developmental lag rather than chronic brain syndrome.

Similarly, a child with a hyperactive syndrome but no independent evidence of neurological dysfunction was classified simply under the title of the syndrome, in accordance with the DSM II nomenclature. When a patient had both a hyperactive syndrome and indices of CNS damage, he was included in the chronic brain syndrome category.

Two children of the matched cases were mentally retarded; this number is in line with the statistical expectation for the general population. Of the neurologically damaged children 27 were mentally retarded, a typical proportion of cognitive disability due to brain damage.

SUMMARY

The relationship between neurological dysfunction and childhood behavioral pathology was examined in the case material of a 19-year child psychiatry consultation practice. Eighty-eight neurologically damaged children were identified out of the total of 1,400 cases seen. Each of these 88 children was matched by age, sex and year of consultation with a neurologically intact patient. Nature and frequency of presenting complaints were compared for the two groups. A comparison was also made of the frequency of presentation of the special symptoms of hyperactivity, short attention span, distractibility, mood oscillation, high impulsivity and perseveration, usually considered to be associated with cerebral dysfunction. Finally, the psychiatric diagnoses of the two groups were compared and the significance of the contrasts discussed.

Perseveration was the sole symptom which was statistically more characteristic of the neurologically damaged children. With this exception, there was close agreement in the number of children in each group with one or two of the special symptoms. However, clustering of 3 or more of the special symptoms was significantly related to neurological damage. The absence of all of these symptoms was highly characteristic of the neurologically intact group.

REFERENCES

BIRCH, H. G.: The problem of brain damage in children. In H. G. Birch (Ed.): *Brain Damage in Children*. Baltimore: Williams & Wilkins, 1964.

CHESS, S.: Psychiatric factors. In M. Bortner (Ed.): *Evaluation and Education of Children with Brain Damage*. Springfield, Ill.: Charles C Thomas, 1968.

CHESS, S.: *An Introduction to Child Psychiatry.* (2nd ed.). New York: Grune & Stratton, 1969.

CLEMENTS, S. D.: *Minimal Brain Dysfunction in Children.* Washington, D. C.: United States Government Printing Office, 1966.

EISENBERG, L.: Behavioral manifestations of cerebral damage. In H. G. Birch (Ed.): *Brain Damage in Children.* Baltimore: Williams & Wilkins, 1964.

WENDER, P. H.: *Minimal Brain Dysfunction in Children.* New York: John Wiley & Sons, 1971.

27

PROPOSED CLASSIFICATION OF CHILDHOOD DEPRESSION

Leon Cytryn, M.D.

*Associate Professor of Pediatric Psychiatry, George Washington
University School of Medicine
Research Associate, Dept. of Psychiatry, Children's
Hospital of the District of Columbia*

and

Donald H. McKnew, Jr., M.D.

*Assistant Clinical Professor of Pediatric Psychiatry
George Washington University School of Medicine
Research Associate, Dept. of Psychiatry, Children's
Hospital of the District of Columbia*

*Neurotic depressive reactions of mid-childhood may be
classified into three distinct categories. Masked depression
is the most frequent, appearing in children whose personality and family display severe psychopathology. Children
suffering acute depression are fairly well adjusted prior to
the traumatic event that precipitates the depression; there
may be mild psychopathology in the family. Chronically
depressed children have a history of marginal premorbid*

Reprinted from the AMERICAN JOURNAL OF PSYCHIATRY, Vol. 129, 1972, pp. 149-155.
Copyright 1972, The American Psychiatric Association.

Read at the 125th annual meeting of the American Psychiatric Association, Dallas,
Texas, May 1-5, 1972. This work was supported by Public Health Service Research
Development grant MH-40796 from the National Institute of Mental Health to
Dr. Cytryn.

*social adjustment, depression, and repeated separations
from important adults; in addition, at least one parent has
a history of recurrent depression.*

In contrast to the interest in depressive states in infants and toddlers,
depression in other children and latency-age children was largely neglected until recently, when an increased interest in depression in this
period became manifest. A review of childhood depressive reaction by
Anthony in 1967 (1) dealt with the evidence for and against the existence of such a disorder.

Anthony attributed the difference between the child and the adult
picture to the "inability of the child to verbalize his affective state, to
the incomplete development of the superego, and to the absence of consistent self-representation." He stated that the picture of prepubertal
depression includes, among other symptoms, "weeping bouts, some flatness of affect, fear of death for self or parents, irritability, somatic
complaints, loss of appetite and energy, varying degrees of difficulty in
school adjustment, and vacillation between clinging to and unreasonable
hostility toward . . . [the] parents." Finally, Anthony postulated that
some children are "predisposed to depression," although he did not
comment on the possible origin of such a predisposition. In 1965 Sandler
and Joffe (2) reported that the syndrome of childhood depression had
several consistent features including sad affect, withdrawal, discontent, a
feeling of being rejected and unloved, passivity, and insomnia.

A change in contemporary thinking about childhood depression is evident in a recent report on *Psychopathological Disorders in Childhood* by
the Group for the Advancement of Psychiatry (3). It states:

> Depression in children and even in adolescents may be manifested
> in ways somewhat different from those manifested by adults. . . .
> The picture of depression may be much more clear and marked,
> particularly when precipitated by an actual, threatened, or symbolic
> loss of a parent or parent substitute. . . . Psychomotor retardation
> is ordinarily less marked than in adults, and, except in young in-
> fants, the same is true of some of the other biologic signs of de-
> pression (p. 236).

A paper describing the various clinical manifestations of childhood
depression has been recently published by Poznanski and Zrull (4).
Glaser, in a recent publication (5), dealt with the problem of a so-called
masked depression in children in which the depressive affect is not a
major component of the clinical picture.

In reviewing the literature, one is gratified to see that the existence of childhood depression is given the recognition it deserves. The aforementioned publications and several others we did not mention (6-8) give excellent descriptions of depressed children. However, the reader is sometimes bewildered by the widly divergent clinical pictures, all subsumed under the heading of childhood depression. In this paper we will attempt to identify and isolate the various types of childhood depression. It is hoped that such a categorization will assist future work in providing a common basis for describing clinical pictures, research work, teaching, and therapeutic endeavors.

For several years we have been involved in a large research study concerning biochemical, psychological, and sociological aspects of depression in children aged six to 12. During the several years of this ongoing program we have studied in depth 37 children, most of whom were referred to us as being depressed, for possible participation in our hospital study of mood disorders in children. The patients were referred from Hillcrest Children's Center in Washington, D. C., social agencies, schools, and the various clinics connected with Children's Hospital of the District of Columbia.

All the children received a thorough work-up, including a detailed family history, social history, and mental status examination, which we conducted with the cooperation of the Social Service Department. Selected children who were severely depressed were hospitalizd in our Clinical Rsearch Center (CRC) for a period of three weeks for extended clinical evaluation and biochemical studies. (The CRC is a well-equipped and well-staffed eight-bed research unit of Children's Hospital.) The follow-up of the more severely disturbed children has been extensive, the psychotherapy ranging from three months to two years as of this writing. Our preliminary findings concerning biochemical changes in depressed children are reported elsewhere (9).

A review of the literature and analysis of our own research material leads us to believe that, phenomenologically, depression in latency-age children may be divided into three distinct categories based on clinical manifestations, family background, duration of illness, premorbid history, and precipitating factors, namely, masked depressive reaction of childhood, acute depressive reaction of childhood, and chronic depressive reaction of childhood.

These three forms of childhood depression differ in several aspects, described in the following case reports.

Case 1. Masked depressive reaction of childhood. A. was a 12-year-old boy who was referred to us by school authorities because of his disruptive behavior. He had a long history of school difficulties that included hyperactivity, aggressive behavior, poor scholastic performance, and marginal social adjustment. His behavior had led to several school suspensions in the past.

The home situation had always been very unstable. The mother was unavailable to the children due to full-time work; at one time she was investigated for child abuse. The father was a chronic alcoholic who frequently beat the patient and assumed no responsibility for the family. There was no history of overt depressive illness in the family.

In the interview situation the patient was in a very depressed mood and was apathetic and sad throughout. He described himself as dumb, as the laughingstock of his schoolmates, and expressed the belief that everyone was picking on him. On the fantasy level the boy showed a strong preoccupation with themes of annihilation, violence, explosions, and death, invariably with a bad outcome for the main figures in those fantasies. It was also evident from both verbal productions and figure drawings that the boy's body image was extremely defective and that he viewed himself as inadequate and helpless, with very little initiative or autonomy.

The patient was hospitalized in the CRC for a period of three weeks, and the overt signs of his depression, except for his sleeplessness, gradually disappeared and gave way to aggressive and impulsive behavior.

The follow-up period of one and one-half years was very stormy. The boy continued to have serious school difficulties, leading finally to his suspension from school and admission to a residential school for delinquent boys.

Comment

The child's acting-out behavior succeeded in masking his depression, which went unrecognized until his admission to the hospital, where it became clearly evident. The depth of depression and the pain of self-denigration as revealed in the interview material may help to explain his defensive use of aggressive and delinquent behavior. Although such a defense is self-destructive, it helps to ward off the unbearable feeling of despair.

Case 2. Active depressive reaction of childhood. B., a six-year-old girl, was referred by the pediatric clinic because of progressive withdrawal, depressed affect, sleep disturbance, lack of appetite, school failure, and separation anxiety sufficient to interfere with all social activities. These symptoms appeared after the rape of her 17-year-old sister three months prior to the referral. Before this incident the sister had served as a mother substitute to the patient because of the mother's relative unavailability due to full-time work. After the incident the sister became withdrawn, preoccupied, and less attentive to the patient. Prior to the present illness the patient had never exhibited signs of depression and had a reasonably good social and scholastic record but was described by relatives and friends as stubborn and negativistic. There was no history of depression in other family members, but the father had been absent for many years and the mother was resentful of the burden she had to carry.

The girl was admitted to the CRC for a period of three weeks. At the time of admission her mood was markedly depressed, as evidenced by a sad and tearful facial expression, slowness of movement, monotone voice, and verbal expressions indicating hopelessness and despair. On the ward her clinical picture changed within several days. She became outgoing and started to eat and sleep regularly, her mood brightened, and she was sociable, active, and alert.

Following her symptomatic improvement, the girl was discharged and followed for a period of two years. According to the mother's report, she maintained her gains and behaved very much as she did before the onset of the presenting complaints.

Comment

The patient's relatively good premorbid adjustment and the history of her depressive episode clearly indicate that the depressive signs and symptoms followed the traumatic event that resulted in a loss of a mother figure. The patient had suffered no such losses in the past, which may help to explain her quick and lasting recovery.

Case 3. Chronic depressive reaction of childhood. C., a seven-year-old girl born out of wedlock, was referred on an emergency basis because of severe depression. She had had insomnia, anorexia, weight loss, and screaming episodes for several months. She told the pediatric resident that she wanted to kill herself; according to the mother she had made suicidal threats repeatedly, claiming that she was "a bad girl" and that nobody loved her. Ten months prior to this episode she had been seen in the Psychiatric Crisis Clinic because of persistent insomnia.

The girl's mother was an immature, helpless woman; she had a tendency toward frequent depressions and was overwhelmed by family responsibilities. She shared with her daughter a passive, helpless attitude toward life as well as poor self-esteem. There is some evidence that the mother had been neglected as a child by her own mother and was exposed to frequent violence in her surroundings. She was hospitalized once with what seems to have been an agitated depression. During our contacts with her she had at least one serious depressive episode, during which she made suicidal threats. She had left home twice for several months, once when the patient was one and one-half years old and again when she was four. Her only marriage was stormy, and at the time of our contact the parents were separated, after the child's stepfather had beaten the child severely.

The father had a long history of delinquent behavior and had had little contact with the girl or her mother following the child's birth. The paternal grandmother, however, kept the child during the day, while the maternal grandmother was maintaining a full-time job as a housekeeper. According to the child's mother the paternal grandmother had been one of the most significant persons in the patient's life. This relationship, however, was abruptly interrupted when at one year of age the child was transferred to the care of a maternal aunt.

As the patient grew up she became shy and retiring, usually withdrawing from stressful situations. At the age of three she would punish herself (whenever she thought she had transgressed) by quitting her play or favorite toy and sitting quietly in the corner until she was told to resume her activities.

When first seen, C. appeared poorly nourished, very small for her age, and passive; she had a sad facial expression. Her withdrawal, apathy, lack of spontaneity, and psychomotor retardation were the most striking features of her behavior. She was admitted to the CRC for a period of three weeks. At first she continued to be depressed, apathetic, and withdrawn, refused most meals, and slept poorly. However, following two episodes of open expression of violent anger, steady improvement began, marked by more spontaneity, improved mood, appetite, and sleep, and increased social interaction. Along with the decrease of overt depression there was an increase in negativism, defiance, and on occasion even hostility.

After her discharge there was much instability in the child's environment. Her mother went back to the stepfather, who in the past had been cruel to the girl, following which the patient again became depressed and developed abdominal cramps and diarrhea. When the mother again separated from the stepfather, these symptoms rapidly disappeared.

After three months of weekly follow-up visits, we lost track of the patient because the mother did not keep appointments. The mother became depressed and threatened suicide during our telephone conversations; she asked for suggestions but did not follow through. She reported the patient as doing well in school and at home, but the reliability of this information is doubtful.

Comment

The most striking features of this patient were the presence of depressed mood and behavior including suicidal ideation very early in childhood, repeated separations from important maternal figures starting in infancy, and the presence of a chronic depression in the mother.

CLINICAL FEATURES

Depressive symptoms, especially sad affect in response to environmental trauma, are very common in children. However, they usually are of short duration and do not interfere substantially with the child's thinking, functioning, and physical health. We think in terms of depressive illness rather than of depressive affect when the depression is of long duration (of at least several months) and is associated with severe impairment of the child's scholastic and social adjustment and with disturbances of the vegetative functions, especially those of food intake and sleep. In more serious cases the child's thinking is affected by feelings of despair and hopelessness, general retardation, and, in the severe form, by suicidal thoughts.

Where depression is more pervasive, it does not usually manifest itself in a clearly recognizable form but instead presents a *masked depressive reaction*. The children afflicted with the latter syndrome may show a variety of emotional disorders, among them hyperactivity, aggressive behavior, psychosomatic illness, hypochondriasis, and delinquency. In such cases the underlying depression is largely inferred from periodic displays of a purely depressive picture and from depressive themes on projective tests such as the Rorschach, Thematic Apperception Test (TAT), figure drawings, and fantasy material.

In addition to the many children with masked depression, there is a group of latency-age children who present a more clearly identifiable depressive syndrome. The symptoms of this syndrome include a persistent sad affect, social withdrawal, hopelessness, helplessness, pychomotor retardation, anxiety, school and social failure, sleep and feeding disturbances, and suicidal ideas and threats but only rarely suicidal attempts. The clinical picture is sometimes preceded by a traumatic event and usually lasts at least two to three months before medical help is sought. The children with this clinical picture can be further subdivided into those with *acute* and *chronic depressive reactions*.

PRECIPITATING CAUSES

In the children with acute reactions we were able to find a precipitating cause in all cases; usually it was a severe trauma associated with object loss. This was sometimes in the form of the death of a loved one. More often, however, it was in the more subtle forms of withdrawal of interest or change in involvement on the part of important persons because of remarriage, new siblings, somebody's moving away, or personal difficulties leading to a diminution of the love and care previously given.

We could not find an immediate precipitating factor in most of the patients with chronic depressive reactions. Rather, in reviewing the backgrounds of these children, we did find a history of many separations and object losses during the child's life, usually beginning in early infancy. Such a history of periodic recurring emotional deprivation was not characteristic of patients suffering from the other forms of depression we studied.

FAMILY HISTORY

The family members of the children with masked depressive reactions often presented a picture of disorganization and severe psychopathology, usually in the form of a character defect, but they gave no history of a clearcut depressive illness.

The close family members of the patients with acute depressive reactions often showed mild to moderate neurotic problems but an absence of gross psychopathology. These families had considerable strength and cohesion, and, again, no clear-cut history of depressive illness could be elicited.

All of the children with chronic depressive reactions had at least one parent (in most instances the mother) with a history of recurrent depressive illness. We noted an interesting phenomenon in the treatment and follow-up of these children. In some cases the depression in the children and the parents started at about the same time. The parents were usually the first to exhibit depressive symptomatology, and the children, to use the words of Anna Freud (10), "produced the mother's mood in themselves." However, in some cases the interaction between the parent's and the child's depression operated in a seesaw fashion, and whenever the patient improved, the parent would develop a depressive episode soon afterward.

The children with the soundest personality structures seemed to be those with acute depressive reactions. These children had been functioning relatively well prior to the precipitating episode; their defenses broke down only under the impact of severe trauma. However, their histories often revealed some maladjustment in the form of exaggerated stubbornness, negativism, and other signs of a passive-aggressive personality structure. .

The children with chronic depressive reactions usually had a history of marginal emotional and social adjustment. They were helpless, passive, clinging, dependent, and lonely and often had had depressive episodes in the past that lasted from several days to several months.

The personality structures of the children with masked depressive reactions contained elements of psychopathology as varied as their clinical pictures. They displayed compulsive, hysterical, and obsessive features as well as character defects with acting-out tendencies.

All of the children we studied displayed intense anger; those with masked depressive reactions displayed it more openly than those with acute and chronic depressive reactions, who displayed it only episodically. Their fantasy material was replete with themes of violence, aggression, explosions, and death, and their self-image, as expressed verbally and as projected in figure drawings, was usually inadequate and damaged.

The children with chronic depressive reactions seemed to lack the protective shield or character armor that the children with reactive and masked depressions had to protect them against normal strains and stresses. In the children with acute depressive reactions it took a serious precipitating event such as death, divorce, or unusual trauma to cause a collapse of their usual defensive maneuvers, resulting in depression. In contrast, in the children with chronic depressive reactions, even a seemingly minor trauma would cause a breakdown of customary defenses and lead to depression.

The children with masked depressive reactions seemed to be able to call upon a variety of defenses even under the most severe stress. We do not wish to make a value judgment about the virtue of the various forms of defenses used by these children. Those used by patients with masked depressive reactions were maladaptive and often led to a serious breakdown in overall functioning, conflict with their environment, or psychosomatic illness, but they did at least ward off depression. Thus, starting with masked depressive reactions and proceeding to acute and chronic depressive reactions, we seem to be dealing with a hierarchy of defense systems, progressively less capable of protecting the children against depression.

DIFFERENTIAL DIAGNOSTIC AND NOSOLOGICAL CONSIDERATIONS

It should be stressed that we are discussing neurotic rather than psychotic types of childhood depression. None of the children we studied showed any signs of psychotic disorder. They had no hallucinations or delusions and no bizarre thoughts, speech, or behavior. Their social withdrawal was clearly different from the autistic aloofness of psychotic children. In the hospital they often improved within days or weeks and then began to relate, function, and verbalize in a normal fashion, which could not possibly occur in psychotic children. The depressed children we studied all attended regular schools and were not grossly retarded. Some may have been of borderline intelligence due to sociocultural deprivation, but their intellectual deficit was definitely not their main problem.

The question can be raised of whether these children were simply having adjustment reactions of childhood. In a broad sense such a designation would be justified, since all these patients reacted to adverse life circumstances. What distinguishes these children, especially those with masked and chronic depressive reactions, from children with the usual adjustment reactions, is the pervasiveness, intensity, and duration of the clinical picture as well as the more lasting personality changes. The latter feature is least applicable to the children with acute depressive reactions.

Another diagnostic category with which the depressed children may be confused is chronic or acute childhood anxiety. As is the case with adults, depressed children usually show signs of anxiety as part of the clinical picture. However, in our patients the depressive symptomatology clearly predominated as the outstanding problem.

In cases of acute depressive reactions and in some cases of masked depressive reactions, one could argue that we are dealing with a prolonged grief reaction since the symptoms followed an acute loss. However, this is clearly not the case with our patients with chronic depressive reactions, for the symptoms were not preceded by an acute loss and had lasted intermittently for many years.

It should be added that masked depressive reaction in children is seen frequently, although it often goes unrecognized. In contrast, children with a clear-cut depression, both of the acute and chronic variety, are seen rather infrequently. For instance, in our clinical setting, which has 220 pediatric beds and a busy outpatient department, we received only ten to 20 such referrals each year. Thus we presumably are dealing with a rare, but clearly recognizable and distinguishable, phenomenon.

We chose the diagnostic labels "acute," "chronic," and "masked depressive reaction" because our patients' depressions bore enough similarity to the the adult types of neurotic depression to justify the use of the official APA diagnostic nomenclature (11). We added, however, the designation "of childhood" in order to underscore the unique features of depression in children.

SUMMARY

Depressive symptoms, especially sad affect, are very common in children. Most of the time, however, they are of short duration and do not interfere substantially with the child's functioning. In those cases where depression is more pervasive, it does not usually manifest itself in a clearly recognizable form but rather presents as masked depressive reaction of childhood. Children afflicted with such depression may show a variety of emotional disorders, among them hyperactivity, aggressive behavior, psychosomatic illness, hypochondriasis, and delinquency. In such cases the underlying depression is largely inferred from periodic displays of a purely depressive picture and from depressive themes on projective tests such as the Rorschach and TAT.

Our survey of the literature on childhood depression, as well as our own studies of clinical and biochemical aspects of childhood depression, leads us to believe that in addition to the many children with masked depression, there is a group of latency-age children who present a clearly identifiable depressive syndrome. This syndrome includes a persistent sad affect, social withdrawal, hopelessness, helplessness, psychomotor retardation, anxiety, school and social failure, sleep and feeding disturbances, and suicidal ideas and threats but rarely suicidal attempts; it usually lasts at least two to three months before medical help is sought. The children with this clinical picture can be further subdivided into those with acute and chronic depressive reactions of childhood.

The children with acute depressive reaction of childhood often have a history of a relatively normal adjustment prior to a traumatic event that is followed by the onset of depression. The close family members may show a mild to moderate degree of psychopathology, but there is usually no depressive illness reported.

The children with chronic depressive reaction of childhood have a history of marginal premorbid social adjustment. They often have had depressive episodes in the past. Their early life is replete with traumatic separation experiences, with loss of significant people. In addition, in our experience, there has always been at least one parent with a history of recurrent depressive illness.

REFERENCES

1. ANTHONY, E. J.: Psychoneurotic disorders. In A. M. Freedman & H. G. Kaplan (Eds.): *Comprehensive Textbook of Psychiatry*. Baltimore: Williams & Wilkins Co., 1967, pp. 1387-1406.
2. SANDLER, J., & JOFFE, W. G.: Notes on childhood depression. *Int. J. Psychoanal.*, 46:88-96, 1965.
3. Group for the Advancement of Psychiatry: Psychopathological Disorders in Childhood, Report No. 62. New York: GAP, 1966.
4. POZNANSKI, E. & ZRULL, J. P.: Childhood depression. *Arch. Gen. Psychiat.*, 23:8-15, 1970.
5. GLASER, K.: Masked depression in children and adolescents. *Amer. J. Psychother.*, 21:565-574, 1967.
6. DIZMANG, L. H.: Loss, bereavement and depression in childhood. *Int. Psychiat. Clin.*, 6:175-195, 1969.
7. MALMQUIST, C. P.: Depressions in childhood and adolescence: I. *New Eng. J. Med.*, 284:887-893, 1971.
8. MALMQUIST, C. P.: Depressions in childhood and adolescence: II. *New Eng. J. Med.*, 284:995-961, 1971.
9. CYTRYN, L. & McKNEW, D. H., JR.: Biochemical correlates of affective disorders in children (submitted for publication).
10. FREUD, A.: *Normality and Pathology in Childhood*. New York: International Universities Press, 1965.
11. American Psychiatric Association: Diagnostic and Statistical Manual of Mental Disorders, 2nd ed. Washington, D. C.: APA, 1968.

DISCUSSION

Edwin Z. Levy, M.D. (Topeka, Kans.)—In their clinical investigative program Drs. Cytryn and McKnew are working to bring order to our biochemical, psychological, and sociological understanding of the various depressive entities of mid-childhood. They rightly point to the confusing array of published clinical descriptions. They could also have said the same thing about all age groups—child and adult. The confusion derives from several sources: problems in description and language, the subjective versus the objective, problems in thinking about etiologies and mechanisms, organic versus psychodynamic, and so forth.

The authors offer us valuable help in classification as a step toward diagnosis. They describe a group of children, ill for at least a few months, whose functioning is interfered with in many areas, who are more disturbed than with a brief mood change or an adjustment reaction, but who are not psychotic. Those whose appearance is depressed, whose defenses have collapsed in response to a clearly identifiable precipitating event, but whose personality and family are relatively sound are termed "acutely depressed." Those whose appearance is depressed, who seem poorly defended against repeated traumata, whose parent or parents are depressed, and whose personality is weak are termed "chronically depressed." Those who are only occasionally depressed, who have a variety of behavioral disruptions, whose family and personality are seriously disturbed in a variety of ways, and whose defenses against feeling (against feeling depressed) are effective, but at considerable cost, are said to have "masked depression."

The authors find that they can accept the views of most of the authors they cite and, in general, can work within the structure of *DSM-II* (referenced in the article). In support of their work I would like to engage in some speculations about where we may be going from here. Our conceptual morass about this subject is intricate. Think for a moment about the variety of issues related to the phenomenon of depression—catecholamines, loss, guilt, failure, anger, personality structure, and so forth. Recall the authors' legitimately felt need not to criticize a child's capacity to protect himself from feeling depression. Contrast this with Klein's view of the child's achievement during the first year of the depressive position as a hallmark of passing beyond the schizoid position.

Depressive feelings are a repeated element in everyone's life experience. Some children (masked type) cannot accept them; some children (acute type) confront and go beyond, integrating the past with new life experience; and some (chronic type) have long been gripped by and identify with depression. But the same seems to be true for people of all ages. Are the authors bringing to child psychiatry ideas long common in adult psychiatry (depressive equivalent, neurotic depression, and endogenous depression) from the child psychiatrist's perspective?

I think their work contains more. I wonder—how do we relate depressive phenomena to developmental phase? For instance, regarding latency, Erikson speaks of industry versus inferiority, the task of latency being to develop a sense of industry—confidence in one's capacity to do. If the child fails in this, his fate includes a sense of inferiority. I suspect that those latency-age children who respond to precipitating events with acute depression (beyond normal grief or mourning) are those children who are struggling with the phase-specific crisis of industry versus inferiority to a degree that renders them vulnerable. A close study of these children may tell us much about the contribution of the latency phase *per se* to depressiveness, just as the work of Abraham and Spitz contributed to our knowledge of the sadistic and anaclitic elements of depression derived from the oral phase.

Children with chronic depression, I will surmise, have already struggled defensively with loss-guilt crises around the trust (oral), autonomy (anal), and initiative (phallic) issues—to use Erikson's terms. The difficult-to-deal-with but more independent children with masked depression undergo a similar experience; I suspect that to understand them we must also look to the earlier developmental phases.

I cannot resist a footnote about language. A lot of our common English words that refer to various aspects of depression seem to fall into groups describing downness, darkness, spiritlessness, sadness, or badness. Some words refer more or less discretely to one or another of these elements; others contain a fusion. It intrigues me how common English describes the same intricacy that technical psychiatry struggles with. You have to hear how a person says "I'm sorry" to know what he means —and even then it may be hard to tell. Similarly, one must pay close attention to the complex messages of the depressed child—our most valuable clues to his or her inner life.

Part VII

CLINICAL STUDIES

As in previous years, the clinical studies cover a number of issues of interest. Money and his colleagues examine the question of the relationship between neglect of children and aberrations in pain awareness in a sample of 32 children. Their findings have implications beyond the syndrome of dwarfism itself.

The so-called feral child has been reported periodically, but his accuracy of history has always been in doubt. Whether these were retarded children initially or whether permanent retardation was secondary to early stimulus deprivation could not be answered from these previous case studies. The well-documented report presented here by Koluchova illustrates a remarkable recovery in intellectual and emotional levels of functioning from social isolation. The commentary on this report by Clarke relates this case to others reported in the literature and considers the factors involved in the children's ability to respond to corrective environmental measures.

Galdston presents a study of 100 children admitted to a surgical ward for severe burns. He delineates the stresses produced by the event, the immediate injuries and the necessities of treatment (debridement, traction, isolation, etc.) and the approach to prevention and treatment of psychological consequences. The case material provides a striking example of the interaction of physical and emotional factors.

Murphy and Pounds investigate the reasons why parents seek new opinions with regard to children diagnosed as retarded. They note that "shopping around" and denial accounted for only a minor proportion of repeat evaluations. They emphasize the part professionals often play in engendering repeat diagnostic workups by their failure to meet the need of child and parents.

Bohman's summary of the prevalence of maladjustment in adopted children in Sweden deals with the often-asked question, are adopted children overrepresented in child psychiatric facilities. His examination of the importance of a number of factors, including the nature of the adoptive situation itself, has implications that appear relevant to other countries.

433

PART VII: CLINICAL STUDIES

28

PAIN AGNOSIA AND SELF-INJURY IN THE SYNDROME OF REVERSIBLE SOMATOTROPIN DEFICIENCY (PSYCHOSOCIAL DWARFISM)

John Money, Ph.D., Georg Wolff, Ph.D. and

Charles Annecillo, Ph.D.

*Department of Psychiatry and Behavioral Sciences
and Department of Pediatrics
The Johns Hopkins University School of Medicine and Hospital*

Hospital and social service records of 32 patients, 23 boys and 9 girls, with reversible behavioral symptoms in a syndrome of dwarfism characterized by reversible inhibition of growth in stature are surveyed and discussed. When first seen, the patients ranged in age from 22 months to 16 years and 2 months. After initial hospitalization, they were discharged to a convalescent home and then to foster homes to experience a prolonged change of domicile and thus continue to grow. Changes in domicile from adverse environments, where growth failure began and persisted, to amelio-

Reprinted from JOURNAL OF AUTISM AND CHILDHOOD SCHIZOPHRENIA, 1972, 2, 2, pp. 127-139. Copyright © 1972 by Scripta Publishing Corporation.

This study was supported by a grant from the Erickson Educational Foundation and by USPHS grants HD 18635, HD 00325, HD 01852 and R.R. 00035 (GCRCP).

The patients in this sample were diagnosed and managed under the supervision of Dr. Robert M. Blizzard. The clinical cooperation of members of the pediatric endocrine clinic and the availability of its medical files are greatly appreciated. Dr. Robert Athanasiou assisted with the statistical reduction of the data. We also thank the staff at Happy Hills Hospital for their excellent cooperation.

rative where catch-up growth took place covaried significantly ($p<.001$) with decreased incidence of physical injury,
severe physical punishment or abuse, self-inflicted injury,
and behavior indicating pain agnosia. It is suggested that
self-injury may counteract cognitional starvation under conditions of sensory deprivation when self-inflicted injury and
pain agnosia coexist.

This paper presents the second of two studies dealing with reversible
behavioral symptoms in a syndrome of dwarfism characterized by reversible inhibition of pituitary growth hormone (somatotropin) secretion
and, therefore, of growth in stature. The syndrome, often referred to as
psychosocial dwarfism, has been variously described by other investigators
(Patton & Gardner, 1962, 1963, 1969; Powell, Brasel, & Blizzard, 1967;
Powell, Brasel, Raiti, & Blizzard, 1967; Silver & Finkelstein, 1967; Capitanio & Kirkpatrick, 1969; Reinhard & Drash, 1969).

Our preceding paper (Wolff & Money, 1972) deals with the relationship
between sleep and growth in 27 patients with psychosocial dwarfism.
The purpose of the present one is to present findings regarding pain
agnosia and self-harming behavior in a sample now increased to 32 patients so diagnosed. Although self-injury as well as lack of pain response
have been discussed by Powell, Brasel, and Blizzard (1967), Silver and
Finkelstein (1967), and Freedman (1969), no systematic survey has
hitherto been made of a group of patients with a focus on manifestations
of these phenomena.

METHODS

Sample

The sample comprised a census of 32 patients, 9 girls and 23 boys
(25 white and 7 black) with a diagnosis of reversible somatotropin deficiency formulated at the pediatric endocrine clinic of The Johns Hopkins Hospital during the period of 1959 to 1971. When first seen, the
patients ranged in age from 22 months to 16 years and 2 months ($M =
73; SD = 38$ mo.). The duration of follow-up ranged from 8 months
to 9 years and 3 months ($M = 43; SD = 30$ mo.). Follow-up was scheduled at biannual intervals.

All patients were initially referred for short stature and admitted to
the hospital for a period of diagnostic evaluation. The diagnosis was
confirmed when the statural growth rate accelerated and growth hormone
levels rose to normal in response to change of domicile from home to
hospital, and in the absence of other treatment.

After the initial evaluation at The Johns Hopkins Hospital most patients were discharged to Happy Hills Hospital, a convalescent home for children. From there, they proceeded to foster homes in order to experience a prolonged change of domicile and thus continue to grow which they would not do if returned to the original domicile. In the latter, severe and at times bizarre forms of behavior typical of the syndrome would also recur.

Procedure

Information was obtained retrospectively from available hospital and social service records, and also from transcripts of interviews performed in the past with parents, guardians, or nurses. The patient's current status was ascertained by direct observation, by talking with each child, and also interviewing appropriate adults. Such interviews always began with open-ended inquiry prior to factual true-false questioning. All office interviews were recorded and transcribed. Notes reflecting pertinent observations during the course of home visits were dictated immediately after such visits.

All sources were pooled to extract and chronologically tabulate data relating to noxious injury, the source of injury (whether accidental, self-inflicted or other), and complaints (or lack of such) concerning hurting and feeling (or not feeling) pain. Chronological classification provided for the time when each child lived in the original domicile of growth failure as well as for that when the child had been relocated.

RESULTS

The distribution of patients, before and after changes in domiciliary environment, who showed signs of physical injury, a history of severe physical punishment or abuse, behavior indicating self-harm, and indications of pain agnosia, is given in Table 1. The *before* and *after* comparisons on all of the four criteria were significantly different with χ^2 significant at less than the .001 level. The high significance of each χ^2 is all the more impressive, because these parameters are based on 3×2 tables with entries for inconclusive data.

Physical Injury

Symptoms of injury are enumerated in Table 1 irrespective of the suspected etiology (i.e., accidental, self-inflicted, or other). Observable signs of physical injury, varying in degree of severity, were noted on hos-

Table 1

Injury and Pain prior to Hospitalization and in Ameliorative Environment in 32 Children with a Diagnosis of Psychosocial Dwarfism

Patients with:		Prior to hospital admission for growth failure			During stay in ameliorative environment			Differences before and after change of domicile		
		Present	Absent	Inconclusive	Present	Absent	Inconclusive	χ^2	df	p
Observable signs of physical injury	N	24	4	4	7	19	6	19.5	2	.001
	Percent	75	12.5	12.5	22	59	19			
History of severe physical punishment and/or questionably authentic accidents	N	22	1	9	1	31	0	56.2	2	.001
	Percent	69	3	28	3	97	0			
Behavior indicating self-injury	N	20	0	12	0	24	8	44.8	2	.001
	Percent	63	0	37	0	75	25			
Behavior indicating pain agnosia	N	14	2	16	5	21	6	21.4	2	.001
	Percent	44	6	50	16	65	19			

Table 2

Types of Self-harming Behavior prior to Hospitalization in
32 Patients with a Diagnosis of Psychosocial Dwarfism

Self-harming behavior	Presence or absence (N of patients)		
	Present	Absent	Not recorded
Head banging	7	3	22
Hair twisting and plucking	6	1	25
Nail-biting and tearing nailbed skin	5	0	27
Falling often and/or bumping frequently into furniture, walls, corners, etc.	10	0	22
Temper tantrums with head banging, self-biting, etc.	9	0	23
Eating indigestible or harmful objects (e.g., stones, drugs from medicine cabinet)	5	0	27
Not protecting with hands when falling	2	0	30
Other self-inflicting injuries (e.g., eating soup that is too hot for other family members)	7	0	25

pitalization in 24 patients (75%). Such symptoms included bruises, scars, bone fractures and/or skin lesions that were not as yet healed.

The incidence of new lesions decreased after removal from the pre-referral domicile so that only 7 patients (22%) were involved—5 while still in the hospital, and 2 while newly placed in a foster home. The occurrence of physical injuries after hospitalization could not be ascertained for one of these patients, as he returned from the hospital to his pre-referral home and was no longer available for follow-up. The remaining 6 patients had no further signs of physical injury after they settled in their new and ameliorative environments. Also, 19 patients (59%) exhibited the same lack of injury while hospitalized as during subsequent placement in other ameliorative environments. Even without including the eventual improvement of the 6, physical injury was recorded significantly less frequently while the patients were in ameliorative environments in comparison with their stay in prehospitalization domiciles of origin ($\chi^2 = 19.5$; $p < .001$).

History of Physical Punishment

Prior to initial hospitalization, 22 patients (69%) had a positive history of severe physical punishment, abuse and/or alleged accidents. More likely, the allegedly accidental injuries had been inflicted by parents. Among the 22, there was only one patient whose injury might have been genuinely accidental as no other history of physical abuse could be authenticated.

Table 1 shows that there was only one recorded instance of unusual physical punishment after change of domicile. This was the case of an 8-year-old girl whose foster mother reported that she had punished her for picking up chewing gum from the street by biting her fingers. The girl appeared indifferent to the intentionally inflicted pain and did not respond to the punishment, much to the foster-mother's frustration.

Generally, the incidence of severe punishment or physical abuse was reduced significantly after transfer to a new domiciliary environment in comparison with such incidence in the domicile of origin ($\chi^2 = 56.2$; $p < .001$).

Self-Injury

Prior to initial hospitalization, 20 of the 32 patients exhibited diverse modes of self-harming behavior detailed in Table 2. Three cases of severe self-harm included a boy, 3 years and 9 months of age, who banged his head on a concrete floor, a girl who at the age of 2 years and 5 months cut off the circulation of her forefinger by twisting hair so tightly around it that it had to be cut free with a razor blade, and a 7-year-old boy who had a history of temper tantrums during which he injuriously bit himself.

After the children were transferred to a new environment for a long-term period, the ameliorative effects of such transfer could be documented in 24 cases by subsequent absence of self-injurious behavior. The change is significant ($\chi^2 = 44.8$; $p < .001$). Onset of change was rapid, being manifested even during the relatively brief initial diagnostic hospital admission, though 2 of the 24 patients did manifest sporadic head banging in the hospital. Also, 2 others in the group of 24 briefly continued mildly self-injurious behavior while settling in a foster home. One was a head banger, and the other contrived to trip over his foster mother's extended foot and fall with a thump.

Pain Agnosia

Despite the injuries suffered or self-inflicted that one would expect to have been painful, it could be retrospectively documented for as many as 14 cases that the children appeared to be hyporeactive to pain. One might define their hypoalgesia as insensitivity or indifference to pain, but a preferable term is nonrecognition of pain, or pain agnosia.

Injuries to which a lack of response was reported in these 14 patients were due to physical punishment, accidents (including, for example, the fracture of a clavicle), self-inflicted traumata, infections or inflammatory illnesses, medical injections, minor surgery, and dental treatment. In addition, the parents or guardians of 11 patients reported that the children never complained about anything, never cried or shed tears when punished, and generally did not react or complain when being hurt or injured.*

The only available information pertaining to periods preceding hospitalization that was positive involved two children who had shown responses to pain. Parental punishment inflicted on these children was excessively traumatic.

For 16 cases (50%), the data were either inconclusive or no record was made regarding reaction to physical injury prior to hospitalization. However, 9 of the 16 had exhibited self-harming behavior of varying severity. They might have also been agnosic for pain from such self-injurious behavior.

After transfer to a new place of domicile, pain agnosia appeared to occur in only five patients, and only for relatively brief, transient periods. For example, 2 of the 5 children failed to react to finger-pricks or injection needles during the first 2 weeks in the hospital. In the 3 other cases, upon arrival in respective foster homes, the children were reported to have shown behavior that indicated pain agnosia. However, during subsequent follow-up (ranging from 16 months to 3 years and 7 months) all 5 were reported to manifest reactions to minor injuries or medical procedures, which indicated that they appropriately experienced pain. These 5 patients are excluded from the 21 who, while living in ameliorative environments, were at no time reported to neglect pain but showed reactions to physical injuries that were indicative of appropriate experience of pain. Despite the exclusion, there is a significant difference ($\chi^2 = 21.4$; p $<$ .001) in the manifestation of pain agnosia before and after transfer to an ameliorative living environment in a hospital or foster home.

---

* At times, such statements reflected puzzlement and surprise at the lack of complaint about hurting.

Return to the Symptom-Producing Domicile

Table 1 does not reveal that the exigencies of case management required that a child be returned at times, albeit temporarily, from the symptom-relieving environment of the hospital to the symptom-producing environment of the original domicile prior to foster home placement.

Twenty-one children returned from the hospital to live for a while in the domicile from which they had been hospitalized. Subsequently, documented signs of physical injury, a history of physical abuse or self-harming behavior, and pain agnosia were again in evidence in 10 of the 21. Four patients in this group exhibited a definite relapse into self-harming behavior with pain agnosia, which had disappeared during the prior period of hospitalization. One of these 4 patients was not available for follow-up in his original domicile where he remained on a permanent basis. The other 3 ultimately went to foster homes or other residential domiciles where they did not exhibit further evidence of self-harming behavior or neglect of pain. One of these 3 is the subject of the following case illustration.

CASE ILLUSTRATION

The patient, Mary G., was placed with an older sister in an emergency shelter home at the age of 2 years and 4 months following physical neglect and abuse by her alcoholic parents. After 3 months, she was transferred with her sister to a foster home, where both girls stayed until they were, respectively, 6 years and 9 months and 8 years and 7 months old.

At 4 years and 2 months of age, the patient was referred by the foster placement agency to the Johns Hopkins Hospital for evaluation of short stature. The child was hospitalized for 3 months, and a diagnosis of reversible somatotropin deficiency was established.

According to the social worker's report, the child would, prior to hospitalization, occasionally "throw herself on the floor in a tantrum . . . she falls down and bangs herself up quite a bit, but this does not seem to bother her at all. She rarely cries and has yet to really cry when she has cut herself severely as she has on many occasions. She has on many occasions hurt herself quite severely. For instance, on two occasions she cut herself with glass. One cut was right beneath her eye and the other one was on her thumb. Both of these cuts required stitches, yet the child did not seem to be upset about them and did not cry. At one time she had a vaginal infection which, according to the doctor, would have been quite painful when she urinated. However, she never mentioned any pain and the infection was only noted by the blood in her underpants.

She has banged up her head and other parts of her body on many occasions and has also broken her collar bone at one time without mentioning any pain or discomfort."

There was no evidence during the initial hospitalization that the patient harmed herself or manifested apparent pain agnosia. A nurse reported one incident when Mary, having slipped while running, cried.

After 3 months in the hospital, the girl had grown 1½ inches as compared with a normally expected ½ inch. When returned to her foster home, she initially continued to grow well, gaining 2 inches in 7 months. During this 7-month period, there were fewer injuries and more normal reactions to pain. By the time the girl was 5 years of age, she cried when given injections, when falling during the course of play, or otherwise hurting herself.

After her fifth birthday, the girl's growth rate had slowed for 10 months in comparison with the preceding 7 that followed discharge from the hospital. Her dentist remarked on his surprise that the child, contrary to expectations, did not show any pain reaction. Mary's foster mother reported: "Before she went in the hospital, it seemed like she was always falling, always hurting herself, and all. Well, she doesn't do this as much. But I still have the feeling that she still will not confide in us completely, if she hurts herself and doesn't feel good."

Concomitantly with a relapse into growth failure and pain agnosia, the girl also manifested a relapse into generally impaired behavior, poor eating and severe insomnia. For investigative as well as therapeutic purposes, sleeping medication (Seconal®, ¾ grain nightly) was prescribed to counteract the insomnia.*

A few days after the onset of treatment, the girl's foster mother reported improvement in sleeping, eating, and general behavior, including more normal reactions to the pain of injury. Two months thereafter the child was still reported to cry and complain when she suffered physical injury. The improvement lasted one additional month, at which time the foster mother became pregnant (possibly to justify her desire to discontinue fostering the two sisters); she also required surgery for a breast cyst.

Once again the child began to manifest self-harming behavior and pain agnosia, as well as a relapse into other symptoms, including excessive masturbation. The foster mother reported that, at times, the girl's pubic area looked raw; she could not understand why the child did not

---

* The medication was prescribed by Dr. Robert M. Blizzard who also supervised the treatment during its 5½ month course.

complain about pain when she took a hot bath. Although the foster mother continued to believe that the child's reactions to pain were otherwise normal, she also mentioned that the girl's legs had been recently covered with bruises. The origin of such bruises could not be explained, as Mary had made no complaints.

In response to the foster parents' requests, the patient and her sister were finally removed from the foster home, when Mary was 6 years and 9 months of age. While she had grown in stature 2.7 inches during the 12 months prior to removal, the girl grew at a rate of 3.3 inches per year during the first 9 months following that removal. Three of these 9 months were spent in two hospitals, and the remaining 6 in a new foster home. During these 9 months, no incidence of self-harming behavior or neglect of pain has been either observed or reported.

DISCUSSION

Pain agnosia was reversible in a short period of time in our patients, concomitantly with reversal of other symptoms subsequent to change of domicile and social environment. This fact takes the symptom of nonresponsiveness to painful stimuli in the syndrome of reversible somatotropin deficiency out of the realm of what might be termed irreversible pain-agnosic, or analgesic syndromes into the realm of syndromes of reversible agnosia.

Analgesic syndromes include (a) analgesia associated with an extra chromosome of the 12-15 group as exemplified in Beçak, Beçak, and Schmidt (1963); (b) congenital analgesia as exemplified by Ford and Wilkins (1938) and Critchley (1956); and (c) analgesia based on neuropathology as exemplified in Ogden, Robert, and Carmichael (1959).

Reversible pain-agnosic syndromes include: pain agnosia secondary to experimental sensorimotor and social deprivation in young animals (Melzack, 1968; Harlow, 1961, 1964; Harlow & Suomi, 1970; Miller, Mirsky, Caul, & Sakata, 1969); pain agnosia sporadically observed in some psychiatric, especially schizophrenic patients (Marchand, 1955, 1959; Petrie, 1967); pain agnosia as a sequel to stress, deprivation and trauma of imprisonment as reported in a description of a Siberian labor camp and inferred from the occurrence of extreme self-mutilation (Martschenko, 1969); and pain agnosia as a short-term sequel to sudden traumatic wounding, as experienced by a soldier in battle.

The three conditions of irreversible pain agnosia, classified as analgesia, share in common the trait of a presumed irreversible dysfunction of the central nervous system. In the four conditions classified as reversible pain agnosia, the central nervous system dysfunction may recover, partially if not completely, after the disappearance of circumstances that precipitate inhibition of the response to pain from which inhibition of pain recognition (pain agnosia) is inferred.

Analgesia syndromes typically are not associated with self-inflicted harm. Pain-agnosic syndromes may be accompanied by self-injury, though not inevitably so, but pain agnosia is not a prerequisite of self-injury. The compulsive self-injury of the Lesch-Nyhan syndrome (Nyhan, 1965), for example, is chronic despite the pain the patient evinces, which suggests that it may somehow be triggered by the biochemical anomaly that underlies the syndrome.

When self-inflicted injury and pain agnosia coexist, self-injury may well function to counteract a condition of cognitional starvation, such as occurs in conditions of sensory deprivation in which the cognitional input from one or more of the exteroceptive sensory sources—eyes, ears, skin, nose, and tongue—is insufficient.

At the mild end of the spectrum, self-harming behavior may take the form of nail-biting, tearing the skin of the nailbed, or plucking out hair. People who engage in such behaviors usually manifest them as replacements for a degree of deficiency in cognitional input from one or more of the senses. The deficiency is typically secondary to enforced inhibition. Thus, self-biting, tearing or plucking may occur when a child has a history of not being permitted to play but of being required to sit still and study instead, of being required to suppress barely controllable rage, or of electing not to talk when under pressure to do so.

More severe forms of self-injury would seem to require a more intense and prolonged history of insufficiency of activity of various types, as in the example of Siberian labor camp inmates mentioned above, and in institutionalized, deprived children (Spitz, 1945; Spitz & Wolf, 1946; Bowlby, 1952). Experimentally imposed social isolation in the young rhesus monkey (Harlow, 1961, 1964; Harlow & Suomi, 1970) suggests that both the severity and chronicity of self-injurious behavior may be related to the timing of social deprivation at a critical period early in development.

The nature of the blockage of pain recognition in either analgesia or pain agnosia cannot be fully specified. The distinction between the two is based on still incomplete knowledge as to the nature and timing of the onset of lack of pain, rather than on full knowledge of etiology.

The special feature of pain agnosia in the syndrome of psychosocial dwarfism, more precisely defined as dwarfism secondary to reversible somatotropin deficiency, is that it is reversible. Its reversal parallels the reversal of other symptoms of the syndrome, including growth failure. In all instances, symptom reversal is secondary to change of domicile and interpersonal environment. The key variable in the change of place to live and people to live with which is responsible for symptom reversal has not yet been identified. Thus, the symptoms of pain agnosia and self-injury, and their reversibility, cannot yet be fully and satisfactorily explained in the syndrome of psychosocial dwarfism. The fact that these and, apparently, all other symptoms of the condition are reversible, despite their severity, presents one with a special challenge, theoretically and empirically.

SUMMARY

In the sample of 32 patients with the syndrome of reversible somatotropin deficiency, changes in domicile from adverse environments where growth failure began and persisted to ameliorative environments, where catch-up growth took place, covaried significantly with decreased incidence of physical injury ($\chi^2 = 19.5$; p $< .001$); severe physical punishment or abuse ($\chi^2 = 56.2$; $p < .001$); self-inflicted injury ($\chi^2 = 44.8$; $p < .001$); and behavior indicating pain agnosia ($\chi^2 = 21.4$; $p < .001$). Corresponding symptoms, or their reversal, have been reported in prisoners of Siberian labor camps, lonely institutionalized infants, young animals experimentally deprived of sensorimotor and social stimulation, in some schizophrenic patients, and in sudden trauma as on the battlefield. When self-inflicted injury and pain agnosia coexist, self-injury may well function to counteract cognitional starvation under conditions of severe or partial sensory deprivation.

REFERENCES

BECAK, W., BECAK, M. L., & SCHMIDT, B. J.: Chromosomal trisomy of group 13-15 in two cases of generalized congenital analgesia. *Lancet*, 1963, 1, 664-665.

BOWLBY, J.: Maternal care and mental health. Geneva: *World Health Organization Monograph Series*, 1952.

CAPITANIO, M. A. & KIRKPATRICK, J. A.: Widening of the cranial sutures. A roentgen observation during periods of accelerated growth in patients treated for deprivation dwarfism. *Radiology*, 1969, 92, 53-59.

CRITCHLEY, M.: Congenital indifference to pain. *Annals of Internal Medicine*, 1956, 45, 737-747.

FORD, F. R., & WILKINS, L.: Congenital universal indifference to pain. *Bulletin of The Johns Hopkins Hospital*, 1938, 62, 448-466.

FREEDMAN, D. A.: The role of early mother/child relations in the etiology of some cases of mental retardation. In G. Farrell (Ed.), *Advances in Mental Science. I: Congenital Mental Retardation*. Austin: University of Texas Press, 1969.

HARLOW, H. F.: The development of affectional patterns in infant monkeys. In B. M. Foss (Ed.). *Determinants of Infant Behavior*. London: Methuen, 1961.

HARLOW, H. F.: Early social deprivation and later behavior in the monkey. In A. Abrams, H. Garner, & J. Toman (Eds.), *Unfinished Tasks in the Behavioral Sciences.* Baltimore: Williams & Wilkins, 1964.

HARLOW, H. F. & SUOMI, S. J.: Induced psychopathology in monkeys. *Engineering and Science,* 1970, 33, 8-14.

MARCHAND, W. E.: Occurrence of painless myocardial infarction in psychotic patients. *New England Journal of Medicine,* 1955, 253, 51-55.

MARCHAND, W. E.: Occurrence of painless acute surgical disorders in psychotic patients. *New England Journal of Medicine,* 1959, 260, 580-585.

MARTSCHENKO, A. T.: Die Waechter schaemen sich. (Trans.: The guards are embarrassed.) *Der Spiegel,* 1969, 23, 140-153.

MELZACK, R.: Early experience: A neuropsychological approach to heredity-environment interactions. In G. Newton & S. Levine (Eds.), *Early Experience and Behavior.* Springfield, Ill.: Charles C Thomas, 1968.

MILLER, R. E., MIRSKY, I. A., CAUL, W. F., & SAKATA, T.: Hyperphagia and polydipsia in socially isolated rhesus monkeys. *Science,* 1969, 165, 1027-1028.

NYHAN, W. L.: A disorder of uric acid metabolism and cerebral function in childhood. *Arthritis and Rheumatism,* 1965, 8, 659-664.

OGDEN, T. E., ROBERT, F., & CARMICHAEL, E. A.: Some sensory syndromes in children: Indifference to pain and sensory neuropathy. *Journal of Neurology, Neurosurgery and Psychiatry,* 1959, 22, 267-276.

PATTON, R. G. & GARDNER, L. I.: Influence of family environment on growth: The syndrome of "maternal deprivation." *Pediatrics,* 1962, 30, 957-962.

PATTON, R. G. & GARDNER, L. I.: *Growth Failure in Maternal Deprivation.* Springfield, Ill.: Charles C Thomas, 1963.

PATTON, R. G. & GARDNER, L. I.: Short stature associated with maternal deprivation syndrome: Disordered family environment as cause of so-called idiopathic hypopituitarism. In L. I. Gardner (Ed.), *Endocrine and Genetic Diseases of Childhood.* Philadelphia: Saunders, 1969.

PETRIE, A.: *Individuality in Pain and Suffering.* Chicago: University of Chicago Press, 1967.

POWELL, G. F., BRASEL, J. A., & BLIZZARD, R. M.: Emotional deprivation and growth retardation stimulating idiopathic hypopituitarism. *New England Journal of Medicine,* 1967, 276, 1271-1278.

POWELL, G. F., BRASEL, J. A., RAITI, S., & BLIZZARD, R. M.: Emotional deprivation and growth retardation simulating idiopathic hypopituitarism. II. Endocrine evaluation of the syndrome. *New England Journal of Medicine,* 1967, 276, 1279-1283.

REINHART, J. B., & DRASH, A. L.: Psychosocial dwarfism: Environmentally induced recovery. *Psychosomatic Medicine,* 1969, 31, 165-172.

SILVER, H. K. & FINKELSTEIN, M.: Deprivation dwarfism. *Pediatrics,* 1967, 70, 317-324.

SPITZ, R. A.: Hospitalism. *Psychoanalytic Study of the Child,* 1945, 1, 53-74.

SPITZ, R. A. & WOLF, K. M.: Anaclitic depression. *Psychoanalytic Study of the Child,* 1946, 2, 313-342.

WOLFF, G. & MONEY, J.: Relationship between sleep and growth in patients with reversible somatotropin deficiency (psychosocial dwarfism). *Psychological Medicine,* 1972, in press.

29

SEVERE DEPRIVATION IN TWINS: A CASE STUDY

Jarmila Koluchova, Ph.D.

Department of Psychology and Psychiatric Clinic, Palacky University
(Olomouc, Czechoslovakia)

CASE HISTORY

The Background of Deprivation

This is a case record of monozygotic twins, two boys *P.M.* and *J.M.*, born on 4 September 1960. Their mother died shortly after giving birth to them and for 11 months they lived in a children's home. According to the records their physical and mental development was normal at that stage. Their father then applied to take them into the care of his sister, but soon afterwards he remarried and the boys were again placed in a children's home until the new household could be established. This new family included 2 natural elder sisters of the twins, and 2 children (a boy and a girl) of the stepmother—6 children altogether, the oldest being 9 years old. The married couple M. bought a house in the suburbs of a small town where nobody knew them. All the subsequent events concerning the twins could only be reconstructed after their discovery in the autumn of 1967.

For 5½ years the twins lived in this family under most abnormal conditions. Some of the neighbors had no idea of their existence, others guessed there were some little children in the family although they had

Reproduced from the JOURNAL OF CHILD PSYCHOLOGY AND PSYCHIATRY, Vol. 13, 1972, pp. 107-114 with the permission of Microforms International Marketing Corp., licensee. © Pergamon Press Journal back files.

never seen them. It is surprising that this could happen in a quiet street of family houses where the environment and social relations are very like those in a village. During the trial, however, the people next door testified that they had often heard queer, inhuman shrieks which resembled howling, and which came from a cellar leading to the back court. The father was once seen beating the children with a rubber hose until they lay flat on the ground unable to move. The neighbors, however, did not interfere in any way because they did not want to risk conflict with the children's stepmother, who was known to be a selfish, aggressive woman, unwilling to admit anyone into her house.

In spite of very good and extensive child welfare services in the country, the true situation of these children was somehow undetected by the authorities concerned. The children had never been medically examined either routinely or because of illness. They were not registered for school attendance at the appropriate age. The relatives of the natural mother of the twins complained that the children were very poorly cared for, but their complaints were never properly investigated by a personal visit to the family from a social welfare officer. It was a quite exceptional case which, because of its severity, was scrutinized very closely by the jury when the matter came to light.

The central figure in the family, and in the tragedy involving the twins, was the stepmother. All the investigations, and especially the trial at the district and regional court, showed that she was a person of average intelligence, but egocentric, remarkably lacking in feeling, possessing psychopathic character traits and a distorted system of values. The father was a person of below average intellect, passive, and inarticulate; the stepmother dominated the family. Her own children (the first of them illegitimate and the second the product of a disturbed marriage which ended in divorce) were reared in early childhood by their maternal grandmother. The stepmother therefore had little experience with small children and showed no interest in them. When the twins joined the family she fed them, but the other aspects of their care were left to their father. This disinterest developed into active hostility towards the twins, and she induced a similar attitude towards them in other members of the family. The other children were forbidden to talk to the twins or to play with them. The father, who worked on the railways, was often away from home and took little interest in the boys. He probably realized that they were not receiving proper care but he was incapable of changing the situation. The twins therefore grew up lacking emotional relationships and stimulation, and were totally excluded from the family. Relationships between the other members of the family were also unnaturally cool due to the mother's abnormal personality. The elder children were well dressed, their homework was supervised and so on, but these measures seemed to have been motivated by the mother's ambitions. She accepted the 2 stepdaughters into the family though she preferred her own children, but with none of the children did she have a genuine maternal relationship.

The boys grew up in almost total isolation, separated from the outside world; they were never allowed out of the house or into the main living rooms in the flat, which were tidy and well furnished. They lived in a small, unheated closet, and were often locked up for long periods in the cellar. They slept on the floor on a polythene sheet and were cruelly chastised. They used to sit at a small table in an otherwise empty room, with a few building bricks which were their only toys. When one of their natural sisters was later examined for another reason, she depicted this scene in a drawing entitled "At Home."

The twins also suffered physically from lack of adequate food, fresh air, sunshine and exercise. At the end of August 1967 the father brought one of the boys to a pediatrician, asking for a certificate that his son was unfit to enter primary school. Because the boy looked as if he were 3 years old rather than 6, hardly walked, and was at first sight severely mentally retarded, the doctor agreed to postpone school entry, but insisted that the twins should be placed in a kindergarten, and that the family situation should be investigated by a social worker and a district nurse. The stepmother objected to these visits, criticized everybody concerned, and stressed that she was overworked at home. Probably anticipating further intervention by the welfare authorities, she tried to remove traces of the way in which the twins had been living.

Gradually it became clear that this was a case of criminal neglect. In December 1967 the twins were removed from the family and placed in a home for preschool children, while legal proceedings were taken against the parents. Several days after their admission to the home it was found that the twins suffered from acute rickets, a disease which has been practically eliminated in modern Czechoslovakia. The children were admitted to an orthopedic clinic and at the same time examined by a multi-disciplinary team.

PSYCHOLOGICAL FINDINGS

On admission to hospital attempts were made to assess the mental status of the twins. It was clear that the improvement in their living conditions during the 3 months prior to hospital admission had allowed some progress to take place. For example, on admission to the kindergarten the twins did not join in any activities but were timid and mistrustful. They had to be brought to the kindergarten in a wheelchair, because they could barely walk, and when given shoes could not walk at all. During their last 3 months with the family they were not locked in the cellar and their little room was better equipped, but at the same time the stepmother's negative attitude towards them became even more acute, because she saw in them the cause of the unwelcome interference from outside.

While in hospital, the children were psychologically examined. They were encouraged to become familiar with the testing room and adapted to it very well. At first it was impossible to use a diagnostic tool which required their direct cooperation, and the preliminary step in assessment was the observation of their spontaneous behavior, and in particular of their free and controlled play. Later it was possible to establish direct contact and to move on to more formal testing in which the author used Gesell's scale and the Terman-Merrill test.

The boys' restricted social experience and very poor general information was most strikingly shown in their reactions of surprise and horror to objects and activities normally very familiar to children of their age— e.g., moving mechanical toys, a TV set, children doing gymnastic exercises, traffic in the street, etc.

However, their inquisitiveness gradually prevailed, the reactions of terror disappeared, and they began to explore their environment, although often they were easily distracted. Their shyness with people was reduced during their stay in the children's home, and in the hospital ward they were the center of interest. They related to adults positively and indiscriminately, in a way that is typical of deprived children. Their reactions with other children were at an immature and uncontrolled level for their age.

The spontaneous speech of the boys was extremely poor. In order to communicate with each other they used gestures more characteristic of younger children. They tried to imitate adult speech, but could repeat only 2 or 3 words at a time with poor articulation. They could not answer questions, even if it was evident from their reactions that they had understood them. It was obvious that they were not used to speech as a means of communication.

Their spontaneous play was very primitive, and predominantly at first it was only the manipulation of objects, but imitative play soon developed. As they became familiar with the toys and with their surroundings in the clinic their play gradually reached more mature levels, but they continued to need adult intervention to initiate and develop a play activity and were unable to join in the play of other children.

A remarkable finding was that the boys could not understand the meaning or function of pictures. It was impossible therefore to measure the extent of their vocabulary by means of pictures, because they had never learned to perceive and understand them. We started therefore with pictures which were of the same size and color as the real objects which they represented. After repeated comparisons of picture and object, understanding of the relationship emerged and extended to a constantly widening range of phenomena.

The author felt that to express the boys' intellectual level in terms of an I.Q. would be quite inadequate. Their I.Q.s at that stage would have been within the range of imbecility, but qualitative analysis of their responses, their total behavior, and their considerably accelerated development since they had been taken away from their family, all unambiguously suggested that this was a case not of a primary defect in the sense of oligophrenia, but of severe deprivation. It seemed more appropriate therefore to consider their mental ages, which in December 1967 varied for both boys around the 3-year level, with a range of ± 1 year for separate component items. At this time their chronological age was 7 years 3 months.

After the period of hospitalization the children returned to the children's home where they made good progress. They began to participate with the children there; this was made easier for them by the fact that the other children in the home were some 2-3 years younger. Relationships with adults and children improved and they acquired much of the knowledge and many of the skills appropriate to preschool children. As their health improved so their motor abilities developed; they learned to walk, to run, to jump, to ride a scooter. Similar progress was also noted in their fine motor coordination.

After 6 months' stay in the children's home the boys were readmitted to the clinic for a short time to enable pediatric, audiological and psychological examinations to be made. Their mental age was by this time approximately 4 years, with a narrower range of passes on the component items than on the previous examination. There was evidence of considerable progress in habit formation, experience, and the development of knowledge.

THE FORENSIC PROBLEM

During the first period of hospitalization the investigating authorities requested a report from a forensic pediatrician, who in turn asked for a consultant psychologist's report. However, the problem of assessment seemed too complex to be handled on the basis of one or more consulting examinations. We therefore asked the investigating authorities to assign an expert psychologist to the case, who would have both the support of the court and the right of a forensic expert as well. The panel of forensic specialists followed the progress of the boys for a period of 6 months while they were in the children's home, and undertook careful control examinations during the second period of hospitalization. The problem for the panel was to assess the total developmental picture presented by the children, and to decide whether their disabilities were likely to have been congenital or acquired. The psychologist, moreover, had also to try to answer the question as to whether the twins were likely to grow up to become mentally and emotionally normal people.

The psychologist's report was of considerable importance in this case. It was necessary to disprove the statement of the defendant that the children had been defective from birth, and to prove that their disabilities were caused by severe neglect and lack of stimulation. For this reason a lengthy period of 6 months' observation was necessary, although it was apparent much earlier that the children were developing more quickly in the environment of the children's home than they ever had in their family home. During the trial, too, we had to refute the statement of the defendant and her husband that the children had had experience of picture material and play opportunities at home.

It was more difficult to answer the question about the future development of the twins. There was no evidence from the literature on deprivation, and because the case was so exceptional we had no personal experience to guide us. We could therefore only outline a probable prognosis and assume that in a good environment the children would develop in every respect, that their developmental deficits would show a tendency to be reduced, but that it was necessary to take into account the possible consequences of such severe deprivation on the development of personality. We pointed out to the judges some of the handicapping effects of this deprivation: entry to school delayed by 3 years, the probable necessity for the boys to attend a school for mentally retarded children, the effects on employment prospects, and the possibility of other difficulties in their social and intellectual development. We recommended that the children be placed as soon as possible in a compensating foster-home, on the grounds that even the best children's home could not be the optimal solution in the long term.

The main trial at the district court lasted for 3 days, all the forensic specialists being present. The defendant did not admit to having damaged the twins in any way. She denied that anything unusual had happened and maintained that they had been handicapped since infancy and that she had done her best for them by cooking and cleaning. She poured out her own troubles and expressed again her sense of being overworked. The court sentenced her to 4 years' deprivation of liberty and both father and stepmother also lost their parental rights.

In his final speech the public prosecutor and the chairman of the senate of judges, in confirming the verdict, emphasized the importance of the experts' reports in their evaluation of the defendant's guilt.

THE FURTHER DEVELOPMENT OF THE CHILDREN

In the school year 1968/1969 the boys remained in the preschool children's home. Their mental development was better than the original prognosis had suggested. Whereas some experts were doubtful about their educability, a psychologist's assessments showed that the retardation was diminishing and that the boys had reached a level of readiness for school. Because of their retarded speech, and relatively poor fine motor coordination and powers of concentration, we thought that a school for mentally retarded children was indicated as an initial step, since there were greater possibilities of individual teaching and a slower pace of learning.

Simultaneously with their starting school we tried to solve the problem of their foster-home placement. A number of families were willing to take the children, but we had to assess the motivation of the applicants very carefully, considering the personalities of the potential substitute parents, and existing family structures. Finally, in July 1969, the boys were placed with a family who have been able to accept them as natural and loved children. After 2 years observation we still consider this to be the optimal placement, although in the conventional sense the family is not a complete family at all. It consists of two unmarried middle-aged sisters, both intelligent, with wide interests, living in a pleasant flat, and capable of forming very good relationships with the children. One of these sisters had already adopted a baby girl some years before, and this child is now an intelligent, well-educated, 13-year-old. The second sister became the foster-mother of the twins. Our observations, and information from many sources, show that deep emotional bonds have been formed between the children and their foster-family, and many of the consequences of deprivation—e.g., a narrow outlook, a small range of emotional expression, etc.—which had remained during their stay in the children's home, are gradually diminishing. The boys have recollections of their original home, and though the foster-family tries to avoid reviving the past, the boys themselves will sometimes begin to talk about it; we also have touched on this during our psychological examinations. Until recently the boys did not have sufficient language ability to describe even in outline their life in their original family. If we compare their story now with the facts established during and before the trial, it is evident that their account is reliable. They have a completely negative attitude to their stepmother, and refer to her as "that lady," or "that unkind lady." They remember the names of their brother and sisters, and they recollect how they used to be hungry and thirsty, how they were beaten about the head (their scalps are badly scarred), and how they used to sit at the small table. The stepmother often carried them into the cellar, thrashed them with a wooden kitchen spoon until it broke, and put a feather-bed over their heads so that no one would hear their screaming.

For a long time they had a dread of darkness. They appreciated the physical warmth of their new home, the good food they received, and the fact that they were no longer beaten. During our first visit to them in the foster-home we had to reassure them that we would not take them away from their foster-mother.

In September 1969 they were admitted to the first class in a school for mentally retarded children. On the basis of our observations of the children in class, the teacher's records, and our further examinations, we found the boys soon adapted themselves to the school environment and began to excel their classmates. Their writing, drawing, and ability to concentrate improved remarkably in the second term, and it became clear that this type of school would not extend them sufficiently. Accepting that there was a risk involved, we recommended a transfer to the second class of a normal school from the beginning of the next school year. In spite of the difference in curriculum and teaching methods, they proved to be capable of mastering the subject matter of the normal school, and did well enough to suggest that they have the ability to complete successfully the basic 9-year school course which, however, they would finish at the age of 18 instead of the normal age of 15. Their schoolmates are 3 years younger, and it remains to be seen how relations between them and the twins develop, particularly as they enter puberty; the effects on the self-confidence and personality of the twins may be considerable but only extended observation will give us the answer to this.

A summary of the psychological test findings shows that in the 15 months from June 1968 to September 1969 the mental age of the twins

TABLE 1
WECHSLER INTELLIGENCE TEST SCORES (WISC)

Twin P. I.Q.		Twin J. I.Q.	
8 yr 4 months			
Verbal	80	Verbal	69
Performance	83	Performance	80
Full scale	80	Full scale	72
9 yr			
Verbal	84	Verbal	75
Performance	83	Performance	76
Full scale	82	Full scale	73
10 yr			
Verbal	97	Verbal	94
Performance	85	Performance	86
Full scale	91	Full scale	89
11 yr			
Verbal	97	Verbal	96
Performance	93	Performance	90
Full scale	95	Full scale	93

increased by 3 years; this was an immense acceleration of development, indicating how the change of living conditions provided a rapidly effective compensation for the consequences of earlier deprivation.

At first the children were assessed using Gesell's Developmental Scale and later the Terman-Merrill Scale in which their verbal level was markedly below non-verbal test items. Since the age of 8 years and 4 months the boys have been examined by means of the Wechsler Intelligence Scale (WISC). The test scores are presented in Table 1 and indicate the low-level verbal response initially, especially in the Twin J, and the consequent improvement over 3 years. Both children now seem to be functioning almost at an average level for their age.

CONCLUSIONS

This is a very exceptional case of deprivation, firstly because of the lengthy period of isolation, and secondly because of the unusual family situation which by outward appearances was a relatively normal and orderly one.

The children suffered from a lack of stimulation and opportunity for psychomotor development. The most severe deprivation, however, was probably their poverty of emotional relationships and their social isolation. The stepmother did not even partially satisfy their need for maternal nurturance. She was on the contrary, as the dominating person in the family, the instigator of hostile attitudes towards the children and an active agent in their physical and mental torment. The influence of the father was confined to occasional repressive actions. The stimulating influence of brothers and sisters was also lacking. Thus we may speak of a combination of outer and inner causes of deprivation, the inner or psychological ones being primary.

We have not found in the literature a similar case of such severe and protracted deprivation in a family. Following Langmeier and Matejcek (1968), we can define the situation of the twins as one of extreme social isolation, where the children are still fed by people, but are almost completely isolated from human society. Cases in the literature differ from ours both in recording a shorter period of social isolation, and in showing more severe consequences of deprivation than we have so far found. We assume, therefore, that the twins were able to bear the onerous situation better than any single child would have done.

Almost 4 years of observation of the twins have shown that in comparison with analogous cases in the literature their mental and social development has been very good. It is, however, difficult to foresee how their intelligence will develop, what the course of their development will be, how their personalities will be formed, and what residual effects of the deprivation will remain. The comparison between these monozygotic twins, living in essentially the same environment, will also be of interest.

SUMMARY

The author reports an unusual case of deprivation. Monozygotic twin boys were reared from age 18 months to 7 years in social isolation by a psychopathic stepmother and an inadequate father. On discovery, their mental age level was 3 years, but after treatment, a period in a children's home and approximately 2 years in a good foster-home, they have made remarkable progress and now appear about average for their age. Forensic aspects of the case are discussed, as are features of the foster-home placement, and the significance of twinship in the recovery. Residual effects of deprivation will be studied by an extended follow-up.

Because of the criminal behavior of the stepmother the children were exposed to living conditions which resembled those of an experimental situation. From the human standpoint, of course, it was an extremely cruel and unrepeatable experiment. From the scientific point of view, however, it was also a very valuable one. It will be important, therefore, to follow up the case over a long period, in the hope of contributing to a solution of some of the problems associated with mental deprivation.

Acknowledgments—In the presentation of this paper, the assistance of Professor A. D. B. Clarke, University of Hull, and Geoffrey A. Dell, Principal Psychologist at the Child Guidance Clinic, Glasgow, is gratefully acknowledged.

REFERENCES

LANGMEIER, J. & MATEJCEK, Z. (1968): *Psychická deprivace v detstvi.* Praha, SZDN.
PELIKAN, K., MORES, A., KOLUCHOVA, J., SIROKY, J., & FARKOVA, H. (1969): Tezky deprivační syndrom u dvojčat po dlouhodobé sociálni izolaci. *Cs. Pediat.,* 24, 980-983.

30

COMMENTARY ON KOLUCHOVA'S "SEVERE DEPRIVATION IN TWINS: A CASE STUDY"

A. D. B. Clarke, Ph.D.

Department of Psychology, The University of Hull (England)

It has long been appreciated that properly conducted studies of children who have suffered prolonged and severe social isolation would yield data of considerable significance for an understanding of human development. Thus, writing in 1801 of earlier and inadequate reports on feral children, Itard observed in very modern terms that "in those unenlightened times so retarded was the progress of science—given up as it was to the mania for explanation, the uncertainty of hypothesis, and to explanation undertaken exclusively in the armchair—that actual observation counted for nothing and that valuable facts concerning the natural history of man were lost . . . (nevertheless) the most striking and most general conclusion . . . is that these individuals were susceptible to no very marked improvement . . . doubtless because the ordinary method of social instruction was applied to their education. . . ."

Most studies of isolated children remain little more than anecdotal, and since these are always functioning at the lowest level, there is commonly the suspicion that they were mentally subnormal in the first place. Indeed, the mothers of such children tend, as did the mother in Koluchova's study, to use this as an excuse for their own conduct. More-

Reproduced from the JOURNAL OF CHILD PSYCHOLOGY AND PSYCHIATRY, Vol. 13, 1972, pp. 103-106 with the permission of Microforms International Marketing Corp., licensee. © Pergamon Press Journal back files.

over, more often than not, stories concerning feral children scarcely bear serious scrutiny (e.g., Ogburn and Bose, 1959) and there are many who believe that there is a good case for regarding these as recently abandoned psychotic or severely retarded children.

The cases so carefully described by Koluchova bear some resemblance to one discussed by Mason (1942) and Davis (1947). It has always been impressive that these two authors wrote their accounts independently and that the testimonies were not discrepant. Even so, the writers, being a speech consultant and sociologist, respectively, failed to ask some obvious psychological questions, the answers to which would have been of great value to developmental theory. Nevertheless, the findings on "Isabella" indicate in a most extreme form the existence of very powerful recovery processes commencing at the age of 6 years, after an almost life-long period of social isolation.

The bare facts were as follows:

In the 1930s, two illegitimate children, each aged about 6 years, who had been kept locked in attics for virtually their whole lives, were discovered in different areas in the United States at about the same time. When rescued, neither could talk, both were rachitic and both functioned at imbecile level. The more deprived of the two did not receive any special treatment and her relative status did not alter; her mother was herself subnormal. The other, "Isabella," had been with her deaf mute mother alone in a darkened attic where both had been imprisoned by her mother's father. She received highly skilled treatment, learned to speak in sentences within 2 months, was reading and writing in 9 months and had a vocabulary of 2000 words after 16 months. Her I.Q. trebled in 18 months, and after two years she was considered intellectually normal. There seems little doubt that on final follow-up at age 14 this girl was considered normal. It seems, then, that 6 years of considerable isolation (though not from a deaf-mute mother) resulting in gross retardation, did not predestine the child to an unalterable condition. Her progress was, indeed, remarkably rapid. The other case was unaltered, but whether because of severer isolation or lack of skilled treatment or because of congenital factors, or a combination of these, is unknown.

Two similar cases of 4- and 5-year-old boys reared in complete isolation by psychopathic parents, have been reported in Poland by Szuman (1958). On discovery, they could not speak, could not stand upright, were rachitic and "gave the impression of being savages." Although the paper did not aim to discuss the subsequent development of the children, and indeed offers a very fragmentary account, it appears that after about a year these boys began to speak in short sentences. On discovery, their condition could "be likened to that of an infant. However, their development proceeded at a much faster rate, e.g., learning to walk." It is not clear whether active psychological treatment was in fact undertaken and, as in some other cases, potentially valuable information was not recorded.

It is possible to make a direct comparison between the case of "Isabella" and the Koluchova twins. In both cases, early history was normal (and the twins spent the first year of life in a children's home followed by 6 months in the care of an aunt) but the subsequent isolation of "Isabella" seems to have been more profound, although within that situation there was no indication of cruelty from the deaf-mute mother. On rescue at the ages of 6 and 7, respectively, the Davis and Koluchova children were all rachitic but "Isabella" showed a greater intellectual deficit and even rudimentary speech was not present. While "Isabella's" initially very low I.Q. trembled in 18 months of very active treatment following discovery, the mental ages of the twins increased from 3 to 8 years in a 2-year period, and I.Q.s from about 40 to 95 and 93 respectively in 4 years, a slower rate of advance but nevertheless indicating an immense acceleration of development. By the age of 10 they appeared already to be approximately to the level of relative ability ascribed to their father and further small I.Q. increments are still occurring up to age 11.

Attention should be particularly drawn to a number of points of great theoretical interest in Koluchova's paper. First, the fact that the twins spent the first 18 months of life in nutritionally normal environments may be relevant. Brain growth is considerable during this period, and evidence from malnutrition in animals, and inferences from human studies (e.g., Cravioto, DeLicardia and Birch, 1966) suggest that protein deficiency may have a direct and irreversible effect upon brain growth during the early months. It is also probable that the bases for perceptual and linguistic development were laid during this period. Second, the failure of the twins to understand the meaning of pictures and their relation to reality, is itself testimony to the length and severity of their deprivation. The successful use of special techniques not unlike those employed by Itard in 1800-1805, showed clearly the role of learning in the development of cognitive processes.

The Koluchova paper is the most detailed account in the literature of the facts surrounding the discovery of isolated children, of their particular deficits and of their response to remedial measures. While in many ways the twins remain impaired, being educated with children 3 years their junior, their changing status has indeed been remarkable. Malnutrition, severe cruelty, neglect and considerable isolation (though not from each other) has not predestined them to a permanent condition of severe subnormality.

In extreme form, these findings are congruent with those on other children following severe but less depriving experiences (e.g., Dennis, 1960; Rathbun, di Virgilio and Waldfogel, 1958). They indicate, among other things, the inadequacy of theories stressing the over-riding importance of early experience in the formation of later characteristics. Indeed, psychological experiences which have anything other than transitory effects must involve learning in its broadest sense. What seems to be important is not so much the early learning as the extent and duration of its subsequent reinforcement or non-reinforcement (Clarke, 1968). The relatively late age of rescue (7 years) from $5\frac{1}{2}$ years of almost unprecedently bad conditions, as well as the responsiveness to remediation, underlines the resilience of these children, and has a bearing on such concepts as critical periods of development. Where studies stress the permanency of the effects of early deprivation one should examine carefully the new situation in which the child finds himself and ask whether it continues to reinforce earlier experiences. Indeed, the pessimism with which the whole area has been surrounded may have itself contributed to a passivity in the subsequent treatment of deprived children.

One awaits with the greatest interest further reports on the progress of the Koluchova twins. The author has the opportunity of conducting a unique long-term study which is already, and will be more so in the future, rich in its implications for our understanding of human development. Although there are many matters about these children which must unfortunately remain unknown, the factual account given does shed some light on the important question of the interaction of constitutional and environmental factors in the development of human characteristics.

SUMMARY

Koluchova's on-going study of twin boys who suffered extreme deprivation between 18 months and 7 years, and who thereafter received remedial treatment, is discussed in the context of relevant literature. Malnutrition, cruelty, neglect and considerable isolation over $5\frac{1}{2}$ years did not predestine them permanently to the condition of severe subnormality which they had manifested on discovery. Their greatly accelerated development confirms similar work and sheds some light on the interaction of constitutional and environmental factors in the formation of human characteristics. Results underline the inadequacy of theories stressing the over-riding importance of early experiences for later growth.

Acknowledgments—I am very grateful to Mr. G. A. Dell, who first brought this report to my notice, and to Mrs. M. M. Radon, who translated Szuman's article for me.

REFERENCES

CLARKE, A. D. B. (1968): Learning and human development—the forty-second Maudsley Lecture. *Br. J. Psychiat.*, 114, 1061-1077.

CRAVIOTO, J., DELICARDIE, E. R. & BIRCH, H. G. (1966): Nutrition, growth and neurointegrative development: An experimental and ecologic study. *Pediatrics*, 39, 319-372.

DAVIS, K. (1947): Final note on a case of extreme isolation. *Am. J. Sociol.*, 45, 554-565.

DENNIS, W. (1960): Causes of retardation among institutional children. *J. Genet. Psychol.*, 96, 47-59.

MASON, M. K. (1942): Learning to speak after years of silence. *J. Speech Hearing Disord.*, 7, 295-304.

OSBORN, W. F. & BOSE, N. K. (1959): On the trail of the wolf-children. *Genet. Psychol. Monogr.*, 60, 117-193.

RATHBUN, C., DI VIRGILIO, L., & WALDFOGEL, S. (1958): The restitutive process in children following radical separation from family and culture. *Am. J. Orthopsychiat.*, 28, 408-415.

SZUMAN, W. (1958): Obraz rozwoju dwóch chlopców ze skrajnej izolacji (bezposrednio po zabraniu ich z domu). *Szkola Specjalna*, XIX, 241-254.

PART VII: CLINICAL STUDIES

31

THE BURNING AND THE HEALING
OF CHILDREN

Richard Galdston, M.D.

Assistant Professor of Psychiatry, Harvard Medical School
Chief, In-Patient Psychiatric Consultation Service,
The Children's Hospital Medical Center (Boston)

*This is a report of the burning and the healing of 100
children who were admitted to the surgical wards of The
Children's Hospital Medical Center between 1964 and 1970.
It comprises a description of the forces and circumstances
which resulted in the burning of these children, and an
account of the process of their healing. All of these children
were burned badly enough to require hospitalization for
periods of weeks to months. All had second or third degree
burns. Four died as a result of their burns.*

In making this study, I first followed 40 consecutive admissions for
burns during 1964-1965, and then studied 60 more cases over the next
five years. All but four of the initial group came from middle-class

Reprinted from PSYCHIATRY: JOURNAL FOR THE STUDY OF INTERPERSONAL PROCESSES,
Vol. 35, February 1972, pp. 57-66. Copyright 1972 by The William Alanson White
Psychiatric Foundation, Inc.

This paper was presented at a Scientific Program in honor of George E. Gardner,
Ph.D., M.D., at the Kresge Auditorium of the Massachusetts Institute of Technology,
Boston, Mass., November 30, 1970. The author wishes to express appreciation to Dr.
Robert E. Gross, Surgeon-in-Chief of Cardiovascular Surgery of The Children's Hospi-
tal Medical Center, for his encouragement, and to Angelo J. Eraklis, M.D., Assistant
Professor of Surgery, Davis S. Trump, M.D., formerly Chief Resident in Surgery, Mrs.
Marilyn Blake, R.N., Misses Carole Arenge, R.N., Eleanor Colcord, R.N., Jane Tundorf,
R.N., Carole Cerusulo, R.N., and Mrs. Mary Gavin Hull, M.S.S.W., for their assistance
in gathering case material.

families which were intact and without evidence of parental neglect. In the cases seen between 1965 and 1970, there was an increase in the number of families with obvious marital, economic, social, and psychological troubles.

The method of study was clinical; 45 of the children and their parents were interviewed upon the day of admission or shortly thereafter. The others were interviewed at some point during their hospitalization. All the children were followed throughout their stay on the surgical wards with frequent observations during the course of their treatment—at times of debridement in tub baths, before and after skin grafting, and during casting or traction to the extremities when necessary. In addition to my direct observations and interviews, reports on experiences with these children were presented at weekly meetings by the nursing staff of the surgical wards, the social workers, and the play ladies; they provide a source of data essential to this study. Only a few of the children have been followed since discharge from the hospital.

The ages of the children ranged from 10 months to 16 and a half years at the time of the burn. There were 68 boys and 32 girls, with more boys than girls in every age group, except that between the ages of one and a half and 3 years there were 14 girls and 10 boys. Two-thirds of the children were below the age of 5 when burned.

Two-thirds of the children were inside their homes when burned— the largest number in the kitchen, and the rest, in this order, in the living room, bathroom, or bedroom. The remainder were burned in their own or neighboring yards, with the exception of 4 adolescent boys who suffered gasoline burns while away from home.

Fourteen children were burned by adults, 10 were burned by other children, and 76 were themselves the immediate cause of their burns.

Of the 14 children burned by adults, 4 were victims of arson, and 5 had been thrust into hot water, stoves, or radiator pipes on purpose. Five appeared to have been burned by accident.

Eight of the 10 children burned by other children were adolescent boys who were fooling around with gasoline or open fires. One was an adolescent girl who was scalded on purpose by her brother. Another was an infant whose plastic baby bottle was ignited by an older sibling.

Of the 76 children who caused their own burns, two-thirds did so by touching hot objects and one-third burned themselves by playing with flames—matches, candles, or open fires. All of the children who burned themselves by touching hot objects were below the age of 6, and all those who burned themselves by playing with open flames were over 16.

THE BURNING

There are a number of features which are peculiar to a burn. It is an event, a happening, which punctuates the child's conduct of his ordinary life. It results in an acute, severe, and unexpected disruption of his state of health, and is in contrast to an illness, which is understood by child and parents to result from forces beyond the ordinary and out of their control.

A burn occurs as the outcome of a lapse in prevention. Our attitude toward thermal power in the conduct of our lives leads to a fail-safe system of protection. Beginning at an early age we caution our children with the word "hot" even before they learn to speak. An awareness of this hazard early becomes an integral part of family life. For the child, a burn is betrayal by his environment. For his parents, it is a lapse, a failure of their protective system to take care of their child. Consequently, both parents and child feel compelled to reconstruct a skein of causality in which to fix the events, the appetites, and the circumstances which led to this disastrous experience.

The burning of a child requires the coincidence of three factors: an agent to cause the burn, the presence of a child for burning, and the absence of protective adult intervention at the moment of burning.

(1) *The Presence of a Burning Agent*

Most of the burns were produced by agents that are commonly available in the home: matches, cigarette lighters, stoves, and hot coffee. Leaf and rubbish fires and outdoor barbecues are a warm-weather hazard. Hot water vaporizers used to treat respiratory illness are a cold-weather danger. The ready availability of electrical appliances in the home and the common use of gasoline for outdoor machinery render the home replete with potential sources of hazards for serious burns as an integral part of common daily life.

(2) *The Presence of a Child*

Most of the younger children were under the supervision of an adult at the time of the burn. Several of them were in the care of an older sibling or a young baby-sitter when they burned themselves. The whereabouts of the older boys who were burned by gasoline were known to their parents, although the parents were unaware of the sons' specific activities. The children who were burned by adults by accident were standing close to them when a hot liquid scalded them or a flammable fluid ignited them.

(3) *The Absence of Parental Intervention*

The presence of parental attention sufficient to provide protective intervention was the most complex of the three elements. There were 73 children from intact homes with a father and a mother living together, and 27 children from homes where the father was absent.

Beyond the issue of the physical presence of both parents, the question of the integrity and viability of the marital relationship of the parents proved to be a significant variable in the vulnerability of the older boys who burned themselves by playing with open flames. All of the 24 boys 6 years and older who were burned by playing with fire came from homes in which there was significant marital strife, as evidenced by statements of the parents or their behavior during the course of the son's hospitalization. Following are examples of this:

While his parents were asleep on New Year's Day, Jeffrey, a boy of 6, the oldest of three children and his mother's pride and joy, ignited his pajamas with a leaky cigarette lighter which his mother had given to his father for Christmas. The mother spoke of the boy in terms befitting a lover—"He's everything I have," "When he's ready for me, I am ready for him,"—and the boy was observed to pat his mother's pregnant abdomen, greeting her, "Hello, Fatso!" Though the home was intact at the time, it appeared that both parents viewed the boy as the man of the house. This child had never been injured until one month previously when his father broke his leg at work and had to remain at home. Shortly thereafter, the boy fell off a cliff, breaking his arm. While still in a cast, he burned himself with his father's lighter. Some months after the boy's discharge, his father left the home.

Peter, an 11-year-old boy, was playing in the yard next door when the neighbor's son ignited a can of gasoline, which he sprayed on Peter, producing serious burns. Peter's father had divorced his mother shortly after his birth and had ceased all contact with them. His mother remarried some years later, but Peter had never accepted his stepfather, whom he always referred to by his first name. Immediately upon being burned, he began to call his stepfather "Daddy" and asked to be adopted by him legally. It is of note that Peter had been severely injured three times previously while playing in the same neighbor's yard, twice by bites from the neighbor's dog, which was a known neighborhood menace and was ultimately exterminated on court order.

Sam, a 16-year-old boy, was badly burned while fooling around by tossing matches on open gasoline which he and a friend were using as a cleaning agent. When queried, he accounted for his actions with: "I thought I could get away with it. Sure, I knew the danger of gasoline but I thought if I moved fast enough, I could make it." Both he and his mother spoke in openly disparaging terms of the father as an ex-drunk, a failure and a no-account.

The absence of parental intervention to protect the younger children who were burned by touching hot objects was of two sorts: that due to absolute neglect in which the child was left exposed to the abuse of other children or to other serious hazards, and that due to a relative decrease from a habitually high level of parental attention. Examples of each type follow:

An example of absolute neglect is provided in the case of Cheryl, an 8-year-old, who was allegedly immersed in a tub of scalding hot water while in the care of a teen-age baby-sitter. It was not clear whether she fell or was pushed, but she suffered severe burns and disfiguring scars. Two years later she was charged with the murder of an 18-month-old sibling by asphyxiation with a plastic bag. Her parents maintained total and constant neglect of her, disowning any responsibility or concern for her.

The relative decrement in parental attention is exemplified in the case of John, age 2, who spilled a pan of hot water on himself while reaching for his plate, which had been put on top of the stove to keep it out of his reach. He had been adopted shortly after birth by a childless, middle-aged couple and never had been out of the sight of one or the other of his parents until this day, when they were resting because they had spent a sleepless night. The day before they had received notification of the court hearing to legalize the adoption. The child had been born out of wedlock to a former girl friend of the husband. The adoptive parents felt their own marriage was questionable because of a difference in their religious backgrounds. Plagued with guilt, anxiety, and fatigue, they lay down to rest, entrusting the care of the child to a visiting relative, whose response to the child's accident was so immediate that she herself was burned by the falling hot water.

Sandra, 2½ years of age, was playing at her mother's side while she was drinking a cup of coffee in the kitchen. The mother, who was two months pregnant, suddenly recalled that she had left the washing machine running in the basement and left abruptly without commenting to her daughter, who promptly climbed up on the table to look in the coffee cup and pulled over the coffee pot, scalding herself.

John, 3 years of age, was playing at his mother's side while she was ironing. The telephone rang and she went to answer it without commenting to the boy, who then reached up onto the board pulling the iron over and burning his hand.

Scott, a 4-year-old boy, was his father's pride and joy and constant companion. He was allowed to stand next to his father while he ignited a faulty camp stove which blew up, badly burning the boy and superficially burning the father. The stove had malfunctioned two weeks previously.

These cases are cited to illustrate the coincidence of the presence of the burning agent and the child and the absence of parental intervention as the outcome of a complex of vectors which derive from intrapsychic, interpersonal, and developmental forces. In a discussion of these forces, the items of curiosity, impulse, and inhibition warrant consideration.

There were 51 children 5 years of age and younger who burned themselves by touching hot objects. In every instance in which it could be ascertained, the burn occurred in a setting in which maternal attention had been diverted abruptly away from the child without the benefit of verbal warning. Recapitulation of the event suggested that the direction of the child's curiosity had been determined by the object which last held the mother's attention.

Curiosity can be defined as the desire to engage the mind with anything novel. The motor response to this appetite of the mind appears to have been held in abeyance by the inhibiting effect of maternal attention. As long as the mother's presence was felt by the child he did not act upon his appetite. Her recognition of his being afforded a barrier between his curiosity and its motor discharge in impulse. For the young child without speech as communication, parental recognition is a visual condition in which the parent sees and can be seen by the child.

Young children will play freely and adventurously in a clinic waiting room or in a park as long as the mother remains seated on a bench. The moment the mother rises to move, the children scoot back to her side. The state of maternal visual surveillance is a source of a sense of security for the young child which appears to derive from his awareness of her capacity to provide inhibition to the impulses pressing to fulfill his curiosity. It is as if the child believed in the adage, "Out of sight, out of mind," which is exemplified in the early childhood game of peek-a-boo.

As the child acquires speech and mobility, parental recognition and its inhibiting function take on an auditory dimension. Mother and child each develop the capacity to monitor the sounds of the other and respond to deviations from the basal level of noise. At this age, inhibition of impulse no longer depends entirely upon the parent's visible presence. It can be communicated through words, the echoes of which reverberate in the child's mind, helping to control the impulsive realization of his curiosity. A mother notes a sudden silence and says to her older daughter, "Go find out what Johnny is doing and tell him to stop!" It is noteworthy that at least 5 of the children over 5 years of age who burned themselves by playing with fire did so in the early morning on a weekend or holiday, igniting their nightclothes while their parents slept.

For the young child, the desire to engage the mind and the impulse to touch with the body are as one. When looking at something he wants, the young child will say, "Gimme that, let me see it *in my hand!*" Sight and action are like a reflex arc with a negligible time lag. Drawing a hot bath, starting a vaporizer, ironing clothes, drinking coffee, placing a dish out of reach above the stove can indicate an object for desire. But the motor response to curiosity is interrupted by the mother's presence in recognition of the child, which itself functions as his inhibition. In her absence, no matter how brief, the object which last held her attention remains as a memento. It is hard to know if the child reaches for the object or the missing mother.

In a consideration of these forces of curiosity, impulse, and inhibition, the role of parental presence in the prevention of burns appears clear. Yet parents leave their children frequently, and in their absence the wonder is that there are not more young children burned. The mothers' leave-taking of our patients was sudden and without comment. The attention of the patients was left in a free-floating state. Without a warning that might stay the child's attention, which had been held by the mother, it appears to have fallen from her onto that which was last hers.

The young child's attention, the source of the raw material for curiosity, can be viewed as the property of a relationship with his mother. Whither she goes, he goes, with her. They enjoy a meeting of the minds about a common object. When she leaves, his attention stays with her or falls onto her things unless she detaches his attention from her with a word in recognition of her leave-taking. Then his attention appears to be fixed, planted, stayed—the process seems similar to that in which a dog can be stayed from wandering by his master's voice.

The inhibitory effect of parental attention depends upon two elements. It requires that the parents have emotional energy available sufficient to identify with the child in empathic anticipation of his particular pattern of curiosity. The degree of this empathic anticipation is highly variable. In some cases the mothers knew what the children were doing all of the time. In others, they were quite casual. It is not the absolute level of anticipation that seems to be important, but rather any significant reduction in that level. It is a reciprocal affair. The child comes to rely upon the mother to anticipate a certain amount of his behavior and he accommodates to that expectation. Any significant decrement in her attention because of preoccupation with grief, guilt, or other personal issues throws an unaccustomed burden upon the inhibitory capacities of the child himself and, without any warning, he is unable to take up the resultant slack in their system of surveillance.

The second element upon which the inhibitory effect of parental attention depends is the ability to recognize the child as he actually is without major distortions about his age, competence, or wisdom, so that the child will hear words chosen to convey an accurate recognition of himself and not another.

The element of parental surveillance was particularly important in the several cases of young children who were burned by their parents while accompanying them in pursuits that were appropriate to parental peers, but not to children. The mother in one case and the fathers in two spoke of their small children as pals and buddies, endowing them with maturity which could not be theirs.

Among the older boys, the parental distortion followed the oedipal rule. Each of these boys viewed himself and was seen by his parents as the man of the house, the special case who would get away with it! The parents of one boy who was home on weekend leave recuperating from gasoline burns allowed him to ride his motorbike while his legs were still in casts!

For the older children, fire as a source of a sense of power presented a compelling appeal to their desire. It is difficult to epitomize the appeal of the open flame. Children are taught to put out the flames of matches and candles long before they are allowed to light them. The forbidden pleasure associated with fire is indicated in the terms used by the parents, "I caught him playing with matches," in the attitudes of the nurses who reported "catching" the children scratching their skin grafts, and in the claims of children that the fires they tried to extinguish were started by "older" boys. At least three of the children who burned themselves with fire did so while trying to control its spread. They were victims of their efforts to control the expression of their impulse rather than the impulse itself. The mental counterpart of their efforts to control their impulses was manifest by their behavior in the hospital, which commanded maximum intervention by the staff. The statements they made and the emotion they expressed served as an admission of defeat in their inability to regulate their impulses and a plea for the substitution of adult inhibition, control, and punishment. There was strong circumstantial evidence to indicate that several of the children who burned themselves by fire did so out of an unconscious sense of guilt at having arrogated a power which they felt was not their due.

It is of interest that none of the children had a history of being fire-setters, although several were the victims of known fire-setters, and a few had played with matches.

THE HEALING

About the healing of the burned child, surgeons and nurses have been heard to say, "There is nothing worse than caring for a burned child." This complaint is made with pride and despair in appreciation of how the need to provide the indispensable functions of being for the child tax and penetrate the depths of one's own being. The outstanding feature of the process is the extent of contact between the caring person and the child.

The healing of burned children in the hospital can be considered in two phases, an acute phase comprising admission and early treatment, and a secondary phase comprising the period up to grafting.

At admission, the child is often in shock. He may feel comparatively little pain because of the destruction of skin and nerve endings. Usually the parents do not appreciate the severity of the burn. Partly this is due to their need to defend against the emotional assault of the trauma with denial. Also, the burned skin initially may appear only reddened, and once the area is covered the child is docile.

The specific treatments employed for these patients varied somewhat, but in all cases the basic surgical principles followed were support of metabolic processes, protection from infection, debridement of wounds with baths and dressing changes, skin grafting, protection from contracture by physiotherapy, and splinting or traction of extremities.

Within five to ten days the child usually has responded to initial therapy aimed at restoring lost electrolytes, overcoming shock, and protecting against sepsis. With the removal of the dressings the parents come to recognize the severity of tissue destruction. Although in general it is desirable to encourage frequent visiting by parents, the stress of beholding the extent of the burn may warrant less frequent visits temporarily to spare the child the extra burden of parental anxiety.

The secondary phase of management commences at this stage with the determination of the severity of tissue destruction, and continues until skin grafting can be begun. The removal of dead tissue is a prerequisite for the grafting of new skin regardless of the specific treatment techniques. Debridement involves the use of frequent baths and the repeated changing of dressings for the burned areas.

The nurse and the child form a couple, charging each other with the task of care and of being cared for. The establishment and maintenance of this exchange is a collaborative enterprise. The nurse and the child contribute increments of activity in accordance with the particular requirements of the task. Their reciprocal accommodation of activity to passivity accomplishes the work of the healing process.

The beginning of the baths, which are usually daily, burdens the child with several specific assaults. The child is obliged to reveal to himself and to others the extent to which the surface which encloses his body has been destroyed. He is required to watch as blackened bits and pieces of himself float away into the bath water. This sight occurs in a setting which is heir to a tradition of intimate pleasures for most children. The use of auxiliary heaters to warm the bathroom, record players, story-telling, and bath toys for diversion have proven helpful in supporting the child, and the attendance of a male physician has been helpful in attenuating the intensity of the experience. The bath is warm and the child is tended by nurses who patiently support him in what once upon a time was an experience of particular closeness between mother and child.

The bathing of the burned child produces intense, rapid, and extreme changes in affect and behavior in the child. The sudden shift from shrieks of anxiety and pain into bouts of joyful water play is perplexing. The change from accusations of attempted murder to cooing proclamations of love is disconcerting.

A 9-year-old boy fought violently while in the tub, screaming, "You are mean. You want to hurt me. You're trying to kill me!" Abruptly he stopped and squirted water into the air with his cupped hands. "Hey, super-nurse, look how high I can squirt the water. Hey, look at me!"

Nor can these changes in affect and behavior be correlated with the pain or the pleasure of the bath.

A 7-year-old boy chattered gaily about his hope that he would get to fight in Viet Nam while his nurse pulled off dried scabs which failed to soak loose. But later, when the nurse approached him with soothing vaseline gauze, he screamed, "Aah, get her out of here, she's trying to kill me!"

The changing of dressings, wet or dry, in or out of the tub, poses a set of stresses peculiar to the burned child. In effect the child must moult his dead skin to make way for the grafting of new skin. Removal of the dressings facilitates this process and is crucial to treatment. The process is painful and causes anxiety because the dressing concealed from the child the extent of his bodily damage. Removal of the dressing confronts him with the visual evidence until it is concealed by the application of a new dressing.

It has proven preferable to have the child pull off his dressings insofar as he is able. This requires patience and sensitivity in establishing a collaboration with the child in which the necessity is held before him by others while the motor response is preserved as his. Regression is reduced when the child can retain the active role in removing the dressing. When the child is the passive member from whom the dressing is pulled off, regression ensues.

An 8-year-old girl who had burned herself while playing with matches dawdled, teased, and played while efforts were made to get her to remove a sticky dressing after her bath. In exasperation her physician suddenly pulled off the dressing she had been guarding, which left several bleeding points. The child became glassy-eyed, and mute, and began to smear the blood with her hands on her face and onto others. The next day when the nurse urged her to become more active, she bit the nurse, and for several days thereafter she spoke baby talk and was incontinent.

The need to guard against infection requires techniques of asepsis. Isolation may be employed for varying lengths of time and poses a special stress on the child. The restriction of contact with other human beings to the touch of surgically gloved hands, usually painful, and to the sight of masked eyes brings loneliness to the child. The extent of the burn often precludes holding or cuddling, resulting in a profound deprivation of sensory stimulation.

The use of volunteers, aides, and others for visits to the isolated child can be very helpful if they are willing to read to the child for long periods of time without expecting any return in understanding or gratitude. It is the voice of a real live present person to which the child responds. The child in isolation can be mute and immobile while a television set blabs away. At the sound of a nurse's voice, even when directed to another nurse, the child becomes animated and cries. Record players, radios, and television are of questionable utility here, except inasmuch as they entertain personnel while they spend time talking to the child.

The child in isolation quickly stops talking and then stops expressing any emotion in any way unless he is directly called by name, whereupon he starts crying out. It appears that personal recognition has become a prerequisite for the letdown and delivery of the expression of emotion.

Reversal of sleep rhythm, with sleep during the day and wakefulness at night, is common. The recurrence of repetitive dreams reenacting the circumstances of the burn is a common experience for these children. Occasionally such dreams will spill over into the waking state as hallucinations or hypnopompic phenomena associated with tremulousness and the facial expression of great fright.

Regression in behavior is the rule with these children. They give up all of the more recently acquired skills. Speech is greatly affected, with a reversion to baby talk and a frequent loss of the distinction between self and others in the child's mind.

A 5-year-old boy said to his nurse during his bath, "I am a bad boy." The nurse replied, "You are a good boy." The child said, "No, you are a bad nurse!"

The nurse asked, "Now who are you?" to which the boy replied, "I am Mrs. Henrietta Jones" [his mother's name].

The severity of regression in behavior correlates clearly with the degree of guilt which the child felt about the circumstances of his burn. Those children who caused their burns by playing with matches or other sources of flames displayed the most profound regression in behavior and presented the greatest difficulty in ward management.

The danger that contractures of the neck or extremities will develop as the result of scarring often necessitates the application of splints and traction. The associated immobilization reduces the child's ability to gratify his desires through his own activity. The child is deprived of the proprioceptive stimulation of active movement and the relief from nervous tension afforded by physical activity.

A 30-month-old male had been deliberately immersed in a tub of scalding water in the second known attempt on his life. The danger of contractures from his burns was such that all four extremities were immobilized in traction. Within several days the child had developed the musculature of an infant Hercules from pulling against the weights. He had worked out four of his teeth from grinding and gnashing his jaws. His struggle was incessant. The provision of a rubber bone to chew on and a rubber and cloth toy to squeeze and the placement of his bed and traction upon rollers so that he could be rocked, afforded some relief from these stresses.

It is important to maintain a positive nutritional balance to promote healing. The child often complains that the smell of his burns takes away his appetite, and efforts to disguise the odor can be useful. With the younger children the use of feeding games and the method of sharing the meal by eating alternate mouthfuls have been effective in overcoming the reluctance to eat. It is also helpful to try not to change dressings near mealtime because the sight and smell inhibit appetite.

The turning point in the healing process is the application of skin grafts. Even though the donor site for the graft adds another denuded area, the children experience significant and predictable relief at this point. They seem to do better in every way once the grafting process can be begun. The quality of surgical attention shifts from the removal of the dead parts to growth of new living parts, and the child is spared the pain and anxiety of debridement.

As the grafts take, they often itch intensely, and the need to guard against scratching perpetuates the intense involvement between nurse and child about his skin.

When the integrity of the grafts is established, the healing process takes on a new dimension in the restoration of mobility as the means of returning to activity. The inhibition of thought and action consequent upon the burn and its healing leaves many of these children severely restricted in their initiative from fear, guilt, and shame. Many of the children retain a hunched-over posture or a shuffled gait long after their physical restrictions could account for it.

Most of these children were lost to psychiatric follow-up at discharge. Some were seen again when readmitted for the release of contractures or for other reasons. From these, and from older burned patients who were not part of this study, the impression is gained that such burns leave a lasting scar upon the child if for no other reason than the intensity of the sensory experience.

DISCUSSION

As Bernstein et al. have stated, "The problems facing the psychiatrist working with severely burned children are complex and require flexible and changing methods of approach . . . the child psychiatrist . . . should involve himself immediately in the care of the burned child and become a member of the therapy team."

Early commitment to the clinical management of the patient affords, the psychiatric consultant the opportunity to acquaint himself with the particular reaction of the child to being burned and hospitalized. These reactions have been described by Long and Cope, Bergman and Freud, Woodward (1959, 1961, 1962), Hamburg et al., and others. The most effective psychiatric intervention can be achieved through the study of the individual child's background, experience, and behavior in the hospital.

In a consideration of the significance of the healing process, the concept of holding as described by Winnicott has been useful. The burn makes holding a child impossible, for the skin has been destroyed and the pleasure of its sensation has been turned to pain. The nurse must provide the child with holding equivalents. Her skill and ingenuity in offering herself to the child as an object of holding fulfills the dual sense of the word—to hold as to comfort, and to hold as to contain.

It is a distressing experience for the child to see his insides outside. The nurse covers his nakedness with dressings until it can be enclosed by new skin. It is distressing for the child to be overwhelmed by emotion beyond his containment. She helps him to reclaim his affects as his own by allowing him to personalize the source of his suffering in accusation of her. This drainage of affect allows the child to regain himself through her recognition of him.

The regression with which these children respond to their experience appears to have two components: (1) regression for relief in flight from pain and suffering, to conserve energies at a simpler level of functioning; (2) regression in acute search of a relationship: to found a new self based upon a holding relationship which will afford protection from falling into pieces.

For these children, in the extremity of their suffering, emotion is sensation, sensation is emotion, and there is nothing else that can be seen. As they recover, emotion takes on the quality that we know it by, half way between flesh and mind, yet ever mindful of its sensory origins.

REFERENCES

BERGMANN, THESI, & FREUD, ANNA: *Children in the Hospital.* Internat. Univ. Press, 1966.

BERNSTEIN, N. R., SANGER, S., & FRAS, I.: The functions of the child psychiatrist in the management of severely burned children. *J. Amer. Acad. Child Psychiatry*, 8:620-635, 1969.

HAMBURG, DAVID A., HAMBURG, BEATRIX, & DEGOZA, SYDNEY: Adaptive problems and mechanisms in severely burned patients," *Psychiatry*, 16:1-20, 1953.

LONG, ROBERT T. & COPE, OLIVER: Emotional problems of burned children. *New England J. Medicine*, 264:1121-1127, 1961.

WINNICOTT, DONALD W.: *The Maturational Processes and the Facilitating Environment*. Internat. Univ. Press, 1965.

WOODWARD, J. M.: Emotional disturbances of burned children. *British Med. J.*, 5128: 1009-1013, 1959.

WOODWARD, J. M.: Parental visiting of children with burns. *British Med. J.*, 5320: 1656-1657, 1962.

WOODWARD, J. M., & JACKSON, D.: Emotional reactions in burned children and their mothers. *British J. Plastic Surgery*, 13:316-324, 1961.

32

REPEAT EVALUATIONS OF RETARDED CHILDREN

Ann Murphy, M.S.W., and Lois Pounds, M.D.

Developmental Evaluation Clinic, The Children's Hospital
Medical Center, Boston

Six types of parental motivation for repeated evaluation
of retarded children are identified. Two reflect parents' use
of evaluations to deny a defect in the child. The remainder
represent inability of professionals to meet the needs of
parent and child. Suggestions are given as to how services
can be adapted to be more effective.

It has been observed that certain persons go from physician to physician, or clinic to clinic, with the same complaint. In the field of mental retardation, this phenomenon is not rare, and is usually attributed to parental denial of the child's basic handicap or the search for a magic cure. In the past these parents have been mentioned recurrently in the literature (1-7), but their characteristics have not been clearly delineated, nor their motivation analyzed. From a purely economic point of view, these parents constitute an over-consumption of resources in their repetitive use of professional time and the cost to themselves. The reponse of professionals varies from dismay that the parents appear not to "accept" the diagnosis, to a feeling of certainty that the current evaluation will be so superior as to end the traveling. This study evaluates some of the

Reproduced by permission from AMERICAN JOURNAL OF ORTHOPSYCHIATRY, Vol. 42, No. 1, January 1972, pp. 103-109. Copyright ©, the American Orthopsychiatric Association, Inc.

family dynamics and situational pressures that produce multiple evaluations, and suggests that denial is not the only mechanism.

METHOD AND MATERIALS

The material in the present report has been obtained from a review of records and interviews of the clinic population in a newly opened university-affiliated mental retardation unit within a large children's hospital. The children were new patients seen from September 1967 to September 1968. Each child was seen for three consecutive out-patient days with studies in approximately twelve professional disciplines. In order of frequency, referrals came from parents, other hospital clinics, private pediatricians, social agencies, and schools. Children are accepted in all age groups if the need for developmental evaluation exists. The parents complete a questionnaire describing the child's development, medical history, their reason for seeking an evaluation, and what expectations they have from the evaluation. Prior to their appointment every effort is made to obtain records of delivery, school work, and previous evaluations. During the year studied, no attempt was made to screen out children who had had competent evaluations elsewhere. The information below encompasses the material from 264 children, of whom 206 had had no previous evaluation except by their personal pediatrician. Fifty-eight families, or 22%, constituted the repeat evaluation population, having been studied at competent facilities on one or more occasions in the past. The average number of prior evaluations was 2.8.

Data were collected on patient age, socioeconomic status, reason for evaluation, and diagnosis, to determine whether those families seeking repeat evaluation could somehow be defined quantitatively from those who did not. Although significant differences were found in age and socioeconomic status, and in some categories of diagnoses, these data were not able to separate the new from the repeat patients clearly enough to be useful. The increased age of children in the re-studied category is obviously related to the time it takes to locate and arrange numerous evaluations, and the younger children in the first category may only indicate that this clinic was the first facility approached. Higher socioeconomic status, based on income, was significantly more frequent among the repeat patients, but again this reflects the ease with which the well-to-do can move about and afford repeated study. The reasons for requesting evaluation do not differ in the two groups, delayed development being the most common, followed by behavioral disturbances, school problems, and physical or sensory handicaps. The diagnoses in the two populations differed significantly in three areas: more normal and educable children in the first admission group and more retarded children with psychiatric disorders among the patients for repeat study.

Since quantitative data were not particularly helpful, a qualitative assessment of the repeating families was undertaken. It was found that these parents fell into six groups. Illustrative examples of each of these groups are given; these, while admittedly dramatic, authentically represent the mechanisms involved.

Twenty-six percent had realistic reasons for seeking re-evaluation. Geographic moves, decisions regarding school placement, the onset of adolescence and the need for different planning seemed appropriate bases for new study. In many of these instances the former facility was unavailable or not equipped to answer the current questions. These parents demonstrated their acceptance of the diagnosis, and were asking for specific planning:

D.A., age 8 years, is an example of a child with realistic reasons for re-evaluation. He was referred by his pediatrician and parents in order to "evaluate his potential to learn and the appropriateness of his present educational placement" in a special class for the retarded, where he was not progressing. At birth a diagnosis of Apert's Syndrome was made and the mother was advised to place the child without seeing him, as his appearance would upset her and his life expectancy was limited. She was told that surgical correction of his deformities was not appropriate, and she had to take the initiative to obtain other opinions that were more hopeful and that proved correct. Family relationships were impaired as the mother was fearful of having other children, and the father withdrew from active participation in decisions for this boy's care. The family was searching for an objective assessment of this boy's ability and some information on which to make a plan for his education. Evaluation indicated his normal intellectual potential but showed his learning to be interfered with by emotional problems. More individualized schooling combined with counseling for parents and child was recommended, and acted upon by the parents.

In direct contrast was another 26%, classified as deniers—not of retardation, but of the extent of it. These were the parents of children with moderate to profound retardation, in whom the handicap was so great that it appeared to be a void that parents desperately tried to fill by repeated evaluation, in lieu of doing nothing. These parents were honest about what they had been told by previous facilities, which often included "put him away," "give him lots of love," and "there is nothing to be done." They focused on specific areas such as speech ("if only he could have speech therapy"), walking ("all he needs is a brace to help him stand"), or other fractions of the problem in order to avoid the unbearable total:

T.M., age 4 years, is a severely retarded child whose parents were seeking evaluation partly to offset the emotional impact of his poor prognosis. He was brought to the clinic with a specific request for "therapy and stimulation." They reported his main problem to be "severe brain damage," which had been diagnosed at six months. They expressed dissatisfaction with previous medical advice, as the only recommendation was that they provide "tender, loving care." T. had been attending a pre-school nursery for the retarded, which had been located by his parents, for one year. The experience outside the home produced a reduction in the frequency of episodes of screaming. Parents had become active in the local parents' association, holding leadership positions. On the advice of friends, they consulted our hospital. Present evaluation found a child who could sit only with support, with functioning estimated at the sixth month level. The father spoke of hopes that T. would be able to attend public school classes for the retarded, but it was evident this was a wish rather than a plan. The mother stated firmly she would keep T. forever, even though placement was not suggested. A program of motor stimulation was offered, and consultation was arranged with a plastic surgeon on the possibility of cosmetic repair of his prominent ears. The parents conscientiously followed the suggestions, and re-evaluation indicated slight acceleration in the child's development. The family then requested referral to another center to see whether he might profit from orthopedic care, such as bracing, to facilitate walking. The mother seemed hopeful that if walking could be accomplished the more basic problem would be resolved. Thus, though traveling continued, it seemed that the family was approaching a new facility with somewhat reduced goals. There were indications that these steps were preliminary to being able consciously to consider placement.

The third group of 22% consisted of those more clearly identified in the past as deniers, those who failed to accept the presence of any deficit, however small. These parents frequently failed to include on the questionnaire the complete list of previous evaluations, and were unable to recall what had been discussed with them by previous examiners. They were more difficult to relate to in the clinic setting, often challenging results of individual examiners or trying to locate discrepancies between what the speech pathologist said and what the physical therapist demonstrated, etc.:

R.B., age 5 years, was the child of professional parents who felt a need to deny the child's intellectual defect. Evaluation was requested, as the parents were "puzzled by her behavior" and suspected that she had a "poor ego and emotional immaturity." They had first noted a problem at age 2 years, when she failed to develop language, although motor milestones were significantly slow, with sitting at ten months. The child had previously been evaluated by several excellent resources, whose reports indicated consistent diagnoses of mild mental retardation, and noted the parents' refusal to permit certain studies that would have allowed more definitive diagnosis of the extent of the child's handicap and its possible genetic origin. The parents' school plan was for regular class, although this had been ruled out by previous evaluators. The child was obese, passive, with poor ability to tolerate frustration or failure. Her upbringing was characterized by a great deal of infantilization coupled with unrealistic expectations and challenges. The current evaluation confirmed the diagnosis of retardation, but the parents requested that the findings not be forwarded to the school. Special class placement was arranged independently by the school, primarily because there was no alternative. The family remained in contact with the clinic through our efforts, rather than because of any rapport established. They continued to describe their daughter as emotionally immature and believe her to be in the wrong class.

Twelve percent of the repeating parents had emotionally disturbed children for whom they were seeking organic diagnoses, or for whom no program could be located:

P.W., a 14-year-old emotionally disturbed boy of borderline intelligence, was brought to our center from another state in order to obtain an evaluation that would determine the "proper medication to enable the boy to follow a more normal course of development." The chief complaint was inability to concentrate. Since he had reached school age, the parents had repeatedly sought evaluation and treatment of the same problem, and the boy had been enrolled in a number of schools for able children. Psychotherapy had been attempted, but was interrupted by the parents. Early reports described the boy as anxious and clinging. The current evaluation indicated many obsessional traits, and a preoccupation with trivia designed to conceal his limitations from himself and others. The father particularly denied knowledge of, or active participation in previous evaluations. However, when an attempt was made to discuss our findings with him, he pulled out a folder containing copies of previous reports, continually challenged and interrupted, and spoke of the boy in depreciatory terms. These people were unable to relate to their child as a person, finding it intolerable that he did not achieve. Consequently, the child was unable to value himself and apply his potential to real learning. The problems had been compounded by inappropriate school placements and the insecurity of constantly seeking a right program.

Nine percent of the repeat evaluations could be attributed to agency misdirection. When a social agency is faced with decisions regarding a shift in placement, lack of an available resource, or no clear plan of action, the response frequently is to delay the decision by getting another evaluation:

W.W., a 3-year-old boy was referred for evaluation of severe hearing loss, hyperactive behavior, and failure to grow. A social agency was responsible for him, as his mother had voluntarily relinquished his care. He had lived in a succession of homes, with relatives and foster parents. He was enrolled in a pre-school nursery for the deaf and had been consistently found to have a profound hearing loss by several other reputable centers. His erratic response to auditory training was reportedly related to shifts and upsets in his environment. This study confirmed previous reports of normal intelligence, profound hearing loss, and the need for a stable home situation. These recommendations were given to the referring agency, offering specific guidance on how they might be implemented. Follow-up contact revealed that no action had been taken, and the child had been shifted to a new foster parent who was totally unaware of the recommendations for care. This agency was failing to recognize the real needs implied by the child's complicated problem, and attempted to resolve their concern about him by securing another evaluation. They had not defined for themselves in any way how new data might alter this situation.

And finally, five percent were considered to be the result of poor medical advice. Many physicians react to the mentally retarded in a stereotyped fashion, and fear becoming involved with the family of a retarded child because of their own feelings of helplessness. Hence, quick referrals may be made without investigating previous workups:

K.P., age 4 years, who provides an example of poor medical advice, was referred to the hospital's medical clinic because of short stature. She had been identified by previous evaluations to be a retarded child and was attending a pre-school for the retarded. The specific request from the referring physician was for an endocrine workup. This was carried out and was normal, but the results were not presented to the parents. The child was then referred to this clinic for a retardation evaluation. This was clearly an unnecessary study for all concerned, but represented the automatic response of the clinic seeing a retarded child. The parents were obliged to come for the evaluation in order to get the results of the endocrine workup.

DISCUSSION

If the assumption is correct that continuity of care is necessary in order to provide a maximum support to the development of a retarded child, a significant number of families fail to develop rapport with a single center to which they can turn for guidance over the years. However, initially it is not unreasonable, in the face of a devastating diagnosis, to offer parents the option of a second opinion. If this is desired, help should be provided to locate a second competent facility, with encouragement for the parents to return to the original clinic for follow-up if the diagnosis is confirmed. Professionals who react with anger to the suggestion that their findings are not the final answer are not likely to establish a useful relationship with parents who are struggling with grief.

Unnecessary repeated studies are an indication of the quality of services offered to the parents of retarded children, as well as a reflection of the family's conflict about the diagnosis. There was no indication that the families in the realistic group would have searched for new facilities if their questions had been answered, and guidelines for constructive action offered. Those who came at the bidding of professional people had little opportunity to exercise their own judgment.

Re-evaluation is frequently used by families as a mechanism for coping with their feelings about the diagnosis, rather than to obtain facts. Those who wish to use it to deny the existence of a defect in their child, or to explain a psychological problem by the substitution of a treatable organic diagnosis, rarely benefit from restudy. Recognition of the real nature of the problem apparently is an overwhelming threat to their self-esteem. Unfortunately, repeated evaluation compounds the child's insecurity about himself, and probably contributes to a high incidence of emotional disturbance in this group. It seems appropriate to question the role professional people play in this dilemma. In fact, they rarely challenge it, and often facilitate it by making the necessary arrangements. Some means should exist for providing a focus on the parents' needs. One method would be to arrange for an interview with the parents in advance of the child's appointment, to attempt to define with them what their questions are, why previous resources failed to provide the answers, and in what way a new evaluation might contribute to their understanding. Even if the decision was to proceed with the evaluation, it is possible that a common understanding of the goals might be established.

The parents of severely retarded children are attempting intellectually and emotionally to make the transition from perceiving their child as normal to that of accepting him as severely impaired. It is not surprising that a frequent defense, utilized to handle their grief, is active mastery rather than passive acceptance. Factors that support various parents in their denial are the normal appearance of the child, highly developed social skills relative to cognitive ability, the lack of an apparent etiology, and the obvious progress of the retarded child with age. Parents may equate mental retardation with failure to do anything, with Down's Syndrome, or with primitive behavior; if their child does not fit these patterns, they cannot see him as retarded. They need the support of professional people to work gradually through a process of assessing the child's potential to develop, and recognition of his deficits and assets. The professional person is fairly immediately aware of the child's handicap, and feels his role is to impress upon the parents the degree and irreversible nature of the problem. Parents find their reports of progress, albeit limited, brushed aside and devalued, and they come up against the professional fear that recognition of forward motion will support the parents in denial of the deficit. Each encounter is apt to be characterized by a conflict of values and aims, rather than an opportunity for development of rapport and mutually established goals. It should be recognized with the parents that the child has a potential to develop, that there will be progress, but that the rate may not permit competitive adult functioning. If the parent focuses on specific aspects of the child's development, such as speech or motor function, consultants should be used to assess whether programs of stimulation in these areas would provide the parents with an active role in enhancing function. The family then would not have to fulfill its needs for activity by shifting to a new clinic, jeopardizing the opportunity for continued relationships.

Parental travel from clinic to clinic cannot be attributed only to the parents or to any one mechanism, but must be faced by those in the field of mental retardation as an individual matter deserving of thoughtful handling. A knowledge of the psychological impact of bearing a retarded child, and the interaction of social and emotional forces that drive these parents, will enable otherwise highly competent evaluation services to carry out their programs with less conflict, and more satisfaction to both parties.

SUMMARY

A review of 264 new patients seen in a university-affiliated mental retardation unit located 58 families who had an average of 2.8 competent previous evaluations elsewhere. The repeat patients did not differ from the total clinic population in terms of reason for referral, but they were characterized by higher socioeconomic level and older age. Qualitative assessments of their families suggested six categories:

1. those seeking guidelines for planning required at a new developmental stage;

2. those complying with the recommendations of physicians who did not wish to deal with a retarded patient;

3. social agencies who were using the evaluation as a way of postponing a difficult decision;

4. those attempting to obtain professional support that no defect existed;

5. those searching for a treatable organic diagnosis rather than an emotional disorder as a basis for the child's problem; and

6. parents of severely impaired children who were coping with their depression by looking for a more positive response from professional people, particularly in the area of remedial measures that might enhance the child's development.

Some suggestions were made for handling of the various patient groups by identifying the real need being expressed. The specialized facility can raise questions with referral sources as to what kind of additional data on the child's handicap will facilitate planning. Initial interviews can be arranged with parents who are suspected of denying the diagnosis to identify how a repeat evaluation will serve the child. A more active and positive response from professional people would foster better clinic-family interaction with parents of the profoundly retarded.

REFERENCES

1. BECK, H. 1969. *Social Services to the Mentally Retarded.* Springfield, Ill.: Charles C Thomas (pp. 53-54).
2. MILLER, L. 1968. Toward a greater understanding of the parents of the mentally retarded child. *J. Ped.*, 73 (5):699-705.
3. OLSHANSKY, S. 1962. Chronic sorrow: A response to having a mentally defective child. *Soc. Casework*, 43:190.
4. RHEINGOLD, H. 1945. Interpreting mental retardation to parents. *J. Cons. Psychol.*, 9:142-148.
5. SHERMO, S. 1951. Problems in helping parents of mentally defective and handicapped children. *J. Ment. Def.*, 56:42-47.
6. SMITH, E. 1952. Emotional factors as revealed in the intake process. *J. Ment. Def.*, 56:806-811.
7. WORCHEL, T. & WORCHEL, P. 1961. The parental concept of the mentally retarded child. *J. Ment. Def.*, 65:782-788.

33

A STUDY OF ADOPTED CHILDREN, THEIR BACKGROUND, ENVIRON- MENT AND ADJUSTMENT

Michael Bohman

Child Psychiatric Department of Karolinska Institutet at St. Göran's Hospital (Stockholm)

This paper summarizes the results of a study of adopted children and their families that was conducted by me during the years 1965-1968 and which has been published elsewhere (2).

Studies on the process of adoption have been stimulated mainly from two quarters: Genetic research and the child welfare authorities of the community. For genetic research the adoptive situation presents a ready-made experiment for testing hypotheses concerning the relative importance of heredity and environment. Such studies were done in the twenties and the thirties by Freeman and co-workers (8), Burks (6), Leahy (17) and more recently by Heston & Denney (10), Kety et al. (15), Rosenthal et al. (21) and Schulsinger (25). On the other hand, the goal of social research into adoption is to determine which factors in the child, the adoptive parents and society influence the adoptive process and to what extent this process can be forecast prior to placement.

It is generally accepted that adoption affords society an instrument for social therapy and the responsibility of placing children without parents is considered to call for a high level of knowledge and decision-making. Despite this, few representative studies have been made to throw light

Reprinted from ACTA PAEDIATRICA SCANDINAVICA, 61, pp. 90-97, 1972.

on the various aspects of adoption. An extensive survey of adoption research by Pringle concerning the years 1948-1965 (20) mentions only three major studies involving non-clinical populations of adopted children, all in the United States. Most studies on adoption (that are not specifically concerned with genetic questions) are on small clinical populations, whose selection is not reported. The majority of studies have been exploratory and designed to tackle some particular aspect of adoption. There are also a good many contradictions between their results, though there seems to be a certain amount of agreement on the following points:

1. Placement of an adoptive child should be undertaken as early as possible though there is still disagreement as to whether this means during the third and fourth weeks of life rather than during the first or even the second year (20).

2. Environmental factors appear to be more important than genetic factors for the development of the child's general character, whereas the greater part of the variation in intelligence among groups of adopted children is attributable to genetic factors (17).

3. The personal characteristics of the adoptive parents and their mutual relations have the greatest bearing on the outcome of an adoption, while their ages, income, socioeconomic group and education appear to be of secondary importance (28).

4. It is agreed that the child should be informed about the situation but opinions differ as to the age at which the child should first learn about its adoptive status (5, 16, 18, 23, 24).

5. Adopted children appear to be overrepresented in various clinical populations and this has been interpreted as indicating that they are more vulnerable to stress than children in general (4, 9, 11, 12, 14, 19, 22, 23, 26, 27).

6. Tests during infancy are seldom able to predict the child's subsequent development (1, 29).

Little research has been done on the importance of genetic, pre-natal and peri-natal factors for the child's development and not much is known about how society's attitudes to adoption affect the adoptive family.

The Follow-Up Study

The purpose of the study was to investigate questions connected with the placement of adopted children and to codify past experience as a foundation for future adoptions and was conducted on 168 adopted children (93 boys and 75 girls), representing all children born during 2

years in the mid fifties and placed in adoptive homes by the Stockholm
Adoption Agency. The children were 10-11 years old at the time of the
follow-up. Most of the families (124) were living in Stockholm and a
smaller group (40) were living in other parts of Sweden; the remaining
4 families were living abroad.

The investigated group of children is the result of many selective factors. For various reasons the agency did not or could not place all
children whose mothers had applied for an adoption. Of all 624 children
born during the 2 years and registered for adoption about a third returned to their mothers, who had changed their minds about adoption,
and lived there at the time of the follow-up 10 years later. Another
third had, because of certain selective factors, been placed in foster-
homes, where some had been legally adopted. This leaves only 27% of
the primary series placed in adoptive homes selected by the agency. Table
1 gives an account of the various placement-groups at the time of the
follow-up. All children were born after an undesired and socially complicated pregnancy and measures of decisive importance for their future
were as a rule taken before they were 1 year old. This similarity made
it interesting to compare the development and the adjustment of children in different placement categories. Consequently the study was
planned so that these other groups were included in certain parts of the
follow-up. The results of these comparative studies will be published
later (3), but some of the results are given also in this paper.

Information was obtained from previous investigations and records
as well as from official registers but chiefly through interviews with
adoptive parents and teachers. The interviews with parents covered 122
of the 124 families living in Stockholm (2 families refused to participate). The interviews with teachers covered all but 5 of the children
in the study. Information was also obtained about the children's school
marks and their general health according to the school health cards. A
control group was obtained in the form of classmates of the same sex and
certain comparisons were also made with all classmates of the same sex.
The information obtained from the adoptive parents was compared with
corresponding data from a representative study of Stockholm boys and
their parents by Jonsson & Kälvesten (13).

Pre- and Perinatal Conditions

The mean and range of the adopted boys' weight at birth displayed
good agreement with a normal Swedish population. On the other hand
the mean birth weight of the adopted girls was significantly lower than

expected. Only 5 children were born prematurely (3%). This unexpectedly low figure was the result of a positive selection, since most prematurely born children in the primary series were not placed in adoptive homes by the agency. Toxemia, including cases with no more than elevated blood pressure, was present in about 20% of the births and appears to have been over-represented in the adoptive series, compared with normal births.

Institutional Care

Prior to placement, all but 6 of the children were cared for at an infants' home for varying lengths of time. Rather more than half of the children had been placed in an adoptive home before they were 6 months old, 10% were placed during the last quarter of their first year and only one was a year old at placement.

The Biological Parents

The majority of the women who had their child adopted were young, unmarried or living alone. Only about one in four of the mothers had a home of her own. About half had previously given birth to one or several children. Financial circumstances and lack of housing were cited by most of the mothers as reasons for having the child adopted, in addition to the purely personal reason that was probably decisive in most cases, namely lack of support from the child's father. About one-fifth considered that a major reason for leaving the child was society's moral condemnation of illegitimate birth.

Information was obtained on 150 fathers, paternity not having been established in the other 18 cases. Most of the fathers were Swedish citizens (85%) and the others belonged to the European ethnic group. Their mean age, 28.55 years, was somewhat lower than in a representative group of fathers. Some idea of the biological fathers' social conduct was obtained by studying the registers concerning abuse of alcohol and crime. The proportion of biological fathers registered for abuse of alcohol, 27%, was somewhat higher than in a representative group of fathers. The proportion of registered criminality was 27% as against 11% in the comparative group. There was also a tendency to greater recidivism compared with "normal" fathers registered for crime and this may have to do with the higher proportion of the present fathers who appeared in both registers, for abuse of alcohol and for crime.

Table 1. *Whereabouts of the 624 children in the primary series at the time of the follow-up. Children 10–11 years*

Whereabouts	No. children
Adopted through the Adoption Agency in Stockholm ("Agency Adoptions")	168
Adopted without Agency assistance	126
Foster home	77
With biological mother	228
At an institution	3
Other placement	6
Dead	14
Unknown	2
Total	624

Table 2. *Adopted children's adjustment to school compared with controls (percentages)*

	Boys		Girls	
Adjustment	Adopted (N 90)%	Controls (N 51)%	Adopted (N 73)%	Controls (N 44)%
1. No symptoms	29	56	62	75
2. Slight symptoms	14	14	15	9
3. Moderate symptoms	35	18	12	11
4. Problem child	20	12	11	5
5. Institutional case	2	0	0	0
Total	100	100	100	100
	A	B	C	D

Diff. A–B: χ^2 11.71 (3 df) $p < 0.01$ Items 4 and 5 combined
Diff. C–D: χ^2 2.84 (3 df) Items 4 and 5 combined
Diff. A–C: χ^2 20.95 (3 df) $p < 0.001$ Items 4 and 5 combined

The Adoptive Parents

When the children were placed in their care, the adoptive parents were about 35 years old on the average and 6-7 years older than a representative group of Stockholm parents. Concerning the occupation of the family provider (usually the adoptive father), there were 34% with professional occupations, 37% with intermediate and 29% with skilled-unskilled occupations (according to the official British classification (7) modified somewhat for circumstances in Sweden). The two most qualified occupational groups were thus heavily overrepresented among the adoptive families. The average educational level of the adoptive parents was higher than that of the fathers in the comparative group and considerably more of them had also advanced socially.

The health of the adoptive parents was assessed from their own or the other parent's statements. Two adoptive fathers and 2 adoptive mothers had died of some disease, while a further adoptive father and an adoptive mother died while the study was in progress. One adopted child in five appears to have had at least one parent whose physical health was impaired. More than one child in four had a parent with a history of mental disturbance that had led to medical consultation "for nerves." The adoptive mothers reported physical or mental trouble more frequently than the adoptive fathers. According to their own statements, however, the physical and mental status of the adoptive parents was better than that of the parents in the comparative group but even so, the number with an impaired physical or mental condition does seem large considering that the adoptive parents as a group were assumed to represent a positive selection in respect of health.

In 19 of the adoptive families the marriage had been dissolved by divorce and in 4 by the death of one of the parents. Two more parents died while the study was in progress. Thus about one adopted child in six had lost one of its adoptive parents. The proportion of incomplete homes due to divorce or death was approximately the same among ordinary Stockholm families in the comparative group. The interviews showed in retrospect that in most of the divorce cases, conflicts and disharmony—expressed, for instance, in problems of sexual adjustment—had already existed when the child was placed. In only a few cases, however, had this state of affairs been noted in the investigation that preceded placement.

The adoptive parents' attitudes to various aspects of their life (marriage, work, financial situation, relatives, religion, leisure etc.) were measured from the interviews on attitude scales and compared with corresponding results for the comparative group of Stockholm families. Most of the adoptive parents had very positive attitudes in the case of prevailing marriages and good agreement was noted between the partners' statements. Similar results were obtained for sexual adjustment. In other respects, too, the majority of adoptive parents indicated an affirmative attitude to life and seldom expressed dissatisfaction with their situation. They differed significantly in most categories from the parents in the comparative group. Social relations and social life were the only aspects that appeared to cause any appreciable dissatisfaction.

Concerning the adoptive parents' own upbringing, 20-50% considered that this had been strict as against 70-75% in the comparative group. Thus, most of the adoptive parents appear to have had a relatively mild upbringing and as a consequence of this only a few of them had a negative attitude to their own upbringing.

The adoptive parents' attitudes to upbringing were measured with a questionnaire comprising seventeen statements that had also been used in the study of the comparative group. On average, the adoptive parents' attitudes to upbringing were "milder" than those of the comparative group. The questions on which the groups differed most concerned corporal punishment and sexual behavior in the child, the adoptive parents expressing more liberal views. The two groups of parents had fairly similar attitudes, on the other hand, concerning obedience and discipline.

Type of Upbringing

The author made a subjective evaluation of the type of upbringing practiced by the parents (level of demands). The demands of the adoptive fathers were relatively high in the case of boys but not girls, whereas the adoptive mothers placed roughly the same, relatively high demands on boys as on girls. A significant relationship was also found between the "level of demands" of the adoptive fathers and their own upbringing as a child, so that fathers who had received a mild upbringing expressed more "adequate" demands than those who had received a strict upbringing.

Disclosure of Adoption

Of the 164 couples who were asked, orally or in writing, whether they had disclosed the fact of adoption to the child, 68% stated that they had done so before the child was 5 years old, 13% between 5 and 7 years and 4% after 7 years. Of the remainder, 7% stated that they had not wished or could not bring themselves to inform the child that it had been adopted and 7% refused to answer the question. Most of the children in the latter group were probably completely or partially unaware that they were adopted.

Infertility

Childlessness was due to infertility in the adoptive mother alone in 45% of the cases and in the adoptive father alone in 15%. Both partners were reportedly infertile in 9%. The cause of childlessness was not known in spite of examinations in 20% of the cases, while only an incomplete or no examination had been undertaken in 6%. In the remaining 5% the childlessness was said to be voluntary owing to the use of contraceptives for medical or genetic reasons. Assuming that male infertility is as common as female, it seems that the considerably higher incidence of infertility among the adoptive mothers may reflect different attitudes to infertility and adoption among men compared with women. In marriages where the husband is infertile, it seems that the problem of childlessness is resolved by an adoption less frequently than when the woman is infertile. In the decade between the placements and the present study 17 live births had taken place in 13 of the families (8%). Five of these children were born to the couples who practiced contraception voluntarily for medical or genetic reasons.

The Adopted Children

Nearly all the adopted children were in good health. Two of them, however, had severely impaired hearing, probably congenital but not diagnosed until after the child had been placed with its adoptive parents.

School Performance

About 6% of the adopted children attended special classes (for slow learners, assistance in reading and writing etc.), which is about the usual frequency among school children in Sweden. None of the children was mentally retarded. The mean marks of the adopted children in Swedish and mathematics were compared with the means for class populations of the same sex. No difference was found in the case of Swedish but in mathematics the adopted children had a lower mean mark. The difference was only significant, however, for the children attending school in the City of Stockholm. No differences were observed between the mean marks of the adopted boys and the adopted girls.

Behavior as Perceived by the Teachers

The occurrence of certain readily-defined behavioral characteristics among the adopted children was studied without the teacher being aware of the subject's identity among classmate populations in the same sex. As perceived by the teachers the adopted boys were significantly more lively than their classmates, were in conflict with their peers more frequently and had a lower status. As regards intelligence, on the other hand, the adopted boys displayed the same distribution as their classmates. The adopted girls deviated considerably less than the boys from the behavior of their classmates. They had conflicts with peers somewhat more often than their classmates of the same sex and were also perceived by the teachers as more industrious and ambitious than the other girls.

Adjustment in School

Among the adopted boys 22% were judged to be maladjusted in the school situation compared with 12% of the controls, while a further

35% had moderate symptoms compared with 18% of the controls. The difference between the groups was significant.

Problems and difficulties of adjustment also occurred more frequently among the adopted girls compared with their class controls but the difference was less pronounced and not significant. It was considered that 11% of the adopted girls were problem cases compared with 5% of the controls. The adopted boys were significantly less well adjusted than the adopted girls. Compared with the controls, a significantly larger proportion of the boys as well as the girls displayed multiple symptoms. The results are summarized in Table 2.

The teachers and the parents differed considerably in their perception of the children's general adjustment as well as in their observation of individual symptoms. Thus, many more symptoms were registered during the interviews with teachers than during those with parents. The adoptive parents were considerably less prone to mention the child's problems even if these existed in the school situation. The differences between the interviews with teachers and with parents were particularly marked in the case of families with internal problems.

Asocial symptoms (truancy, vagrancy, lying, stealing and pilfering, destructiveness) were reported relatively seldom by the adoptive parents or teachers and do not appear to have been more common among the children than in a normal group of children. The boys who were "problem children" were chiefly characterized by a cluster of the following symptoms: psychomotor hyper-activity, inability to concentrate, disturbed relations with peers, defiance and aggressiveness.

GENERAL ANALYSIS

Before ascertaining the data outlined above, numerous hypotheses had been set up in accordance with certain theories that attempt to explain variations in the adjustment and behavior of children as being dependent on different background variables. Briefly, test of these hypotheses produced the following results:

1. Conditions registered during pregnancy and birth displayed no significant relationship with the children's adjustment or school marks. Complications during pregnancy did, however, show a significant relationship with difficulties in reading and writing. The children who were classified as maladjusted also had wider variations in weight at birth than the other children but the differences were not significant.

2. The time spent at an infant's home showed no significant relationship with the children's adjustment. A regression analysis revealed a weak

linear relationship between the duration of institutional care and the number of symptoms registered. Difficulties in reading and writing were more common among boys who had spent more than 6 months at an infants' home than among those whose stay had been shorter ($p < 0.05$, one-tailed test).

3. A weak, positive correlation was found between the mothers' education and the girls' marks in Swedish ($p < 0.05$, one-tailed test). Psychological or social insufficiency in the biological mothers was not significantly associated with the adjustment among the children.

4. The occurrence of the biological fathers in the registers of crime or abuse of alcohol was not related to the children's adjustment. It may be concluded that the children's social heritage so far had been neutralized in their new adoptive homes. The results do not confirm or exclude that genetic factors may be of etiological importance for the development of nervous symptoms in children. That genetic factors may be of some importance was shown in the study of those children from the primary series who were placed in foster homes or had returned to their biological mothers. In these groups I found a significant correlation between the adjustment of girls and the criminality of their biological fathers. On the other hand there was no such correlation between the boys and their fathers.

5. The education and occupational group of the adoptive parents were not correlated as expected with the children's school performance; if anything the results pointed in the opposite direction. The children who had been placed with the most qualified adoptive parents had lower mean marks than other children.

6. Neither the age nor the socio-economic circumstances of the adoptive parents correlated with the adjustment of the adopted children.

7. The adoptive mothers' attitude to marriage co-varied significantly with the adjustment among the children but this was not true of the attitude of the adoptive fathers. The attitudes of both parents to social contacts (friends, acquaintances) also co-varied significantly with the children's adjustment. The mental status of the adoptive mothers showed a weak correlation with the boys' adjustment.

8. The adoptive parents' own upbringing as children did not display the expected relationship with the children's adjustment. In the case of the adoptive fathers the results pointed, if anything, in the opposite direction—the fathers who had had a "mild" upbringing had less well adjusted children than those who had been brought up strictly. The attitudes of the adoptive parents to upbringing were not significantly associated to the adjustment of the children. A significant association was

observed, on the other hand, between the adoptive parents' type of upbringing (level of demands) as estimated at the interviews and the adjustment of the boys, but not with the adjustment of the girls.

9. Maladjustment was significantly more common among boys who were the only child than among the other boys but this was not true of the adopted girls.

In conclusion it may be noted that the adjustment of the children appeared to be relatively independent of the background variables investigated. Neither the environmental factors studied nor those connected with the biological background displayed very clear correlations with the children's adjustment or school performance. There is reason to suppose that the over-representation of behavioral disturbances observed among the boys in particular may be connected with the adoptive situation itself and the disturbances that this involves in the relationship between parents and child. It is conceivable that these disturbed relationships were connected with an uncertainty on the part of adoptive parents in their attitude to adoption, expressed by many of them in a desire to adopt a girl rather than a boy.

REFERENCES

1. BAYLEY, N.: Mental growth during the first three years. *Genet. Psychol. Monogr.*, 14:1, 1933.
2. BOHMAN, M.: *Adopted Children and Their Families.* Proprius, Stockholm 1970.
3. BOHMAN, M.: A comparative study of adopted children, foster children and children in their biological environment born after undesired pregnancies. *Acta Paediat. Scand.*, Suppl. 221, 1971.
4. BORGATTA, E. F. & FANSHEL, D.: *Behaviour Characteristics of Children Known to Psychiatric Outpatient Clinics with Special Attention to Adoption Status, Sex and Age Groupings.* Child Welfare League of America, Inc., New York, N. Y. 1965.
5. BRENNER, R. F.: *A Follow-up Study of Adoptive Families.* Child Adoption Research Committee, Inc., New York 1951.
6. BURKS, B. S.: The relative influence of nature and nurture upon mental development. *27th Yearbook Nat. Soc. Stud. Educ.*, 1:219, 1928.
7. *Classification of Occupations.* Her Majesty's Stationary Office, London, 1951.
8. FREEMAN, F. N., HOLZINGER,, K. J., & MITCHELL, B. C.: The influence of environment on the intelligence, school achievement and conduct of foster children. *27th Yearbook Nat. Soc. Stud. Educ.*, 1: 1928.
9. GOODMAN, J. D., SILBERSTEIN, R., & MANDELL, W.: Adopted children brought to child psychiatric clinic. *Arch. Gen. Psychiat.*, 9:451, 1963.
10. HESTON, L. L. & DENNEY, D.: Interaction between early life experience and biological factors in schizophrenia. In D. Rosenthal & S. S. Kety (Eds.): *The Transmission of Schizophrenia.* Oxford: Pergamon Press, 1968, p. 363.
11. HUMPHREY, M. & OUNSTED, C.: Adoptive families referred for psychiatric advice. Part I: The children. *Brit. J. Psychiat.*, 109-599, 1963.
12. JAMESON, G. K.: Psychiatric disorders in adopted children. *Texas Med.*, 63:83, 1967.

13. JONSSON, G. & KÄLVESTEN, A.-L.: *222 Stockholmspojkar*. Almqvist & Wiksell, Uppsala, 1964.
14. JOHNSSON, G.: Delinquent boys. *Acta Psychiat. Scand.*, Suppl. 195, 1967.
15. KETY, S. S., ROSENTHAL, D., WENDER, P. H., & SCHULSINGER, F.: The types and prevalence of mental illness in the biological and adoptive families of adopted schizophrenics. In D. Rosenthal & S. S. Kety (Eds.): *The Transmission of Schizophrenia*. Oxford: Pergamon Press, 1968, p. 345:
16. KIRK, H. D.: *Shared Fate. A Theory of Adoption and Mental Health*. The Free Press of Glencoe, London, 1964.
17. LEAHY, A.: A study of adopted children as a method investigating nature-nurture. *J. Amer. Stat. Ass.*, Vol. 30, Suppl. 281, 1935.
18. McWHINNIE, A. M.: *Adopted Children, How They Grow Up*. London: Routledge & Kegan Paul, 1967.
19. PRINGLE, M. L. KELLMER: The incidence of some supposedly adverse family conditions and of left-handedness in schools for maladjusted children. *Brit. J. Educ. Psychol.*, 31, Part 2: 183, 1961.
20. PRINGLE, M. L.: KELLMER, ET AL.: *Adoption—Facts and Fallacies. A Review of Research in USA, Canada and Great Britain 1948-1965*. Studies in Child Development. London: Longmans, 1967.
21. ROSENTHAL, D., WENDER, P. H., KETY, S. S., SCHULSINGER,, F., WELNER, J., & ØSTERGAARD, L.: Schizophrenics' offspring reared in adoptive homes. In D. Rosenthal & S. S. Kety (Eds.): *The Transmission of Schizophrenia*. Oxford: Pergamon Press, 1968, p. 377.
22. SCHECHTER, M. D.: Observations on adopted children. *Arch. Gen. Psychiat.*, 3:45, 1960.
23. SCHECHTER, M. D., CARLSON, P. V., SIMMONS, J. Q., & WORK, H. H.: Emotional problems in the adoptee. *Arch. Gen. Psychiat.*, 10:37, 1964.
24. SCHECHTER, M. D.: Psychoanalytic theory as it relates to adoption. *J. Amer. Psychoanal. Ass.*, 15:695, 1967.
25. SCHULSINGER,, F.: Psychopathy—heredity and environment. To be published in: *Int. J. Ment. Health*, 1971.
26. SWEENEY, D. M., GASBARRO, D. T., & GLUCK, M. R.: A descriptive study of adopted children seen in a child guidance center. *Child Welfare*, 42:345, 1963.
27. TOUSSIENG, P. W.: Thoughts regarding the etiology of psychological difficulties in adopted children. *Child Welfare*, 41:59, 1962.
28. WITMER, H. L., HERZOG, E., WEINSTEIN, E. A., & SULLIVAN, M. E.: *Independent Adoptions*. New York: Russell Sage Foundation, 1963.
29. WITTENBORN, J. R.: *The Placement of Adoptive Children*. Springfield, Illinois: C. C Thomas, 1957.

Part VIII

CHILDHOOD PSYCHOSIS

The subject of childhood psychosis justifiably attracts great interest despite the fact that it represents such a small proportion of child psychopathology. Understanding severe disorders often leads to comprehension of normative processes. In addition, the chronicity of such disorders gives it importance beyond the number of children involved.

This interest is reflected in the large number of studies summarized in the review by Hingtgen and Bryson. Churchill and Bryson present a specific study of one of the phenomena usually considered a cardinal sign of autism and offer a surprising finding.

34

RECENT DEVELOPMENTS IN THE STUDY OF EARLY CHILDHOOD PSYCHOSES: INFANTILE AUTISM, CHILDHOOD SCHIZOPHRENIA AND RELATED DISORDERS

Joseph N. Hingtgen, Ph.D.

Associate Professor, Dept. of Psychiatry
Indiana University School of Medicine

and

Carolyn Q. Bryson, M.S.

Staff Psychologist, Mark-Alpern Clinic (Indianapolis)

The research literature on psychotic disturbances of early childhood has rapidly expanded in the last 6 years. Since the appearance of Rimland's review of infantile autism in 1964 and the annotated bibliography on childhood schizophrenia done by Tilton, DeMyer, and Loew 2 years later, publications relevant to early childhood psychoses have numbered more than 400 articles and six books,[1] making it increasingly difficult to keep abreast of current research trends. Recent investigations have

---

Reprinted from SCHIZOPHRENIA BULLETIN, Issue #5, Spring, 1972, pp. 8-53.

[1] For a complete listing of these references, see: C. Q. Bryson, and J. N. Hingtgen, *Early Childhood Psychosis: Infantile Autism, Childhood Schizophrenia, and Related Disorders. An Annotated Bibliography, 1964-1969.* Rockville, Md.: National Institute of Mental Health, DHEW Publication No. (HSM) 71-9062, 1971. 127 pp.

been characterized by renewed interest in the development of treatment procedures, attempts at more adequate description of perceptual processes, intelligence, and language, and a search for neurobiological correlates. In this review we shall summarize some of these newer directions in research, with the hope of clarifying a number of critical issues and further stimulating the design of systematic research strategies and effective therapeutic methodologies.

Any paper on childhood psychoses must address the problem of differential diagnosis, a topic which has generated much heated discussion among various investigators. Numerous attempts have been made to delineate specific syndromes within the general classification of childhood psychosis (Alderton 1966, Bender 1967, Eisenberg 1966 and 1968, Fish and Shapiro 1965, Gold and Vaughn 1964, Goldfarb 1961, Kanner 1968, Mahler 1965, Perron 1964, Rimland 1964, Rutter 1965 and 1968, and Rutter et al. 1969) and to define their relationships to such other childhood disturbances as acute deprivation, pseudoschizophrenic negativism (O'Gorman 1967), elective mutism, retrolental fibroplasia (Wing 1966), developmental aphasia (Rutter 1965a and b, Savage 1968, and Wing 1966), and congenital dysphasia (Alderton 1966). Despite widespread agreement about the behavioral characteristics of psychotic children (see table 1), much controversy revolves around the following three major issues:

(1) *Should children with clearly established mental retardation (with or without signs of organicity) be included or excluded from the category of psychotic children?* Even though many psychotic children have severely subnormal intellectual levels, most investigators clearly distinguish between psychosis and mental retardation, and many consider the two diagnoses mutually exclusive. This view is based on observations that psychotic children generally look intelligent, have normal motor development and little or no physical stigmata, but do have grossly impaired relationships with people (Alderton 1966, Creak 1964, Menolascino 1965a, O'Gorman 1967, Rimland 1964, Rutter 1965a and b, and Wing 1966). Using Rimland's diagnostic checklist for infantile autism (1964), Douglas and Sanders (1968) were able to distinguish, without overlap, between autistic and retarded children. Nonetheless, several clinicians would diagnose retardates as psychotic if they manifested this disorder's characteristic behavioral symptoms (Creak 1964, Menolascino 1965b, Rutter 1965a, 1965b, and 1968, and Taft and Goldfarb 1964). A recent proposal, aimed at eventually eliminating this "either/or" diagnostic problem, suggests that psychotic behavior and intellectual functioning be considered as independent dimensions in

the classification of all childhood disturbances (Rutter et al. 1969). Thus, a child could be diagnosed as psychotic, psychotic/retarded, or retarded.

(2) *Is infantile autism a type of childhood schizophrenia or a distinct diagnostic category?* Some investigators contend that autism and childhood schizophrenia form a single diagnostic category of childhood psychosis, characterized by similar symptoms and outcome (Creak 1964, Eaton and Menolascino 1967, Gorman 1967, Ornitz and Ritvo 1968b, Rutter 1965a and b, and Taft and Goldfarb 1964). Others view autism as one of several distinguishable types of childhood schizophrenia (Alderton 1966, Bettelheim 1967, Dundas 1964, Ferster 1961, Fish and Shapiro 1965, Mahler 1965, Ruttenberg 1971, Salk 1968, Schopler 1965, Smolen 1965, Stroh and Buick 1964, White, DeMyer, and DeMyer 1964, and Zaslow 1967). A third contingent of investigators regards autism as a syndrome distinctly different from childhood schizophrenia (Eisenberg 1966 and 1968, Kahn and Arbib 1968, Kanner 1965 and 1968, Rimland 1964, and Rutter 1967), although both are considered psychotic disturbances.

(3) *Is childhood schizophrenia an early manifestation of adult schizophrenia?* Here again, one faction sees childhood schizophrenia as being on a continuum with adult schizophrenia (Bettelheim 1967, Edelson 1966, Mahler 1965, Salk 1968, and Smolen 1965), while another regards autism (as well as other childhood psychoses) as a separate entity (Rimland 1964 and Rutter 1965a, 1965b, and 1968).

Because much of the conflict between classification systems stems from a too heavy emphasis on theoretical considerations, further progress in resolving the problem of differential diagnosis will require additional descriptive studies, perhaps making use of factor-analytic techniques. *For the purposes of this review, we have focused our attention on psychotic children who manifest most of the behavioral symptoms listed in table 1, regardless of diagnosis.*

DESCRIPTIVE STUDIES

PREVALENCE

There have been few studies of prevalence rates of early childhood psychosis, but figures reported for the United States and England range from 2/10,000 to 4.5/10,000 (Lotter 1966a, Treffert 1970, Wing 1966, and Wing, O'Connor, and Lotter 1967). Although it is frequently mentioned that autism occurs primarily in first-born males, no clear relationship to birth order has been demonstrated (Lotter 1967, Lowe 1966, Rutter and Lockyer 1967, Wing 1966, and Wing, O'Connor, and Lotter

1967). Most authors do agree, however, that autism occurs more frequently in males than in females, with male/female ratios ranging from 2/1 to 4.25/1 (Lotter 1966a, Lowe 1966, Rimland 1964, Rutter and Lockyer 1967, Treffert 1970, Ward and Hoddinott 1965, Wing 1966, and Wing, O'Connor, and Lotter 1967).

Although Rimland (1964), Kanner (1965), and Eisenberg (1966 and 1968) would limit the diagnosis of autism to children manifesting autistic behaviors from birth, many investigators include cases with onset prior to age 3, following periods of normal development. Age of onset has also been suggested as a basis for a classification system, with the diagnosis of infantile autism limited to cases with onset before age 2, that of childhood schiophrenia applied to cases with onset after age 8, and cases with onset and regression between ages 3 and 8 considered to be a heterogeneous group of organic psychoses (Rutter 1967). Where series of psychotic children have been studied, proportions with gradual onset from birth have been reported as 50 percent (Wolff and Chess 1964), 54 percent (Rutter and Lockyer 1967), and 69 percent (Lotter 1966a and Wing, O'Connor, and Lotter 1967). Behavioral symptoms tend to be most pronounced at about age 3, with decreases in symptom severity frequently occurring between ages 5 and 6, suggesting a maturational factor (Rimland 1968 and Wing 1966).

The parents of psychotic children are often described as being cold, aloof, introverted, and mechanical in their relationships with people (Alanen, Arajärvl, and Viitamäki 1964, Alderton 1966, Eisenberg 1968, Kanner 1968, Polan and Spencer 1969, and Rimland 1964 and 1968); but when actual comparisons have been made—either with the general population or other clinical groups—the data have proved inconclusive. Although some investigators have reported the parents of psychotic children to be of higher intellectual, educational, and socioeconomic status than parents of other clinical groups (Gibson 1968, Lotter 1967, Lowe 1966, Rimland 1968, Rutter and Lockyer 1967, Von Brauchitsch and Kirk 1967, and Wing, O'Connor, and Lotter 1967), others have found no differences (Alanen, Arajärvi, and Viitamäki 1964, Levine and Olson 1968, McDermott et al. 1968, and Wolff and Chess 1964). There is no evidence of increased paternal age, and evidence regarding maternal age is mixed (Lotter 1967, Lowe 1966, and Wing, O'Connor, and Lotter

1967). Indications of a lowered incidence of broken homes (Lowe 1966) and of an unelevated and lower incidence of familial psychosis (Alderton 1966, Gittelman and Birch 1967, Lotter 1967, Polan and Spencer 1959, Rimland 1964, Rutter and Lockyer 1967, and Wing, O'Connor, and Lotter 1967) than in other emotionally disturbed groups are fairly conclusive; however, a higher incidence of other nonpsychotic affective disturbances has been reported in the families of psychotic children (Lotter 1967 and Wing, O'Connor, and Lotter 1967).

Although many clinicians have speculated about psychopathology in the parents of psychotic children, there have been relatively few objective investigations of this issue. Moreover, results of the studies which *have* been conducted are far from consistent. While Rice, Kopecs, and Yahalom (1966) reported that mothers of childhood schizophrenics were rated by therapists as less competent than mothers of emotionally disturbed children, and Lordi and Silverberg (1964) described abnormal mother-child relationships, Pitfield and Oppenheim (1964) found no evidence of deviant child-rearing attitudes in the mothers of psychotic children. Similarly, Schopler and Loftin (1969a and b) failed to identify a thought disorder specific to these parents, and Block (1969) found no differences between parents of neurotic and psychotic children, although the combined groups demonstrated more psychopathology than parents of asthmatic and congenitally ill children. Thus, the conception of a "schizophrenogenic" or "refrigerated, mechanical" mother who produces psychotic children is not well supported. Of interest may be the personal reports by parents of their experiences with autistic children (Eberhardy 1967, Kysar 1968, Lauder 1966, Park 1967, and Wilson 1968).

FOLLOWUP STUDIES

The results from recent followup studies indicate a continuing poor prognosis for childhood psychosis. As the children mature, psychotic behaviors remain dominant or evidence of organic damage or retardation increases; there are few reports of complete remission. In a 1- to 7-year followup of 17 nonreactive child psychotics, only two (12 percent) were judged nonpsychotic (Alanen, Arajärvi, and Viitamäki 1964); in a 6-year followup of 43 childhood schizophrenics, 58 percent remained schizophrenic, while 33 percent were diagnosed as mentally defective (Gittelman and Birch 1967); and in a 30-year followup of 12 cases, 75 percent remained schizophrenic, while 25 percent were classified as mentally defective (Bennett and Klein 1966). Although somewhat more

Table 1. Behavioral characteristics of early childhood psychosis.

Key: A—infantile autism; P—childhood psychosis; S—childhood schizophrenia; 1—primarily children with speech retardation; 2—poor motor development; 3—not regarded as a characteristic peculiar to early childhood psychosis.

	Kanner (1948)	Polan and Spencer (1959)	Creak (1964)	Goldfarb (1964)	Taft and Goldfarb (1964)	Rimland (1964)	White, DeMyer, and DeMyer (1964)	Wolff and Chess (1964)	Alderton (1966)	Lotter (1966a)	Ruttenberg et al. (1966)	Wing (1966)	O'Gorman (1967)	Rutter and Lockyer (1967) (Compared with controls)
1) Extreme self-isolation, aloofness, or withdrawal, noticeable in infancy	A	A				A	A		A		A	A	P	P
2) Do not anticipate being picked up, unresponsive to mother	A	A	S	S		A	A	A, S	A		A	A		
3) Insensitivity to pain			S					A, S				A		
4) Lack or avoidance of eye contact, looking through or past people	A	A				A	A		A	A	A	A	P	P
5) Try to maintain sameness in a) objects and their placement	A	A	S	S	S	A		A, S	A	A	A	A	P	P
b) behavior patterns	A	A	S	S	S	A		A, S			A	A	P	P
6) Pay more attention to objects than to people	A	A				A	A		A		A	A		
7) Repetitive manipulation of objects Little recognition of function	A	A	S			A	A	A, S	A		A	A	P	P
8) Fail to develop speech, mute	A	A	S	S	S	A	A	A, S	A		A	A	P	P
9) Limited speech or echolalia, without communication Immediate and delayed echolalia	A	A	S	S	S	A	A	A, S	A	A	A	A	P	P

10) Pronominal reversal	A	S		A	S	A		A	A	A	A	A	A	P
11) Repetitive body movement, rocking, hand flapping, posturing	A	S	S	S	A,S	A,S		A	A	A	A	A	P	P
12) Self-mutilation, head banging	S	S		A	A	A		A	A	A	A	A	P	P
13) Laughing or smiling, crying or tantrums for no apparent reason.				A		A		A		A	A	A	P	3
14) Impression of normal intelligence: Retardation with islets of normal functioning	A	S		A	A	A		A	A	A	A	A	P	1
15) In some cases, short period of normal development followed by regression		S				S		A	A	A	A	A	P	P
16) Normal motor development	A	S		A	S	A		A	A		2	A	P	P
17) Empty clinging	A	S		S	A,S	S		S		S			P	
18) Difficulty in playing with other children	A	S		A	A	A		A	A	A	A	A	P	P
19) Abnormal responses to stimuli, avoidance, hypo- or hyper-sensitivity, especially to sound	A	S		A	A	A		A	A	A	A	A	P	P
20) Little or no comprehension of language	A				3			A			A			
21) Use people as objects or tools	A	S		A	A,S	A		A		A	A	A	P	
22) Problems with feeding, sleeping, toileting refusals, fads	A		A,S	A,S	A	A,S.		A		A	A	A	P.	3
23) Abnormal fears or lack of appropriate sense of fear	A	S		A	A,S	A		A		A	A	A	P	3
24) Unusual abilities, e.g., rote memory, musical, reading, spatial	A	S		A	A,S	A		A		A	A	A	P	
25) Hyperkinesis, hypokinesis	A	S									A	A		
26) Serious or sad facial expression	A			A	A,S	A				A		A	P	
27) Extreme negativism, no imitation of others				A							A	A		
28) Short attention span with less distractibility														P

optimistic results were reported for a group of 129 "atypical children," the proportion of autistic or schizophrenic children in the sample is unknown (Reiser and Brown 1964). Menolascino and Eaton's report (1967) that 55 percent of their psychotic brain-syndrome cases had received initial diagnoses of childhood schizophrenia, which were modified as a result of later neurological findings, indicates that the age at which children are first seen may be an important factor in diagnosis and prognosis. In a predictive study, three infants under 1 year of age (out of a sample of 16) were judged "vulnerable" to schizophrenia on the basis of uneven development; by age 10, all three were emotionally disturbed, although only one was considered schizophrenic (Fish et al. 1965).

Although such behavioral symptoms as rituals and resistance to change tend to diminish with age, the childhood psychotic's social adjustment generally remains poor. In a 5- to 15-year followup of 63 such children, Rutter, Greenfeld, and Lockyer (1967) reported that only one had achieved normal relationships with adults. When childhood psychotics were compared with a matched nonpsychotic emotionally disturbed group, 3 percent of the psychotics (compared to 64 percent of the controls) had good or fair social adjustment, while 61 percent (compared to 36 percent of the controls) had poor or very poor social adjustment (Rutter 1966 and Rutter, Greenfeld, and Lockyer 1967). Mittler, Gillies, and Jukes (1966), in a followup of 27 psychotic, 21 borderline psychotic, and 25 subnormal cases, found that, in those cases where frequency of psychotic symptoms could be obtained, 35 percent of psychotics, 18 percent of borderline psychotics, and only 6 percent of subnormals demonstrated ritualistic and obsessional behavior; and 70 percent of psychotics, 36 percent of borderline psychotics, and, again, only 6 percent of subnormals had abnormal relationships with people. Bennett and Klein (1966) also reported that only one of 12 childhood schizophrenics was able to make a marginal social adjustment over a 30-year-followup period. The only study reporting an improved rate of social adjustment involved many cases with much later onset (Lempp and Vogel 1966).

There are also high rates of continued institutionalization for psychotic children—e.g., 92 percent of 12 cases (Bennett and Klein 1966), 35 percent of 43 cases (Gittelman and Birch 1967), 44 percent of 63 cases (Rutter, Greenfeld, and Lockyer 1967), 74 percent of 27 cases (Mittler, Gillies, and Jukes 1966), and 100 percent of three autistic cases, 33 percent of nine schizophrenic cases, and 40 percent of five chronic psychotic cases (Alanen, Arajärvi, and Viitamäki 1964).

Although one might expect intellectual and language development to increase as symptom severity decreases, there is little or no evidence of such a relationship. In their 1967 followup study, Rutter, Greenfeld, and Lockyer reported that only 3 percent of the psychotics but 23 percent of the emotionally disturbed children were employed and that less than 50 percent of the 63 psychotics had received 2 years of public schooling. Similarly, Wing, O'Connor, and Lotter (1967) reported that only 50 percent of 32 autistic children between the ages of 8 and 10 had received any schooling, and Mittler, Gillies, and Jukes (1966) reported that only 30 percent of their series of 27 psychotics had attended school for more than 1 year. Alanen, Arajärvi, and Viitamäki (1964) also reported that only one of 17 autistics, schizophrenics, or chronic psychotics had attended school, while five of six reactive psychotics had. In the Rutter, Greenfeld, and Lockyer (1967) sample, only 16 percent of the psychotics achieved a normal level of speech development. Of the 32 psychotics without speech at age 5, however, 22 percent subsequently developed some speech. In the 20 psychotic cases of Mittler, Gillies, and Jukes (1966) on whom such data could be obtained, 45 percent had no speech and 30 percent demonstrated echolalia or pronominal reversals at followup. In the Menolascino and Eaton (1967) sample of seven autistic or schizophrenic and 22 psychotic brain-syndrome cases, 41 percent had no language development, and only one case achieved normal language deveolpment. These authors also reported that, although 24 percent of the children were initially untestable and 41 percent had marked motor performance discrepancies suggestive of higher potential, none of the children subsequently showed improved test performance, despite improvement in cooperation. Sixty-two percent of the cases demonstrated severe mental retardation, and none achieved normal intellectual development.

Outcome does not appear to be related to duration or type of treatment (Eaton and Menolascino 1967, Eisenberg 1968, Rimland 1964, and Rutter, Greenfeld, and Lockyer 1967), sex, abrupt or gradual onset, evidence of brain injury, or family situation (Rutter, Greenfeld, and Lockyer 1967). Nor are there any differences in eventual outcome among brain-damaged psychotic, schizophrenic, or autistic children (Eaton and Menolascino 1967). Outcome has, however, been found to be related to speech development, IQ, amount of schooling, and original severity of symptoms (Eisenberg 1968, Gittelman and Birch 1967, Mittler, Gillies, and Jukes 1966, Rimland 1964, and Rutter, Greenfeld, and Lockyer 1967). On the basis of followup data, Rutter (1966) has suggested that, if marked improvement is to occur, it is usually evident by age 6 or 7.

BEHAVIORAL CHARACTERISTICS

Self-mutilation

A relatively high proportion of childhood schizophrenics engage in self-mutilative behaviors: 40 percent of 70 cases (Green 1967), and 38 percent of 58 cases (Shodell and Reiter 1968). Although Green (1967) found more self-mutilation in girls than boys (61 percent vs. 33 percent), Shodell and Reiter (1968) found no sex differences. Occurrence appears to be unrelated to IQ and cerebral dysfunction but related to histories of infantile headbanging (Green 1967) and parental physical abuse (Green 1968). This behavior is more frequent in nonverbal (47 percent) than verbal (19 percent) children (Shodell and Reiter 1968). Although behavior-modification techniques have been successful in decreasing self-mutilation in some cases (Lovaas 1966, Simmons and Lovaas 1969, Tate and Baroff 1966), they have been unsuccessful in producing prolonged cessation in others (Churchill and Bryson 1968). The data suggest that self-mutilative behaviors may originate as rhythmic behaviors which are then utilized as adaptive responses by children lacking other means of responding to their environment.

Toy Play

The toy play of psychotic children has been compared with that of normals, retardates, brain-damaged, and nonpsychotic emotionally disturbed children through direct observations (Haworth and Menolascino 1967, Hutt and Hutt 1970, Hutt et al. 1965, and Tilton and Ottinger 1964) and through maternal interviews (DeMyer 1967). It has been found that psychotics demonstrate less combinational, appropriate, constructive, and functional uses of toys, have more restricted repertoires of toy play, and engage in more repetitive manipulations of toys and their own bodies. Evidence regarding oral contacts is mixed, and there are some indications that autistic children also engage in less appropriate gross motor activity than normals (DeMyer et al. 1967). Of particular interest is the finding that toy play is related to amount of stereotypy. Hutt et al. (1965) found that autistics with predominant stereotypy played with toys only when actively engaged by an adult, while autistics without predominant stereotypy played with blocks even when an adult was not present. In a later study, Hutt and Hutt (1970) found that exploratory play occurred only after a decrease in stereotyped movements in response to a novel stimulus. It has also been noted that normal and emotionally disturbed children frequently use their toy play as a means of interacting with an adult, while the play of autistic children is less related to an adult's presence (Churchill and Bryson 1967 and Hutt et al. 1965).

Looking, Social

Because psychotic children engage in so little spontaneous social behavior, few controlled observations of social behavior have been attempted. In repeated observations of four autistic children, Boer (1968) reported that adult-directed behavior was absent except when initiated by an adult and that only one child engaged in any measurable amount of child-directed behavior. These results are similar to those found by Hutt et al. (1965). Hermelin and O'Connor (1963), in comparing autistics and retardates, found that psychotics demonstrated more alternating approach-avoidance behavior and produced fewer verbal responses to an adult than did retardates. It has also been demonstrated, however, that appropriate social behavior can be increased through the use of behavior-modification techniques.

Although lack of eye-to-eye contact is a frequently mentioned symptom, the evidence is mixed on this point. While Hutt and Ounsted (1966) found that autistics spent more time attending to environmental fixtures and less time attending to human faces than did other emotionally disturbed children, conflicting data have been reported by other investigators. On items tapping visual avoidance, Spivack and Levine (1964) found no significant differences between children who were schizophrenic and those with brain damage or personality disorders. Hermelin (1967b) found that autistics demonstrated the same preferences as retardates and normals for faces over other stimuli and for an actual face over a photograph. Churchill and Bryson (1967) also found no differences among autistics, schizophrenics, and normals in amount of time spent looking at or in close proximity to a preoccupied or attentive adult. And no differences were found between autistics and retardates in physical contact or proximity to an adult (Hermelin 1966 and O'Connor and Hermelin 1963a). It has been found, however, that autistic children do engage in more undirected gazing and show fewer visual fixations on either objects or persons than do emotionally disturbed children (Hutt et al. 1965), retardates, or normals (O'Connor and Hermelin 1967b). When looking and avoidance were measured as a function of success or failure on sign-language tasks, there were large individual differences in looking behavior, while avoidance responses were related to both the condition and duration of failure (Churchill 1970). It thus appears that lack of visual fixation is characteristic of *all* autistic behavior (rather than a specific response to persons) and that avoidance responses may be related to inability to perform required tasks.

Repetitive Behaviors

Several studies have been specifically directed to the measurement of ritualistic or repetitive behavior. Although individual differences in quantities and patterns of repetitive behaviors have been found among psychotic children, their individual behavioral patterns remained stable over both prolonged and repeated observations, and variations in quantities were unrelated to elapsed time or environmental events (Boer 1968, Ritvo, Ornitz, and LaFranchi 1968, and Sorosky et al. 1968). Boer reported that almost 80 percent of the spontaneous behavior of the autistic children involved the manipulation of objects, while Ritvo, Ornitz, and LaFranchi (1968) found differences among children in relative proportions of repetitive perceptual or motor behaviors. Ritvo's group further suggested that repetitive gross body movements were of a different nature than rapid flapping, clapping, hitting, and oscillating objects. Some of the difficulties encountered in trying to distinguish between responses to specific external stimuli and self-generated behavior are discussed by Spurgeon (1967).

Significant differences among clinical groups have also been found. Hutt et al. (1965) reported that autistic children engaged in more body manipulations but less manipulation of environmental fixtures than emotionally disturbed children. Hermelin and O'Connor (1963) observed significantly more self-generated behavior in autistics than in retardates, who remained relatively stable over repeated sessions; there was no difference between these two groups in amount of responding to environmental events. In another comparison of autistic and retarded children, Hutt and Hutt (1970) found that both the rate and duration of stereotypies were significantly higher in the autistic children; moreover, retardates showed less stereotypy with increased environmental complexity, while autistics showed more. Additional evidence of a relationship between self-stimulation and environmental complexity was reported by Churchill (1970), who observed that self-stimulation generally increased with both the condition and duration of failure on sign-language tasks.

Parental Reports of Early Symptomatology

Using retrospective questionnaires completed by parents, Wing (1969) compared the occurrence of abnormal behaviors in the early childhood of autistic, normal, mongol, aphasic, and partially blind/partially deaf children. While behaviorally different from the normal and mongol groups, the autistic group was quite similar to the partially blind/ partially deaf group in overall patterns of abnormalities and resembled both the receptive and executive aphasic groups in areas specifically related to perceptual and language disabilities.

In summary, the analyses of spontaneous behavior all indicate that when psychotic children are observed, either for prolonged periods or repeated sessions, their behavior remains remarkably stable and relatively unaffected by environmental events or fatigue. In general, psychotic children are relatively inattentive to either adults or children and engage in little constructive play; their behavior is characterized by a large amount of repetitive, nonfunctional manipulation of objects, environmental fixtures, and their own bodies—including self-injurious behaviors. There are, however, stable individual differences among children in the proportion of time spent in various activities, and recent evidence suggests that both avoidance and stereotyped behaviors may be related to the success/failure ratio in structured task situations. The major discrepancy between studies centers on whether autistic children selectively avoid eye-to-eye or eye-to-face contact; at present, evidence on this question is inconclusive. It does appear, however, that autistic children look less at all environmental objects, including adults, than do their normal counterparts. When they *do* look at adults, they do so without the accompanying behavioral responses usually considered indicative of attention in normal children.

INTELLIGENCE

Psychotic children are thought to be untestable by standardized psychological tests, but are frequently assumed to have normal or above normal intelligence—an assumption based on such negative indicators as lack of cooperation, lack of attention to test materials, absence of physical stigmata, and relatively normal gross motor skills. More and more children *are* being tested, however, and evidence of severe deficits in many areas of social, intellectual, and perceptual functions is accumulating.

The Vineland Social Maturity Scale does not require the direct cooperation of the child and has proved useful as an indicator of the nursery school performance of young psychotic children. But even on this test, the performance of autistic children remains low. Social quotients (SQ)[2]

---

[2] Social quotient = social age (as obtained from the scale) ÷ chronological age × 100.

ranging from 36 to 87 were reported for a group of 12 young psychotics (Allen and Toomey 1965), and a mean SQ of 40 was reported for a group of 28 child psychotics of mean chronological age (CA) 8-6, with 29 percent below SQ 29, 50 percent between SQ 30 and 49, 18 percent between SQ 50 and 69, and only 4 percent between SQ 70 and 79 (Gillies 1965). Social ages (SA) ranging from 1-1 to 5-0 for a group of 14 autistic children of CA 3-7 to 7-4 were reported by Alpern (1967) and a mean SA of 3-6 for a group of 40 child psychotics of mean CA 8-6 was reported by Whittam, Simon, and Mittler (1966).

To avoid the use of standardized tests, Ruttenberg et al. (1966) developed the Behavior Rating Instrument for Evaluating Autistic Children (BRIAC), and DeMyer, Norton, and Barton (1971) devised a structured interview. Although good interrater reliabilities and descriptions of both methods were reported, no data on the children were given for the BRIAC in this study, and only factored group profiles were described for the DeMyer interview. DeMyer, Norton, and Barton did report, however, that interview ratings on the adaptive age and personal/social age of a group of autistic children were highly correlated with independently obtained Vineland Social Ages and Cattell-Binet IQ scores as reported by Alpern and Kimberlin (1970). In a later study, Wenar et al. (1967) used the BRIAC to evaluate three methods of treatment.

The assumptions that psychotic children are untestable or that obtained IQ scores are not representative of true potential have not been supported by actual testing. Although Goldfarb, Goldfarb, and Pollack (1969) reported IQ increases of at least 10 points over a 3-year treatment period in 11 out of 26 childhood schizophrenics, Menolascino and Eaton (1967) found no improvement in test performance despite enhanced cooperation. The administration of infant items appears to reduce lack of responding (Alpern 1967 and Alpern and Kimberlin 1970). Employing an adaptation of the Cattell Infant Scale with autistic children ranging in CA from 3-7 to 7-4, Alpern (1967) obtained highly reliable scores which correlated with Vineland SA scores and clinical ratings but which could not be readily transformed to standardized mental age (MA) or IQ scores. When a short-form Cattell-Binet Intelligence Test was given to a group of 32 autistics, IQ scores, which ranged from 4 to 78, were highly reliable and correlated with clinical ratings (Alpern and Kimberlin 1970).

Using only the Seguin Formboard or the Wallen Pegboard with 28 psychotics of mean CA 8-6, Gillies (1965) reported that 11 percent scored below IQ 29, 36 percent between IQ 30 and 49, 36 percent between

IQ 50 and 69, and 18 percent between IQ 70 and 89. When standardized tests requiring higher levels of functioning are attempted, reports of untestability increase and obtained scores remain low. Of her series of 28 psychotics of mean CA 8-6, Gillies found 61 percent untestable on any part of the Wechsler Intelligence Scale for Children (WISC) Performance Scale, 60 percent untestable with the Goodenough Draw-a-Man test, and 50 percent untestable on the Peabody Picture Vocabulary Scale. Based on obtained scores or assigned basal scores on the Peabody, 71 percent scored below vocabulary quotient (VQ) 29, 21 percent between VQ 30 and 49, 8 percent between VQ 50 and 69, and none above VQ 70. Hermelin and O'Connor (1964a) also encountered difficulty in using the Peabody, finding 16 out of 32 autistic children of mean CA 11-5 untestable. When Peabody scores were later obtained on 12 autistics, ranging in CA from 8-0 to 14-5, MA scores ranged from 2-6 to 10.8 (1967b). In another group of 43 child psychotics, the Peabody was considered applicable for only 23. Of these 23, eight were untestable, and 12 scored under the test floor of 21 months. The obtained mean Peabody MA was 3-3 for these children of mean CA 8-6 (Whittam, Simon, and Mittler 1966).

Although the large majority of psychotic children tend to score at extremely low levels, higher levels of functioning and large variations in obtained scores have been observed both within and between groups. IQ ranges of from 50 to 129 for 30 cases (Schopler 1966), from 54 to 125 for 26 cases (Goldfarb, Goldfarb, and Pollack 1969), from 15 to 60 for 24 cases (Gibson 1968), and from 20 to 102 for four cases (Krall 1967) have been reported. Spivack and Levine (1964) found a median IQ of 45 for 17 cases, and Alanen, Arajärvi, and Viitamäki (1964) found that mean WISC verbal and performance IQ scores for four groups of psychotic children ranged from 45 to 87, with autistics and schizophrenics scoring lower than chronic and reactive child psychotics.

Where investigators have designated the proportions of children scoring within given ranges, it is evident that few psychotic children score above IQ 90. Gittelman and Birch (1967) reported that, of 97 psychotic children, 18 percent scored above IQ 90, 26 percent scored between IQ 70 and IQ 90, and 56 percent scored below IQ 69. Lotter (1966b) found that, of 32 autistic children, 15.6 percent scored above IQ 80, 15.6 percent scored between IQ 55 and 79, and 68.8 percent scored below IQ 55 or were untestable. In a study of seven autistic cases, 14 percent scored between IQ 70 and 90, and 86 percent scored below IQ 70 (Fish and Shapiro 1965). Rutter (1966) reported that, of 63 psychotic children, 11 percent scored above IQ 90, 18 percent scored between IQ 70 and 89, 30 percent scored between 50 and 69, and 41 percent scored below IQ 50 or were untestable. Despite the variety of investigators and tests employed and the use of somewhat different diagnostic criteria, the results of all these studies show a remarkable consistency.

Both short- and long-term reliabilities of test scores are high—correlations of .97 for a 1-week test-retest interval (Alpern and Kimberlin 1970), .90 and .92 for a 2-year test-retest interval (Gittelman and Birch 1967), and .80 for a 5- to 10-year test-retest interval (Rutter 1965a). IQ scores have been related to outcome (Gittelman and Birch 1967, Rutter, Greenfeld, and Lockyer 1967, and Rutter and Lockyer 1967), to presence of neurological signs and age of referral (Gittelman and Birch 1967), and to later educational outcome (Mittler 1966). Furthermore, IQ scores for severely psychotic children were found to predict educational outcome as well as or somewhat better than test scores for groups of borderline psychotic and nonpsychotic subnormal children (Mittler 1966).

Reports of extreme scatter among subtest scores are common, with autistics performing at higher levels on manipulation of visual-motor tasks than on verbal comprehension items (Gold 1967, Rutter and Lockyer 1967, and Wassing 1965). Gillies (1965) observed more subtest scatter for psychotics than retardates within the WISC Performance Scale, while Rutter (1966) found subtest scatter to be most characteristic of psychotics with continuing speech retardation. Although Whittam, Simon, and Mittler (1966) found that Peabody scores were significantly lower than Seguin Formboard or Wallen Pegboard scores for a group of 39 psychotics, the obtained mean performance MA was 4-7 for children of mean CA 8-6, indicating a large deficit even in the performance tasks. Safrin (1964), however, found no differences in performance on visual-motor tasks between psychotics and nonpsychotics when MA was controlled, indicating neither elevated nor depressed visual-motor skills in her group.

In comparing the test results of 28 psychotics and 28 subnormals matched for CA and nonverbal MA, Gilles (1965) found that the psychotics were significantly lower than the subnormals on Peabody vocabulary and Vineland SA. The discrepancy between the verbal and nonverbal scores was greater for the psychotics than subnormals; while the nonverbal and social scores of the subnormals were equal, the psychotics' social scores were lower than their nonverbal scores. When only Peabody-testable psychotics were considered, however, there were no differences between groups, and both groups had lower verbal than nonverbal or

TABLE 2

STUDIES OF SPEECH ABNORMALITIES IN PSYCHOTIC CHILDREN

Investigator	Sample Size	Mute Percent	Adequate or normal speech Percent
Fish, Shapiro, & Campbell (1966)	28	61	*
Gittelman & Birch (1967)	97	36	*
Gold (1967)	7	29	0
Lotter (1966 a & b)	32	28	16
Pronovost, Wakstein, & Wakstein (1966)	14	57	43
Rimland (1968)	24	42	*
Rutter, Greenfeld, & Lockyer (1967)	63	46-50	16
Ward & Hoddinott (1965)	39	36	31
Wolff & Chess (1965)	14	28	28

* Not reported.

social scores. To more fully investigate the language deficits of autistic children, Tubbs (1966) administered the Illinois Test of Psycholinguistic Abilities (ITPA) to autistic, subnormal, and normal children roughly matched on MA. Although standardized ITPA scores were not reported, autistics were found to score significantly lower than normals on five of the nine scales and significantly lower than subnormals on three of the nine scales.

The increasing administration of standardized psychological tests indicates that: 1) infantile psychotic children are testable if low-level items are employed; 2) relatively few psychotic children obtain IQ scores within the normal range, and most function at a severely retarded level; 3) IQ scores are remarkably stable over either brief or prolonged periods of time, regardless of clinical changes in behavior; 4) scatter within subtest scores tends to be largely a function of poor language comprehension and does not diminish the validity of total IQ scores; and, finally, 5) obtained IQ scores are predictive of later adjustment. More comparisons between psychotic and other clinical groups on standard and specially designed tests will be necessary, however, in order to determine whether the test patterns reported are specific to childhood psychosis.

LANGUAGE

While there are some reports of adequate or normal speech development in psychotic children, speech abnormalities are usually present in the form of failure to develop speech, immediate and delayed echolalia, or impaired communicative function. As shown in table 2, the incidence of mutism in psychotic children reported in various studies ranges from 28 to 61 percent; adequate or normal speech development occurs in 5 to 43 percent of the reported cases.

Immediate or delayed echolalia is the most common characteristic of psychotic children who do speak. Rutter (1965b) reported that 75 percent of the speaking children in his study exhibited echolalia and 25 percent exhibited pronominal reversal. Although pronominal reversal has previously been considered a sign of psychopathology and confusion of personal identity, it is now generally thought to be a type of echolalia (Cunningham 1966, Kanner 1968, Rutter 1965b, and Wing 1966). There appears to be no difference in degree of communication between echolalic and mute children (Kanner 1968). Echolalia is used both for communication and as repetitive or ritualistic behavior (Wing 1966 and Wolff and Chess 1965). In psychotic children it is related to lack of comprehension and is qualitatively different from the developmental echolalia of normal children (Fay 1969), with the articulation of echolalic phrases tending to be at a higher level than original speech productions (Pronovost, Wakstein, and Wakstein 1966 and Ruttenberg and Wolf 1967). The degree of echolalia is negatively correlated with level of language development— —.61 between echoisms and sentence length— (Cunningham 1966); it has also been reported that previously echolalic children progress to the use of more complex and spontaneous speech faster than previously mute children (Lovaas 1966a).

Other speech characteristics have been described by several investigators (Cunningham 1966, Goldfarb, Goldfarb, and Scholl 1966, Rutter 1965b, Ward and Hoddinott 1968, and Wolff and Chess 1965) and have been compared with the speech of aphasic (de Hirsch 1967, Rutter 1966, Savage 1968, and Wing 1966), nonpsychotic emotionally disturbed (Fish et al. 1968, Shapiro and Fish 1969, Weber 1965, and Weiland and Legg 1964), brain-damaged (Weiland and Legg 1964), mentally retarded (Cunningham 1968), and normal children (Cunningham 1966 and Goldfarb, Goldfarb, and Scholl 1966). Although there may be overlap with other clinical groups in some respects, the speech of psychotic children is generally characterized by low developmental level, lack of questions and informative statements, few personal pronouns, greater use of imperatives, limitations in verbal output, and more frequent idiosyncratic uses of words. There is little comprehension of the speech of others, little gestural reinforcement of speech, and there are many deviations in articulation, pitch, stress, rhythm, and inflection, as well as poor coordination of speaking and breathing.

The several methods of speech evaluation which have been employed are usually based on spontaneous or elicited speech productions during free play or structured observation sessions. Ruttenberg and Wolf (1967) developed scales within the BRIAC to evaluate communication and verbalization; Shapiro and Fish (1969) described scales for rating developmental and functional levels of speech development; Davis (1967) presented a method of evaluating inner, receptive, and expressive language; and Cunningham (1966 and 1968), Wolff and Chess (1965), Ward and Hoddinott (1968), and Weiland and Legg (1964) investigated the proportions of types of words used.

Since speech production and comprehension are the primary forms of communication between individuals, the relationship between speech development and other variables is especially important. It has been found that speech development is closely related to: 1) IQ (Fish et al. 1968, Gittelman and Birch 1967, Lotter 1966a, Rutter, Greenfeld, and Lockyer 1967, and Spivack and Levine 1964); 2) degree of improvement in response to placebo and drug treatment (Fish et al. 1968); and 3) development of relationships with people (Ruttenberg and Wolf 1967). Wolff and Chess (1965) reported that not only was clinical status highly related to speech development, but specifically, clinical status was more highly correlated with ratio of original to repetitive speech (tau = .78) than with ratio of communicative to noncommunicative speech (tau = .54). It has also been found that nonspeaking children demonstrate less verbalization in infancy (Ruttenberg and Wolf 1967), are less alert and less responsive to sound in infancy, manifest more autistic behaviors (Rimland 1968), engage in more self-mutilative behaviors (Shodell and Reiter 1968), and show more evidence of other perceptual deficits (Hermelin and O'Connor 1965 and Pronovost, Wakstein, and Wakstein 1966). It is thus clear that difficulties in language development are not an isolated phenomenon but, rather, relate to difficulties in other areas of functioning and characterize lower-functioning psychotic children.

The basic nature of the language deficit, however, is still a subject of controversy. Rubin, Bar, and Dwyer (1967) feel that children must pass through each stage of speech development in succession (babbling, echolalia, words, phrases, and finally sentences), while Wing (1966) does not consider the speech anomalies to be merely a delay in normal development, and Fay (1969) stresses the difference between autistic and normal developmental echolalia. Rutter (1965b) and Pronovost, Wakstein, and Wakstein (1966) consider the speech abnormalities to be primary rather than due to emotional disturbance, while Ruttenberg and Wolf (1967), Rubon, Bar, and Dwyer (1967), and Morrison, Miller, and Mejia (1969) stress disturbances in interpersonal relationships. Goldfarb, Goldfarb, and Scholl (1969) implicate inadequate maternal speech models, but their data are questioned by Klein and Pollack (1966). Cunningham (1968) attributes speech peculiarities to lack of maturity, lack of empathy, and poor discrimination of social reinforcers, and de Hirsch (1967) attributes the language disturbances of schizophrenia to psychopathology and those of aphasia to CNS impairment, even though she notes that the speech characteristics of both groups are similar. It has been further suggested that, because deviations in language development reflect and can be used to measure deviations or retardation in ego development (Shapiro and Fish 1969 and Weiland and Legg 1964), they might prove more useful than the usual psychiatric classifications as indicators of prognosis (Fish et al. 1968).

Methods of speech training are, of course, related to concepts of causation. Those investigators who regard lack of communicative speech as a function of withdrawal stress the development of relationships as the primary treatment approach and report that language improves concomitantly with improved relationships. Those who consider lack of speech to be another type of behavioral deficit tend to use behavior-modification techniques as the primary means of increasing speech production and report successful results. Weiss and Born (1967), however, distinguish between speech training and language development and point out that, while behavior-modification techniques are successful in training speech, there appear to be little generalization from the training context and little increase in spontaneous or creative speech. They further note that, while speech training is facilitated by the development of relationships, the children remain retarded in language development. Their position is that techniques such as those used with aphasic children might prove more productive. Rutter (1966), however, notes that even with the use of techniques other than operant procedures, when psychotic children show some improvement in language development, their speech still remains mechanical and concrete. Savage (1968) suggests that, although the distinction between operantly trained speech and normal language development is a relevant point, the former at least provides a basis for language development and gives the child a chance to develop language that he may never gain through other methods.

PERCEPTION

Data from a number of recent studies have suggested a basic perceptual dysfunction in many psychotic children. Although the exact nature of the deficit has not yet been clearly demonstrated, the evidence is sufficiently impressive to warrant serious consideration as a possible etiological factor.

Goldfarb (1964) and Schopler (1965) suggest that psychotic children tend to avoid the distance receptors of vision and hearing and make relatively greater use of the proximal receptors of touch, taste, and smell. Because both vision and hearing are so directly involved in communication and most other higher-order adaptive acts, the question of receptor preferences has important implications for understanding early childhood psychoses.

In a factor analysis of the Devereux Scales, Spivack and Levine (1964) found mixed evidence of impaired sensory receptivity in schizophrenic children; factors tapping deviant sensory receptivity were related to IQ as well as diagnosis. When the visual and tactile preferences of schizophrenics, retardates, and normals were compared, the schizophrenics were observed to spend less time with *all* stimuli than retardates or normals; moreover, even though schizophrenics spent less time with the visual stimuli than either of the control groups, they did not compensate with increased tactile exploration (Schopler 1966). When the auditory volume preferences of autistics, schizophrenics, and normals were compared, it was found that autistics preferred higher volumes than schizophrenics or normals, while the schizophrenics were more variable in their preferences than the other groups (Metz 1967). Interpretation of these data is difficult because position responses were present in all groups, and the effect of the pretraining required by the autistics is unknown. In addition, since a light was always present in the position of highest volume, the autistics may have been responding to the light rather than auditory intensities.

In a series of experiments, Hermelin and O'Connor (1964b) compared the responsivity of autistic and retarded children to light, sound, and tactile stimuli presented in pairs. When every response was rewarded, both groups responded more frequently to light than to the other two stimuli. When only sound and touch were paired, the autistics responded more frequently to touch, while the retardates responded more frequently to sound. And when only responses to sound and touch were rewarded when paired with light, both groups responded equally to sound and touch correctly and to light incorrectly. Thus, in both groups, light dominance was decreased but not eliminated when conflicting responses were rewarded. Then light, sound, and touch stimuli were presented singly rather than in pairs, and the children were required to point to the side where sound and touch occurred (orientation) and to point to the side opposite from light (inhibition). The performance of the retardates was similar for both tasks, while the autistics had more difficulty with the inhibition than orientation task. Inhibition to sound and touch was not tested, however, so the question remains whether the autistics' failure to inhibit responses is a generalized deficit or specific to light stimuli.

O'Connor and Hermelin (1965a) then paired light with a tone or verbal command ("come here") and varied the relative intensities of the stimuli. All responses, regardless of modality of presentation, were rewarded. Autistics, mongols, and nonmongols were all significantly different in responsivity. The autistics demonstrated predominant position responses and thus did not respond differentially to stimulus intensity, modality of presentation, or type of auditory stimulus. Both mongols and nonmongols demonstrated light dominance and intensity dominance, but only the nonmongols differentiated between the types of auditory stimuli. In addition, responsivity to the vocal stimulus was correlated with Peabody IQ scores across all three groups.

The empirical data thus indicate that, while autistics may make fewer responses to incoming stimuli, there is no evidence that they *selectively* avoid either auditory or visual stimuli or that they compensate for this avoidance by increased responsivity to tactile stimulation. Further, presentation conditions strongly influence responding, and the general lack of responsivity appears to be more directly related to problems of information utilization than to the affective tone of the stimuli.

VISUAL-MOTOR SKILLS

It has been frequently reported that the variability in the intellectual functioning of psychotic children is characterized by relatively higher performance scores than verbal scores and, particularly, by higher scores on the Block Design and Object Assembly subtests of the WISC (Rutter and Lockyer 1967 and Wassing 1965). The fact that these subtest scores, along with formboard scores, have often been used as the only obtainable estimates of the intellectual potential of autistic children suggests that, of all areas of functioning, visual-motor skills are the most intact.

Visual-motor skills are not above average, however, for when MA was controlled (mean MA 8-8), Safrin (1964) found no differences in performance between psychotic and normal children on either reproduction or visual recognition tasks, which included the WISC Block Designs. Somewhat different results were reported by Birch and Walker (1966), who compared the reproduction and recognition performances of brain-damaged psychotics and schizophrenics of unknown etiology (CA range 6-5 to 11-11, mean IQ 80). They found that the schizophrenics' recognition performance was disrupted by failures in reproduction, which, by contrast, had relatively little effect on the performance of either brain-damaged psychotics or a previously tested group of cerebral palsied children. Thus, the visual-motor skills of the schizophrenics were not so independent of other skills as those of the two types of brain-damaged children.

Bryson (1970b) reports that a younger group of six low-functioning autistic children (CA range 4-8 to 8-8, MA range 1-11 to 4-4) performed below average on tests involving a variety of simple tasks. She found that the children who performed at a level of at least 2 years below CA did much more poorly on reproduction than on visual matching-to-sample tasks. Gillies (1965) also reported low formboard and peg-board scores for her children. There may be further important differences between autistic and retarded or normal children in the types of information utilized in performing visual-motor tasks. When their performances were compared on fitting and tracking tasks in which the amount of available visual information was varied, it was found that normals used visual information more efficiently than autistics, while autistics made the most efficient use of kinesthetic or motor cues (Frith and Hermelin 1969). Thus, it appears that the general description of autistic children as having well-developed visual-motor skills may no longer be appropriate and may, in fact, be misleading, unless the specific skills in each task are evaluated.

VISUAL DISCRIMINATION SKILLS

A relatively large amount of data is available to demonstrate the poor visual discrimination skills of psychotic children, even though visual acuity appears to be within normal limits. In comparing a group of schizophrenic and normal children matched for CA (mean CA 5-6), Ottinger, Sweeney, and Loew (1965) found that, while the normals were able to solve simple two-choice discrimination problems almost immediately, five of the 11 schizophrenics performed at chance levels throughout the maximum of 200 trials. Hermelin and O'Connor (1965) also found that retardates performed significantly better than autistics on a series of two-choice visual discriminations and, further, that nonspeaking autistics performed more poorly than normals matched for MA on a visual length-discrimination task, although they were able to learn a position discrimination as well as the normal controls (Hermelin and O'Connor 1967a).

When visual-to-visual-matching-to-sample, rather than visual-discrimination procedures were employed, however, the performances of young autistic children (CA range 4-8 to 8-8) were generally within normal chronological age expectations (Bryson 1970b), suggesting that it may be the memory factor inherent in standard discrimination-training procedures rather than the difficulty of the visual stimuli, *per se,* which depresses visual discrimination performance.

AUDITORY DISCRIMINATION SKILLS

Only one study has investigated the auditory discrimination skills of autistic children without requiring association between the auditory stimuli and specific visual, vocal, or fine motor responses. Hingtgen and Coulter (1967), using operant procedures, attempted to train four autistic children (CA range 5-9 to 8-3) to discriminate among five pairs of auditory stimuli. Only one of the children learned to discriminate between words, and one of the children failed to learn the discrimination between music and silence in over 13 hours of training. This evidence of serious deficits in the processing of auditory information has been supported by a number of investigators who require more specific responses.

CROSS-MODAL INFORMATION PROCESSING

Visual-to-Tactile

It has been found that psychotic children are similar to retardates and normals in performing poorly on a tactile-to-visual coding task (O'Connor and Hermelin 1965b) and in showing more transfer from visual-to-tactile than from tactile-to-visual stimuli when a simple fitting task is employed (Hermelin and O'Connor 1964a).

Auditory-to-Vocal

Echolalia is a frequent behavioral symptom of autism, and auditory-to-vocal tasks are essentially measures of the accuracy of echolalia. Tubbs (1966), in administering the ITPA, found that verbal rote memory was the only task on which autistic children approached a near normal level of performance. Bryson (1970b) also found that immediate echolalia of single words was quite good in five out of six children tested. However, both studies demonstrated that echolalia was not predictive of ability to use auditory cues or provide vocal responses under other conditions.

Aside from the behavior-modification studies which describe the methods and amounts of training required to produce vocal imitation in mute psychotic children (see below), Hermelin and O'Connor (1967b) and O'Connor and Hermelin (1965b) provide the most complete data comparing the auditory-to-vocal performance of children who are autistic, retarded, and normal (Peabody MA range 1-11 to 10-8). In presenting sequences of words arranged randomly and in sentences, they found that: 1) autistics repeated the sequences as accurately as normals and more accurately than retardates but were less affected by the method of presentation; 2) retardates recoded the sequences as accurately as normals ingful arrangements more frequently than autistics; and 3) autistics demonstrated more marked recency effect than the normal controls. Thus, while the quantity of words accurately repeated did not differ among groups, the retardates and normals utilized the meanings of the words more frequently than the autistics.

Auditory-to-Visual

There is a large amount of evidence that autistic children have particular difficulty in understanding language and in making simple auditory-to-visual associations (see Peabody scores above). Cowan, Hoddinott, and Wright (1965) found that only two out of 12 autistic children were able to associate simple shape or color labels with visual stimuli initially and that, after an additional 120 trials of training, six of the remaining 10 children continued to perform at chance levels. Bryson (1970b) also found that auditory-to-visual associations were more difficult for her six children than either visual-to-visual matching or auditory-to-vocal responding with the same stimuli.

Auditory-to-Fine Motor

Many investigators have mentioned that a large proportion of autistic children appear unable to comprehend instructions, but aside from the behavior-modification studies little testing has been done in this area. Bryson (1970b) found that fine motor performances decreased when auditory rather than visual stimuli were presented, even though the children had received previous training with the stimuli under other conditions.

Visual-to-Vocal

The lack of communicative speech in psychotic children has been amply described and demonstrated in clinical interviews, direct observations of spontaneous behavior, and behavior-modification studies. Only one study with a limited group of six autistic children has been undertaken to test more formally whether the identical words available in an echolalic repertoire could be used for providing labels for previously discriminated visual stimuli (Bryson 1970b). Of the six children tested, two were unable to make any visual-to-vocal associations, and the scores of the other four children were below those obtained on the auditory-to-visual and auditory-to-vocal tests.

MEMORY

Although psychotic children are frequently described as having surprisingly good rote memory skills, the small amount of empirical information available in this area is contradictory. In comparing the auditory-to-vocal memory abilities of autistics and retardates, Hermelin and O'Connor (1967b) found no differences between groups in the quantity of words recalled. A comparison of auditory and visual short-term memory skills of autistics and normals also failed to uncover quantitative differences between groups (O'Connor and Hermelin 1965b). Both of these studies support the hypothesis that what is impaired is the ability to attach meaning to incoming stimuli, *per se*. Contradictory results were obtained earlier by O'Connor and Hermelin (1965b) when nonspeaking psychotics were found to have lower performances than speaking psychotics, retardates, or normals on a visual-to-visual size-matching task involving a 3-second delay interval, and later by Bryson (1970a), who found severe short-term memory disabilities in her sample of seven autistic children, under both visual-to-visual and auditory-to-visual matching-to-sample and sequencing tasks. She noted that, although there were large individual differences among children, in general, delay produced a more marked decrement in performance under the visual-to-visual condition than under the auditory-to-visual condition, even though simultaneous visual-to-visual matching and sequencing were superior to simultaneous auditory-to-visual performances. The apparent conflict in results raises an important question concerning the relationship of meaning, memory, and modality in autistic children, for the data appear both to support and negate the hypothesis that autistic children have unusual, or at least unimpaired, short-term memory abilities.

Although the careful and systematic testing of the abilities of psychotic children is a relatively recent development, there is already strong evidence of impaired intellectual and perceptual functioning—impairments which would also interfere with language development. Visual-motor, visual-discrimination, and auditory-discrimination skills all tend to be below age level; of even greater significance, however, are the data indicating especially severe deficits in short-term memory and most cross-modal information processing. Whether these patterns are unique to psychotic children or are also characteristic of other low-functioning children will remain an unresolved question until further research involving comparison groups is completed.

NEUROBIOLOGICAL STUDIES

Since many of the current theories of early childhood psychosis allow for possible organic involvement, it is not surprising that over 40 studies of neurobiological correlates have appeared since 1964. However, the results of these investigations do not present a unified picture, since there are few testable hypotheses indicating what physiological and biochemical measures should be made. In spite of these shortcomings, most of the studies strongly suggest that neurobiological factors may be implicated in some types of childhood psychoses.

EEG STUDIES

A number of recently published studies have reported the results of various types of electroencephalographic (EEG) investigations with psychotic children. Three of the earlier studies found no difference in the sleeping and dreaming patterns of autistic and normal children (Onheiber et al. 1965, Ornitz, Ritvo, and Walter 1965a and b, and Roffwarg, Dement, and Fisher 1964). Subsequent studies (Ornitz and Ritvo 1968a and Ornitz et al. 1968), however, have presented data suggesting that the normal phasic inhibition of the auditory evoked response during rapid-eye-movement (REM) stages of sleep is overridden in autistic children. Autistic children under 5 years of age showed significantly larger responses than controls when amplitudes during eye-movement bursts were compared to ocular quiescent phases of REM sleep and also when amplitudes during either REM sleep or its ocular quiescent phase were compared to stage 2 sleep. The authors postulated a disruption of the equilibrium between phasic excitation and phasic inhibition during the REM sleep of autistic children which might carry over into the waking state. A variety of additional differences between the REM sleep of autistic and normal children have also been reported (Ornitz et al. 1969).

Studies of waking state (rather than sleep) EEG's have also suggested possible deviations in psychotic children. White, DeMyer, and DeMyer (1964) examined records of 162 children who were divided into five groups: autistic, chronic undifferentiated early childhood schizophrenic, nonpsychotic with acting-out behavior disorders, neurotic, and psychiatrically normal. None of the psychiatrically normal children and only one of the 10 neurotic children showed abnormal EEG activity, but 51 percent of the other three groups demonstrated abnormal EEG's, most frequently characterized by irregular paroxysmal spike-and-wave complexes.

Hutt et al. (1964 and 1965) also found differences in their group of 10 autistic children, reporting statistically unusual EEG records which demonstrated a low voltage irregular activity without any established rhythm. Since a "flat" record was found in only one of 60 nonpsychotic, psychiatrically disturbed children, the "flat" records appeared to be identified with childhood psychosis. Fish and Shapiro (1965) also found a higher incidence of abnormal EEG's in their autistic group than in a control group of psychiatrically disturbed children.

Considering alpha waves as indicators of arousal states in darkness, Hermelin and O'Connor (1968) found no differences between autistics and normals for light stimulation but did find a significantly greater degree of arousal for auditory stimuli in the autistic children. Walter et al. (1971) compared 30 children (13 autistic and 17 with autistic features) to a group of institutionalized controls and found that the disturbed group had fewer mature EEG interaction patterns following visual and auditory stimulation. When Small (1971) studied averaged sensory evoked responses and slow potential shifts in autistic and control children, she observed that responses of lower and more stable amplitude followed visual stimuli presented to autistic children, whereas auditory stimuli appeared to initiate less complex evoked responses in these children.

In general, EEG studies indicate that large numbers of psychotic children vary significantly from normal controls in demonstrating more positive signs of neuropathology. Of course, not all psychotic children manifest abnormal EEG's; nor do these findings suggest any one specific type of organicity. What is apparent is that more thorough neurological examinations with appropriate followup tests are indicated for all cases of childhood psychoses, including autism.

DRUG STUDIES

The limited number of drug studies performed in recent years with psychotic children has not produced dramatic results in terms of consistent or marked improvement but has strongly suggested differences in pharmacological reactivity in psychotic and control children. Mixed results have been obtained with a variety of different drugs. When trifluoperazine was administered (Fish, Shapiro, and Campbell 1966), the most severely impaired autistic children not only showed greater improvement than the control group but also required and tolerated larger doses of the drug, while the less severely impaired either showed no improvement or became worse. Fish and Shapiro (1965) found no response to placebo treatment in a group of early childhood schizophrenics, whereas about 50 percent of another psychiatrically disturbed group of children improved; but psychotics did improve following chlorpromazine and Benadryl treatments. Metrazole convulsive therapy facilitated remission in a group of schizophrenic boys when given during puberty but had no effect on a group of autistic boys (Bender 1964). Some improvement in both behavioral and EEG measures was also found when a combination of diphenylhydantoin and thioridazine was administered to a group of behaviorally disturbed children that included schizophrenics (Itil, Rizzo, and Shapiro 1967).

Simmons et al. (1966) found transient but significant effects in two autistic twins who were treated with LSD. During a standard test situation, the children demonstrated an increase in eye-to-face contact, laughing, and smiling and a decrease in self-stimulatory behavior following LSD. Bender and coworkers (Bender 1966, Bender et al. 1966, and Faretra and Bender 1964) reported no undesirable side effects from LSD given daily over an average period of 9 months to a group of childhood schizophrenics. She observed overall behavioral improvement with qualitative, but not quantitative, changes in the Vineland Social Maturity Scale. It was concluded that LSD potentiates the reactions of the sympathetic nervous system and either lowers or has a less marked effect on the parasympathetic system.

Abramson (1967), in reviewing some of the earlier LSD studies, reported that large doses of LSD and Sansert may be safely administered to psychotic children for long periods of time, with no obvious brain damage and some general improvement. Mogar and Aldrich (1969) reviewed seven independent studies in which psychedelic agents were used with psychotic children; they concluded that, since the results consistently indicated some improvement, these drugs should be more extensively used with this population.

Attempting to devise a better methodology for assessing improvement in psychotic children following drug treatment, Rolo et al. (1965) used film ratings made by a number of objective raters who had observed one child treated with LSD. They failed to report any noticeable improvement following drug treatment.

In terms of immediate therapeutic value, psychopharmacological studies of childhood psychosis have not been very encouraging to date. A few of these studies, however, in demonstrating basic dose-response differences among groups of psychotic and control children, have provided further data indicating a possible role for neurobiological factors in these disorders.

PHYSICAL CHARACTERISTICS

Although gross physical stigmata have not been demonstrated, indications of physical and metabolic abnormalities have been seen in psychotic children. In a study of the growth patterns of 25 psychotic males (CA 6 to 20), Dutton (1964) found evidence of depressed growth and skeletal development and suggested a metabolic cause for the disturbance. When 34 psychotic children were compared to the standard growth patterns of normal children (Simon and Gillies 1964), the psychotic group was significantly below normal in weight and bone age and contained an excess of children below the 10th percentile for height; these differences could not be explained in terms of diet or social class. Brambilla, Viani, and Rossotti (1969) studied endocrine functions in 16 psychotic children and found that 87 percent of the subjects exhibited metabolic imbalance. The most dramatic alterations, appearing in the pituitary gland, consisted of reduced secretions of gonadotropin, corticotropin, and thyrotropin. Severity of the endocrine imbalance appeared to be positively related to degree of psychotic disturbance.

Shapiro (1965) noted a distinctive indentation between thumb and first finger of both hands of 11 severely autistic children (CA 3 to 8) which resembled the configuration of the hand in normal children up to about CA 3. Silver and Gabriel (1964) found primitive postural responses and decreased muscle tone in 30 of 39 schizophrenic children (CA 8 to 12), while they found this same disorder in only one of 39 normal, two of 13 borderline schizophrenic, one of nine reading-disability and two of 16 brain-damaged children. All these studies indicate that some psychotic children have definite atypical physical characteristics.

CELL STUDIES

Cytogenetical examinations by Book, Nichtern, and Gruenberg (1963) failed to show any significant deviations from normal in the chromosome counts or karyotypes of sex chromatins in cell cultures of normal and autistic children. Although Judd and Mandell (1968) were also unable to find significant or consistent chromosomal abnormalities in 11 autistic children, Fowle (1968), in studying three large groups of children, found that several atypical types of lymphocytes and cells of the plasmacyte series occurred at a higher frequency in smears of psychotic than in normal children—22.9 percent in psychotic compared to 9.3 percent and 7.8 percent in siblings and normals, respectively. Two of the types of atypical cells were similar to those associated with antibody production, one resembling response to virus infections and another resembling immature lymphocytes. Total cell counts of proplasmacytes were considered the best criteria to use in comparing smears of normal and schizophrenic children and in relating blood-cell patterns to severity of illness.

NEUROCHEMICAL STUDIES

In an early study, Seller and Gold (1964) found that the cerebrospinal fluid of schizophrenic children produced seizures in mice more rapidly than control fluids. These same investigators noted in 1965 that the injection of the serum of psychotic children into mice produced effects which were more severe and of shorter onset than those for control serum. A followup study (Gold 1967) reported that larger numbers of animals died when injected with psychotic serum than with control serum. Although this latter study found no differences in seizure time, it verified the presence of epileptogenic factors in the serum of psychotic children. Heeley and Roberts (1965) found that nine of 16 psychotic children had a tryptophan metabolism defect. All children with the defect had deviant behavior from an early age whereas children who regressed later had normal metabolism. Because of reports that magnesium imbalance produces abnormal behavior, Gittelman and Cleeman (1969) studied serum magnesium levels in hospitalized normal and psychotic children but found no differences between the groups.

CASE-HISTORY EXAMS, PREGNANCY STUDIES, AND MORBIDITY STUDIES

A number of investigators have intensively perused the case histories of psychotic children and their parents in the hope of uncovering some clue to the possible organic basis for this disease. In a study of the records of 97 noninstitutionalized childhood schizophrenics, Gittelman and Birch (1967) furnished support for the view that neurological damage, or the risk of such damage, is frequently encountered in a large group of these children. Over 50 percent of the children had subnormal IQ's, which were frequently associated with 1) clinical findings of neurological dysfunction, 2) perinatal complications and abnormalities, and 3) earlier age of onset of symptomatology. Both age of onset and IQ were found to be good indicators of prognosis. No relationship was established, however, between occurrence of CNS pathology and either parental psychopathology or familial history of mental disorders. In the followup group, over 25 percent of the children had been rediagnosed as mentally subnormal and/or had been given a subsequent diagnosis consistent with chronic brain disorder. In general, CNS pathology was evident in 80 percent of the children.

Increased incidence of a variety of prenatal, perinatal, and postnatal abnormalities in the development of psychotic children has been reported, supporting the hypothesis that at least a subgroup of these children is organically damaged. In a review of five controlled studies, Pollack and Woerner (1966) noted a significantly higher incidence of prenatal complications in psychotics than in control groups, with the most frequently reported complications being toxemia, vaginal bleeding, and severe maternal illness. Taft and Goldfarb (1964) reported that prenatal complications were particularly characteristic of male psychotic children. The data regarding prematurity are contradictory: Zitrin, Ferber, and Cohen (1964) found a higher incidence of prematurity, while other investigators have reported no differences between psychotic and control groups (Pollack and Woerner 1966 and Terris, Lapouse, and Monk 1964). There is, however, an increased incidence of stillbirths or abortions among mothers of schizophrenics (Pollack and Woerner 1966 and Terris, Lapouse, and Monk 1964). A higher incidence of perinatal or postnatal difficulties has also been reported (Pollack and Woerner 1966 and Whittam, Simon, and Mittler 1966), particularly among males (Taft and Goldfarb 1964). Leonberg and Bok (1967) found organic patterns in their case study. The overall pattern of the findings, except for the factor of prematurity, is similar to data reported for cerebral palsy, epilepsy, and mental deficiency. In reviewing the literature on neurological involvement in the siblings of psychotic children, Pollack and Gitelman (1964) found evidence of neurological deviancy in the siblings, along with the predominantly male sex pattern. A later comparison of psychotic children and their siblings led to the conclusion that psychotic children demonstrated more "hard" and "soft" neurological signs, lower IQ's, lower SQ's, and probably represented a heterogeneous group with chronic brain syndromes (Pollack et al. 1970).

Although no specific factor has yet been identified, the accumulative evidence strongly suggests that there may be physiological involvement in the mother which could interfere with normal fetal development and produce organic impairment in the infant. Exhaustive work in this area is needed to verify this possibility.

MISCELLANEOUS STUDIES

A number of studies have uncovered some interesting neurobiological abnormalities in specific cases of early childhood psychosis. Ritvo et al. (1969) found that autistic children differed from their controls in that they had a significantly shorter postrotatory nystagmus than normals when tested with eyes open in a lighted room after rotary stimulation induced by the Bárány chair. There was no significant difference when subjects were rotated in a dark room with a blindfold. The authors suggested that their results supported the hypothesis that such children have a unitary organic disease which becomes apparent with the presentation of multiple stimuli (rotation plus visual input).

In a preliminary report of their psychophysiological studies on autistic children, Bernal, Simmons, and Miller (1969) state that their psychotic children had a uniformly lower GSR responsivity when compared to normals, regardless of the stimulus modality tested—a finding which is functionally consistent with those patterns reported for retardates.

Using measures of dietary intake, DeMyer, Ward, and Lintzenich (1968) found that, although 11 early childhood schizophrenics ingested the same percentage of carbohydrates, proteins, and fats as four control children, their caloric intake was 35 percent less than the control group's. Since the controls were taken from lower socioeconomic families, this finding is very tentative.

Although the diverse studies cited above do not conclusively point to the involvement of a neurobiological factor in childhood psychoses, they strongly suggest such a possibility. Atypical EEG records occur in sufficient numbers to indicate neurological dysfunction; certain gross physical characteristics and cell abnormalities point toward organic or biochemical disturbances; and, finally, prenatal, perinatal, and postnatal factors indicate that there are sufficient disturbances in maternal physiological condition to have produced some organic changes in the infant. Certainly all these possibilities should be more extensively investigated.

Traditional methods of analytically oriented psychotherapy have been generally unsuccessful with young psychotic children. Rimland (1964) summarizes early studies to demonstrate that psychotherapy did not lead to significant improvement in autistic behavior beyond spontaneous recovery rates. In fact, children who received no intensive psychotherapy often showed a better recovery rate than those receiving therapy. This failure of conventional therapy has stimulated the development of new therapeutic approaches for the psychotic child, including body stimulation techniques, group therapy, educational programs, and behavior therapy.

PSYCHOTHERAPY

In spite of Rimland's conclusions, the use of traditional therapeutic methods with psychotic children is still reported (Des Lauriers 1967, Dundas 1964 and 1968, Ekstein 1966, King 1964, King and Ekstein 1967, Langdell 1967, Maslow 1964, Miller 1969, Rice and Klein 1964, Tessman and Kaufman 1967, and Thomas 1966). Perhaps the most prominent advocate of the intrapsychic approach is Bettelheim (1967), who believed that autistic children must be removed from the home atmosphere and be treated in a residential school setting. Since he feels that autistic children have fled from the real world because it is too threatening, the therapist makes no demands and waits for the child to emerge from his own private world. Some of the academic aspects of Bettelheim's program may resemble the educational methods described below, but the major emphasis of his approach is directed toward uncovering postulated underlying psychodynamic mechanisms.

BODY STIMULATION

Many of the newer therapeutic approaches incorporate various forms of bodily stimulation to make the first contact with the psychotic child. The necessity of early tactile stimulation in helping autistic children react with their environment has been stressed by Schopler (1962 and 1964). He suggested that the improvement seen in children following stimulation with contact techniques indicated that they were forming a central body image which had previously been lacking. Postulating that aversion to body stimulation is a primary symptom of autism, Freides and Pierce (1968) proposed a program similar to that of Schopler. Kemph (1964 and 1966) and his co-workers (Kemph, Harrison, and Finch 1965) also used tactile stimulation in association with oral gratification to bring a child out of his autistic withdrawal during the initial stage of therapy; the next two stages involved the strengthening of ego functioning and the resolution of intrapsychic conflicts. Alpert and Pfeiffer (1964) reported general behavioral improvement following muscle and rhythmic stimulation of a psychotic child. When body stimulation is used, Wilson (1966) feels that the therapist must approach the child rather than wait for the child to make the initial move toward bodily contact.

In their treatment program for autistic children, Des Lauriers and Carlson (1969) pointed out the importance of sensory-affective experiences (tactile, kinesthetic, and proprioceptive stimulation) which are pleasurable and gratifying to the child. The therapist provided this affective climate until the child began to "experience his own humanity" and expressed the need for more stimulation. These initial learning experiences, even at such a primitive level, then led to more complex situations in which the child's curiosity and striving for mastery were further reinforced. Des Lauriers and Carlson—in contrast to Bettelheim—stress the need for training parents as therapeutic educational agents, a position also supported by Schopler and Reichler (1971). In addition to parents, other nonprofessionals have also been used effectively in training psychotic children in daycare centers (Belz, Drehmel, and Silvertsen 1967 and Reiser and Sperber 1969).

GROUP THERAPY

A number of therapists have tried group techniques with psychotic children. Utilizing materials chosen to increase interactions with the environment, Lifton and Smolen (1965) treated children in small groups which met for 7-12 hours weekly (Smolen and Lifton 1966). The therapist actively invited contact with subjects, conveyed expectations, and interpreted the hidden feelings of the children. Although improvements in ego integration and self-control and decreases in psychotic fantasies were observed, Lifton and Smolen were least successful with those most severely autistic children who had not had any period of normal development. Similar success with group methods was obtained by Speers and Lansing (1964 and 1965) and Coffey and Wiener (1967).

EDUCATIONAL PROGRAMS

Many therapists who work with psychotic children regard training in specific tasks as necessary for behavioral improvement. They feel that these children should be helped to develop basic skills—or at least a means of communication. Such broad programs of remedial education resemble behavior-modification techniques (see below), but descriptions of them usually make no direct reference to the use of reinforcement methods.

Elgar (1966) considers psychotic children as handicapped rather than emotionally disturbed; she directs her efforts towards alleviating their deficiencies in speech and visual learning through the use of special classroom methods. Similarly, the Wings (Wing and Wing 1966a, Wing 1966, and Wing and Wing 1966b) look upon education and training— especially in the areas of speech and visual discrimination—as essential to any effort to help psychotic children. They feel that the environment must be highly structured rather than permissive and that emphasis should be placed on effective training rather than relationship formation.

While not deemphasizing the importance of establishing relationships with the child, Harper (1967) cites the necessity of stimulating the child and providing him with as many learning experiences as possible, using whatever he is interested in to entice him into the world. Dubnoff (1965) and Chambers (1966) direct their attention to ego development through mastery of tasks and they allow only appropriate behaviors to be gratified. Wolf and Ruttenberg (1967) initiated a training program beginning with simple imitative tasks and advancing to work in the area of speech therapy. Although their treatment program was based on the concepts of psychosexual development and ego dysfunction, the methods themselves were quite similar to those used by some of the reinforcement therapists presented below. Other types of educational programs have been suggested by Garcia and Sarvis (1964), Weiland (1964), Weiland and Rudnik (1961), and Goldfarb (1965).

The need for educational facilities for psychotic children in the home as well as the school has been pointed out by Lotter (1966b). Weston (1965) gives parents and teachers some practical suggestions for effectively teaching autistic children. Other authors cite the need for attention to the problems of the parents (Cohen 1964, Connell 1966, and Schulman 1963).

OTHER METHODS

Two unusual methods for treating infantile autism have been reported by Schechter et al. (1969) and Robertson (1966 and 1969). In the former study, psychotic children were perceptually isolated for a period of 6-12 weeks. Each child was individually placed in a sensory isolation room void of all furniture except for a mattress; food was given on an irregular schedule, as was contact with the therapist. During isolation, demands and novel stimuli were gradually introduced. Based on clinical judgment, all three children showed improved social interaction and eye contact after leaving the room. Using a technique she refers to as shadow therapy, Robertson feels that it is easier for the therapist to "reach" an autistic child in a darkened room than in a normally lighted setting.

BEHAVIOR THERAPY

The first study in which direct behavior modification techniques were applied to psychotic children was that reported by Ferster and DeMyer in 1961. Since that time almost 100 papers have appeared in which reinforcement methods have been used. Although the early work involved reinforcing mechanical responses under automated laboratory conditions (Ferster 1964 and Ferster and DeMyer 1961), later studies have been directed toward developing behaviors necessary for the psychotic child to function more effectively in a real life environment. An initial study of this latter type was conducted by DeMyer and Ferster (1962). It was found that ward attendants were able to modify some general behaviors of eight psychotic children using only social reinforcers (attending, physical contact, verbal praise, and other signs of affection). Subsequent to this study, Ferster continued using behavior-modification techniques with psychotic children outside of the laboratory (Ferster 1966 and Ferster and Simons 1966). These early research efforts pointed the way for dozens of other studies in which reinforcement methods have been used to modify the behavior of children with psychotic disorders.

Attending Responses

Lack of attention to relevant cues is a characteristic of many psychotic children which makes efforts to shape new behaviors extremely time-consuming. Although most therapists develop attending responses as the first step in a behavior modification program, a few have specifically concentrated on developing an attentive set.

Brooks, Morrow, and Gray (1968) worked with a 19-year-old autistic deaf mute and successfully increased visual attending responses using food reinforcers. When reinforcement was discontinued, response rates decreased but were quickly reinstated when reinforcement was again made contingent on visual attention. In another study, McConnell (1967) used praise and smiling to reinforce eye-to-eye contact with an autistic boy (CA 5). When the social reinforcers were removed, the eye contact decreased but was reinstated during reconditioning. The frequency of attending responses in psychotic children has also been increased by the use of reinforcers such as playback tape recordings (Marr, Miller, and Straub 1966), electric shock, and spanking (Simmons and Lovaas 1969).

General Behavioral Repertoire

Many studies using operant conditioning methods have attempted to increase the general behavioral repertoire of psychotic children. In an early study, Wolf, Risley, and Mees (1964) applied operant conditioning over a 7-month period to one autistic child (CA 3½). Training parents and teachers to use food and isolation as reinforcers, they increased wearing of glasses and verbal behavior and decreased temper tantrums. In a followup study of the same child, Wolf and Risley (1967) modified other behaviors so that eventually the child was able to make adequate progress in a special public school class. Davison (1964, 1965a, and 1965b) described a program in which he taught undergraduates and teachers to use reinforcement techniques with autistic children to increase the frequency of socially acceptable behaviors and a number of academic and preacademic skills. In one case, Davison found that after 7 weeks of treatment a child followed 17 of 17 commands, whereas previously she had followed only one command.

Brawley et al. (1969), using food and social reinforcers over a 3-month period with a 7-year-old autistic child, were able to decrease nonappropriate behaviors and increase such appropriate behaviors as simple imitative and more complex tasks of a social and vocal nature. During a reinforcement reversal period, the behavior also reversed but was quickly reinstated once the schedule was reestablished, indicating that the schedule was maintaining control over the behavior. Metz (1965) and Hingtgen, Coulter, and Churchill (1967) successfully established imitative sets by reinforcing general imitative behavior in autistic children.

Speech Development

One of the most dramatic uses of behavior modification with psychotic children has been in the area of speech, especially with mute psychotics. Since 1964, over 25 studies have used reinforcement therapy in attempts to expand the verbal repertoires of psychotic children. Although there are no reports of complete success in developing creative speech in a mute psychotic child, in contrast to echolalic children, the methods do appear effective in developing at least low level communication skills in many previously nonspeaking children.

The most basic type of work in this area involves increasing the frequency of simple vocalizations. Kerr, Myerson, and Michael (1965) were able to train a 3-year-old psychotic within a few hours to vocally respond to one-word vocal cues by reinforcing his vocalizations with singing and rocking on the knee. Similar successes with increasing rates of nonspecific vocalizations were obtained by Salzinger et al. (1965) and Hingtgen and Trost (1966). In the latter study, pairs of psychotic children were required to make a vocal response combined with mutual physical contact to obtain candy. Fineman (1968) used changing visual color displays as reinforcers for vocalizations.

One of the first studies in which actual speech was developed was that reported by Hewett in 1965. Over an 18-month period, food was used as a reinforcer for general imitative behavior, then imitative verbal behavior, and finally generalized language in a 4-year-old psychotic boy. Hewett (1964 and 1966) and his group (Hewett, Mayhew, and Rabb 1967) have also been able to develop reading skills in autistic children. Davison (1964) found increases in communicative speech after a limited treatment program was established for one autistic child. Later he (1965a) extended this program to the home where the parents reinforced appropriate speech.

Some of the most important work in the area of speech development with psychotic children has been done by Lovaas and his coworkers. They initially reinforced two schizophrenic children (CA 6) with food following any spontaneous vocalizations (1966a). Gradually, through successive approximations, imitative vocalizations were shaped and subsequently only appropriate imitative vocal responses were rewarded. Many sounds and words were acquired very rapidly, but others took weeks of daily sessions. After both subjects had developed imitative speech, Lovaas tested whether a generalized set was formed. He found that his subjects would imitate words without extrinsic rewards, indicating that imitation in itself had become rewarding. Later this imitative vocabulary was used to develop more spontaneous speech (Lovaas 1966a and 1971).

Risley and Wolf (1966) taught the parents of an autistic child to use successive approximation and fading techniques for shaping both imitative and more complex speech in many situations. These same investigators also developed spontaneous speech in four echolalic autistic or brain-damaged children (CA 7-0 to 12-0) by using verbal prompts and fading (1967). There are numerous other reports of these techniques being used to facilitate speech development (Brawley et al. 1969, Churchill 1969, Colligan and Bellamy 1968, Gardner et al. 1968, Gray and Fygetakis 1968, Hingtgen, Coulter, and Churchill 1967, Jensen and Womack 1967, Matheny 1968, and Shaw 1969).

Two additional studies of special interest are those of Martin et al. (1968) and Ney (1967). In the former, language development was carried out in a classroom situation in which seven of 10 psychotic children significantly improved. And in the latter, *matched* groups of schizophrenic children, divided into play-therapy and operant-conditioning groups, received 50 45-minute sessions directed toward developing speech; the group receiving behavior therapy showed more improvement in speech and in Vineland scores than did the play-therapy group.

Although behavior therapy has led to substantial improvements in the speech of psychotic children, the extent to which these techniques can develop spontaneous language, especially in mute subjects, is still unclear. Hingtgen and Churchill (1969 and 1971), who used reinforcement methods during an extensive training period to develop vocal responses in four mute psychotic children, reported a wide variation in results. Although all subjects developed imitative speech, two of the children were never able to make the initial auditory-visual and visual-vocal associations necessary for spontaneous speech. Other investigators have questioned whether mute psychotic children can ever develop more than rote speech (Weiss and Born 1967). It is too early at this stage of research to accept such a possibility, but, even if true, most clinicians would regard rote speech as better than no speech. Nelson and Evans (1968) have suggested that a combination of traditional speech-therapy techniques and operant-conditioning principles might be most effective in establishing functional speech.

Social Behavior

A major characteristic of childhood psychosis is a deficiency of social behavior. One of the earliest attempts to develop social behavior in psychotic children was carried out by DeMyer and Ferster (1969), who reinforced eight children for initiating peer and adult interactions. Simple cooperative social behaviors in early childhood schizophrenics were shaped by Hingtgen, Sanders, and DeMyer (1965), who required three pairs of children to manipulate various devices in order to receive reinforcement. Not only did the mechanical cooperative behavior increase under these circumstances but other appropriate social behaviors that were not directly rewarded increased as well. While these social behaviors did not extend beyond the experimental room, a followup study (Hingtgen and Trost 1966), in which social behaviors involving physical contact were directly reinforced, did result in some transfer to the ward and home situations.

Lovaas (1966b) and Lovaas, Schaeffer, and Simmons (1965) used the elimination of electric shock as a reinforcer for social behavior in one set of identical autistic twins (CA 5-0); the twins could escape shock by approaching an adult and hugging or kissing him. A later study from Lovaas' group (1966b and 1967) provided food rewards for increases in such socially appropriate behaviors as participating in preschool games.

In a 5-week treatment program, Carlin and Armstrong (1968), working with brain-damaged and psychotic children, used token reinforcers to shape social interaction and responsibility during group play. They found a reduction in disruptive behaviors and an increase in playing together which carried over to the ward situation. Similarly, Metz (1966) was able to establish a token reinforcement program in which 11 emotionally disturbed children (some of whom were autistic) earned their tokens for self-help skills and social behaviors (e.g., holding hands, giving other children tricycle rides, and playing games together).

Using a behavior-therapy program in a kindergarten class setting, Martin et al. (1968) succeeded in developing socially appropriate behaviors in 10 autistic children by assigning one reinforcing adult for each child. Many other studies have used behavior modification to increase social interaction both on the hospital ward and in the home. All report some degree of success in expanding the social repertoires of psychotic children (Brawley et al. 1969, Gardner et al. 1968, Jensen and Womach 1967, Johnson and Brown 1969, Maes 1969, Means and Merrens 1969, Patterson and Brodsky 1966, Sussman and Sklar 1969, Wetzel et al. 1966, and Wolf and Risley 1967).

Aversive Conditioning

A number of controversial (Breger 1965) studies have appeared which employed electric shock to control the behavior of psychotic children (Baroff and Tate 1968, Lovaas 1966b, Lovaas et al. 1965a, Lovaas, Schaeffer, and Simmons 1965, Risley 1968, Simmons and Lovaas 1969, and Tate and Baroff 1966). Because these drastic measures are effective in rapidly eliminating self-mutilative behaviors, their use appears justified. Whether shock should be used to manipulate other behaviors is highly questionable. Certainly, the substantial improvements reported by the great majority of studies using positive reinforcement would suggest that electric shock is neither necessary nor appropriate when the goal is to develop new behaviors.

Other Studies

Three other studies employing reinforcement methods deserve special mention. Hudson and DeMyer (1968) found that the initial use of food as a medium during occupational therapy sessions facilitated the later manipulation of regular craft media by psychotic children. A successful toilet training program for autistic children has been designed by Marshall (1966). Goodwin and Goodwin (1969) employed the Edison Responsive Environment (a cubicle enclosing a multiphase electric typewriter, projector, and programming device designed to respond to or direct the user in a variety of ways) in a large study of children with learning disabilities, including some diagnosed as psychotic. Following various amounts of exposure to the apparatus, most children demonstrated general behavioral improvement and decreases in disruptive behavior and hyperactivity. Additional data on the use of behavior modification with psychotic children are included in four recent review articles (Gelfand and Hartmann 1968, Leff 1968, Werry and Wollersheim 1967, and Yates 1970).

TREATMENT OUTCOME STUDIES

Although treatment studies of childhood psychoses are typically based on small numbers of subjects with no comparison groups, there have been a few large-scale outcome reports. Wenar et al. (1967) found that a small daycare center with a 1:1 adult-child ratio was most effective in bringing about improvement in the areas of relationship, mastery, and psychosexual development, when compared to milieu therapy in a custodial-care institution or a modern well-staffed State institution. In the latter two situations there was little difference in the progress made. None of the treatment procedures, however, produced significant improvement in communication and vocalizations. In a long-term followup of children who had been hospitalized for various lengths of time, Levy (1969) reported that schizophrenics with low IQ's had the poorest prognosis, regardless of the length of hospitalization.

Several studies have compared residential and daycare treatment programs. Davids, Ryan, and Salvatore (1968) found no large differences between these approaches, but Kemph (1966b) in a 3-year followup of 51 subjects reported that the greatest improvement occurred in the group that had received the most intensive therapy. In a series of studies Goldfarb and coworkers (Goldfarb and Goldfarb 1965, Goldfarb, Goldfarb, and Pollack 1969, and Goldfarb and Pollack 1964) matched 26 schizophrenic children for age, sex, IQ, and neurological findings and divided them into organic, nonorganic and unscorable (IQ) groups. Half of each group received daycare treatment and half received residential treatment. The unscorable group showed no improvement in either daycare or residential treatment; the organic group showed equal improvement in the two types of therapy; and the nonorganic children showed more improvement in residential than daycare treatment.

No firm conclusions can be drawn from this very limited number of outcome studies. The data do suggest, however, that in some cases psychotic children show greater improvement under conditions of intensive therapy.

EVALUATION OF TREATMENT

The treatment picture of childhood psychotic disorders has dramatically changed in the last 6 years. In contrast to the very pessimistic view presented by Rimland in 1964, therapists are now reporting greater success in working with psychotic children, even of the mute type. Although the introduction of more effective therapeutic techniques (body stimulation, group therapy, educational programs, and behavior modification) could account for this altered outlook, other contributing factors might include the following: 1) therapists and trained ancillary workers (e.g., parents, teachers, and ward attendants) are spending much more time in working with the children; 2) almost all forms of therapy now involve some training in basic perceptual-motor skills, even when the orientation remains essentially psychodynamic; and 3) therapeutic goals are often limited, resembling more closely those set for nonpsychotic retarded and brain-damaged children. The relative importance of these variables has not yet been determined, but they must be considered in any study of therapeutic procedures.

Regarding the comparative effectiveness of the new types of therapy, no objective assessment has been made to date. This problem is especially difficult since there are similarities in actual practice among the the therapies, in spite of their different rationales. Body stimulation, group therapy, and educational programs all involve techniques that could be interpreted in terms of behavioral techniques. On the other hand, behavior therapists do form relationships with the children, and such interpersonal responding cannot be ignored as irrelevant to the behavioral changes observed (Weiland 1971).

Despite these difficulties, outcome studies comparing various therapeutic approaches are sorely needed. These investigations will require clear and detailed descriptions of methodology as applied to matched groups of subjects (including appropriate control groups) for fixed periods of time. In addition, pre- and post-therapy evaluation procedures, plus adequate followups, should be provided (Fish 1964 and Yates 1970). Now that a number of promising treatments for childhood psychotic disorders have been proposed, it is not too early to submit them to a more precise appraisal.

While the therapeutic outlook has brightened considerably, the general prognosis for most childhood psychotics is still poor in terms of developing levels of normal functioning. Significant expansion of their behavioral repertoires can be achieved, but spontaneity may remain absent, especially in the area of speech. At an even lower level many of these children do not seem able to make various types of simple cross-modal associations. Whether these major therapeutic roadblocks can be eliminated will be answered by further intensive study. What is clear at this point is that abilities vary widely from child to child, no matter what the diagnosis. Until each child's specific limitations of learning are objectively determined, all methods of proven effectiveness must be used to enable him to reach his highest level of performance. At best, these therapeutic approaches could allow the child to function well in home and school settings; at the very least, they could provide for the construction of prosthetic environments, designed for the individual child according to his maximum abilities.

THEORY

The progress of experimental studies of early childhood psychoses has been relatively independent of formal theoretical considerations, since all current theories share a major weakness—they generate few testable hypotheses. In addition, many are fragmentary, dealing with only selected aspects of psychotic behavior in children. Specification of the diagnostic categories to which the theories refer is also frequently unclear. In spite of these heuristic limitations, a large number of theories of psychotic disorders of childhood have been proposed, with new ones appearing every few months. They may be divided into three types according to the etiological factors emphasized in each: nonorganic, organic-experiential interaction, and organic.

Most nonorganic theories are psychodynamically oriented, assume that the infant is physically normal at birth, and attribute the development of psychotic behavior to pathological personality characteristics and behaviors in the parents. They differ, however, in the interpretations of the deviant parent-child interactions and their suggestions of specific critical periods during which time the children are assumed to be unusually susceptible to parental mishandling.

Bettelheim (1967), one of the leading proponents of a psychogenic theory, interprets autistic behavior as denial of self in defense against threats of total destruction from a world perceived as hostile and rejecting. Pathological characteristics within the parents, particularly the mother, lead to pathogenic under- or over-stimulation, which prevents the child from effectively acting on his environment. Thus, the child is blocked from experiences necessary for developing a concept of self. Similar interpretations of autistic behavior as withdrawal from a hostile and threatening world are proposed by Griffith and Ritvo (1967) and Haworth and Menolascino (1968), although they differ on whether the underlying mechanism is one of fixation or deviant development.

In contrast, Zaslow (1967) attributes autistic behavior to the combined effects of stimulus deprivation (as a result of inadequate tactile-kinesthetic handling) and the mother's inappropriate tolerance and reduction of the infant's rage reactions. All schizophrenic reactions, ranging from autism to adult schizophrenia, are mourning reactions to the perceived loss of maternal love according to Edelson (1966).

Somewhat different pathological mother-child relationships are postulated by Lordi and Silverberg (1964) and Speers and Lansing (1964). Lordi and Silverberg speculate that the breakdown of the mother-child relationship is due to an extension of, and reaction to, early narcissistic injury in the mother, coupled with a dependent personality in the father. Speers and Lansing, on the other hand, regard the parents, as well as the child, as committed to a symbiotic relationship because of their own unresolved dependency conflicts. They feel that the mother identifies with the child's dependency needs and projects her own undesirable impulses onto the child. In a later revision of their theory, Speers and Lansing (1968) suggest that psychobiological functioning of the mother during gestation may be a causative factor. This position would put them more in the organic-experiential class of theories.

Whereas most nonorganic theories are psychodynamically oriented, Ferster (1961 and 1966) presents a purely behavioral interpretation of autistic etiology. He sees parents as failing to sufficiently pair primary reinforcements with a wide variety of behaviors. Thus, parental responses which are social in nature do not become conditioned or generalized reinforcers and the child develops little or no appropriate social behavior. Ferster further postulates that atavisms, because of their aversive effects, are frequently reinforced by parents. In addition, repetitive, self-stimulative behaviors are maintained by continuous reinforcement through their immediate and direct effects on the environment and the child's own body.

ORGANIC-EXPERIENTIAL

The organic-experiential interaction theories may be subdivided into those which are similar to the psychodynamic nonorganic theories in emphasizing pathological mother-child relationships, while allowing for some unspecified vulnerability in the child, and those which are similar to the organic theories in stressing deviations in the child for which the mother does not compensate.

The interaction theories that emphasize breakdowns in the mother-child relationship postulate a basic failure to develop real object relationships. They differ, however, in their interpretation of the underlying mechanisms. For example, while Smolen (1965), Soddy (1964), and Garcia and Sarvis (1964) all consider the autistic disturbance to be due to a combination of organic predisposition and maternal deficiency, Soddy specifically implicates inadequate feeding satisfaction patterns, and Garcia and Sarvis suggest that a paranoid reaction, directed at the mother, is the basic core of autism.

Ruttenberg (1971) and his group (1966) make a distinction between primary autism, which is considered to be largely due to innate or congenital organic brain damage, and secondary autism, which is considered to be largely a response to an inadequate environment. In both types, the development and severity of autistic behavior are thought to be determined by the interaction between degree of organic damage and degree of environmental stress, and the basic mechanism is interpreted as developmental arrest at the preoral level of psychosexual development as a defense against mothering behavior which is perceived as noxious or overwhelming. Goldfarb (1961) also distinguishes between organic and nonorganic childhood schizophrenia on the basis of the relative contributions of congenital brain damage and environmental inadequacy, resulting in severe deficits of ego development.

A somewhat similar system has been proposed by Ward (1970), who makes an additional distinction between early infantile autism and childhood schizophrenia. While the childhood schizophrenic is thought to have a fragmentary body ego, the autistic child is seen as having a defensively developed behavioral ego. Ward believes that autism basically results from the lack of experience of a varied and stimulating patterned environment which may result from one of three conditions: 1) an organically based, abnormally high stimulus barrier, 2) an organically based hypersensitivity to external stimuli, or 3) a nonnurturant, non-stimulating, nonpatterned home environment.

Weiland (1964 and 1966) and Mahler (1965) distinguish between autism and symbiosis, although both syndromes are thought to originate in the early mother-child relationship. Both investigators suggest that autism stems from a basic failure to associate the mother as an external object with internal need gratification, with resulting lack of development of elementary ego functions (Weiland 1964) and retraction of affective contact (Mahler 1965). Their conceptions of autism differ in that Weiland does not consider anxiety to be a factor, while Mahler sees autism as a defense against anxiety. Both investigators agree that symbiosis reflects chronic separation anxiety: Weiland (1966) postulates a circular relationship between failure to develop object relationships and employment of symbiotic behavior, while Mahler suggests that the infant associates all need gratification with the mother and never generalizes tension reduction to other objects, with the result that any break in the symbiotic relationships produces overwhelming anxiety. Although the authors attribute both autism and symbiosis to the combined effects of central-nervous-system pathology and/or environmental stress, Mahler places somewhat more emphasis on constitutional vulnerability.

While O'Gorman (1967) also traces autism to the basic failure to develop a normal relationship with the mother, and hence to become involved with reality, he suggests a variety of possible causes—an excessively stressful environment, a genetic predisposition, and anatomic, metabolic, or physiologic diseases.

The preceding interactional theories all stress disruptions in the mother-child relationship which prevent the development of object relationships, while those that follow tend to emphasize the constitutional limitations of the child.

Kanner (1963)[3] postulates an inborn defect in relatedness, *per se*, which is aggravated by lack of emotional involvement in the parents;

---

[3] See, also, Chambers 1969.

thus, he suggests that, although the determining factor in autism is the interaction between the inborn defect and lack of environmental compensation, the development of the syndrome could be avoided by more intense parental involvement. By contrast, Eaton and Menolascino (1967) view the psychotic base as a more general process which prevents or interferes with all integrative functions, and Gibson (1968) interprets autistic symptoms as an organically damaged child's defensive reactions to unrealistic parental expectations.

Several authors are more specific in their emphasis on perceptual dysfunctions for which the environment fails to compensate. For example, Kirk (1968) postulates that unrecognized perceptual defects in the child lead to a circular relationship between the child's learning handicaps and the parents' difficulties in developing appropriate responses. Stroh and Buick (1964) suggest that constitutional and/or environmental deficiencies result in arrested perceptual development and that autistic behaviors represent the child's attempt to adapt to the environment and integrate incoming stimuli within his limited perceptual system. Salk (1968) speculates that these children are unusually vulnerable to insufficient sensory stimulation and that lack of compensation with adequate sensory stimulation during the first few days of life may produce irreversible damage. Schopler (1965) postulates a specific dysfunction in the arousal and inhibition of sensory processes, which takes the form of hyposensitivity in autism and of hypersensitivity in childhood schizophrenia. Attempting to isolate a specific causal event, Glavin (1966) proposes that a rapid decrease in oxygen tension in the blood produces both retrolental fibroplasia and autism; he attributes the differences in behavior between the two groups to differences in interaction between environmental variables and the extent of the underlying brain damage.

ORGANIC

Organic theories also take many different forms, ranging from those suggesting diffuse organic damage to those postulating more specific sites of impairment.

Bender (1966b and 1967) attributes childhood schizophrenia to an uninherited vulnerability and believes it is characterized by a lag in maturation at the embryonic level, which results in embryonic plasticity in all areas of functioning, particularly those which are integrated by the central nervous system. Because the child is consequently unable to perceive reality and experience clearly defined patterns of sensation, anxiety is produced. In Bender's conception, autistic behaviors are merely one group of a variety of defense mechanisms which could be employed to cope with the anxiety.

Stressing the behavioral similarities between autism and developmental aphasia, Rutter (1965a, 1965b, and 1971) and Wing (1966) both postulate an underlying general brain damage occurring before or very soon after birth which disrupts speech, perceptual, and cognitive development. Autistic symptomatology is considered to be an adaptation to lack of comprehension of the environment. Gittelman and Birch (1967) also postulate that the inappropriate behaviors of autism result from primary disorders in the sensory and response systems—rather than representing defense mechanisms against pathological environmental or parental factors.

A number of authors hypothesize that innate defects in the arousal mechanisms interfere with the psychotic child's ability to process incoming information. Hutt and Hutt (1968), for example, suggest that there is a chronically high level of cortical arousal in these children. Autistic behaviors, particularly stereotypies, are thought to serve an arousal-reducing function by producing repetitive endogenous stimulation and blocking sensory input.

Rimland (1964 and 1968) contends that a malfunction of the reticular formation which produces inadequate arousal to incoming stimuli results in the child's inability to relate new stimuli to remembered experience, or, at the infant level, to associate biological rewards with social, particularly maternal, relationships. Rimland further speculates that the malfunction of the reticular formation results from genetic homozygosity in the gene related to the ability to focus attention and ignore distractions—the gene which he suggests would contribute to high intelligence in heterozygous individuals.

Des Lauriers and Carlson (1969) postulate that there is an imbalance between the ascending reticular activating system (Arousal I) and the limbic reward system (Arousal II), such that Arousal I dominates or inhibits Arousal II. Thus, because of his chronically high state of arousal, the child cannot form stimulus-reward relationships, and the majority of all impinging stimuli remain forever new and novel to him. A similar hypothesis is presented by Freides and Pierce (1968), who suggest that, because of a chronic imbalance between the nonspecific and specific somasthetic processing systems, somasthetic stimulation is channeled largely through nonspecific pathways with direct connection to the reticular formation rather than through specific pathways projecting to the cortex via thalamic centers. Again, the result is that the child is in a chronically high state of arousal which interferes with information processing. Freides and Pierce suggest, however, that aversion to body stimulation is the primary symptom and that other autistic behaviors are derivatives.

Ornitz and Ritvo (Ornitz 1969 and Ornitz and Ritvo 1968a and b) postulate an innate failure of homeostatic regulation within the CNS, such that environmental stimuli are either inadequately modulated or unevenly amplified, resulting in perceptual inconstancy and an inability to organize internal and external stimuli. The physiological equilibrium between facilitatory and inhibitory systems is disrupted, and, on the basis of comparisons with REM sleep, they hypothesize that the defect lies within the vestibular system.

Using analogies with computer programing, Kahn and Arbib (1968) suggest an inborn neurochemical defect resulting in the failure of processes to integrate analogic (emotional) and digital (logical) information. The breakdown in development occurs when the child cannot make systematic digital associations between the mother and tension relief, with the result that the homeostatic mechanisms dealing wih input or feedback become highly restrictive. Their organic hypothesis refers only to autism, since they attribute childhood schizophrenia to environmental factors in the form of inadequate or confusing information.

DEFECTS IN THEORIES

Nonorganic theories, whether psychodynamic or behavioral, are similar in their emphasis on parental, especially maternal, pathology as the primary cause of behavioral deficits in the child. The assumption is that maternal over protection, rejection, emotional deprivation, improper somasthetic stimulation, or inappropriate reinforcement can be so severe or traumatic that a child who is biologically or physically normal at birth is prevented from effectively interacting with his social and physical environment. One would expect that such deviant behavior on the part of the parents would be relatively easy to identify. In recent studies, however, there appears to be little or no evidence of parental psychopathology. On the contrary, they demonstrate low incidences of familial psychosis, broken homes, and sibling pathology, compared to control groups.

Most nonorganic theories also postulate the occurrence of critical periods, during which time the child is especially susceptible to parental mishandling. As yet, critical periods of this type have never been demonstrated in man; nor is there any evidence that stresses actually occurred during such periods. In addition, these theories do not account for the fact that other children subjected to severe environmental stress during this same time develop into normal adults.

Since organic-experiential theories allow for interaction between organic vulnerability and environmental stress, they are less weakened than nonorganic theories by the lack of demonstrated severe parental pathology. But the interactional theories are vague in defining either the nature of the underlying vulnerability, the nature of the environmental stress, or the degree to which each factor contributes to pathology. Also, if the severe behavioral deficits observed in childhood psychotics can result from moderate amounts of stress, one might expect to see a much higher incidence of these disorders.

Organic theories allow for a wide variety of types of damage, including defects in the arousal and integrative mechanisms. Until more information on the normal functioning of these systems is obtained, however, the hypotheses of malfunction cannot be adequately tested. Recent experimental data would indicate that there is neurobiological damage in a large number of psychotic children, but the evidence does not tend to support one organic theory over another. Furthermore, none of the organic theories provide an acceptable explanation for the fact that most organically damaged children are not psychotic.

CURRENT STATUS

Two major hypotheses have guided much of the early work with psychotic children. In the first, the childhood psychoses were thought to represent the earliest manifestations of adult schizophrenia. Therefore, the identification of etiological factors and the development of effective treatment procedures for disorders of childhood were expected to broaden understanding of adult schizophrenia. In the second hypothesis, psychotic children were believed to be *potentially* capable of normal functioning in all areas of development. If disruptive, environmentally caused emotional difficulties could be resolved, it was postulated, these disturbed children might become normal adults with little or no residual impairment. Unfortunately, the evidence available from current research provides little support for either of these initial hypotheses.

Contrary to the theory of normal "potential," the large majority of psychotic children demonstrate severe deficits in intellectual, perceptual, and language development. Followup studies indicate that, even when bizarre behaviors diminish and social relatedness increases, gross deficits in other areas of functioning remain. Many recent reports also indicate that, regardless of the treatment program followed, these children show more improvement in affective contact than in intellectual, perceptual, and language skills. Thus, it now appears that their deficits in social behavior are less a cause than a reflection of deviations in other areas of development.

While the concept of a link between childhood and adult psychoses is still accepted, on theoretical grounds, by a small number of investigators, data from epidemiological and followup studies suggest that there are few similarities between childhood and adult psychotics in terms of family characteristics or psychopathology. On the other hand, there are many similarities in symptomatology between psychotic and brain-damaged children.

If there is little or no relationship between childhood and adult psychosis, and if the children diagnosed as psychotic are more similar to brain-damaged or retarded children than to psychotic adults, one might wonder how childhood schizophrenics can be differentiated from other atypical children. Although some agreement exists regarding childhood schizophrenia's identifiable symptomatology, more progress could be made in answering this question if investigators were more thorough in describing subjects and routinely made comparisons with control groups. At present, individual investigators employ differing classification systems, which often are not readily communicable to the rest of the research community. For this reason, a number of investigators have proposed a tri-axial classification system for all childhood disorders (including aphasias, hyperkinesis, and minimal brain damage). The proposed system would have behavioral rather than interpretive descriptions of symptoms as one axis, test-derived estimates of intellectual and language functioning as a second independent axis, and the results of neurological examinations as the third axis. By eliminating the controversy as to whether psychotic children are retarded and/or brain-damaged, this system would provide a better means for obtaining comparison group data. Until this system is more widely accepted, however, it is to be hoped that—as a minimum requirement—all reports (regardless of the classification system used) should provide adequate descriptions (i.e., profiles of CA, MA, social behavior, speech development, organicity indicators, and other relevant data) for each individual or group of subjects.

There has been an encouraging increase in the number of objective studies of the behavioral, intellectual, perceptual, language, and neurobiological characteristics of psychotic children. The majority of these studies indicate that psychotic children have moderate to severe dysfunctions in almost every area of development explored. Although there are many individual differences, most psychotic children seldom interact with either adults or other children, exhibit little constructive play, and engage in many repetitive behaviors (nonfunctional manipulations of objects, environmental fixtures, and their own bodies). Recent evidence suggests that many of their avoidance and stereotyped behaviors may be related to success/failure ratios in structured task situations.

Although psychotic children have frequently been considered "untestable," renewed efforts in administering standardized psychological tests have indicated that they can be reliably tested when low-level items are employed. Most function at moderately to severely defective levels, and their scores tend to remain quite low regardless of concurrent improvements in cooperation and social behavior. When subtest scatter occurs, it is generally associated with poor language development rather than unusual psychopathology. Therefore, the low intelligence test scores characteristic of childhood schizophrenics do not appear to be an ephemeral reflection of emotional disturbance; instead they seem to represent remarkably stable and useful predictors of later social adjustment and educational achievement.

Severe language abnormalities are frequently the first readily identifiable symptoms of childhood psychosis. In addition to their characteristic failure to develop communicative speech, most psychotic children demonstrate severe comprehension deficits under controlled testing conditions. Although some schizophrenic children have adequate or normal speech development, muteness and noncommunicative echolalia are frequent hallmarks of childhood psychosis. Despite the heavy emphasis speech training receives in almost all therapeutic programs, regardless of theoretical orientation, success in developing spontaneous or creative speech has been limited and appears to be directly related to the children's initial levels of social and intellectual functioning.

While systematic testing of perceptual processes in psychotic children is a relatively recent research development, many types of perceptual dysfunction have already been demonstrated. Below age level in visual and auditory discrimination and visual-motor skills, many of the children appear to be especially deficient in short-term memory and cross-modal information processing. Only in the development of early gross motor skills do these children meet normal expectations. At present, most standardized psychological tests are not designed to provide detailed deficit profiles for low functioning children. Moreover, because experimental procedures have varied from study to study, it is difficult either to contrast their performance with normative data on nonpsychotic children. A more thorough investigation of the perceptual deficiencies of psychotic children will be necessary if we are to assess their contribution to deviant social, intellectual, and language development and their possible etiological significance. To accomplish this goal will require greater employment of control groups (e.g., retarded, aphasic, and brain-damaged children) as well as further standardization of testing procedures. Finally, to answer the question of whether test-item failure is due to low motivational levels (including negativism) or inability to perform, techniques for increasing and maintaining high motivational levels (such as those used in behavior modification) should be implemented during testing periods.

The data on neurobiological correlates do not present a unified picture of organic involvement in childhood psychoses. Although many indicators of organicity have been found in different groups of psychotic children—for example, abnormal EEG records, cell abnormalities, unusual drug responses, deviant physical characteristics, metabolic deviations, and prenatal, perinatal, and postnatal difficulties—no one particular type of organic dysfunction has yet been found in *all* psychotic children. Nonetheless, large proportions of these children demonstrate many varieties of neurobiological involvement. Technological limitations in measuring physiological and biochemical parameters and the paucity of information regarding the neurobiology of the normal developing child create special difficulties for this type of research, but preliminary evidence justifies an intensified search for solutions to these problems.

The picture of psychotic children which has emerged from recent research investigations is dramatically different from that which earlier prevailed. Once considered normal except for severe emotional problems, psychotic children have now been shown to have severe deficits in all other areas of development: behavioral, intellectual, perceptual, language, neurobiological, and social. Unfortunately, the lack of interaction between theory and experimentation in this field has produced a situation in which research efforts have not been particularly systematic or efficient and most theories of etiology have not been modified to accommodate the recent empirical data.

Nonorganic theories stress faulty environmental conditions as the primary cause of behavioral deficits in psychotic children. In tracing the development of pathology, both the psychodynamic and behavioral theories implicate parental (particularly maternal) pathology, either in the form of the parents' unresolved emotional problems or their failure to provide sufficient reinforcement. If we assume—as do proponents of nonorganic theories—that psychotic children were biologically normal at birth, we should also expect that parental deviations severe enough to have produced such profound and pervasive behavioral defects would be readily identifiable. But when actual comparisons have been made—whether with the general population or other clinical groups—parents of psychotic children do not appear to be unusually deviant, either in their own personality organization or their child-rearing practices. Moreover, the fact that some therapists have successfully trained parents to serve as adjunct therapists suggests that any previously observed "pathological" behaviors may merely have reflected their confusion and uncertainty in dealing with severely damaged children. Unfortunately, much of the popular press emphasizes parental responsibility in producing these children. It has taken decades of educational effort to alleviate parental guilt in the case of retarded and brain-damaged children, and, in the case of psychotic children, where the physical stigmata are not so obvious, the educational task will be much more difficult.

In organic-experiential theories, the childhood schizophrenic's disturbance is attributed to a combination of organic vulnerability and environmental stress. While suggesting less severe parental pathology than the nonorganic theories, organic-experiential theories are generally quite vague in defining the nature of either "organic vulnerability" or "environmental stress" and frequently tend to emphasize the parental contribution. Many of these theories also employ the concept of critical periods during which the child is particularly susceptible to environmental mishandling—a notion which was extrapolated from animal studies and which has received little empirical support from studies with human infants. Given the long period of dependency and plasticity in child development, as well as the wide range of developmental milestones accepted as normal, it remains highly speculative that such critical periods exist in man.

Hypotheses of organic defects are more congruent with the existing empirical data which demonstrate many types of neurobiological impairment as well as a variety of severe intellectual, perceptual, and language dysfunctions in these children. There is no conclusive evidence supporting one organic theory over another, however, and the data strongly suggest that there may be many forms of organic damage present which result in similar maladaptive behaviors.

Although some progress has been made, most etiological theories are untestable in their present form, and are often based on an extremely selective portion of the available data. This is due partly to the relative recency of the organic hypotheses, partly to the lack of detailed knowledge concerning many aspects of early normal development (particularly in the neurobiological area), and partly to the lack of systematic research strategies designed to reject or support precisely defined alternative hypotheses. It may be that efforts to develop comprehensive theoretical systems are premature at this stage, particularly since the necessary descriptive and experimental data comparing psychotic and control groups are not yet available.

Not all advances in therapeutic procedures depend upon theoretical advances or the uncovering of etiological substrates (for example, the use of psychopharmacological agents in the treatment of adult schizophrenia or of special training techniques with retarded children). Even in the absence of clear statements of etiology, some progress has been made in the treatment of psychotic children. Conventional therapy is still used with these children occasionally, but the major concentration of recent efforts has been directed toward a number of new approaches— for example, body stimulation, group therapy, educational programs, and behavior modification.

In brief, the body-stimulation therapists use various types of tactile stimulatory procedures to provide the child with sensory experiences presumed to be lacking in his earlier development, while the group therapists attempt to remedy his social deficiencies by developing interactions within small groups. Educational and behavior therapy programs have achieved encouraging results by focusing on specific target behaviors, rather than general therapeutic goals. Although some educational programs are based on psychodynamic theories, both the educational and behavior therapy techniques emphasize training in specific academic or preacademic skills (for example, speech and language development, perceptual discriminations, and perceptual-motor tasks), as well as attempting to increase overall attention and social behaviors.

Because of difficulties in obtaining adequate descriptions of initial clinical state and subsequent behavioral change, relatively few attempts have been made to compare the effectiveness of differing treatment approaches. Some standardization of reporting procedures is badly needed. Used in conjunction with appropriate control groups, pre- and post-therapy evaluation scores (from standardized tests, rating scales, or structured observations) would be extremely valuable in determining degree of clinical improvement. If objective profiles of differential changes in behavior following therapeutic intervention were routinely provided, these data could prove most helpful in drawing diagnostic and etiological conclusions.

The new therapeutic approaches have not only been successful in developing new behaviors in psychotic children but also in uncovering previously underestimated areas of severe deficit. Their effectiveness in developing new responses stems from their emphasis on actively eliciting and rewarding specific behaviors, rather than waiting for the child's hypothesized emotional disturbance to be resolved and for these new behaviors to spontaneously emerge. Surprisingly, the so-called "autistic barrier" appears to be the easiest obstacle to overcome, and at least minimal social relationships are established fairly quickly. But in spite of increased social interaction and elevated motivational levels (as demonstrated by consistent and reliable responding) there are many areas of behavioral development in which very limited progress has been made —perception, cognition, language, and the development of spontaneous behaviors. Although greater improvement is achieved with children who exhibited some minimal social development and communicative speech before therapy began, most of the children rather rapidly reach developmental plateaus or "low ceilings" in these areas. Only further work will determine whether these limitations can be overcome.

SUMMARY

Recent developments in the study of early chldhood psychoses are reviewed in terms of description, diagnosis, intellectual functioning, language characteristics, perceptual processes, neurobiological research, therapeutic procedures, and theoretical position. Despite the variety of diagnostic classification systems, actual descriptions of symptomatology appear remarkably similar for all forms of childhood psychoses. There is increasing evidence that the great majority of psychotic children demonstrate moderate or severe intellectual retardation, serious communication deficits, gross disturbances of perceptual processes, and various types of neurobiological dysfunction. Studies of family characteristics tend to rule out parental psychopathology as a causative factor. The introduction of body-stimulation, group-therapy, special educational, and behavior-modification techniques offers hope for more effective treatment, but controlled outcome studies comparing the various therapies are needed. Many theories of limited heuristic value have been proposed, including those stressing nonorganic, organic-experiential interaction, or organic factors. The growing evidence of perceptual and neurobiological involvement suggests that research in these areas should be intensified.

ACKNOWLEDGMENT

Preparation of this paper was supported by the National Institute of Mental Health, PHS, Grant No. 05154-09 and the LaRue D. Carter Memorial Hospital, Indianapolis,

Ind. We thank Drs. M. K. DeMyer, J. I. Nurnberger, and D. F. Moore for their support and Phil Enz, Judith Smith, and Janet Allen of the LaRue Carter Medical Library for their assistance in obtaining the necessary references. Special thanks are due Lynn Jenkins for her outstanding technical skill during all stages of the preparation of this review.

REFERENCES

ABRAHAMSON, H. A.: The use of LSD (d-lysergic acid diethylamide) in the therapy of children. *The Journal of Asthma Research*, 5:139-143, 1967.

ALANEN, Y. O., ARAJÄRVI, T., & VIITAMÄKI, R. O.: Psychoses in childhood. *Acta Psychiatrica Scandinavica*, 40: Supplement 174, 1964.

ALDERTON, H. R.: A review of schizophrenia in childhood. *Canadian Psychiatric Association Journal*, 11:276-285, 1966.

ALLEN, C. E. & TOOMEY, L. C.: Use of the Vineland Social Maturity Scale for evaluating progress of psychotic children in a therapeutic nursery school. *American Journal of Orthopsychiatry*, 35:152-159, 1965.

ALPERN, G. D.: Measurement of "untestable" autistic children. *Journal of Abnormal Psychology*, 72:478-486, 1967.

ALPERN, G. D. & KIMBERLIN, C. C.: Short intelligence test ranging from infancy levels through childhood levels for use with the retarded. *American Journal of Mental Deficiency*, 1:65-71, 1970.

ALPERT, A. & PFEIFFER, E.: Treatment of an autistic child: Introduction and theoretical discussion. *Journal of the American Academy of Child Psychiatry*, 3:591-616, 1964.

ASPERGER, H.: On the differential diagnosis of early infantile autism. *Acta Paedopsychiatrica*, 35:136-145, 1968.

BAROFF, G. S. & TATE, B. G.: The use of aversive stimulation in the treatment of chronic self-injurious behavior. *Journal of the American Academy of Child Psychiatry*, 7:454-460, 1968.

BELZ, J. F., DREHMEL, V. W., & SILVERTSEN, A. D.: "Volunteer: The Community's Participant in Treatment of Schizophrenic Children in a Day Care Program." Paper presented at the American Orthopsychiatric Association, 1967.

BENDER, L.: A twenty-five year view of therapeutic results. In: P. H. Hoch and J. Zubin (Eds.): *The Evaluation of Psychiatric Treatment*. New York: Grune and Stratton, Inc., 1964.

BENDER, L.: D-lysergic acid in the treatment of the biological features of childhood schizophrenia. *Diseases of the Nervous System*, 7:43-46, 1966a.

BENDER, L.: The concept of plasticity in childhood schizophrenia. In: P. H. Hoch and J. Zubin (Eds.): *Psychopathology of Schizophrenia*. New York: Grune and Stratton, Inc., 1966b.

BENDER, L.: Childhood schizophrenia: A review. *Journal of Hillside Hospital*, 16:10-22, 1967.

BENDER, L., FARETRA, G., COBRINIK, L., & SANKAR, D. V.: The treatment of childhood schizophrenia with LSD and UML. In M. Rinkel (Ed.): *The Biological Treatment of Mental Illness*. New York: L. C. Page and Co., 1966.

BENNETT, S. & KLEIN, H. R.: Childhood schizophrenia: 30 years later. *American Journal of Psychiatry*, 122:1121-1124., 1966.

BERNAL, M. E., SIMMONS, J. Q., III, & MILLER, W. H.: Psychophysiological studies of autistic children (progress report). *California Mental Health Research Digest*, 7:151-152, 1969.

BETTELHEIM, B.: *The Empty Fortress: Infantile Autism and the Birth of the Self*. New York: The Free Press, 1967.

BIRCH, H. G. & WALKER, H. A.: Perceptual and perceptual-motor dissociation. Studies in schizophrenic and brain-damaged psychotic children. *Archives of General Psychiatry*, 14:113-118, 1966.

BLOCK, J.: Parents of schizophrenic, neurotic, asthmatic, and congenitally ill children: A comparative study. *Archives of General Psychiatry*, 20:659-674, 1969.

BOER, A. P.: Application of a simple recording system to the analysis of free-play behavior in autistic children. *Journal of Applied Behavior Analysis*, 1:335-340, 1968.

BOOK, J., NICHTERN, S., & GRUENBERG, E.: Cytogenetical investigations in childhood schizophrenia. *Acta Psychiatrica Scandinavica*, 39 (2):309-323, 1963.

BRAMBILLA, F., VIANI, F., & ROSSOTTI, V.: Endocrine aspects of child psychoses. *Diseases of the Nervous System*, 30:627-632, 1969.

BRAWLEY, E. R., HARRIS, F. R., ALLEN, K. E., FLEMING, R. S., & PETERSON, R. F.: Behavior modification of an autistic child. *Behavioral Science*, 14:87-97, 1969.

BREGER, L.: Comments on "building social behavior in autistic children by use of electric shock." *Journal of Experimental Research in Personality*, 1:110-113, 1965.

BROOKS, B. D., MORROW, J. E., & GRAY, W. F.: Reduction of autistic gaze aversion by reinforcement of visual-attention responses. *Journal of Special Education*, 2:307-309, 1968.

BRYSON, C. Q.: *Short-Term Memory Deficits in Young Autistic Children*. Research Report No. 4, Clinical Research Center for Early Childhood Schizophrenia, Indianapolis, Ind., 1970a.

BRYSON, C. Q.: Systematic identification of perceptual disabilities in autistic children. *Perceptual and Motor Skills*, 31:239-246, 1970b.

CAIN, A.: Special "isolated" abilities in severely psychotic young children. *Psychiatry*, 32:137-149, 1969.

CARLIN, A. S. & ARMSTRONG, H. E.: Rewarding social responsibility in disturbed children: A group play technique. *Psychotherapy: Theory, Research and Practice*, 5:169-174, 1968.

CHAMBERS, C. H.: Leo Kanner's concept of early infantile autism. *British Journal of Medical Psychology*, 42:51-54, 1969.

CHURCHILL, D. W.: Psychotic children and behavior modification. *American Journal of Psychiatry*, 125:1585-1590, 1969.

CHURCHILL, D. W.: *The Effects of Success and Failure on Psychotic Children*. Indianapolis, Ind.: Research Report No. 5, Clinical Research for Early Childhood Schizophrenia, 1970.

CHURCHILL, D. W. & BRYSON, C. Q.: *Looking and Approach Behavior of Psychotic and Normal Children as a Function of Adult Presentation*. Indianapolis, Ind.: Research Report No. 1, Clinical Research Center for Early Childhood Schizophrenia, 1967.

CHURCHILL, D. W. & BRYSON, C. Q.: *Analysis of Self-Hitting Behavior in a Six-Year-Old Boy*. Indianapolis, Ind.: Research Report No. 2, Clinical Research Center for Early Childhood Schizophrenia, 1968.

COFFEY, H. S. & WIENER, L. L.: *Group Treatment of Autistic Children*. Englewood Cliffs, N. J.: Prentice-Hall, Inc., 1967.

COHEN, R. S.: Some childhood identity disturbances: Educational implementation of a psychiatric treatment plan. *Journal of the American Academy of Child Psychiatry*, 3:488-497, 1964.

COLLIGAN, R. C. & BELLAMY, C. M.: Effects of a two-year treatment program for a young autistic child. *Psychotherapy: Theory, Research and Practice*, 5:214-219, 1968.

CONNELL, P. H.: Medical treatment. In J. K. Wing, (Ed.): *Early Childhood Autism: Clinical, Educational, and Social Aspects*. London: Pergamon Press, Inc., 1966.

COWAN, P. A., HODDINOTT, B. A., & WRIGHT, B. A.: Compliance and resistance in the conditioning of autistic children: an exploratory study. *Child Development,* 36: 913-923, 1965.

CREAK, M.: Schizophrenic syndrome in childhood: Further progress report of a working party. *Developmental Medicine and Child Neurology,* 6 (5):530535, 1964.

CUNNINGHAM, M. A.: A five-year study of the language of an autistic child. *Journal of Child Psychology and Psychiatry,* 7:143-154, 1966.

CUNNINGHAM, M. A.: A comparison of the language of psychotic and nonpsychotic children who are mentally retarded. *Journal of Child Psychology and Psychiatry,* 9:229-244, 1968.

DAVIDS, A., RYAN, R., & SALVATORE, P. D.: Effectiveness of residential treatment of psychotic and other disturbed children. *American Journal of Orthopsychiatry,* 38: 469-475, 1968.

DAVIS, B. J.: A clinical method of appraisal of the language and learning behavior of young autistic children. *Journal of Communication Disorders,* 1:277-296, 1967.

DAVIDSON, G. C.: A social learning therapy programme with an autistic child. *Behaviour Research and Therapy,* 2:149-159, 1964.

DAVIDSON, G. C.: An intensive long-term social learning treatment program with an accurately diagnosed autistic child. *Proceedings of the 73rd Annual Convention of the American Psychological Association,* 1965a, pp. 203-204.

DAVIDSON, G. C.: The training of undergraduates as social reinforcers for autistic children: In L. P. Ullman and L. Krasner (Eds.): *Case Studies in Behavior Modification.* New York: Holt, Rinehart and Winston, Inc., 1965b.

DE HIRSCH, K.: Differential diagnosis between aphasic and schizophrenic language in children. *Journal of Speech and Hearing Disorders,* 32 (1):3-10, 1967.

DeMYER, M. K. & FERSTER, C. B.: Teaching new social behavior to schizophrenic children. *Journal of the American Academy of Child Psychiatry,* 1:443-461, 1962.

DeMYER, M. K., MANN, N. A., TILTON, J. R., & LOEW, L. H.: Toy-play behavior and use of body by autistic and normal children as reported by mothers. *Psychological Reports,* 21:973-981, 1967.

DeMYER, M. K., NORTON, J. A., & BARTON, S. Social and adaptive behaviors of autistic children as measured in a structured psychiatric interview. In D. W. Churchill, G. D. Alpern, and M. DeMyer (Eds.): *Infantile Autism: Proceedings of the Indiana University Colloquium (1968).* Springfield, Ill.: Charles C Thomas, Publisher, 1971.

DeMYER, M. K., WARD, S. D., & LINTZENICH, J.: Comparison of macronutrients in the diets of psychotic and normal children. *Archives of General Psychiatry,* 18:584-590, 1968.

DES LAURIERS, A.: The schizophrenic child. *Archives of General Psychiatry,* 16 (2):194-201, 1967.

DES LAURIERS, A. M. & CARLSON, C. F. *Your Child Is Asleep: Early Infantile Autism.* Homewood, Ill.: The Dorsey Press, 1969.

DOUGLAS, V. I. & SANDERS, F. A.: A pilot study of Rimland's Diagnostic Check List with autistic and mentally retarded children. *Journal of Child Psychology and Psychiatry,* 9:105-109, 1968.

DUNOFF, B.: The habilitation and education of the autistic child in a therapeutic day school. *American Journal of Orthopsychiatry,* 35:385-386, 1965.

DUBNOFF, B. & CHAMBERS, I. "Perceptual Training as a Bridge to Conceptual Ability: A Multifaceted Approach." Paper presented at the Council for Exceptional Children Conference, 1966.

DUNDAS, M. H.: Autistic children. *Nursing Times,* 60:138-139, 1964.

DUNDAS, M. H.: The one-to-one relationship in the treatment of autistic children. *Acta Paedopsychiatrica,* 35:242-245, 1968.

DUTTON, G.: The growth patterns of psychotic boys. *British Journal of Psychology,* 110:101-103, 1964.

EATON, L. & MENOLASCINO, F. J.: Psychotic reactions of childhood: A follow-up study. *American Journal of Orthopsychiatry*, 37:521-529, 1967.

EBERHARDY, F.: The view from "the couch." *Journal of Child Psychology and Psychiatry*, 8:257-263, 1967.

EDELSON, S. R.: A dynamic formulation of childhood schizophrenia. *Diseases of the Nervous System*, 27:610-615, 1966.

EISENBERG, L.: Classification of psychotic disorders in childhood. In L. D. Eron (Ed.): *Classification of Behavior Disorders*. Chicago: Aldine Publishing Company, 1966.

EISENBERG, L.: Psychotic disorders in childhood. In R. E. Cooke (Ed.): *The Biologic Basis of Pediatric Practice*. New York: McGraw-Hill, Inc., 1968.

EKSTEIN, R.: *Children of Time and Space, of Action and Impulse*. New York: Appleton-Century-Crofts, 1966.

EKSTEIN, R. & CARUTH, E.: Distancing and distance devices in childhood schizophrenia and borderline states: Revised concepts and new directions in research. *Psychological Reports*, 20:109-110, 1967.

ELGAR, S. Teaching autistic children. In J. K. Wing (Ed.): *Early Childhood Autism: Clinical, Educational, and Social Aspects*. London: Pergamon Press, Inc., 1966.

FARETRA, G. & BENDER, L.: Autonomic nervous system responses in hospitalized children treated with LSD and UML. In J. Wortis (Ed.): *Recent Advances in Biological Psychiatry*, Vol. 7. New York: Plenum, 1964.

FAY, W. H.: On the basis of autistic echolalia. *Journal of Communication Disorders*, 2:38-41, 1969.

FERSTER, C. B.: Positive reinforcement and behavioral deficits of autistic children. *Child Development*, 32:437-456, 1961.

FERSTER, C. B.: Psychotherapy by machine communication. *Disorders of Communication*, 42:317-333, 1964.

FERSTER, C. B.: The repertoire of the autistic child in relation to principles of reinforcement. In L. Gottschalk and A. H. Auerbach (Eds.): *Methods of Research in Psychotherapy*. New York: Appleton-Century-Crofts, 1966.

FERSTER, C. B.: Arbitrary and natural reinforcement. *Psychological Record*, 17:341-347, 1967a.

FERSTER, C. B.: The transition from the animal laboratory to the clinic. *Psychological Record*, 17:145-150, 1967b.

FERSTER, C. B. & DeMYER, M. K.: The development of performances in autistic children in an automatically controlled environment. *Journal of Chronic Diseases*, 13:312-345, 1961.

FERSTER, C. B. & DeMYER, M. K.: A method for the experimental analysis of the behavior of autistic children. *American Journal of Orthopsychiatry*, 32:89-98,

FERSTER, C. B. & SIMONS, J. Behavior therapy with children. *Psychological Record*, 16:65-71, 1966.

FINEMAN, K. R.: Visual-color reinforcement in establishment of speech by an autistic child. *Perceptual and Motor Skills*, 26:761-762, 1968.

FISH, B.: Evaluation of psychiatric therapies in children. In P. H. Hoch and J. Zubin (Eds.): *The Evaluation of Psychiatric Treatment*. New York: Grune and Stratton, Inc., 1964.

FISH, B. & SHAPIRO, T.: A typology of children's psychiatric disorders: I. Its application to a controlled evaluation of treatment. *Journal of the American Academy of Child Psychiatry*, 4:35-52, 1965.

FISH, B., SHAPIRO, T., & CAMPBELL, M.: Long-term prognosis and the response of schizophrenic children to drug therapy: A controlled study of trifluoperazine. *American Journal of Psychiatry*, 123:32-39, 1966.

FISH, B., SHAPIRO, T., CAMPBELL, M., & WILE, R.: A classification of schizophrenic children under five years. *American Journal of Psychiatry*, 124:1415-1423, 1968.

FISH, B., SHAPIRO, T., HALPERN, F., & WILE, R. The prediction of schizophrenia in infancy: III. A ten-year follow-up report of neurological and psychological development. *American Journal of Psychiatry*, 121:768-775, 1965.

FISH, B., WILE, R., SHAPIRO, T., & HALPERN, F. The prediction of schizophrenia in infancy: II. A ten-year follow-up report of predictions made at one month of age. In P. H. Hoch and J. Zubin (Eds.): *Psychopathology of Schizophrenia*. New York: Grune and Stratton, Inc., 1966.

FOWLE, A. M.: Atypical leukocyte pattern of schizophrenic children. *Archives of General Psychiatry*, 18:666-680, 1968.

FREIDES, D. & PIERCE, P. S. On the neuropsychology of the Kanner-Rimland syndrome: Hypothesis and case report. *Proceedings of the 76th Annual Convention of the American Psychological Association*, 3:477-478, 1968.

FRITH, U. & HERMELIN, B.: The role of visual and motor cues for normal, subnormal and autistic children. *Journal of Child Psychology and Psychiatry*, 10:153-163, 1969.

FURER, F.: The development of a preschool symbiotic psychotic boy. *Psychoanalytic Study of the Child*, 19:448-469, 1964.

GARCIA, B. & SARVIS, M. A.: Evaluation and treatment planning for autistic children. *Archives of General Psychiatry*, 10:530-541, 1964.

GARDNER, J. E., PEARSON, D. B., BERCOVICI, A. N., & BRICKER, D. E.: Measurement, evaluation, and modification of selected social interactions between a schizophrenic child, his parents and his therapist. *Journal of Consulting and Clinical Psychology*, 32:537-542, 1968.

GELFAND, D. M. & HARTMANN, D. P.: Behavior therapy with children: A review and evaluation of research methodology. *Psychological Bulletin*, 69:204-215, 1968.

GIBSON, D.: Early infantile autism: Symptom and syndrome. *Canadian Psychologist*, 9:36-39, 1968.

GILLIES, S.: Some abilities of psychotic children and subnormal controls. *Journal of Mental Deficiency Research*, 9 (2):89-101, 1965.

GITTELMAN, M. & BIRCH, H. G.: Childhood schizophrenia: Intellect, neurologic status, perinatal risk, prognosis, and family pathology. *Archives of General Psychiatry*, 17:16-25, 1967.

GITTELMAN, M. & CLEEMAN, J.: Serum magnesium level in psychotic and normal children. *Behavioral Neuropsychiatry*, 1:51-52, 1969.

GOLD, S.: Further investigation of a possible epileptogenic factor in the serum of psychotic children. *Australian and New Zealand Journal of Psychiatry*, 1:153-156, 1967.

GOLD, S. & SELLER, M. J.: An epileptic factor in the serum of psychotic children. *The Medical Journal of Australia*, 2:876-877, 1965.

GOLD, S. & VAUGHN, G. F.: Classification of childhood psychoses. *The Lancet*, 11:1058-1059, 1964.

GOLDFARB, W.: *Childhood Schizophrenia*. Cambridge, Mass.: Harvard University Press, 1961.

GOLDFARB, W.: An investigation of childhood schizophrenia. *Archives of General Psychiatry*, 11:620-634, 1964.

GOLDFARB, W.: Corrective socialization: A rationale for the treatment of schizophrenic children. *Canadian Psychiatric Association Journal*, 10:481-494, 1965.

GOLDFARB, W. & GOLDFARB, N.: Evaluation of behavioral changes of schizophrenic children in residential treatment. *American Journal of Psychotherapy*, 19:185-204, 1965.

GOLDFARB, W., GOLDFARB, N., & POLLACK, R. C.: Treatment of childhood schizophrenia. *Archives of General Psychiatry*, 14:119-128, 1966.

GOLDFARB, W., GOLDFARB, N., & POLLACK, R. C.: Changes in I.Q. of schizophrenic children during residential treatment. *Archives of General Psychiatry*, 21:673-690, 1969.

GOLDFARB, W., GOLDFARB, N., & SCHOLL, H. H.: The speech of mothers of schizophrenic children. *American Journal of Psychiatry*, 122:1220-1227, 1966.

GOLDFARB, W. & POLLACK, R. C.: The childhood schizophrenic's response to schooling in a residential treatment center. In P. H. Hoch and J. Zubin (Eds.): *The Evaluation of Psychiatric Treatment*. New York: Grune and Stratton, Inc., 1964.

GOODWIN, M. S. & GOODWIN, T. C.: In a dark mirror. *Mental Hygiene*, 53:550-563, 1969.

GORDON, N. & TAYLOR, I. G.: Assessment of children with difficulties of communication. *Brain*, 87:121-140, 1964.

GRAY, B. B. & FYGETAKIS, L. Mediated language acquisition for dysphasic children. *Behavior Research and Therapy*, 6:263-280, 1968.

GREEN, A. H.: Self mutilation in schizophrenic children. *Archives of General Psychiatry*, 17:234-244, 1967.

GREEN, A. H.: Self-destructive behavior in physically abused schizophrenic children. *Archives of General Psychiatry*, 19:171-179, 1968.

GRIFFITH, R. J. & RITVO, E. R.: Echolalia: Concerning the dynamics of the syndrome. *Journal of the American Academy of Child Psychiatry*, 6:184-193, 1967.

HACKETT, J. D.: Schizophrenia: A different but comparable model. *Diseases of the Nervous System* (Supplement), 5:133-143, 1968.

HALEY, J.: Testing parental instructions to schizophrenic and normal children: A pilot study. *Journal of Abnormal Psychology*, 73:559-565, 1968.

HARPER, J.: Further aspects in the treatment of autistic children. *Australian Occupational Therapy Journal*, 14:16-30, 1967.

HAWORTH, M. R. & MENOLASCINO, F. J.: Video-tape observations of disturbed young children. *Journal of Clinical Psychology*, 23:135-140, 1967.

HAWORTH, M. R. & MENOLASCINO, F. J.: Some aspects of psychotic behavior in young children. *Archives of General Psychiatry*, 18:355-359, 1968.

HEELEY, A. F. & ROBERTS, G. E.: Tryptophan metabolism in psychotic children. *Developmental Medicine and Child Neurology*, 7:46-49, 1965.

HERMELIN, B.: Recent psychological research. In J. K. Wing (Ed.): *Early Childhood Autism: Clinical, Educational, and Social Aspects*. London: Pergamon Press, Inc., 1966.

HERMELIN, B. & O'CONNOR, N.: The response and self-generated behavior of severely disturbed children and severely subnormal controls. *British Journal of Social and Clinical Psychology*, 2:37-43, 1963.

HERMELIN, B. & O'CONNOR, N.: Crossmodal transfer in normal, subnormal, and autistic children. *Neuropsychologia*, 2:229-235, 1964a.

HERMELIN, B. & O'CONNOR, N.: Effects of sensory input and sensory dominance on severely disturbed, autistic children and on subnormal controls. *British Journal of Psychology*, 55:201-206, 1964b.

HERMELIN, B. & O'CONNOR, N.: Visual imperception in psychotic children. *British Journal of Psychology*, 56:455-460, 1965.

HERMELIN, B. & O'CONNOR, N. Perceptual and motor discrimination in psychotic and normal children. *Journal of Genetic Psychology*, 110:117-125, 1967a.

HERMELIN, B. & O'CONNOR, N.: Remembering of words by psychotic and subnormal children. *British Journal of Psychology*, 58.213-218, 1967b.

HERMELIN, B. & O'CONNOR, N.: Measures of the occipital alpha rhythm in normal, subnormal and autistic children. *British Journal of Psychiatry*, 114:603-610, 1968.

HEWETT, F. M.: Teaching reading to an autistic boy through operant conditioning. *The Reading Teacher*, 17:613-618, 1964.

HEWETT, F. M.: Teaching speech to an autistic child through operant conditioning. *American Journal of Orthopsychiatry*, 35:927-936, 1965.

HEWETT, F. M.: The autistic child learns to read. *Slow Learning Child*, 13:107-121, 1966.

HEWETT, F. M., MAYHEW, D., & RABB, E.: An experimental reading program for neurologically impaired, mentally retarded, and severely emotionally disturbed children. *American Journal of Orthopsychiatry,* 37:35-48, 1967.

HINGTGEN, J. N. & CHURCHILL, D. W.: Identification of perceptual limitations in mute autistic children: Identification by the use of behavior modification. *Archives of General Psychiatry,* 21:68-71, 1969.

HINGTGEN, J. N. & CHURCHILL, D. W.: Differential effects of behavior modification in four mute autistic boys. In D. W. Churchill, G. D. Alpern, and M. DeMyer (Eds.): *Infantile Autism: Proceedings of the Indiana University Colloquium (1968).* Springfield, Ill.: Charles C Thomas, Publisher, 1971.

HINGTGEN, J. N. & COULTER, S. K. Auditory control of operant behavior in mute autistic children. *Perceptual and Motor Skills,* 25:561-565, 1967.

HINGTGEN, J. N., COULTER, S. K., & CHURCHILL, D. W.: Intensive reinforcement of imitative behavior in mute autistic children. *Archives of General Psychiatry,* 17: 36-43, 1967.

HINGTGEN, J. N., SANDERS, B. J., & DEMYER, M. K.: Shaping cooperative responses in early childhood schizophrenics. In L. P. Ullman and L. Krasner (Eds.): *Case Studies in Behavior Modification.* New York: Holt, Rinehart and Winston, Inc., 1965.

HINGTGEN, J. N. & TROST, F. C., JR.: Shaping cooperative responses in early childhood schizophrenics: II. Reinforcement of mutual physical contact and vocal responses. In R. Ulrich, T. Stachnik, and J. Mabry (Eds.): *Control of Human Behavior.* Glenview, Ill.: Scott Foresman and Company, 1966.

HUDSON, E. & DEMYER, M. K.: Food as a reinforcer in educational therapy of autistic children. *Behaviour Research and Therapy,* 6:37-43, 1968.

HUTT, C. & HUTT, S. J.: Stereotypies and their relation to arousal: A study of autistic children. In C. Hutt and S. J. Hutt (Eds.): *Behaviour Studies in Psychiatry.* Oxford: Pergamon Press, Ltd., 1970, pp. 175-204.

HUTT, C., HUTT, S. J., LEE, D., & OUNSTED, C.: Arousal and childhood autism. *Nature,* 204:908-909, 1964.

HUTT, C. & OUNSTED, C.: The biological significance of gaze aversion with particular reference to the syndrome of infantile autism. *Behavioral Science,* 11:346-356, 1966.

HUTT, S. J. & HUTT, C. Stereotypy, arousal and autism. *Human Development,* 11:277-286, 1968.

HUTT, S. J., HUTT, C., LEE, D., & OUNSTED, C.: A behavioral and electroencephalographic study of autistic children. *Journal of Psychiatric Research,* 3:181-197, 1965.

ITIL, T. M., RIZZO, A. E., & SHAPIRO, D. M.: Study of behavior and EEG correlation during treatment of disturbed children. *Diseases of the Nervous System,* 28:731-736, 1967.

JENSEN, G. D. & WOMACK, M.: Operant conditioning techniques applied in the treatment of an autistic child. *American Journal of Orthopsychiatry,* 37:30-34, 1967.

JOHNSON, S. M. & BROWN, R. A.: Producing behavior change in parents of disturbed children. *Journal of Child Psychology and Psychiatry and Allied Disciplines,* 10:107-121, 1969.

JUDD, L. L. & MANDELL, A. J. Chromosomes studies in early infantile autism. *Archives of General Psychiatry,* 18:450-457, 1968.

KAHN, R. M. & ARBIB, M. A.: "A Cybernetic Approach to Mental Development, With Some Comments on Infantile Autism and the Childhood Schizophrenias." Paper presented at the American Orthopsychiatric Association, Chicago, March, 1968.

KAMP, L. N. J.: Autistic syndrome in one of a pair of monozygotic twins. *Psychiatria, Neurologia, Neurochirurgia,* 67:143-147, 1964.

KANNER, L.: Infantile autism and the schizophrenias. *Behavioral Science,* 10:412-420, 1965.

KANNER, L.: Autistic disturbances of affective contact. *The Nervous Child,* 2:217-250, 1943. Reprinted in *Acta Paedopsychiatrica,* 35:98-136, 1968.

KEMPH, J. P.: Communicating with the psychotic child. *International Psychiatry Clinics,* 1:53-72, 1964.

KEMPH, J. P.: Brief hospitalization in treatment of the psychotic child. *Psychiatry Digest,* 27:35-43, 1966a.

KEMPH, J. P.: Psychotic children treated in a child guidance clinic. *Diseases of the Nervous System,* 27:317-320, 1966b.

KEMPH, J. P., HARRISON, S. I., & FINCH, S. M.: Promoting the development of ego functions in the middle phase of treatment of psychotic children. *Journal of the American Academy of Child Psychiatry,* 4:401-412, 1965.

KERR, N., MEYERSON, L., & MICHAEL, J.: A procedure for shaping vocalizations in a mute child. In L. P. Ullmann and L. Krasner (Eds.): *Case Studies in Behavior Modification.* New York: Holt, Rinehart and Winston, Inc., 1965.

KING, P. D.: Theoretical considerations of psychotherapy with a schizophrenic child. *Journal of the American Academy of Child Psychiatry,* 3:638-649, 1964.

KING, P. D. & EKSTEIN, R. The search for ego controls: Progression of play activity in psychotherapy with a schizophrenic child. *The Psychoanalytic Review,* 54:639-648, 1967.

KIRK, R. V.: Perceptual defect and role handicap: Missing links in explaining aetiology of schizophrenia. *British Journal of Psychiatry,* 114:1509-1521, 1968.

KLEIN, D. L. & POLLACK, M.: Schizophrenic children and maternal speech facility. *American Journal of Psychiatry,* 123:232, 1966.

KRALL, V.: "Measures of Developmental Change in Autistic Children." Paper presented at the American Psychological Association, Washington, D. C., September, 1967.

KYSAR, J. E.: The two camps in child psychiatry: A report from a psychiatrist-father of an autistic and retarded child. *American Journal of Psychiatry,* 125:103-109, 1968.

LANGDELL, J. I.: Family treatment of childhood schizophrenia. *Mental Hygiene,* 51:387-392, 1967.

LAUDER, M.: An autistic child. In J. K. Wing (Ed.): *Early Childhood Autism: Clinical, Educational, and Social Aspects.* London: Pergamon Press, Inc., 1966.

LEFF, R.: Behavior modification and the psychoses of childhood: A review. *Psychological Bulletin,* 69:396-409, 1968.

LEMPP, R. & VOGEL, B.: Research into childhood schizophrenia. *Acta Paedopsychiatrica,* 33:322-331, 1966.

LEONBERG, S. C., JR. & BOK, J. B.: Childhood schizophrenia: Organic or psychogenic? *Diseases of the Nervous System,* 28:686-687, 1967.

LEVINE, M. & OLSON, R. P. Intelligence of parents of autistic children. *Journal of Abnormal Psychology,* 73:215-217, 1968.

LEVY, E. Z.: Long-term follow-up of former inpatients at the children's hospital of the Menninger Clinic. *American Journal of Psychiatry,* 125:1633-1639, 1969.

LIFTON, N. & SMOLEN, E.: "Group Psychotherapy with Schizophrenic Children." Paper presented at the Annual Conference of the American Group Psychotherapy Association, January, 1965.

LORDI, W. M. & SILVERBERG, J.: Infantile autism: A family approach. *International Journal of Group Psychotherapy,* 14:360-365, 1964.

LOTTER, V.: Epidemiology of autistic conditions in young children: 1. Prevalence. *Social Psychiatry,* 1:124-137, 1966a.

LOTTER, V.: Services for a group of autistic children in Middlesex. In J. K. Wing (Ed.): *Early Childhood Autism: Clinical, Educational, and Social Aspects.* London: Pergamon Press, Inc., 1966b.

LOTTER, V.: Epidemiology of autistic conditions in young children: II. Some characteristics of the parents and children. *Social Psychiatry*, 1:163-173, 1967.

LOVAAS, O. I.: A program for the establishment of speech in psychotic children. In J. K. Wing (Ed.): *Early Childhood Autism: Clinical, Educational, and Social Aspects*. London: Pergamon Press, Inc., 1966a.

LOVAAS, O. I.: "Learning Theory Approach to the Treatment of Childhood Schizophrenia." Paper presented at the meeting of the American Orthopsychiatric Association, San Francisco, April, 1966b.

LOVAAS, O. I.: Considerations in the development of a behavioral treatment program for psychotic children. In D. W. Churchill, G. D. Alpern, and M. DeMyer, (Eds.): *Infantile Autism: Proceedings of the Indiana University Colloquium (1968)*. Springfield, Ill.: Charles C Thomas, Publisher, 1971.

LOVAAS, O. I., BERBERICH, J. P., PERLOFF, B. F., & SCHAEFFER, B.: Acquisition of imitative speech by schizophrenic children. *Science*, 151:705-707, 1966a.

LOVAAS, O. I., FREITAG, G., GOLD, V. J., & KASSORLA, I. C. Experimental studies in childhood schizophrenia: Analysis of self-destructive behavior. *Journal of Experimental Child Psychology*, 2:67-84, 1965a.

LOVAAS, O. I., FREITAG, G., GOLD, V. J., & KASSORLA, I. C. Recording apparatus and procedure for observation of behaviors of children in free play settings. *Journal of Experimental Child Psychology*, 2:108-120, 1965b.

LOVAAS, O. I., FREITAG, G., KINDER, M. I., RUBENSTEIN, B. D., SCHAEFFER, B., & SIMMONS, J. Q.: Establishment of social reinforcers in two schizophrenic children on the basis of food. *Journal of Experimental Child Psychology*, 4:109-125, 1966b.

LOVAAS, O. I., FREITAS, L., NELSON, K., & WHALEN, C.: The establishment of imitation and its use for the development of complex behavior in schizophrenic children. *Behaviour Research and Therapy*, 5:171-181, 1967.

LOVAAS, O. I., SCHAEFFER, B., & SIMMONS, J. Q.: Building social behavior in autistic children by use of electric shock. *Journal of Experimental Research in Personality*, 1:99-109, 1965.

LOWE, L. H.: Families of children with early childhood schizophrenia: Selected demographic information. *Archives of General Psychiatry*, 14:26-30, 1966.

MAES, J.: Modifying behavior: The case of Alice. *Journal of Psychiatric Nursing and Mental Health Service*, 7:89-90, 1969.

MAHLER, M. S.: On early infantile psychosis: The symbiotic and autistic syndromes. *Journal of the American Academy of Child Psychiatry*, 4:554-568, 1965.

MARR, J. N., MILLER, E. R., & STRAUB, R. R. Operant conditioning of attention with a psychotic girl. *Behaviour Research and Therapy*, 4:85-87, 1966.

MARSHALL, G. R.: Toilet-training of an autistic eight-year-old through conditioning therapy: A case report. *Behaviour Research and Therapy*, 4:242-245, 1966.

MARTIN, G. L., ENGLAND, G., KAPROWY, E., KILGOUR, K., & PILEK, V.: Operant conditioning of kindergarten-class behaviour in autistic children. *Behaviour Research and Therapy*, 6:281-294, 1968.

MASLOW, A. R.: A concentrated therapeutic relationship with a psychotic child. *Journal of the American Academy of Child Psychiatry*, 3:140-150, 1964.

MATHENY, A. P., JR.: Pathological echoic responses in a child: Effect of environmental mand and tact control. *Journal of Experimental Child Psychology*, 6 (4):624-631, 1967.

McDERMOTT, J. F., JR., HARRISON, S. I., SCHRAGER, J., LINDY, J., & KILLINS, E.: Social class and mental illness in children: The question of childhood psychosis. In S. Chess and A. Thomas (Eds.): *Annual Progress in Child Psychiatry and Child Development*. New York: Brunner/Mazel Publishers, 1968.

MEANS, J. R. & MERRENS, M. R.: Interpersonal training for an autistic child. *Perceptual and Motor Skills*, 28:972-974, 1969.

MENOLASCINO, F. J.: Autistic reactions in early childhood: Differential diagnostic considerations. *Journal of Child Psychology and Psychiatry*, 6:203-218, 1965a.

MENOLASCINO, F.: Psychoses of childhood: Experience of a mental retardation pilot project. *American Journal of Mental Deficiency*, 70:83-92, 1965b.

MENOLASCINO, F. J. & EATON, L.: Psychoses of childhood: A five year follow-up of experiences in a mental retardation clinic. *American Journal of Mental Deficiency*, 72:370-380, 1967.

METZ, J. R.: Conditioning generalized imitation in autistic children. *Journal of Experimental Child Psychology*, 2:389-399, 1965.

METZ, J. R.: Conditioning self-help and social skills of emotionally disturbed children. *The Quarterly of Camarillo*, 2:3-11, 1966.

METZ, J. R.: Stimulation level preferences of autistic children. *Journal of Abnormal Psychology*, 72:529-535, 1967.

MILLER, B. M.: "Communication, Verbal and Non-verbal, with Emotionally Disturbed Children: The Search for Meaning." Paper presented at the American Orthopsychiatric Association, New York, 1969.

MITCHELL, K.: Concept of "pathogenesis" in parents of schizophrenic and normal children. *Journal of Abnormal Psychology*, 74:423-424, 1969.

MITTLER, P.: The psychological assessment of autistic children. In J. K. Wing (Ed.): *Early Childhood Autism: Clinical, Educational, and Social Aspects*. London: Pergamon Press, Inc., 1966.

MITTLER,, P., GILLIES, S., & JUKES, E.: Prognosis in psychotic children: Report of follow-up study. *Journal of Mental Deficiency Research*, 10:73-83, 1966.

MOGAR, R. E. & ALDRICH, R. W.: The use of psychedelic agents with autistic schizophrenic children. *Behavioral Neuropsychiatry*, 1:44-52, 1969.

MORRISON, D., MILLER, D., & MEJIA, B.: "Comprehension and Negation of Verbal Communication in Autistic Children." Paper presented at the American Association of Psychiatric Clinics for Children, 1969.

NELSON, R. O. & EVANS, I. M. The combination of learning principles and speech therapy techniques in the treatment of non-communicating children. *Journal of Child Psychology and Psychiatry*, 9:111-124, 1968.

NEY, P.: Operant conditioning of schizophrenic children. *Canadian Psychiatric Association Journal*, 12:9-15, 1967.

O'CONNOR, N. & HERMELIN, B.: Measures of distance and motility in psychotic children and severely subnormal controls. *British Journal of Social and Clinical Psychology*, 3:29-33, 1963a.

O'CONNOR, N. & HERMELIN, B.: Sensory dominance in autistic children and subnormal controls. *Perceptual and Motor Skills*, 16:920, 1963b.

O'CONNOR, N. & HERMELIN, B. Sensory dominance in autistic imbecile children and controls. *Archives of General Psychiatry*, 12:99-103, 1965a.

O'CONNOR, N. & HERMELIN, B.: Visual analogies of verbal operations. *Language and Speech*, 8:197-207, 1965b.

O'CONNOR, N. & HERMELIN, B.: Auditory and visual memory in autistic and normal children. *Journal of Mental Deficiency Research*, 11:126-131, 1967a.

O'CONNOR, N. & HERMELIN, B.: The selective visual attention of psychotic children. *Journal of Child Psychology and Psychiatry*, 8:167-179, 1967b.

O'GORMAN, G.: *The Nature of Childhood Autism*. London: Butterworth and Co., Ltd., 1967.

ONHEIBER, P, WHITE, P. T., DEMYER, M. K., & OTTINGER, D. R.: Sleep and dream patterns of child schizophrenics. *Archives of General Psychiatry*, 12:568-571, 1965.

ORNITZ, E. M.: Disorders of perception common to early infantile autism and schizophrenia. *Comprehensive Psychiatry*, 10:259-274, 1969.

ORNITZ, E. M. & RITVO, E. R.: Neurophysiologic mechanisms underlying perceptual inconstancy in autistic and schizophrenic children. *Archives of General Psychiatry*, 19:22-27, 1968a.

ORNITZ, E. M. & RITVO, E. R.: Perceptual inconstancy in early infantile autism. *Archives of General Psychiatry*, 18:76-98, 1968b.

ORNITZ, E. M., RITVO, E. R., BROWN, M. B., LAFRANCHI, S., PARMELEE, T., & WALTER, R. D.: The EEG and rapid eye movements during REM sleep in normal and autistic children. *Electroencephalographic and Clinical Neurophysiology*, 26:167-175, 1969.

ORNITZ, E. M., RITVO, E. R., PANMAN, L. M., LEE, V. H., CARR, E. M., & WALTER, R. D.: The auditory evoked response in normal and autistic children during sleep. *Electroencephalography and Clinical Neurophysiology*, 25:221-230, 1968.

ORNITZ, E. M., RITVO, E. R., & WALTER, R. D.: Dreaming sleep in autistic and schizophrenic children. *American Journal of Psychiatry*, 122:419-424, 1965a.

ORNITZ, E. M., RITVO, E. R., & WALTER, R. D.: Dreaming sleep in autistic twins. *Archives of General Psychiatry*, 12:77-79, 1965b.

OTTINGER, D. R., SWEENEY, N., & LOEW, L. H. Visual discrimination learning in schizophrenic and normal children. *Journal of Clinical Psychology*, 21:251-253, 1965.

PARK, C. C.: *The Siege*. New York: Harcourt, Brace & World, Inc., 1967.

PATTERSON, G. R. & BRODSKY, G.: A behaviour modification programme for a child with multiple problem behaviours. *Journal of Child Psychology and Psychiatry*, 7:277-295, 1966.

PERRON, L.: The psychoses of childhood. *Canadian Nurse*, 60:42-43, 1964.

PITFIELD, M. & OPPENHEIM, A. N: Child rearing attitudes of mothers of psychotic children. *Journal of Child Psychology and Psychiatry*, 5:51-57, 1964.

POLAN, C. G. & SPENCER, B. L.: A check list of symptoms of autism of early life. *West Virginia Medical Journal*, 55:198-204, 1959.

POLLACK, M. & GITTELMAN, R. K.: The siblings of childhood schizophrenics: A review. *American Journal of Orthopsychiatry*, 34:868-873, 1964.

POLLACK, M., GITTELMAN, M., MILLER, R., BERMAN, P., & BAKWIN, R.: "A Developmental, Pediatric, Neurological, Psychological and Psychiatric Comparison of Psychotic Children and Their Sibs." Paper presented at the American Orthopsychiatric Association, 1970.

POLLACK, M. & WOERNER, M. G.: Pre- and peri-natal complications and "childhood schizophrenia": A comparison of five controlled studies. *Journal of Child Psychology and Psychiatry*, 7:235-242, 1966.

PRONOVOST, W., WAKSTEIN, M. P., & WAKSTEIN, D. J.: A longitudinal study of the speech behavior and language comprehension of fourteen children diagnosed atypical or autistic. *Exceptional Children*, 33:19-26, 1966.

REISER, D. E. & BROWN, J. L.: Patterns of later development in children with infantile psychosis. *Journal of the American Academy of Child Psychiatry*, 3:650-667, 1964.

REISER, M. & SPERBER, Z.: "Utilizing Nonprofessional Case Aides in the Treatment of Psychotic Children at an Outpatient Clinic." Paper presented at the American Orthopsychiatric Association, 1969.

RICE, G., KEPECS, J. G., & YAHALOM, I.: Differences in communicative impact between mothers of psychotic and nonpsychotic children. *American Journal of Orthopsychiatry*, 36:529-543, 1966.

RICE, G. & KLEIN, A.: Getting the message from a schizophrenic child. *Psychiatry*, 27:163-169, 1964.

RIMLAND, B.: *Infantile Autism: The Syndrome and Its Implications for a Neural Theory of Behavior*. New York: Appleton-Century-Crofts, 1964.

RIMLAND, B.: On the objective diagnosis of infantile autism. *Acta Paedopsychiatrica*, 35:146-161, 1968.

RISLEY, T. & WOLF, M. Experimental manipulation of autistic behaviors and generalization into the home. In R. Ulrich, T. Stachnik, and J. Mabry (Eds.): *Control of Human Behavior.* Glenview, Ill.: Scott, Foresman and Company, 1966.

RISLEY, T., and WOLF, M. Establishing functional speech in echolalic children. *Behaviour Research and Therapy,* 5:73-88, 1967.

RITVO, E. R., ORNITZ, E. M., EVIATAR, A., MARKHAM, C., BROWN, M., & MASON, A.: Decreased postrotatory nystagmus in early infantile autism. *Neurology,* 19:653-658, 1969.

RITVO, E. R., ORNITZ, E. M., & LAFRANCHI, S.: Frequency of repetitive behaviors in early infantile autism and its variants. *Archives of General Psychiatry,* 19:341-347, 1968.

ROBERTSON, M. F.: Shadow image perception: A communicative device in therapy. *American Journal of Psychotherapy,* 20:655-663, 1966.

ROBERTSON, M. F.: Shadow therapy with children. *American Journal of Psychotherapy,* 23:505-509, 1969.

ROFFWARG, H. P., DEMENT, W. C., & FISHER, C.: Preliminary observations of sleep-dream pattern on neonates, infants, children and adults. In E. Harms (Ed.): *Monographs on Child Psychiatry: No. II. Problems of Sleep and Dream in Children.* New York: Pergamon Press, Inc., 1964.

ROLO, A., KRINSKY, L. W., ABRAMSON, H. A., & GOLDFARB, L.: Preliminary method for study of LSD with children. *International Journal of Neuropsychiatry,* 1:552-555, 1965.

ROSENBERGER, L. & WOOLF, M.: Schizophrenic development of two children in the 4-6 age group. *Psychoanalytic Review,* 51:469-530, 1964.

RUBIN, H., BAR, A., & DWYER, J. H.: An experimental speech and language program for psychotic children. *Journal of Speech and Hearing Disorders,* 32:242-248, 1967.

RUTTENBERG, B. A.: A psychoanalytic understanding of infantile autism and its treatment. In D. W. Churchill, G. D. Alpern, and M. DeMyer (Eds.): *Infantile Autism: Proceedings of the Indiana University Colloquium (1968).* Springfield, Ill.: Charles C Thomas, Publisher, 1971.

RUTTENBERG, B. A., DRATMAN, M. L., FRAKNOI, J., & WENAR, C.: An instrument for evaluating autistic children. *Journal of the American Academy of Child Psychiatry,* 5:453-478, 1966.

RUTTENBERG, B. A. & WOLF, E. G.: Evaluating the communication of the autistic child. *Journal of Speech and Hearing Disorders,* 32:314-324, 1967.

RUTTER, M.: Intelligence and childhood psychiatric disorder. *British Journal of Social and Clinical Psychology,* 3:120-129, 1964.

RUTTER, M.: Classification and categorization in child psychiatry. *Journal of Child Psychology and Psychiatry,* 6:71-83, 1965a.

RUTTER, M.: The influence of organic and emotional factors on the origins, nature and outcome of childhood psychosis. *Developmental Medicine and Child Neurology,* 7:518-528, 1965b.

RUTTER, M. Prognosis: Psychotic children in adolescence and early adult life. In J. K. Wing (Ed.): *Early Childhood Autism: Clinical, Educational, and Social Aspects.* London: Pergamon Press, Inc., 1966.

RUTTER, M.: Psychotic disorders in early childhood. In A. Coppen and A. Walk (Eds.): *Recent Developments in Schizophrenia: A Symposium.* London: Royal Medico-Psychological Association, 1967.

RUTTER, M.: Concepts of autism: A review of research. *Journal of Child Psychology and Psychiatry,* 9:1-25, 1968.

RUTTER, M.: The description and classification of infantile autism. In D. W. Churchill, G. D. Alpern, and M. DeMyer (Eds.): *Infantile Autism: Proceedings of the Indiana University Colloquium (1968).* Springfield, Ill.: Charles C Thomas, Publisher, 1971.

RUTTER, M., GREENFELD, D., & LOCKYER, L.: A five to fifteen year follow-up study of infantile psychosis: II. Social and behavioral outcome. *British Journal of Psychiatry*, 113:1183-1199, 1967.

RUTTER, M., LEBOVICI, S., EISENBERG, L., SNEZNEVSKIJ, A. V., SADOUN, R., BROOKE, E., & LIN, T. Y.: A tri-axial classification of mental disorders in childhood: An international study. *Journal of Child Psychology and Psychiatry*, 10:41-61, 1969.

RUTTER, M. & LOCKYER, L.: A five to fifteen year follow-up study of infantile psychosis. I. Description of sample. *British Journal of Psychiatry*, 113:1169-1182, 1967.

SAFRIN, R. K.: Differences in visual perception and in visual-motor functioning between psychotic and non-psychotic children. *Journal of Consulting Psychology*, 28:41-45, 1964.

SALK, L.: On the prevention of schizophrenia. *Diseases of the Nervous System*, 29: 11-15, 1968.

SALZINGER, K., FELDMAN, R. S., COWAN, J. E., & SALZINGER, S.: Operant conditioning of verbal behavior of two young speech-deficient boys. In L. Krasner and L. P. Ullman (Eds.): *Research in Behavior Modification*. New York: Holt, Rinehart and Winston, 1965.

SAVAGE, V. S.: Child autism: A review of the literature with particular reference to the speech and language structure of the autistic child. *British Journal of Disorders of Communication*, 3:75-87, 1968.

SCHACHTER, M.: Evolution and prognosis of early infantile autism. *Acta Paedopsychiatrica*, 35:188-199, 1968.

SCHECHTER, M. D., SHURLEY, J. T., SEXAUER, J. D., & TOUSSIENG, P. W.: Perceptual isolation therapy: A new experimental approach in the treatment of children using infantile autistic defenses: A preliminary report. *Journal of the American Academy of Child Psychiatry*, 8:97-139, 1969.

SCHELL, R. E. & ADAMS, W. P.: Training parents of a young child with profound behavior deficits to be teacher-therapist. *Journal of Special Education*, 2:439-454, 1968.

SCHOPLER, E.: The development of body image and symbol formation through bodily contact with an autistic child. *Journal of Child Psychology and Psychiatry*, 3:191-202, 1962.

SCHOPLER, E.: The relationship between early tactile experience and the treatment of an autistic and a schizophrenic child. *American Journal of Orthopsychiatry*, 34:339-340, 1964.

SCHOPLER, E.: Early infantile autism and receptor processes. *Archives of General Psychiatry*, 13:327-335, 1965.

SCHOPLER, E.: Visual versus tactual receptor preference in normal and schizophrenic children. *Journal of Abnormal Psychology*, 71:108-114, 1966.

SCHOPLER, E. & LOFTIN, J.: Thinking disorders in parents of young psychotic children. *Journal of Abnormal Psychology*, 74:281-287, 1969a.

SCHOPLER, E. & LOFTIN, J.: Thought disorders in parents of psychotic children: A function of test anxiety. *Archives of General Psychiatry*, 20:174-181, 1969b.

SCHOPLER, E. & REICHLER, R. J.: Psychobiological referents for the treatment of autism. In D. W. Churchill, G. D. Alpern, and M. DeMyer (Eds.): *Infantile Autism: Proceedings of the Indiana University Colloquium (1968)*. Springfield, Ill.: Charles C Thomas, Publisher, 1971.

SCHULMAN, J. L.: Management of the child with early infantile autism. *American Journal of Psychiatry*, 120:250-254, 1963.

SELLER, M. J. & GOLD, S.: Seizures in psychotic children. *The Lancet*, 1:1325, 1964.

SHAPIRO, T.: Hand morphology in some severely impaired schizophrenic children. *American Journal of Psychiatry*, 122:432-435, 1965.

SHAPIRO, T. & FISH, B.: A method to study language deviation as an aspect of ego organization in young schizophrenic children. *Journal of the American Academy of Child Psychiatry*, 8:36-56, 1969.

SHAW, W. H.: Treatment of a schizophrenic speech disorder by operant conditioning in play therapy. *Canadian Psychiatric Association Journal,* 14:631-634, 1969.

SHODELL, M. J. & REITER, H. H.: Self-mutilative behavior in verbal and nonverbal schizophrenic children. *Archives of General Psychiatry,* 19:453-455, 1968.

SILVER, A. & GABRIEL, H. P.: The association of schizophrenia in childhood with primitive postural responses and decreased muscle tone. *Developmental Medicine and Child Neurology,* 6:495-497, 1964.

SIMMONS, J. Q., III, LEIKEN, S. J., LOVAAS, O. I., SCHAEFFER, B., & PERLOFF, B.: Modification of autistic behavior with LSD-25. *American Journal of Psychiatry,* 122: 1201-1211, 1966.

SIMMONS, J. Q., III & LOVAAS, O. I.: Use of pain and punishment as treatment techniques with childhood schizophrenics. *American Journal of Psychotherapy,* 23: 23-35, 1969.

SIMON, G. B. & GILLIES, S. M.: Some physical characteristics of a group of psychotic children. *British Journal of Psychiatry,* 110:104-107, 1964.

SMALL, J. G.: Sensory evoked responses of autistic children. In D. W. Churchill, G. D. Alpern, and M. DeMyer (Eds.): *Infantile Autism: Proceedings of the Indiana University Colloquium (1968).* Springfield, Ill.: Charles C Thomas, Publisher, 1971.

SMOLEN, E. M.: Some thoughts on schizophrenia in childhood. *Journal of the American Academy of Child Psychiatry,* 4:443-472, 1965.

SMOLEN, E. & LIFTON, N.: A special treatment program for schizophrenic children in a guidance clinic. *American Journal of Orthopsychiatry,* 36:736-742, 1966.

SODDY, K.: The autistic child. *The Practitioner,* 192:525-533, 1964.

SOROSKY, A. D., ORNITZ, E. M., BROWN, M. B., & RITVO, E. R.: Systematic observation of autistic behavior. *Archives of General Psychiatry,* 18:439-449, 1968.

SPEERS, R. W. & LANSING, C.: Group psychotherapy with preschool psychotic children and collateral group therapy of their parents: A preliminary report of the first two years. *American Journal of Orthopsychiatry,* 34:659-666, 1964.

SPEERS, R. W. & LANSING, C.: Some genetic-dynamic considerations in childhood symbiotic psychosis. *Journal of the American Academy of Child Psychiatry,* 7:328-349, 1968.

SPIVACK, G. & LEVINE, M.: The Devereux Child Behavior Rating Scale: A study of symptom behaviors in latency age atypical children. *American Journal of Mental Deficiency,* 68:700-717, 1964.

SPURGEON, R. K.: Some problems in measuring nonverbal behavior of autistic children. *Nursing Research,* 16:212-218, 1967.

STROH, G. & BUICK, D.: Perceptual development and childhood psychosis. *British Journal of Medical Psychology,* 37:291-299, 1964.

SUSSMAN, S. & SKLAR, J. L.: The social awareness of autistic children. *American Journal of Orthopsychiatry,* 39:798-806, 1969.

TAFT, L. T. & GOLDFARB, W.: Prenatal and perinatal factors in childhood schizophrenia. *Developmental Medicine and Child Neurology,* 6:32-43, 1964.

TATE, B. G. & BAROFF, G. S.: Aversive control of self-injurious behavior in a psychotic boy. *Behaviour Research and Therapy,* 4:281-287, -966.

TERRIS, M., LAPOUSE, R., & MONK, M. A.: The relation of prematurity and previous fetal loss to childhood schizophrenia. *American Journal of Psychiatry,* 121:476-481, 1964.

TESSMAN, L. H. & KAUFMAN, I.: Treatment techniques, the primary process, and ego development in schizophrenic children. *Journal of the American Academy of Child Psychiatry,* 6:98-115, 1967.

THOMAS, R.: Comments on some aspects of self and object representation in a group of psychotic children. *The Psychoanalytic Study of the Child,* 21:527-580, 1966.

TILTON, J. R., DeMYER, M. K., & LOEW, L. H.: *Annotated Bibliography on Childhood Schizophrenia: 1955-1964.* New York: Grune and Stratton, Inc., 1966.

TILTON, J. R. & OTTINGER, D. R.: Comparison of the toy-play behavior of autistic, retarded, and normal children. *Psychological Reports,* 15:967-975, 1964.

TREFFERT, D. A.: The epidemiology of infantile autism. *Archives of General Psychiatry,* 22:431-438, 1970.

TUBBS, V. K.: Types of linguistic disability in psychotic children. *Journal of Mental Deficiency Research,* 10:230-240, 1966.

VON BRAUCHITSCH, H. K. & KIRK, W. E.: "Childhood Schizophrenia and Social Class." Paper presented at the American Orthopsychiatric Association, 1967.

WALTER, W. G., ALDRIDGE, V. J., COOPER, R., O'GORMAN, G., McCULLUM, C., & WINTER, A. L.: Report on: Neurophysiological correlates of apparent defects of sensorimotor integration in autistic children. In D. W. Churchill, G. D. Alpern, and M. DeMyer (Eds.): *Infantile Autism: Proceedings of the Indiana University Colloquium (1968).* Springfield, Ill.: Charles C Thomas, Publisher, 1971.

WARD, A. J.: "Early Infantile Autism: An Etiological Hypothesis." Paper presented at the American Association of Psychiatric Clinics for Children, Boston, 1969.

WARD, J. J.: Early infantile autism: Diagnosis, etiology and treatment. *Psychological Bulletin,* 73:350-362, 1970.

WARD, T. F. & HODDINOTT, B. A.: A study of childhood schizophrenia and early infantile autism. Part I. Description of the sample. *Canadian Psychiatric Association Journal,* 10:377-382, 1965.

WARD, T. F. & HODDINOTT, B. A.: A study of childhood schizophrenia and early infantile autism. Part II: Selection of a group for inpatient treatment. *Canadian Psychiatric Association Journal,* 10:382-386, 1965.

WARD, T. F. & HODDINOTT, B. A.: The development of speech in an autistic child. *Acta Paedopsychiatrica,* 35:199-215, 1968.

WASSING, H. E.: Cognitive functioning in early infantile autism: An examination of four cases by means of the Wechsler Intelligence Scale for Children. *Acta Paedopsychiatrica,* 32:122-136, 1965.

WEBER, J. L.: The speech and language abilities of emotionally disturbed children. *Canadian Psychiatric Association Journal,* 10:417-420, 1965.

WEILAND, I. H.: Development of object relationships and childhood psychosis. *Journal of the American Academy of Child Psychiatry,* 3:317-329, 1964.

WEILAND, I. H.: Considerations on the development of symbiosis, symbiotic psychosis, and the nature of separation anxiety. *International Journal of Psychoanalysis,* 47:1-5, 1966.

WEILAND, I. H.: Summary of treatment approaches. In D. W. Churchill, G. D. Alpern, and M. DeMyer (Eds.): *Infantile Autism: Proceedings of the Indiana University Colloquium (1968).* Springfield, Ill.: Charles C Thomas, Publisher, 1971.

WEILAND, I. H. & LEGG, D. R.: Formal speech characteristics as a diagnostic aid in childhood psychosis. *American Journal of Orthopsychiatry,* 34:91-94, 1964.

WEILAND, I. H. & RUDNIK, R.: Considerations of the development and treatment of autistic childhood psychosis. *Psychoanalytic Study of the Child,* 16:549-563, 1961.

WEISS, H. H. & BORN, B.: Speech training or language acquisition? A distinction when speech training is taught by operant conditioning procedures. *American Journal of Orthopsychiatry,* 37:49-55, 1967.

WENAR, C., RUTTENBERG, B. A., DRATMAN, M. L., & WOLF, E. G.: Changing autistic behavior. *Archives of General Psychiatry,* 17:26-35, 1967.

WERRY, J. S. & WOLLERSHEIM, J. P.: Behavior therapy with children: A broad overview. *Journal of the American Academy of Child Psychiatry,* 6:346-370, 1967.

WESTON, P. T. B., (Ed.): *Some Approaches to Teaching Autistic Children.* London: Pergamon Press, Inc., 1965.

WETZEL, R. J., BAKER, J., RONEY, M., & MARTIN, M.: Outpatient treatment of autistic behavior. *Behaviour Research and Therapy*, 5:169-177, 1966.

WHITE, P. T., DeMYER, W., & DeMYER, M.: EEG abnormalities in early childhood schizophrenia: A double-blind study of psychiatrically disturbed and normal children and their sibs. *Developmental Medicine and Child Neurology*, 8:552-560, 1966.

WHITTAM, H., SIMON, G. B., & MITTLER, P. J.: The early development of psychotic children and their sibs. *Developmental Medicine and Child Neurology*, 8:552-560, 1966.

WILLIAMS, C. E.: Behavior disorders in handicapped children. *Developmental Medicine and Child Neurology*, 10:736-740, 1968.

WILSON, L.: *This Stranger, My Son*. New York: G. P. Putnam's Sons, 1968.

WILSON, M. D.: Problems in providing education. In J. K. Wing (Ed.): *Early Childhood Autism: Clinical, Educational, and Social Aspects*. London: Pergamon Press, Inc., 1966.

WING, J. K.: Diagnosis, epidemiology, aetiology. In J. K. Wing (Ed.): *Early Childhood Autism: Clinical, Educational, and Social Aspects*. London: Pergamon Press, Inc., 1966.

WING, J. K., O'CONNOR, N., & LOTTER, V.: Autistic conditions in early childhood: A survey in Middlesex. *British Medical Journal*, 3:389-392, 1967.

WING, J. K. & WING, L.: A clinical interpretation of remedial teaching. In J. K. Wing (Ed.): *Early Childhood Autism: Clinical, Educational, and Social Aspects*. London: Pergamon Press, Inc., 1966a.

WING, L.: Counseling and the principles of management. In J. K. Wing (Ed.): *Early Childhood Autism: Clinical, Educational, and Social Aspects*. London: Pergamon Press, Inc., 1966.

WING, L.: The handicaps of autistic children. A comparative study. *Journal of Child Psychology and Psychiatry*, 10:1-40, 1969.

WING, L. & WING, J. K.: The prescription of services. In J. K. Wing (Ed.): *Early Childhood Autism: Clinical, Educational, and Social Aspects*. London: Pergamon Press, Inc., 1966b.

WOLF, E. G. & RUTTENBERG, B. A.: Sound acceptance in autistic children. *Journal of Special Education*, 2:353-359, 1968.

WOLF, E. G. & RUTTENBERG, B. A.: Communication therapy for the autistic child. *Journal of Speech and Hearing Disorders*, 32:331-335, 1967.

WOLF, M. & RISLEY, T.: Application of operant conditioning procedures to the behavior problems of an autistic child: A follow-up and extension. *Behaviour Research and Therapy*, 5:103-111, 1967.

WOLF, M., RISLEY, T., & MEES, H.: Application of operant conditioning procedures to the behavior problems of an autistic child. *Behaviour Research and Therapy*, 1:305-312, 1964.

WOLFF, S. & CHESS, S.: A behavioral study of schizophrenic children. *Acta Psychiatrica Scandinavica*, 40:438-466, 1964.

WOLFF, S. & CHESS, S.: An analysis of the language of fourteen schizophrenic children. *Journal of Child Psychology and Psychiatry*, 6:29-41, 1965.

YATES, A. J.: The psychoses: Children. *Behavior Therapy*. New York: John Wiley & Sons, Inc., 1970,pp. 246-272.

ZASLOW, R. W.: "A Psychogenic Theory of the Etiology of Infantile Autism and Implications for Treatment." Paper presented at the California Psychological Association, 1967.

ZITRIN, A., FERBER, P., & COHEN, D.: Pre- and para-natal factors in mental disorders of children. *Journal of Nervous and Mental Disease*, 139:357-361, 1964.

35

LOOKING AND APPROACH BEHAVIOR OF PSYCHOTIC AND NORMAL CHILDREN AS A FUNCTION OF ADULT ATTENTION OR PREOCCUPATION

Don W. Churchill, M.D. and Carolyn Q. Bryson, M.S.

Department of Psychiatry, Indiana University Medical Center

Lack of eye to eye contact and disinterest in or withdrawal from interpersonal relationships are two of the most commonly described characteristics of psychotic children, particularly those diagnosed as autistic (1-7). Whether the symptoms are explained as manifestations of underlying CNS pathology (6, 8, 9) or as reflecting emotional withdrawal from a threatening world (10, 11), most clinicians rely heavily on these criteria for the diagnosis of infantile autism. In addition, the casual observations of parents and hospital personnel suggest that autistic and schizophrenic children actively avoid, rather than passively ignore, human contact. While clinical reports may emphasize the significance of social withdrawal or avoidance, the relatively few attempts to measure

Reprinted by permission of Grune and Stratton, Inc. and the author, from COM-PREHENSIVE PSYCHIATRY, Vol. 13, No. 2 (March), 1972, pp. 171-177.

Supported in part by PHS Grant MH05154 07 and in part by LaRue D. Carter Memorial Hospital, State of Indiana, Indianapolis, Ind. Computations were performed at Indiana University Medical Center Research Computation Center, which is supported in part by PHS Grant FR 00162.

We are indebted to Dr. James Norton for help with the statistical analyses, and to Mrs. Carolyn Fisher and Miss Beth Zimmerman for technical assistance.

such behavior under controlled conditions have yielded equivocal results. Although Hutt and Ounsted (2) found that autistic children demonstrated more gaze aversion than normals in response to human faces, O'Connor and Hermelin (12, 13) found that psychotics did not differ from retardates or normals in their visual preference for social stimuli.

The present study was designed to further investigate the validity of these cardinal signs as diagnostic criteria for differentiating psychotic from normal children. The looking and approach behaviors of psychotic and normal children were observed and recorded in controlled situations where an unfamiliar female adult was either preoccupied or attentive. It was hypothesized that if these signs were valid diagnostic criteria, then: (1) psychotic children would spend less time in the presence of and looking at the adult than the normal controls; (2) psychotic children would avoid the attentive adult more than the preoccupied adult, while normal children would prefer the attentive adult; and (3) within the psychotic group, autistic children would demonstrate more avoidance behavior than schizophrenic children.

MATERIALS AND METHODS

Subjects: The experimental group consisted of 14 children, ranging in age from 3 to 7 years, and diagnosed as autistic (five boys, three girls) or early childhood schizophrenic (three boys, three girls) according to the DeMyer classification (14). They had been hospitalized at the Clinical Research Center for Early Childhood Schizophrenia for periods ranging from 3 days to 3 years. The control group consisted of 14 non-hospitalized normal children matched for age, sex, and socioeconomic status.

Procedure: Experimental sessions were conducted in an observation room containing a one-way mirror along one wall (Fig. 1). A small cubicle, just large enough to provide room for a seated adult, was constructed directly in front of the mirror. The remainder of the room was divided into four zones which radiated from the cubicle. The inside of the cubicle could be viewed or entered from zones 2 and 4 only; thus a child occupying zone 2 could see and be seen by the adult, and if the child entered zone 4, physical contact was possible. In zones 1 and 3, the child could not see or be seen by the adult; zone 3 contained the entrance door, and zone 1 contained a covered window. Three simple and identical sets of toys were placed in zones 1, 2, and 3: a large plastic dump truck, four plastic snap beads, and a set of nesting barrels. From behind the one-way mirror, two observers continuously and simultaneously recorded the child's position in the room and the number and dura-

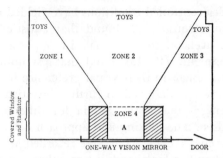

FIG. 1. Floor plan of observation room.

tion of looks at the adult's face by means of a remote Esterline-Angus Recorder.

Each child was observed on one day for three consecutive weeks (day and time of day held constant for each child). On each experimental day there were three 10-minute sessions. Prior to each session, the child spent 20 minutes in a free play situation on the children's ward, during which a variety of toys and adult and peer contacts were freely available. At the beginning of each session, the child was brought to the observation room, where he was positioned near the wall opposite the cubicle and facing the adult, with the comment, "Now you may play in here for a little while." Following the completion of all three sessions on each day, the normal children were allowed their choice of several inexpensive gifts (e.g., crayons, clay, miniature candy bars) and the psychotic children were given miniature candy bars.

During the first session of each day, the child was left in the observation room with no adult present (NA). During the second and third conditions, an unfamiliar female adult was seated in the cubicle in an attentive (AA) or preoccupied (PA) attitude. When attentive, the adult was seated facing into the room, responding with smiles or other expressions of friendly interest considered appropriate to the child's activities; at no time did the adult speak or gesture to or physically interact with the child. When preoccupied, the adult was seated sideways in the cubicle working a cross-word puzzle and presenting only a profile view to the child; all behaviors of the child were ignored. Half of the experimental-control pairs were randomly assigned to each of the two possible initial sequences; the sequences were then reversed for the second week, and the initial sequence was repeated for the third week. Thus every child participated in three NA, three AA, and three PA conditions and was exposed to each sequence at least once over the three-week period.

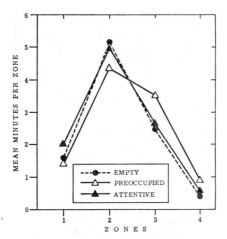

FIG. 2. Distribution of time spent in
each zone by all children.

The following measures of approach and attention behavior were recorded for each child: (1) amount of time spent in each zone; (2) number of looks at the adult's face; (3) duration of looks; and (4) percentage of time in zones 2 and 4 spent looking. At the conclusion of each session both observers also wrote behavioral records to supplement the specific response measures.

RESULTS

Interobserver reliability was established at 0.99 for position in room and between 0.83 and 0.97 for occurrence and duration of looking. Preliminary analyses indicated that the sequence of adult presentation (e.g., AA followed by PA, or PA followed by AA) produced no differential effects; therefore sequence was ignored in all further analyses. Matched-pairs analyses of variance were performed for each of the response measures to compare: (1) all psychotics with all normals; (2) autistics with their normal controls; and (3) schizophrenics with their normal controls. Additional analyses of variance omitting the control groups were also performed for the autistic and schizophrenic subgroups separately. (Summaries of all analyses may be obtained from the authors upon request.) The analyses of the three looking measures yielded nearly identical results; therefore, only the measure of percentage of time in zones 2 and 4 spent looking is discussed here.

The results of the analysis of approach behavior (time spent in each zone) are displayed in Fig. 2. There were no differences in approach

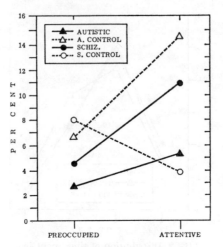

FIG. 3. Percentage of time in zones 2
and 4 spent looking at adult's face.

behavior between groups, either when the entire psychotic and normal
groups were compared or when the autistic and schizophrenic subgroups
were separately compared with their matched controls. A significant
zone effect ($p < 0.005$) reflected the fact that *all* groups of the children
spent the largest amount of time in zone 2 (where they could see and be
seen by the adult) and the least amount of time in zone 4 (where they
could have physical contact with the adult). A significant zone × condition interaction was obtained when the entire psychotic and normal
groups were compared ($p < 0.005$) and when autistics and normals were
compared ($p < 0.01$), and a significant zone × condition × week interaction ($p < 0.025$) was obtained when schizophrenics were compared
with their matched controls. In each case mean values indicated that
time in zone 2 decreased slightly when the adult was preoccupied and
ignoring the child. Zone × condition effects were not found when the
autistic and schizophrenic subgroups were analyzed individually, suggesting that the normal children were somewhat more responsive to
changes in the experimental conditions.

Results of the analysis of attention behavior (percentage of time in
zones 2 and 4 spent looking) are displayed in Fig. 3. When the entire
psychotic and normal groups were compared, only the condition effect
was significant ($p < 0.05$), reflecting the fact that most of the children
looked more at the attentive than the preoccupied adult. However, in
contrast to physical approach behavior, differences between groups did

appear when the subgroups of schizophrenic and autistic children were compared with their own control groups. When autistics were compared with their controls, only the condition effect was significant ($p < 0.05$) and there were no group differences. The condition effect did not reach significance when autistics were considered alone, although there was a strong tendency for autistics to look more at the attentive adult. When the schizophrenics were compared with their controls, a significant group × condition interaction ($p < 0.005$) was obtained, reflecting the fact that the schizophrenics looked more at the attentive than the preoccupied adult, while their normal controls looked more at the preoccupied than attentive adult. This was the reverse of the behavior predicted. When the schizophrenics were considered alone, the significant condition effect ($p < 0.05$) was obtained.

Despite the similarity between the experimental and control children with respect to their looking and approach behavior, obvious qualitative differences between the groups in their style of play and interpersonal contact were reflected in the behavior notes of both observers. As individuals and as a group, the normal children displayed a much wider range of affective responses toward the experimental situation than did the psychotic children. Similarly, their use of the toys and their methods of interacting with (or even ignoring!) the adult were varied, imaginative, often cunning, and regularly had an easily inferred purpose. This was true regardless of whether the normal child's reaction to the situation was one of pleasure, boredom, or distress. Aggressive behavior, when it appeared, was observed almost exclusively in the normal children. The varied strategies of the normal children were reflected in such direct verbal communications by different children as: "There's not much toys. . . . Why don't you talk? . . . Let me out of here. . . . Did you see *that?* . . . I want some people. . . . I need to blow my nose." In contrast, the verbalizations of the psychotic children, when they occurred, had little or no obvious communicative intent. Even when direct verbal communication with the adult was not attempted, much of the toy play of the normal children was used either as a means of expressing feelings about the experimental situation in general (as when a child who seemed annoyed by the confinement repeatedly and violently rammed a truck against the door), or as a means of indirect communication with the adult in particular (as when a child would make toy constructions, stealing glances at the adult each step of the way, or would make "offerings" to the adult). The toy play of the psychotic child was more repetitive, desultory, and had little or no clearly communicative meaning. Even when the behavioral range of the younger normal children was most narrowly limited by distress, they did not demonstrate the stereotyped or ritualistic behavior or the seemingly aimless wandering that was noticed in most of the psychotic children.

DISCUSSION

Under the conditions of this study, the looking and approach behaviors of psychotic children increased in response to an adult's attention in a similar manner as those of normal children of the same chronological age, sex, and socioeconomic status. No support was found for the hypotheses formed from casual observation and from clinical practice that adult attention actually "drives away" autistic or schizophrenic children. Rather, the reverse was found. These findings were unexpected and might still give rise to astonishment in the light of common experience and belief. Many people would still attest that most schizophrenic children and virtually all autistic children look away when looked at and withdraw when approached. Indeed, an unusually active and instructive approach to psychotic children has long been advocated in the literature (15-18) in order to break through the "autistic barrier" or overcome the child's resistance to interpersonal contact.

In attempting to explain the variance of the present findings from common belief, one question which arises is the effect of the experimental group's familiarity with the hospital. Although this factor cannot be entirely eliminated, it does not appear to be an adequate explanation. Several of the psychotic children were newly admitted to the hospital, and there was no indication of a familiarization effect in the normal children over the 3-week period. The female adult who was in the room with the children was a stranger to both groups, as was the observer who brought the children to the observation room and returned them to the ward.

An additional question is whether the unexpected findings might be accounted for by the unnatural conditions of the experiment. This really requires two answers. Although the adult's responsiveness was limited and was unusual in its lack of verbal communication with the child, the attentive and preoccupied conditions still represented situations relevant to the everyday lives of the children. At any rate, the experimental conditions preserved all of the gross and readily recognizable qualitative differences between the two groups, while still providing a set of independent variables which were readily discriminable and responded to in the same way by both groups. Secondly, however, it is acknowledged that a differential response between the two groups might have appeared if the attentive adult had been more "natural" in the sense of actively responding to or seeking out the children. If one conceptualizes a gradient of increasing adult intrusiveness or demand upon *any* child, it is reasonable to suppose that a "breaking point" is reached where the child, rather than returning the adult's attention, actively avoids it. If this were so, it might be argued that the conditions of the present experiment were located below such a breaking point for *both* groups. Further along the gradient, a group differential response might appear, while still further along, beyond the breaking point of the normal group, the groups might again become indistinguishable if considered by their responses along these measures alone. Some behavioral effects of this gradient of adult intrusiveness or demandingness, translated into success:failure ratios, recently have been reported (19).

However, in spite of any postulated demand-gradient, the present results cast doubt on the validity of the avoidance of eye contact and interpersonal relationships as criteria in establishing a diagnosis of autism or early childhood schizophrenia, particularly in a nonstandardized interview in which the demands placed on the child are not objectively evaluated. These avoidance behaviors may simply be a reflection of the type or amount of the interviewer's interaction with the child, or the difficulty level of the responses which the interviewer is attempting to elicit from the child, rather than a generalized affective response by the child to all or most of the adults in the world around him. This is not to say that there are not easily observed differences between psychotic and nonpsychotic children. However, we would agree with the others (12, 20) who have found, upon measurement, that common statements concerning psychotic children's lack of social responsiveness require modification. Perhaps the terms describing such children need to be more accurately or functionally defined. It may be that other aspects of such children's behavior provide the cues from which such things as withdrawal or lack of eye contact are inferred. In particular, the qualitative differences in the toy play behavior of psychotic and normal children were readily apparent to both observers. The toy play of the psychotic children was restricted, repetitive, and generally had no reference to the adult, while the play of the normal children was more directly aimed at eliciting adult responses. Further, when the normal children looked at the adult, their looking was reflected in more attentive postural responses (e.g., cessation of unrelated motor activity, turning of the entire torso toward the adult, etc.); these postural accommodations did not accompany the looking by the psychotic children.

The results of the present study indicate that lack of eye to eye contact and physical distance *per se* are not characteristics unique to psychotic children and cannot be considered pathognomic of childhood psychosis as, in practice, they sometimes are. The repeated interpretation of these behaviors as generalized emotional responses unique to psychotic children may impede the more complete evaluation of behavioral, perceptual, or cognitive deficits.

SUMMARY

Fourteen autistic and schizophrenic children with matched normal controls were found not to differ significantly in their behavior of looking at and of approach toward strange adults, although gross differences in other aspects of their behavior were observed. Both groups responded significantly more to an attentive than to a preoccupied adult. Some implications of these findings for the diagnosis and psychopathology of autism and early childhood schizophrenia are discussed.

REFERENCES

1. CREAK, M.: Schizophrenic syndrome in childhood. Progress report of a working party. *Brit. Med. J.*, 2:889, 1961.
2. HUTT, C. & OUNSTED, C.: The biological significance of gaze aversion with particular reference to the syndrome of infantile autism. *Behav. Sci.*, 11:346, 1966.
3. KANNER, L.: Autistic disturbances of affective contact. *Nerv. Child*, 2:217, 1943.
4. KANNER, L.: Problems of nosology and psychodynamics of early infantile autism. *Amer. J. Orthopsychiat.*, 19:416, 1949.
5. KANNER, L.: *Child Psychiatry* (ed. 2). Springfield, Ill.: C. Thomas, 1957, p. 719.
6. RIMLAND, B.: *Infantile Autism*. New York: Appleton-Century-Crofts, 1964, p. 8.
7. WING, J. K. (Ed.): *Early Childhood Autism*. London: Pergamon, 1966, p. 11.
8. BENDER, L.: Childhood schizophrenia. *Psychiat. Quart.*, 27:663, 1953.
9. SCHOPLER, E.: Early infantile autism and receptor processes. *Arch. Gen. Psychiat.* (Chicago), 13:327, 1965.
10. BETTELHEIM, B.: *The Empty Fortress*. New York: Free Press, 1967.
11. ZASLOW, R. W.: A psychogenic theory of etiology of infantile autism and implications for treatment. Paper read at California State Psychological Association, San Diego, 1967.
12. O'CONNOR, N. & HERMELIN, B.: Measures of distance and motility in psychotic children and severely subnormal controls. *Brit. J. Soc. Clin. Psychol.*, 3:29, 1963.
13. O'CONNOR, N. & HERMELIN, B.: The selective visual attention of psychotic children. *J. Child Psychol. Psychiat.*, 8:167, 1967.
14. WHITE, P. T., DeMYER, W., & DeMYER, M.: EEG abnormalities in early childhood schizophrenia: A double-blind study of psychiatrically disturbed and normal children during promazine sedation. *Amer. J. Psychiat.*, 120:950, 1964.
15. BETZ, B. J.: A study of tactics resolving the autistic barrier in the psychotherapy of the schizophrenic personality. *Amer. J. Psychiat.*, 104:267, 1947.
16. DesLAURIERS, A. M.: *The Experience of Reality in Childhood Schizophrenia*. New York, International Universities Press, 1962, p. 63.
17. DesLAURIERS, A. M. & CARLSON, C. F.: *Your Child Is Asleep: Early Infantile Autism*. Homewood, Ill.: Dorsey, 1969, Chapter V.

18. DESPERT, J. L.: Treatment of child schizophrenia. In G. Bychowski and J. L. Despert (Eds.), *Specialized Techniques in Psychotherapy*. New York: Basic, 1952, p. 158.

19. CHURCHILL, D. W.: The effects of success and failure in psychotic children. *Arch. Gen. Psychiat.* (Chicago), 25:208, 1971.

20. HERMELIN, B. & O'CONNOR, N.: The response and self-generated behavior of severely disturbed children and severely subnormal controls. *Brit. J. Soc. Clin. Psychol.*, 2:37, 1963.

Part IX

DRUG STUDIES

The use of drugs is becoming an increasingly accepted form of therapy for many clinical syndromes in children. Thus, the need for careful studies of new drugs, comparisons of the effectiveness of different drugs for the same condition and follow-ups of the long-term effects of specific medications has become essential.

Campbell and her colleagues discuss the comparative effects of lithium, a relatively new drug, and chlorpromazine in terms of their immediate influence on the behavior of deviant children. McAndrew and his co-authors consider the long-term effects of phenothiazines. They provide data about both the advantages and the risks of prolonged medication.

587

Part IX

DRUG STUDIES

36

LITHIUM AND CHLORPROMAZINE: A CONTROLLED CROSSOVER STUDY OF HYPERACTIVE SEVERELY DISTURBED YOUNG CHILDREN

Magda Campbell, M.D., Barbara Fish, M.D., Julius Korein, M.D., Theodore Shapiro, M.D., Patrick Collins, Ph.D., and Celedonia Koh, M.D.

New York University Medical Center

A controlled crossover study of lithium and chlorpromazine involving 10 severely disturbed children, 3 to 6 years of age, of which 6 were schizophrenic and 1 autistic, is reported in detail. Patients were matched for motor activity (hyper- and hypoactivity) and prognosis. More symptoms diminished on chlorpromazine than on lithium. However, improvements were only slight on both, except in one child whose autoaggressiveness and explosiveness practically ceased on lithium (nonblind evaluations). Blind ratings indicated no statistically significant difference between the two drugs as well as absence of statistically significant change from

Reprinted from JOURNAL OF AUTISM AND CHILDHOOD SCHIZOPHRENIA, 1972, 2, 3, pp. 234-263. Copyright © 1972 by Scripta Publishing Company.

This study was supported in part by Public Health Service Grant MH-04465 from the National Institute of Mental Health and in part by a grant from the Harriett Ames Charitable Trust. The authors wish to thank Dr. Sam Gershon for his valuable comments and suggestions, and Ms. M. Kalmijn, R. Bensimhon, H. Von Hedrich, L. Levidow, and P. Mikel for technical assistance.

Dr. Fish is now Professor of Psychiatry at the University of California (L.A.).

baseline to treatment with either. Lithium diminished the severity of individual symptoms, though not statistically significant, such as explosiveness, hyperactivity, aggressiveness, and psychotic speech. Its effect in adult schizophrenia is compared to responses of schizophrenic children. Also discussed is the relationship of EEG to clinical improvement and toxicity, and effect of lithium on hyperactivity and aggressiveness. It is suggested that lithium may prove of some value in treatment of severe psychiatric disorders in childhood involving aggressiveness, explosive affect and hyperactivity.

This study was designed to explore the effects of lithium in hyperactive psychotic and nonpsychotic children of preschool age and to compare such effects with those of chlorpromazine. In adults, lithium therapy has a well-established role in the manic phase of recurrent manic-depressive illness, which is probably nonexistent under 10 years of age. As yet, the role of lithium ion has not been established in the treatment of psychiatric disturbances of childhood (Schou, 1972) and its use for children is relatively recent. At the initial stage of our study, we were aware of Van Krevelen and Van Voorst's (1959) case report, of Frommer's (1968) experience with lithium in depressed children, and of Annell's (1969a, 1969b) unpublished (at that time) work on lithium in school-age children and adolescents. Since then, a few additional reports on the use of lithium in psychiatric disorders of childhood have been published. However, none of these studies attempted to compare lithium with another standard effective drug. Moreover, the patients' diagnoses were not always well defined.

The case study reported by Van Krevelen and Van Voorst (1959) was focused on a 14-year-old retarded boy whose hospitalization was prompted by onset of alternating depressive and hypomanic states; the etiology remained unclear. The boy failed to respond to other drugs such as chlorpromazine, but responded well to lithium (the initial daily dose was 1,200 mg., subsequently reduced to 600 mg.). Only incidental mention was made in Frommer's (1968) detailed paper on childhood depression that good results were obtained with lithium, alone, or when lithium was combined with other antidepressants in "hypomanic" and depressed patients. The children, 4 to 14 years of age and treated in an outpatient clinic, received small doses (50 to 250 mg. per day). Frommer believed that "a depression without truly endogenous and disruptive mood swings is almost certainly made worse by lithium salts in children."

Annell's patients represented several psychiatric diagnostic categories with multiple etiologies. She began to use lithium in 1965, at first for older adolescents with "typical manic conditions," and later for younger patients exhibiting periodic conditions other than mania, whose relatives had a high incidence of periodic psychoses (including manic depression). In 1969 Annell presented data on 12 patients ranging in age from 9 to 18 years. All but one (including two who were probably schizophrenic) showed mild to moderate improvement on long-term maintenance therapy (900 to 1800 mg. per day, serum level 0.6 to 1.2 mEq/l).

It is difficult to evaluate the efficacy of lithium in the two children reported by Dyson and Barcai (1970), since neither chlorpromazine nor any other major tranquilizer that might have been as effective, or possibly better if tried, was in use. Also, the results were obscured because one child received lithium and amphetamine simultaneously. Both patients had "lithium responder" parents with manic-depressive episodes. The first patient, an 8-year-old hyperactive and depressed boy with a poor school record, did not respond to amphetamine treatment. Marked improvement in all areas of behavior was noted first on a combination of amphetamine (12.5 mg. per day) and lithium carbonate (1,500 mg. per day) and later on lithium therapy alone. The other child, a 13-year-old hyperactive boy, failing in school and suffering from outbursts of bad temper followed by episodes of depression, also did not respond to dextroamphetamine sulfate (20 mg. per day). He improved on 1500 mg. of lithium carbonate per day, manifesting decreased hyperactivity, increased attention span and good academic performance. The symptoms of both patients recurred after lithium was discontinued.

Rifkin, Quitkin, Carillo, and Klein's (1972) doubleblind crossover study compared lithium to placebo in 21 adolescents. Their patients represented the diagnostic category of "emotionally unstable character disorder" (EUCD), with chronic maladaptive behavior patterns and usually nonreactive depressive and hypomanic mood swings. Lithium was found to be statistically significantly better than placebo, using a global measure of mood swings. On the basis of these results, Rifkin and his associates concluded that EUCD is related to affective illness, that lithium is as valuable as chlorpromazine in the treatment of this condition, and perhaps even more valuable because it lacks the sedative effect that is objectionable to adolescents.

Although in adults lithium is the most specific psychoactive agent for mania, it has been tried in the past 2 decades in other psychiatric conditions, including those associated with hyperexcitability. However, the statement made by Gershon and Yuwiler (1960) still holds true:

> The literature indicates a fundamental improvement in cases of mania and a symptomatic improvement in controlling psychomotor activity in a variety of conditions ranging from behavioral disorders to catatonic excitement.

Cade (1949) was the first to use lithium in psychiatric subjects (10 manic patients, 3 melancholics and 6 with dementia praecox). Although there was no change in the schizophrenic symptomatology, three schizophrenics "who were usually restless, noisy and shouting nonsensical abuse" became quiet and manageable for the first time in years. Cade suggested that lithium has a strong quieting effect on excitement of nonmanic chronic psychotics since the restlessness returned after discontinuation of lithium treatment.

This action of lithium on hyperexcitability, reported throughout the literature, led us to investigate its possible therapeutic effects on our population of severely disturbed children. To our knowledge, this is the first and only controlled study of lithium against an effective drug in children; it comprises a part of an ongoing research program in psychopharmacology for preschool-age schizophrenic and autistic children.

SUBJECTS

The 10 patients, 8 boys and 2 girls, were 3 to 6 years of age ($M = 4.9$). All attended the nursery of the children's psychiatric inpatient service of Bellevue Hospital. Six were childhood schizophrenics, one had a chronic organic brain syndrome with a withdrawing reaction of childhood (and Turner's syndrome) and two had severe behavior disorders. The intellectual functioning of these patients ranged from average to severely retarded as shown in Table 1.

The children were hospitalized for a minimum of two months prior to the commencement of our study and given placebo while baseline evaluations and laboratory work were in process. None had a history of seizure disorder. General physical examination and laboratory studies revealed no systematic abnormalities; there was no evidence of neurological or motor deficit (except as noted above).

METHODS

The 10 children were matched for motor activity (hyper- and hypoactivity) and prognosis, using severity of language impairment and

Table 1

Age, Classification, Intellectual Functioning and Diagnosis of Ten Patients

Name	CA (years)	Classi-fication	Level of intellectual functioning	Diagnosis
Harry	6	E	mental age[a] = +3; IQ = 83	childhood schizophrenia (florid psychosis)
Mike	5	E	motor DQ[b] = 77 adaptive DQ = 77 language DQ = 54 personal-social DQ = 46	childhood schizophrenia[d]
Carl	4	E	language DQ[b] = 75	childhood schizophrenia[d]
Peter	5	C	motor DQ[b] = 57 adaptive DQ = 44 language DQ = 25 personal-social DQ = 42	early infantile autism
Mary	6	E_1	full scale IQ[c] = 58 verbal IQ = 69 performance IQ = 54	organic brain syndrome, chronic (Turner's syndrome) with withdrawing reaction
Rose	5	E	mental age[a] = 2.9; IQ = 36	childhood schizophrenia
Sam	5	E	motor DQ[b] = 88 adaptive DQ = 98 language DQ = 66 personal-social DQ = 83	childhood schizophrenia
John	5	E_1	full scale IQ[c] = 94 verbal IQ = 91 performance IQ = 99	behavior disorder of childhood (hyperkinetic reaction)
Kevin	3	E_1	mental age[a] = 3.8; IQ = 98	behavior disorder of childhood (withdrawing reaction)
William	5	E	motor DQ[b] = 53 adaptive DQ = 51.7 language DQ = 41.7 personal-social DQ = 61.7	childhood schizophrenia

Note.—Classification of children is based on criteria delineated in Fish et al. (1968). C = Speech absent, minimal comprehension, minimal adaptive skills. E = Speech present, psychotic, vocabulary above 33DQ. E_1 = Nonpsychotic subgroup, speech present, vocabulary above 33DQ, good comprehension. [a]Based on Stanford-Binet Intelligence Scale, Form L-M. [b]Based on Gesell Developmental Schedules. [c]Based on Wechsler Preschool and Primary Scale of Intelligence. [d]In remission.

Table 2

Ten Patients Matched for Motor Activity and
Prognosis

First drug lithium, hyperactive children	First drug chlorpromazine, hypoactive children
Harry	Mary
Mike	Carl
Peter[a]	Rose[b]
Sam	William
John	Kevin

[a] Hypoactive. [b] Hyperactive.

stereotypy as criteria (Fish, Shapiro, Campbell, & Wile, 1968), as given in
Table 1. One of each matched pair was started on lithium carbonate
(Rowell Laboratories) and the other on chlorpromazine as shown in
Table 2. Each drug was administered in three divided daily doses. Additional fluids and sodium chloride were supplied with lithium tablets.
The increments were one weekly. Doses were individually regulated by
the nonblind research psychiatrist to determine the maximum tolerated
dose. The children were maintained from 7 to 10 weeks on each drug
($M = 8.7$), including the 3 to 8 weeks ($M = 4.6$) maintenance on the
maximum tolerated ("optimal") dose. There was a 4-week drug-free
period between the two treatment periods. Lithium was administered to
the patients for 7 to 10 weeks ($M = 8.4$), starting with 450 mg. per day,
and increasing weekly. The highest dose explored was 1350 mg. per day
(0.91 to 2.075 mEq/1). Lithium blood level was monitored twice a
week during the drug regulation period and weekly during the period
of maximum tolerated dose.

All children were placed on chlorpromazine. One who developed an
intermittent rash (which appeared to be due to sensitivity or allergy
to chlorpromazine), received instead a daily maintenance dose of 3 mg.
thiothixene. Chlorpromazine was administered to the other 9 children
for 8 to 10 weeks ($M = 8.8$). Doses were individually regulated, starting
with 15 mg. per day. The highest daily dose that was explored amounted
to 90 mg.

The research psychiatrist who functioned as the blind observer independently rated the children on CGI* and on symptom severity scales

* CGI = Clinical Global Impressions.

developed for such patients (Fish 1968),* using examination procedures described elsewhere (Fish et al., 1968). Ratings were done on placebo immediately prior to initiation of each drug treatment and during the last week of treatment. Global improvements, total symptom scores and individual symptoms were subjected to statistical analysis. Ratings performed immediately prior to treatment were compared with final ratings on "optimal" doses of each drug.

All children had a routine baseline EEG. Six had their records performed without sedation while 4 who required sedation received chloral hydrate (1.25 to 2 gms P.O. or rectally). In order to obtain comparable conditions of recording, EEG was repeated under conditions similar to baseline records during the last week on "optimal" doses of lithium or chlorpromazine (i.e., sedation was repeated only if the patient required it for the baseline record). Following discontinuation of each drug and after the 4-week "wash-out" period, the EEG was again repeated. Thus, an attempt was made to perform 5 EEGs on each patient (3 were "drug free" and 2 performed while on "optimal" dose of each drug) under approximately the same conditions of recording. Final evaluation was repeated after all recordings were completed without knowledge of clinical improvement and/or toxicity. Reliable comparisons were deemed possible if the following conditions were satisfied: (1) the patient's condition and state of consciousness had to be consistent during each EEG, and (2) if the patient was receiving sedation, the EEG effect of such sedation had to appear relatively constant in "drug free" records (i.e., EEGs during which a patient received chloral hydrate but not lithium or chlorpromazine). If the records were comparable, all "drug free" EEGs were evaluated together for each patient to determine whether or not they were normal. Unequivocally abnormal records were determined using the conservative criteria that were previously established for evaluation of children's EEGs (Korein, Fish, Shapiro, Gerner, & Levidow, 1971), but allowing for differences in age.

RESULTS

Response to Lithium

Maximum tolerated doses of lithium carbonate ranged from 450 to 900 mg. per day (lithium blood level 0.25-1.19 mEq/l; $M = 0.672$). Toxic symptoms on daily doses as low as 450 mg. ranged from subjectively feeling "tired and miserable" or "feeling sick" (at lithium plasma level

---

* This scale has 14 items which assess social, language, affective and motor behavior, as well as a global rating of improvement.

of 0.325 to 0.45 mEq/1), some difficulties in articulation (0.6 mEq/1) to motor retardation, motor excitation, irritability or pallor (0.45 to 0.8 mEq/1).

At the end of treatment, according to the nonblind psychiatrist, one of the 10 children showed marked improvement, 4 slight improvement, 4 no change and one a deterioration as shown in Table 3.

Generally, not many symptoms decreased with lithium and the improvements were slight, except in the case of Harry whose autoaggressiveness (self-mutilating behavior) and explosiveness practically ceased. Although 5 of the 10 children were hyperactive and aggressive, these symptoms decreased in only 2 (also slightly in one). In this group, Harry was the only hyperactive child with explosive affect; 3 hyperactive children had blunted affect and one was not psychotic with mild excitability.

Harry was a 6-year-old boy, with a life long history of irritability, explosiveness, hyperactivity, and aggressiveness turned against his own body. He was extremely impulsive, and unable to sit in one place for even very short periods of time. The boy always walked on his toes. Movements were usually jerky and even speech had an explosive quality; he also stammered. Harry's frustration tolerance was very low and he reacted to the slightest provocation with outbursts of rage and violent temper tantrums. Headbanging resulted in frontal bossing; he kept scratching and hitting himself and also biting his forearms which were covered with old scars. Harry was a withdrawn child who lived in a world of fantasy, preoccupied with world destruction and people and things that were falling apart. As early as on the 4th day of lithium treatment (on 450 mg. per day; blood level 0.7 mEq/1), there was a marked decrease in autoaggressiveness, self-mutilating behavior, as well as a slight decrease in impulsivity and hyperactivity. Stammering also improved. On 600 mg. per day there was a marked decrease in impulsivity and hyperactivity; his attention span improved and selfmutilating behavior and tantrums practically ceased. Harry's preoccupation with world destruction decreased markedly. On his "optimal" daily lithium dose of 600 mg. (blood level 0.593-0.760 mEq/1), he became less withdrawn, more playful and often laughed responsively. All such gains disappeared after discontinuation of lithium.*

---

* Incidentally, Harry was on 6 different drugs, including trifluoperazine, tritluperidol and thiothixene; although all had strong antipsychotic properties, none exhibited the antiaggressive effect of lithium.

Table 3

Global Improvements, Maximum Tolerated Dose and Blood Level in Ten Patients on Lithium Carbonate[a]

Name	Motor activity, aggressiveness, and affect	Global improvement	"Optimal" dose[b] (in mg. per day)	Blood level on "optimal" dose (in mEq/1)
Harry	very hyperactive, (auto) aggressive, very explosive	marked	600	0.593-0.760
Mike	hyperactive, aggressive, blunted	slight	900	0.48-0.65
Carl	hypoactive, blunted	slight	900	0.625-1.190
Peter	hypoactive, blunted	slight	600	0.65-0.75
Mary	hypoactive, blunted	slight	900	0.65-0.85
Rose	very hyperactive, aggressive, blunted	no change	600	0.55-0.90
Sam	hyperactive, aggressive, blunted	no change	450	0.25-0.35
John	very hyperactive, aggressive, mildly excitable	no change	900	0.90-1.05
Kevin	hypoactive, blunted	no change	600	0.5-0.7
William	hypoactive, very irritable	worse	900	0.45-0.70

[a]Nonblind evaluations. [b]Maximum dose tolerated.

Other effects seen in the 10 children on "optimal" doses of lithium included decrease in stereotypy (in 5 patients), decrease in withdrawal and gains in verbal production (in 4), decrease in irritability and nega-tivism (in 3), decrease in psychotic speech and increase in vocabulary and effective responsiveness (in 3), and increase in attention span (in 2). Positive changes occurred as early as on the 2nd, 3rd and 4th day of

Table 4

Global Improvement in Ten Patients on
Lithium Carbonate and Chlorpromazine[a]

| Name | Global improvement | |
	Lithium carbonate	Chlorpromazine
Harry	marked	slight
Mike	slight	slight
Carl	slight	slight
Peter	slight	slight
Mary	slight	marked
Rose	no change	slight[b]
Sam	no change	slight
John	no change	no change
Kevin	no change	marked
William	worse	marked

[a] Nonblind evaluations. [b] Patient received thiothixene
instead of chlorpromazine.

treatment, on daily doses as low as 450 mg. (blood levels ranged from
0.145 to 0.7 mEq/1; the latter found in Harry). All symptoms noted
prior to administration of lithium have reappeared after discontinuation.

Response to Chlorpromazine

Maximum tolerated doses ranged from 9 to 45 mg. per day ($M = 17.3$).
Five of the 9 children required only 9 mg. per day, or 0.2 mg. per lb.
(body weights ranged from 35 to 57 lbs.; $M = 46.7$). Signs and symptoms
of excess chlorpromazine on daily doses as low as 9 to 15 mg. included
excessive sedation, motor excitation, irritability, insomnia, worsening of
psychosis and catatonic-like states.

Ratings of the nonblind psychiatrist at the end of treatment period
indicated marked improvement in 3 of the 9 children,** slight improvement in 6, and no change in one. Table 4 details the various responses of patients to chlorpromazine and lithium.

A goodly number of symptoms decreased on "optimal" doses of chlorpromazine, but in most cases only to a slight degree. We saw decrease
in psychotic speech (in 8 patients) and withdrawal, increase in affective

** The 10th patient (Rose) who was on thiothixene showed only slight improvement.

responsiveness and vocabulary (in 7), decrease in stereotypy, improvements in attention span and initiation of speech (in 6).

On the last week on "optimal" dosage, the blind psychiatrist's ratings of global improvement on CGI indicated no statistically significant difference between the effects of lithium and chlorpromazine (Mann-Whitney U Test). In fact, only 4 patients in the chlorpromazine group and 3 in the lithium group showed improvement (minimal on the global improvement scale); in the other patients, there was either no change or a worsening of symptomatology.

Global improvement ratings on CGI were supported by absence of statistically significant changes in overall severity from pre- to active drug treatment with either chlorpromazine or lithium (Wilcoxen Matched-Pairs Signed Ranks Test). The order of drug treatment had no significant effect on global improvement nor on changes in symptom severity (Mann-Whitney U Test).

With respect to severity of individual symptoms, no significant changes occurred under either drug treatment.* However, with lithium treatment, there was improvement (though not statistically significant) in such areas as explosiveness, hyperactivity, aggressiveness, and psychotic speech.**

Toxic Symptoms and Side Effects

Signs and symptoms of excess lithium during regulation appeared on daily doses as low as 450 mg. (blood level 0.31 to 0.8 mEq/1). They were seen on such low doses in all diagnostic categories (in 2 with childhood schizophrenia, in both cases of behavior disorder, and in the girl with Turner's syndrome) as early as the second or third day of drug administration. The most frequent sign of excess lithium was motor retardation seen in 7 patients on 450-1350 mg. per day (blood level 0.91-1.46 mEq/1). Worsening of psychosis was noted in 3 children (600-900 mg. per day; blood level up to 1.16 mEq/1).

The signs of excess lithium on "optimal" doses (450 to 900 mg. per day; blood level 0.31 to 1.025 mEq/1) included, among others, complaints of "feeling sick," gastrointestinal disturbances, transient polydipsia, polyuria, transient motor excitation, and irritability.

The highest explored daily dose of lithium was 1350 mg.

---

* Matched-pair t-tests were performed since the number of zero changes precluded appropriate nonparametric statistics.

** The blind psychiatrist's ratings were statistically tested twice—once with the patient on thiothixene and once without; there were no significant differences between the two.

Table 5
Toxic Symptoms and Side Effects of Lithium Carbonate on Ten Patients

Toxic symptoms and side effects	T	Minimum doses on which toxic symptoms or side effects had occurred (in mg. per day)	Lithium blood level (in mEq/1)	Number of patients with toxic symptoms or side effects	
				Total	On "optimal dose"
EKG changes		900		2	2
Leukocytosis with lymphocytopenia		600-1350	0.30-0.95	4	4
Decrease of T4		600-900	0.55-1.05	2	2
Pallor	X	900	0.90-1.15	2	1
Pallor		450-1350	0.45-1.16	4	
Rings under eyes		450-450	0.6		
Vomiting	X	450-900	0.450-1.275	4	1
Decreased appetite		900	1.225	1	
Loss of appetite	X	600-900	0.8-0.9	2	1
Loss of weight	X	900	1.15	1	
Loose bowel movements	X	600-1350	0.550-1.483	2	1
Diarrhea	X	900-1350	1.15-?	2	
Polydipsia	X	900	0.475	1	1
Polydipsia		450-1350	0.375-2.075	3	
Urinary frequency		900	1.16	1	
Polyuria		600-900	0.475-1.160	3	1
Diurnal enuresis		600	?	1	1
Achy lower extremities		1350	1.46	1	
Feeling "dizzy"		1350	?	1	
Feeling "tired and miserable" or "sick"		450-1350	0.325-1.460	3	1
Fine tremor	X	1350	?	1	
Intention tremor		1350	?	1	
Ataxia	X	1350	?	2	
Ataxia		1350	?-1.483-?	3	
Slightly slurred speech	X	1350	?	2	
Slurred speech		1350	?	1	
Articulation less clear		450	0.6	1	
Drooling		1350	1.95	1	
As if in a daze		450-1350	?-0.91-?	4	
Lethargy	X	900	1.15	1	
Motor retardation	X	450-1350	0.80-1.08	4	
Motor retardation		450-1350	?-0.91-1.46	7	
Excessive sedation	X	900-1350	1.375-2.075	2	
Excessive sedation		900	0.95	1	
Motor excitation	X	450-900	?	3	1
Motor excitation		600-900	0.111-?	4	
Irritability	X	450-900	0.55-?	4	1
Irritability		450-1350	0.45-1.09-?	4	
Insomnia		1350	0.91	1	
Worsening of psychosis		600-900	?-1.16	3	

T = transient

Table 6

Toxic Symptoms and Side Effects of Chlorpromazine on Ten Patients

Toxic symptoms and side effects	T	Minimum doses on which toxic symptoms or side effects had occurred (in mg. per day)	Number of patients with toxic symptoms or side effects	
			Total	On "optimal dose"
Intermittent skin rash		5	1	
Pallor	X	9-30	2	1
Pallor		30-45	5	
Rings under eyes		15-30	3	
Loss of appetite		30	1	
Increased appetite		30	1	
Weight gain		15	1	
Feeling tired		30	1	
Motor retardation	X	30-45	3	2
Motor retardation		15-60	8	
Excessive sedation	X	9-45	3	
Excessive sedation		15-60	8	
Motor excitation	X	45	1	
Motor excitation		9-15	4	2
Irritability	X	30-45	3	1
Irritability		9-60	7	1
Insomnia		9-15	2	2
Euphoria	X	15	1	
Euphoria		15	2	2
Episodes of positive and negative stimulation		60	1	
Worsening of psychosis		15	1	
As if in a daze		15-45	4	
Catatonic-like state		15-30	3	
Drooling		30	1	
Slurred speech	X	30	1	1
Slurred speech		30-45	2	
Ataxia		30-60	3	
Worsening of strabismus		30	1	
Diurnal enuresis		9	1	1
Diurnal and nocturnal enuresis		15	1	

T = transient

Table 7

Comparison of EEGs During "Drug-free" and "Optimal" Lithium Dose Periods

Name	"Drug-free" EEG		"Optimal" dose period-lithium				
	Description	Sedation	Blood level (mEq/1)	mg. per day	EEG changes	Global improvements*	Persistent Toxicity
Harry	NL	chloral hydrate	0.593-0.760	600	not done	marked	none
Mike[a]	NL	none	0.48-0.65	900	decrease of alpha frequency, increase slowing (Δ)	slight	none
Carl	NL	none	0.625-1.190	900	not comparable	slight	none
Peter	abnormal focal spikes	chloral hydrate	0.65-0.75	600	decreased focal spikes	slight	none
Mary	abnormal focal slowing	none	0.65-0.85	900	increased diffuse slowing (Δ)	slight	polydipsia
Rose	NL	chloral hydrate	0.55-0.90	600	not comparable	no change	enuresis polyuria polydipsia
Sam[b]	abnormal focal spikes	none	0.25-0.35	450	increased amt. and amplitude of focal spikes	no change	subjectively feeling sick periods of hypoactivity
John[c]	minimal abnormal focal paroxysmal	none	0.90-1.05	900	increased amt. and amplitude of focal spikes	no change	EKG changes
Kevin	NL	none	0.5-0.7	600	no change	no change	none
William	abnormal focal spikes	chloral hydrate	0.45-0.70	900	increased amt. and amplitude of focal spikes	worse	polyuria, dec. verbal production and vocab., inc. of withdrawal EKG changes

Note. NL = normal. *Nonblind evaluations; [a]Fig. 1.; [b]Fig. 2.; [c]Fig. 3.

John, a most hyperactive, aggressive and distractible child with very short attention span but normal intelligence, had a diagnosis of behavior disorder. He showed the first therapeutic changes on this high daily dose of 1350 mg. (blood level 1.95 mEq/l) after 3 weeks of maintenance. The therapeutic changes were transient, comprising decrease in aggressiveness and hyperactivity, and stimulation in social, verbal and affective areas of behavior. They were followed by irritability and hypoactivity, and complaints of feeling tired and thirsty (on 2.075 mEq/l). This child showed no change on his "optimal" daily dose of 900 mg. (0.1-1.05 mEq/l).

However, other patients were quite toxic on 1350 mg. per day (on 0.91-2.075 mEq/l), manifesting pallor, insomnia, polydipsia, diarrhea, tremor, ataxia and slurred speech. They felt dizzy or achy in the lower extremities. Side effects, particularly those of a neurological nature, often lasted for periods below 30 minutes to a few hours. All undesirable effects of lithium noted in the 10 children are listed in Table 5.

On chlorpromazine, behavioral or other side effects of excess drug (pallor, motor retardation, sedation, motor excitation, irritability, insomnia, worsening of psychosis and catatonic-like state) were seen on daily doses as low as 9 to 15 mg. Most frequent among the side effects were motor retardation, sedation and irritability. Table 6 shows all toxic symptoms and side effects of chlorpromazine observed in 9 patients.

EEG Findings and Changes

Evaluation of "drug free" EEGs revealed that 5 of the 10 children had unequivocally abnormal records with focal asymmetrics indicating organic cerebral dysfunction. Two had asymmetrical or focal slowing (Mary and Peter) while focal spike activity was noted in 3 (Sam, John and William). Tables 7 and 8 detail the comparison of all EEG findings with clinical and persistent toxic changes. The frequency of such findings is not unusual in similar child populations, and subtle impairment of the CNS might be an important factor in the etiology of childhood schizophrenia (Bender, 1947; Goldfarb, 1961, 1970; Rutter, 1967; Vorster, 1960).

In one child (Kevin), the normal "drug-free" EEG remained unchanged on the "optimal dose" of lithium; in another (Mike), as shown in Figure 1, there was a slowing of α and increased diffuse slow activity ($\triangle$). EEGs of 2 patients were not comparable because of altered state of consciousness and sedation effects. Regretfully, Harry's EEG was not

Table 8

Comparison of EEG's During "Drug-free" and "Optimal" Chlorpromazine Dose Periods

| Name | "Drug-free" EEG | | "Optimal" dose period-chlorpromazine | | | |
	Description	Sedation	mg. per day	EEG changes	Global improvements*	Persistent Toxicity
Harry	NL	chloral hydrate	45	not comparable	slight	none
Mike[a]	NL	none	30	decreased alpha frequency, increased slowing (Δ)	slight	none
Carl	NL	none	9	no change	slight	none
Peter	abnormal focal spikes	chloral hydrate	9	not comparable	slight	insomnia, hyperactivity, aggressiveness, enuresis
Mary	abnormal focal slowing	none	15	decreased focal asymmetry	marked	euphoria
Rose	NL	chloral hydrate	3†	not comparable	slight†	none
Sam[b]	abnormal focal spikes	none	9	decreased focal spikes	slight	increased negativism, irritability, and aggressiveness
John[c]	minimal abnormal focal paroxysmal	none	15	minimal diffuse fluctuating changes	no change	increased aggressiveness and impulsivity
Kevin	NL	none	9	decreased alpha frequency, increased slowing (Δ)	marked	none
William	abnormal focal spikes	chloral hydrate	15	not comparable (awake, no spikes)	marked	insomnia, euphoria

Note. NL = normal. *Nonblind evaluations: †Thiothixene; [a]Fig. 1.; [b]Fig. 2.; [c]Fig. 3.

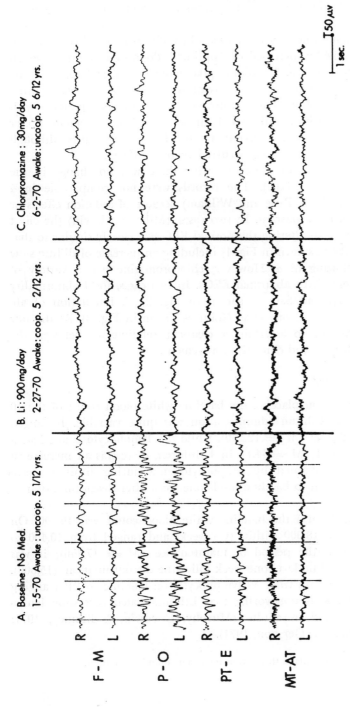

FIG. 1. Effect of lithium and chlorpromazine on EEG activity of a 5-year-old hyperactive schizophrenic patient (Mike). Initial EEG (A) was performed when the patient was not medicated for more than one month, and considered normal. Records (B) and (C) were taken during the last week of optimal therapy on lithium and chlorpromazine, respectively. In (B) lithium level was 0.48–0.65 mEq/l. The effects of chlorpromazine and lithium were similar, with increased diffuse slow activity and decreased amplitude, amount and frequency of alpha activity. The patient was in comparable waking state during the 3 recordings. Slight psychiatric improvement and lack of persistent toxic side effects on either drug were noted.

performed while the boy was on lithium for reasons that were not related to his behavior.

In all 3 patients who had focal spikes in their "drug-free" record, such
spikes were markedly increased on "optimal" doses of lithium as shown
in Fig. 2 (Sam) and Fig. 3 (John). Spike activities did not appear to be
related to lithium blood levels. Behaviorally, one child was worse while
two other children showed no improvement.* In the two patients with
focal slow activity who manifested slight behavioral improvement (Peter
and Mary) lithium did not accentuate the focal abnormality although
some diffuse increased slowing occurred in one (Mary).

On "optimal" doses of chlorpromazine there was no change in the
EEG of one patient (Carl). The records were not comparable in 4
patients (Harry, Peter, Rose and William) because of sedation effects or
altered states of consciousness. In two cases (Mike and Kevin) the effect
of chlorpromazine in altering the normal EEG was clearly similar to that
of lithium (Mike as shown in Fig. 1) including an increase of diffuse slow
activity and slowing of α. However, chlorpromazine had a variety of
effects on patients with abnormal EEGs. In two cases, focal abnormality
decreased (Mary, and Sam as shown in Fig. 2). A fluctuation of abnormalities occurred in one case (John as shown in Fig. 3). At the low
doses, it is difficult to ascertain a clear-cut relationship between the
type of EEG changes and clinical improvement.

Laboratory Findings

As before, while on placebo, the baseline white blood count of the 10
children prior to lithium administration was quite variable. It ranged
from 5,500 to 21,400 ($M = 12,230$), while the lymphocyte count had a
range from 15 to 61 ($M = 44.1$). In 4 children, there was an increase in
white count accompanied by lymphocytopenia during lithium maintenance and a return to baseline levels one week after discontinuation of
treatment.

In one child (Mary) the baseline white blood count was 15,500. On
lithium, it rose to 18,000 within two weeks and ranged from 10,400 to
23,600 throughout the period of maintenance ($M = 17,850$); it was
lowered to its baseline level one week following discontinuation (15,600).
Also, there was a drop from 39 lymphocytes on baseline to 21 (ranging
from 21 to 30). It is noteworthy that lithium-related reversible leukocytosis was reported in adults (Murphy, Goodwin, & Bunney, 1971;
Shopsin, Friedman, & Gershon, 1971).

---

* All global improvements in this section refer to nonblind evaluations.

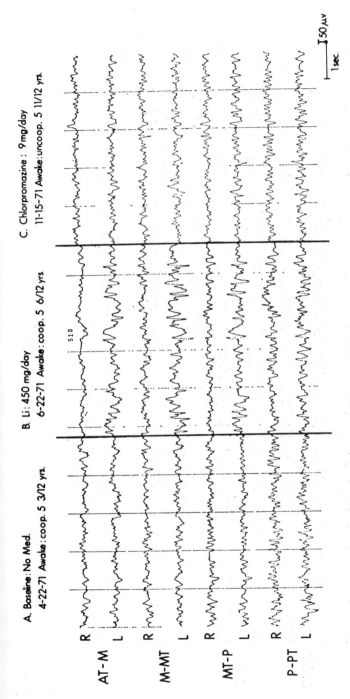

FIG. 2. Effect of lithium and chlorpromazine on EEG activity of 5-year-old hyperactive schizophrenic patient (Sam) whose "drug free" records were considered minimally abnormal because of infrequent asymmetrical sharp waves and minimal persistent asymmetries. Most of the baseline record was relatively normal (A). He became toxic on relatively low blood levels of lithium (0.25-0.35 mEq/l). Maintenance on 450 mg. per day yielded no improvement. EEG changed significantly with high voltage focal spikes on the left side, most prominent in the parietal and mid temporal regions (B). Such spikes persisted after lithium was discontinued but were less marked. He improved slightly on chlorpromazine and although the abnormality was less marked, the left sided spikes and slow activity were still present with some shifting (C). On chlorpromazine, some evidence of persistent toxicity was noted. This focal left sided spiking persisted beyond 2 months after discontinuation of all medication.

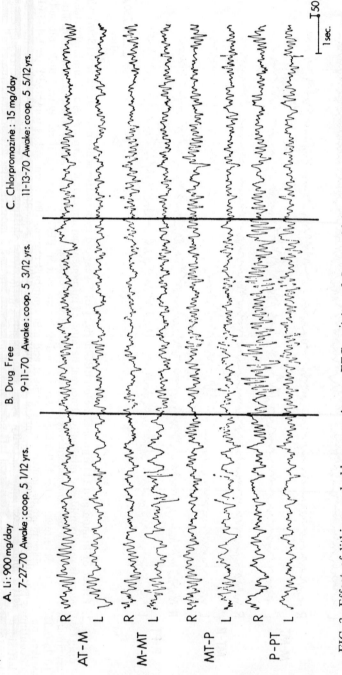

FIG. 3. Effect of lithium and chlorpromazine on EEG activity of 5-year-old hyperactive child with a behavior disorder (John). Baseline EEG was minimally abnormal with asymmetry and rare paroxysmal activity. On 900 mg. of lithium per day (0.51-1.05 mEq/l) with no psychiatric improvement, he developed high voltage focal spikes accentuated in the left parietal and mid temporal regions (A). During this time, lithium toxicity was manifested by persistent EKG alterations. Repeat "drug free" EEG when the patient was off medication for one month, again revealed asymmetries which were considered abnormal (B). On chlorpromazine (15 mg. per day) EEG's changed slightly with minor accentuation of asymmetries, generalized decrease of amplitude, and occasional sharp waves. There was no improvement and some persistent toxic side effects were noted.

Two children (Rose and John), both very hyperactive, had somewhat elevated levels of thyroxine-iodine (7.7 and 7.0, respectively)* on baseline, prior to lithium treatment. During lithium maintenance, the level dropped from 7.7 to 5.5 and from 7.0 to 4.6, increasing to 6.2 in both children four weeks after the drug was discontinued.** It appears that lithium has an antithyroid action (Schou, Amdisen, Jensen, & Olsen, 1968; Rogers & Whybrow, 1961). In our study, all other patients had normal thyroxine-iodine values before, during and after treatment with lithium. Sizes of thyroid glands, also monitored in all patients, remained unchanged.

Two children, both on 900 mg. per day, had EKG changes. William had a mild right ventricular conduction delay (lithium blood level 0.575 mEq/l) and John had sinus arrhythmia, possibly an A-V nodal rhythm (lithium blood level 1.025 mEq/l). These changes disappeared within one week after discontinuation of lithium. Reversible T-wave changes were found during lithium treatment in adults (Demers & Heninger, 1971).

All other laboratory tests, including urinalysis, hemotocrit and BUN, remained within normal limits on lithium.

Laboratory findings during chlorpromazine maintenance, including the results of urinalysis, WBC, differential cell count, SGOT, SGPT, and alkaline phosphatase, remained within normal limits in all patients. However, unlike on lithium, there was a slight tendency in most patients toward decreases in total white counts. One child developed an intermittent papular and erythematous skin rash on cheeks, chin and hands, and swelling of lips. This occurred on the 49th day of treatment with chlorpromazine, on 30 mg. per day.

DISCUSSION

A Comparison of Lithium to Chlorpromazine

The results of this study indicate that in general neither lithium nor chlorpromazine were good psychotropic agents for a severely disturbed group of children.

In lithium as well as in chlorpromazine, the margin between toxic and "optimal" doses was very narrow. Five out of the 10 children showed some signs of lithium toxicity and 5 out of 9 had signs of excess chlorpromazine on "optimal" doses. Thus, higher doses were not in use.

---

* Thyroxine-iodine (by column chromatography) values determined by Bio-Science Laboratories, Van Nuys, California, normal range 2.9 to 6.4.

** Incidentally, neither child improved on lithium.

Some of our previous studies have indicated that chlorpromazine, despite its clear antipsychotic properties, produced fewer and less marked improvements than other neuroleptics (Fish, Campbell, Shapiro & Floyd, 1969; Campbell, Fish, Shapiro, & Floyd, 1970, 1971) chiefly due to excessive sedation produced even by small doses. Sedative effects interfere, detract from and limit improvements in these young, chronic psychiatric patients. The slight effectiveness of chlorpromazine in schizophrenic children was comparable to that in other diagnostic categories. Nonblind ratings indicated that lithium was even less effective than chlorpromazine. However, the number of patients in this study was small and no statistically significant difference between the two drugs was found by the blind psychiatrist.

Possible Differential Response to Lithium

The nonblind psychiatrist believed that lithium was better for schizophrenic children than for children with behavior disorders.* However, again this sample was too small to draw any such conclusions. Harry, who showed the best response to lithium, was a grossly psychotic schizophrenic, extremely hyperactive and impulsive, and with autoaggressive, self-mutilating behavior (Campbell & Hersh, 1971). His excitement, impulsivity, hyperactivity, and particularly violent behavior directed against his own body showed much greater signs of improvement than the psychosis. The boy's bizarre fantasies persisted, even though they reflected less violence. The other schizophrenic children with slight signs of improvement (Mike and Carl) were no longer as floridly psychotic and bizarre when placed on lithium as they were on admission. Both had previously responded to most other drugs tried in the past.

Opinions on the effects of lithium in adult schizophrenia are divided. Australian investigators, Cade (1949) and Glesinger (1954), found lithium to be useful in the treatment of chronic schizophrenics with excitement. In the Soviet Union, Vartanian (1959) studied the effects of lithium on 33 psychiatric subjects with psychomotor excitation, irrespective of the diagnosis. Twenty of the 33 were schizophrenics who were so diagnosed for periods ranging from one month to 18 years. Eight of the 9 schizophrenics exhibiting "manic excitement" showed good results on lithium carbonate. Four of the 6 catatonics (with catatonic excite-

---

* Three out of the 6 schizophrenic patients improved while the condition of both boys with behavior disorder (one hyperactive and the other hypoactive) remained unchanged.

ment) showed no significant improvement, and there was no change in the hebephrenics.

Mosketi, Belskaya, and Muratova (1963) have administered lithium to 127 psychiatric subjects who represented 9 diagnostic categories. This group of patients included 56 schizophrenics whose illness was on record for periods up to 10 years. Ten showed "good results" (complete disappearance of psychopathological phenomena resulting in discharge from hospital), 21 no significant improvement (improvement, requiring further hospitalization), 25 remained unchanged; and none became worse. Gershon and Yuwiler (1960) reported cases with catatonic and acute schizophrenic excitement who showed marked improvement on lithium treatment.

However, well controlled studies on the effects of lithium on acute or chronic schizophrenic patients with acute symptomatology yielded opposite results (Johnson, Gershon, & Hekimian, 1968; Shopsin, Johnson, & Gershon, 1970; Shopsin, Kim, & Gershon, 1971). Lithium exacerbated the disturbance and, instead of the usual signs of lithium side-effects or toxicity seen in patients in the manic phase of the manic-depressive illness, the schizophrenic subjects appeared to develop organic brain syndromes often accompanied by EEG changes (Johnson, Maccario, Gershon, & Korein, 1970). Such deteriorations occurred at lithium blood levels which are associated with improvement in manic patients. It was suggested (Shopshin et al., 1971) that "schizophrenic patients have a decreased threshold tolerance or sensitivity for the lithium ion, which exposes them to central nervous system toxicity at moderate to low levels of serum lithium."

Our preschool-age schizophrenics, representing the youngest with such disorder, show little clinical resemblance to the newly hospitalized schizophrenics of Gershon, Johnson and Shopsin. Their response to psychopharmacologic agents is also quite different. In certain clinical aspects and in responses to drugs, they tend to resemble, to a degree, the most chronic adult schizophrenics (Fish, 1960; Fish, Shapiro, & Campbell, 1966; Campbell et al., 1970, 1971). Such children are generally very resistant to available treatments, including drugs. They might thus be more comparable to the subjects reported by the Australian and Soviet authors. This difference in schizophrenic populations may explain why our clinical results with lithium, although not too promising, were not as poor as the results in the acute adult patients reported by the NYU group (Johnson et al., 1968; Shopsin et al., 1971). It may also explain the reason why our schizophrenics did not respond as well to chlorpromazine as those in the aforementioned controlled studies.

The Relationship Between EEG and Clinical Improvement

Numerous studies have been published on the effects of psychoactive agents on behavior, neurotoxicity and EEG (Korein & Musacchio, 1968; Korein et al., 1971; Johnson et al., 1970). But similar studies involving pre-school age severely disturbed children are scarce due to many inherent complexities and problems. In the uncooperative, hyperactive and disorganized child a baseline EEG may not be feasible and the difficulties in evaluating EEGs insurmountable. Age is known to be a significant factor in a young child's EEG. If the child is sedated, such additional factors as altered state of consciousness and nature of the sedative effect of medication on his EEG must be considered (Laguna & Korein, 1972).*

Such limitations and the significant number of uncomparable records notwithstanding, a pattern seems to emerge which, while not statistically significant, has speculative value in terms of future work. A review of findings in "drug-free" EEGs, EEG changes related to lithium and chlorpromazine, and clinical improvements** detailed in Tables 7 and 8, yielded the following observations: (1) five out of 10 patients have unequivocally abnormal focal EEGs indicative of organic cerebral dysfunction, and (2) the results suggest a correlation between behavioral changes and EEG changes on drug.

There is probably an appreciable difference in therapeutic responses to psychoactive agents between severely disturbed children whose EEGs show focal abnormalities and those with normal EEGs. If the drug (in this case lithium) accentuates the focal abnormality, there is a probability that behavior will either deteriorate or not change. On the other hand, improvement may occur if the focal abnormality is decreased by lithium. Such relationships between focal EEG abnormality and clinical improvement applied to lithium as well as to chlorpromazine.

In contrast, some behavioral improvement is more likely to occur in patients with normal EEGs when medication causes such changes as diffuse slowing and slower α, rather than no changes in EEG. Similar findings were reported in other studies of children and adults. However, most frequently the major factor related to changes in EEG was toxicity. In the present study, persistent toxicity on the "optimal" dose does not appear to be a major factor except in patients with evidence of organic cerebral dysfunction as manifested by focally abnormal EEGs. On chlor-

---

* Therefore, major comment will be limited to those "drug-free" and medication EEGs in this study that were performed without sedation and under comparable conditions.

** All global improvements in this section refer to nonblind evaluations.

promazine, all five children with EEGs evidencing focal cerebral dysfunction had some evidence of persistent drug toxicity on their "optimal" doses. On lithium, 4 of these 5 had evidenced persistent toxicity and their focal EEG abnormalities became significantly worse.

Effects of Lithium on Hyperactivity and Aggressiveness

No consistent pattern of motor activity was in evidence in our study. Of the 5 children who showed improvement, 2 were hyperactive and, interestingly enough, 3 hypoactive and anergic.

Whitehead and Clark (1970), who alternated lithium carbonate, placebo and thioridazine in hyperactive children, found no difference between the motor activity level and behavior on lithium or placebo. On thioridazine a slight decrease in hyperactivity was noted. The 7 children in Whitehead and Clark's study, 5 to 9 years of age, included 1 autistic child and 1 psychotic who was not autistic. Gram and Rafaelsen's (1972) controlled clinical trial of lithium (sustained-release tablets) in 18 psychotic subjects in 5 diagnostic categories, including 9 with "infantile psychosis" (8 to 22 years of age), disclosed "no general pattern" of lithium effect on specific symptoms, even though 11 were rated improved on lithium, and only 2 on placebo. There was no correlation between diagnosis and clinical effects of lithium. Parents reported decrease in aggressivity and hyperactivity, and elevation of depressed mood. In the special school where all these patients were observed, greatest improvements were noted in disturbed speech and stereotypies, and also some in hyperactivity and aggressiveness.

Dostal (1972) found that lithium had a significant "affect-damping and antiaggressive effect" in a group of 14 boys, 11-17 years of age ($M = 14$), who were the most aggressive and hyperactive, phenothiazine-resistant inmates of an institution for mentally retarded juvenile males. Dostal's patients were placed on lithium durules for 8 months and in the course of the last 4, lithium plasma level ranged from 0.7 to 1.2 mEq/1 ($M =$ 0.9). Not unlike in our blind and nonblind evaluations, the greatest improvements were found in affectivity, aggressivity, psychomotor activity, restlessness and "undisciplined behavior," except that in Dostal's work such improvements were statistically significant.

> The most marked improvement was achieved in patients with preponderant excitability, and impulsive infantile manifestations of aggressivity. . . . Patients with hyperkinetic behavior lacking affective accompaniment (spastic irritability, continual restlessness of the whole body, repetitive minute automutilations and stereotypic ritual movements), exhibited practically no response to lithium.

In our hyperactive patient with autoaggressive behavior who showed marked improvement on lithium, a pronounced affective component (explosiveness) was in evidence. In the hyperactive and aggressive children who showed only slight improvement or no change, affect was blunted, except in John (behavior disorder) whose affect was mildly excitable.

The effects of lithium in counteracting aggression were established in animal work. Weischer (1969) found that lithium abolished intraspecies aggressiveness in Siamese fighting fish, mice, and golden hamsters; all other behavior, including motor activity, was unaffected. Aggressiveness reappeared after lithium was discontinued. We were interested in the disclosure that marked individual differences in the animals' sensitivity to lithium were present, particularly in mice. While aggressive behavior ceased on low lithium plasma (and brain) levels in some, aggressiveness in other animals disappeared only at high concentrations. "Poor responders" had a narrow therapeutic margin; if the lithium dose was elevated above the "antiaggressive" dose level, intoxication followed rather rapidly. This was similar to the action on our patient John.

Lithium was found to have anti-aggressive actions in experimental animals (Sheard, 1970a), in animals pretreated with p-chlorphenylalanine, a tryptophan hydroxylase inhibitor (Sheard, 1970b), as well as in aggressive inmates of a maximum-security state prison (Sheard, 1971a). Tupin and Smith (1972) also found lithium to be effective in controlling aggressive violent behavior of prisoners who did not respond with respect to that symptom to phenothiazines. While Sheard's subjects received lithium for only 4 weeks, the patients in Tupin's study were maintained on that drug for periods up to $1\frac{1}{2}$ years. There was a substantial and satisfactory control of violent behavior, a statistically significant decrease in the number of violent disciplinary actions, and a reduction in security classifications based on independent though nonblind reports during this long-term maintenance.

Animal experiments have shown that lowering of brain serotonin increases aggressiveness and affects other behaviors (Ferguson, Henriksen, Cohen, Mitchell, Barchas, & Dement, 1970). At the present time, there is no consensus and considerable disagreement on the effect of lithium on brain serotonin and its metabolism (Blass & Ailion, 1970; Ho, Loh, Craves, Hitzemann, & Gershon, 1970; Perez-Cruet, Tagliamonte, Tagliamonte, & Gessa, 1971; Sheard & Aghajanian, 1970). If lithium increases the rate of synthesis of brain serotonin (Perez-Cruet et al., 1971) it could explain observations that its administration decreases aggressiveness, both in animals and humans.

Blood serotonin has been found elevated in some psychotic children by several authors (Schain and Freedman, 1961; Ritvo, Yuwiler, Geller, Ornitz, Saeger, & Plotkin, 1970). However, decreases in serotonin levels on L-dopa yielded no clinical improvement in such patients (Ritvo, Yuwiler, Geller, Kales, Rashkis, Schicor, Plotkin, Axelrod, & Howard, 1971). We did not study serotonin levels, uptake or release in our patients during this crossover study. Future investigations may reveal differences in serotonin levels in various subcategories of autistic and schizophrenic children.

Our small sample of 10 patients represented 4 clinically delineated diagnostic categories and included a sex chromosome anomaly (XO). Even within each diagnostic group, there were subcategories with differences in motor activity, affectivity and presence and/or mode of expression of aggressiveness. Sheard (1971b) similarly distinguished more than one group with differing clinical responses to lithium among his adult subjects with exaggerated aggressive drive. Our patients were not only different in terms of chronological age, but also different with respect to stage of development and state of psychiatric condition, ranging from floridly psychotic to schizophrenic in remission.

The clinical profiles and states may correlate with different biochemical profiles and these, in turn, with ability to respond to pharmacologic agents or other therapies. We plan to pursue this worthwhile course of investigation.

CONCLUSION

The action of lithium in hyperexcitability prompted us to investigate its possible therapeutic effects on severely disturbed children. Our effort represented the first controlled study of lithium *versus* an effective drug in this age group. The blind psychiatrist's ratings of global improvement in our 10 patients indicated no statistically significant difference between the effects of lithium and chlorpromazine. However, lithium treatment yielded improvement, though not statistically significant, in explosiveness, aggressiveness, hyperactivity and psychotic speech. All such findings were similar to those of the nonblind observer. Our study shows that lithium merits further exploration as it might prove of some value in the treatment of severe psychiatric disorders in childhood. It may be effective in certain diagnostic subcategories with a cluster of symptoms (hyperactivity, aggressivity, explosive affect), and possibly normal baseline EEGs. We can hypothesize that *not only* the child's behavioral profile, *but also* his baseline EEG and EEG response to lithium as well as biochemical profile (the level of neurotransmitters, their precursors or certain enzymes) might be of assistance in developing reliable predictors defining "lithium responders."

REFERENCES

ANNELL, A. L.: Manic-depressive illness in children and effect of treatment with lithium carbonate. *Acta Paedopsychiatrica,* 1969, 36, 292-361. (a)

ANNELL, A. L.: Lithium in the treatment of children and adolescents. *Acta Psychiatrica Scandinavica,* 1969, 207, 19-30. (Supp.) (b)

BENDER, L.: Childhood schizophrenia. Clinical study of one hundred schizophrenic children. *American Journal of Orthopsychiatry,* 1947, 17, 40-56.

BLISS, E. L. & AILION, J.: The effect of lithium upon brain neuroamines. *Brain Research,* 1970, 24, 305-310.

CADE, J. F. J.: Lithium salts in the treatment of psychotic excitement. *Medical Journal of Australia,* 1949, 2, 349-352.

CAMPBELL, M., FISH, B., SHAPIRO, T., & FLOYD, A., JR.: Thiothixene in young disturbed children. A pilot study. *Archives of General Psychiatry,* 1970, 23, 70-72.

CAMPBELL, M., FISH, B., SHAPIRO, T., & FLOYD, A., JR.: Study of molindone in disturbed preschool children. *Current Therapeutic Research,* 1971, 13, 28-33.

CAMPBELL, M., & HERSH, S. P.: Observations on the vicissitudes of aggression in two siblings. *Journal of Autism and Childhood Schizophrenia,* 1971, 1, 398-410.

DEMERS, R. G., & HENINGER, G. R.: Electrocardiographic T-wave changes during lithium carbonate treatment. *Journal of American Medical Association,* 1971, 218, 381-386.

DOSTAL, T.: Antiaggressive effect of lithium salts in mentally retarded adolescents. In A. L. Annell (Ed.), *Depressive States in Childhood and Adolescence.* Stockholm: Almquist & Wiksell, 1972, 491-498.

DYSON, W. L., & BARCAI, A.: Treatment of children of lithium-responding parents. *Current Therapeutic Research,* 1970, 12, 286-290.

FERGUSON, J., HENRIKSEN, S., COHEN, H., MITCHELL, G., BARCHAS, J., & DEMENT, W.: "Hypersexuality" and behavioral changes in cats caused by administration of p-chlorophenylalanine. *Science,* 1970, 168, 499-501.

FISH, B.: Drug therapy in child psychiatry: Pharmacological aspects. *Comprehensive Psychiatry,* 1960, 1, 212-227.

FISH, B.: Methodology in child psychopharmacology. In D. H. Efron, J. O. Cole, J. Levine, & J. R. Wittenborn (Eds.), *Psychopharmacology, Review of Progress* (Public Health Service Publication No. 1836). Washington, D.C.: United States Government Printing Office, 1968.

FISH, B., CAMPBELL, M., SHAPIRO, T., & FLOYD, A., JR.: Comparison of trifluperidol, trifluoperazine and chlorpromazine in preschool schizophrenic children: The value of less sedative antipsychotic agents. *Current Therapeutic Research,* 1969, 11, 589-595.

FISH, B., SHAPIRO, T., & CAMPBELL, M.: Long-term prognosis and the response of schizophrenic children to drug therapy: A controlled study of trifluoperazine. *American Journal of Psychiatry,* 1966, 123, 32-39.

FISH, B., SHAPIRO, T., CAMPBELL, M., & WILE, R.: A classification of schizophrenic children under five years. *American Journal of Psychiatry,* 1968, 124, 1415-1423.

FROMMER, E.: Depressive illness in childhood. In A. Coppen & A. Walk (Eds.), *Recent Developments in Affective Disorders. A Symposium. British Journal of Psychiatry,* 1968, Special Publication No. 2, 117-136.

GERSHON, S. & YUWILER, A.: Lithium ion: A specific psychopharmacological approach to the treatment of mania. *Journal of Neuropsychiatry,* 1960, 1, 229-241.

GLESINGER, B.: Evaluation of lithium in treatment of psychotic excitement. *Medical Journal of Australia*, 1954, 41, 277-283.

GOLDFARB, W.: *Childhood Schizophrenia*. Cambridge, Mass.: Harvard University Press, 1961.

GOLDFARB, W.: Childhood psychosis. In P. H. Mussen (Ed.), *Carmichael's Manual of Child Psychology*. Vol. 2 (3rd ed.) New York: John Wiley & Sons, 1970.

GRAM, L. F., & RAFAELSEN, O. J.: Lithium treatment of psychotic children: A controlled clinical trial. *Acta Psychiatrica Scandinavica*, 1972, in press.

HO, A. K. S., LOH, H. H., CRAVES, F., HITZEMANN, R. J., & GERSHON, S.: The effect of prolonged lithium treatment on the synthesis rate and turnover of monoamines in brain regions of rats. *European Journal of Pharmacology*, 1970, 10, 72-78.

JOHNSON, G., GERSHON, S., & HEKEMIAN, L. J.: Controlled evaluation of lithium and chlorpromazine in the treatment of manic states: An interim report. *Comprehensive Psychiatry*, 1968, 9, 563-573.

JOHNSON, G., MACCARIO, M., GERSHON, S., & KOREIN, J.: The effects of lithium on EEG, behavior and serum electrolytes. *Journal of Nervous and Mental Disease*, 1970, 151, 273-289.

KOREIN, J., FISH, B., SHAPIRO, T., GERNER, E. W., & LEVIDOW, L.: EEG and behavioral effects of drug therapy in children. Chlorpromazine and diphenhydramine. *Archives of General Psychiatry*, 1971, 24, 552-563.

KOREIN, J. & MUSACCHIO, J. M.: LSD in focal cerebral lesions. Behavioral and EEG effects in patients with sensory defects. *Neurology*, 1968, 18, 147-152.

LAGUNA, J. F., & KOREIN, J.: Differential effects of diazepam in diagnostic EEG: Depression of secondary cortical and peripheral activity. *Archives of Neurology*, 1972, 26, 265-272.

MOSKETI, K. V., BELSKAYA, G. M., & MURATOVA, I. D.: Experience in the use of iodinated lithium for the treatment of some psychotic states. *Zhurnal Nevropatologii i Psihiatrii Imeni S. S. Korsakova*, 1963, 63, 92-95.

MURPHY, D. L., GOODWIN, F. K., BUNNEY, W. E., JR.: Leukocytosis during lithium treatment. *American Journal of Psychiatry*, 1971, 127, 1559-1561.

PEREZ-CRUET, J., TAGLIAMONTE, A., TAGLIAMONTE, P., & GESSA, G. L.: Stimulation of serotonin synthesis by lithium. *Journal of Pharmacology and Experimental Therapeutics*, 1971, 178, 325-330.

RIFKIN, A., QUITKIN, F., CARILLO, C., & KLEIN, D. F.: Lithium in emotionally unstable character disorder. *Archives of General Psychiatry*, 1972, in press.

RITVO, E. R., YUWILER, A., GELLER, E., KALES, A., RASHKIS, S., SCHICOR, A., PLOTKIN, S., AXELROD, R., & HOWARD, C.: Effects of L-dopa in autism. *Journal of Autism and Childhood Schizophrenia*, 1971, 1, 190-205.

RITVO, E. R., YUWILER, A., GELLER, E., ORNITZ, E. M., EAEGER, K., PLOTKIN, S.: Increased blood serotonin and platelets in early infantile autism. *Archives of General Psychiatry*, 1970, 23, 566-572.

ROGERS, M. P. & WHYBROW, P. C.: Clinical hypothyroidism occurring during lithium treatment: Two case histories and a review of thyroid function in 19 patients. *American Journal of Psychiatry*, 1971, 128, 158-163.

RUTTER, M.: Psychotic disorders in early childhood. In A. Coppen & A. Walk (Eds.), *Recent Developments in Schizophrenia. A Symposium. British Journal of Psychiatry*, 1967, Special Publication No. 1, 133-158.

SCHAIN, R. J. & FREEDMAN, D. X.: Studies on 5-hydroxyindole metabolism in autistic and other mentally retarded children. *Journal of Pediatrics*, 1961, 58, 315-320.

SCHOU, M.: Lithium in psychiatric therapy and prophylaxis. A review with special regard to its use in children. In A. L. Annell (Ed.), *Depressive States in Childhood and Adolescence*. Stockholm: Almquist & Wiksell, 1972.

SCHOU, M., AMDISEN, A., JENSEN, S. E., & OLSEN, T.: Occurrence of goitre during lithium treatment. *British Medican Journal*, 1968, 3, 710-713.

SHEARD, M. H.: Effect of lithium on foot shock aggression in rats. *Nature*, 1970, 228, 284-285. (a)

SHEARD, M. H.: Behavioral effects of p-chlorophenylalanine in rats: Inhibition by lithium. *Communications in Behavioral Biology*, 1970, 5, 71-73. (b)

SHEARD, M. H.: Effect of lithium on human aggression. *Nature*, 1971, 230, 113-114. (a)

SHEARD, M.: The effect of lithium on behavior. *Communications in Contemporary Psychiatry*, 1971, 1, 1-6. (b)

SHEARD, M. H. & AGHAJANIAN, G. K.: Neuronally activated metabolism of serotonin: Effect of lithium. *Life Sciences*, 1970, 9, 285-290.

SHOPSIN, B., FRIEDMAN, R., & GERSHON, S.: Lithium and leukocytosis. *Clinical Pharmacology and Therapeutics*, 1971, 12, 923-928.

SHOPSIN, B., JOHNSON, G., & GERSHON, S.: Neurotoxicity with lithium: Differential drug responsiveness. *International Pharmacopsychiatry*, 1970, 5, 170-182.

SHOPSIN, B., KIM, S. S., & GERSHON, S.: A controlled study of lithium vs. chlorpromazine in acute schizophrenics. *British Journal of Psychiatry*, 1971, 119, 435-440.

TUPIN, J. P. & SMITH, D. B.: The long-term use of lithium in aggressive prisoners. Paper presented at the meeting of the Early Clinical Drug Evaluation Unit, Psychopharmacology Research Branch, NIMH, Baltimore, Maryland, June 1972.

VAN KREVELEN, D. A., & VAN VOORST, J. A.: Lithium in the treatment of a crypto-genetic psychosis in a juvenile. *Zeitschrift der Kinderpsychiatrie*, 1959, 26, 148-152.

VARTANIAN, M. E.: Experience of treatment of agitated states with lithium carbonate. *Zhournal Nevropatologii i Psihiatrii Imeni Korsakova*, 1959, 59, 586-589.

VORSTER, D.: An investigation into the part played by organic factors in childhood schizophrenia. *Journal of Mental Science*, 1960, 106, 494-522.

WEISCHER, M. L.: On the antiaggressive effect of lithium. *Psychopharmacologia*, 1969, 15, 245-254.

WHITEHEAD, P. L. & CLARK, L. D.: Effect of lithium carbonate, placebo, and thiorida-zine on hyperactive children. *American Journal of Psychiatry*, 1970, 127, 824-825.

PART IX: DRUG STUDIES

37

EFFECTS OF PROLONGED PHENOTHIAZINE INTAKE ON PSYCHOTIC AND OTHER HOSPITALIZED CHILDREN

John B. McAndrew, M.D., Quentin Case, and
Darold A. Treffert

Winnebago State Hospital, Wisconsin

Four related studies of infrequently recognized side effects (weight changes, tardive dyskinesia, impaired learning, and ocular changes) of prolonged phenothiazine intake by children with severe disorders of behavior are presented and discussed. The retrospective investigation involving 86 hospitalized boys and 39 girls, 4 to 16 years of age, covered a 5-year period. Weight gains in 29 out of 30 patients were significantly related to Thioridazine intake. Tardive dyskinesia occurred in 10 children receiving high doses of phenothiazines over prolonged periods. Discontinuation of Thioridazine prompted accelerated learning in 3 boys as evidenced by their periodically measured Stanford Achievement Test scores. Lens stippling occurred in 2 patients whose cumulative Chlorpromazine intake was below 200 grams, and in 3 with higher doses of phenothiazines. Judicious use of phenothiazines in long-term treatment of mentally ill children may be facilitated by routine individual double blind procedures involving patients as their own controls.

Reprinted from JOURNAL OF AUTISM AND CHILDHOOD SCHIZOPHRENIA, 1972, 2, 1, pp. 75-91. Copyright © 1972 by Scripta Publishing Corporation.

While mental hospitals in America have emptied dramatically of adults in the past 10 years, admissions of children and adolescents to these facilities have risen alarmingly (Treffert, 1969). In fact, admissions of patients in this age group to all state and county hospitals in the United States rose 150% during the past decade. At our Winnebago State Hospital, this national trend was mirrored by a 110% increase in child-adolescent admissions so that currently 43% of the hospital's 600 patients are under 21 years of age and 11% are younger than 12.

Whatever the reasons, one concomitant of this increased presence of young people in hospitals is their anticipated continued exposure to both the therapeutic and hazardous effects of phenothiazines. However, while tens of thousands of articles have appeared in print to add to our knowledge of the use of psychotropic agents, relatively few, in fact less than 500 published papers, are focused on uses in children (DiMascio, 1971). One useful overview was provided by Eveloff (1966) who reviewed the literature on pediatric psychopharmacology. A more recent clinical overview discusses indications and limitations of drug treatment in disturbed children. By highlighting the different responses of children and adults to the same drugs, it gives again credence to the treatment axiom that children are not simply miniature adults (Fish, 1968). However, the literature is relatively silent and incomplete with respect to certain long-term side effects in children exposed to psychopharmacologic treatment.

The purpose of this retrospective study is to report the occurrence of four side effects in 125 hospitalized children with behavioral disorders (including 52 psychotic) exposed to phenothiazine treatment during the course of a recent 5-year period in our hospital. The investigation focuses on weight changes (Study 1), tardive dyskinesia (Study 2), impaired learning (Study 3), and ocular changes (Study 4), all rarely recognized as serious complications and rather inadequately studied and documented in the literature on children.

THE SELECTED SIDE EFFECTS

Weight Changes

Weight increases accompanying phenothiazine intake in adults have been well documented (Caffey, 1961; Gordon & Groth, 1964; Klett & Caffey, 1960), and individual gains have been reported to average 7 or 8 pounds during the first 3 months of treatment with Chlorpromazine (Caffey & Klett, 1961). Weight losses usually occurred when phenothiazines have been discontinued (Amdisen, 1964; Singh, DeDios, & Kline,

1970). Although the exact cause of weight gain has not been ascertained, it is thought, at least in the case of Thioridazine, that the drug brings about its effect by action on the hypothalmic pituitary axis (Castelnuovo-Tedesco, Tanguay, Kraut, & Burgess, 1963). Sletten, Mou, Cazenave, and Gershon (1967), whose patients on Chlorpromazine lost weight while on a 1000 calorie diet, generally lend support to the hypothesis that weight gain on Chlorpromazine is due to increased calorie intake or fluid and electrolyte retention. Gordon and Groth (1964), however, were unable to separate drug from milieu effects, hypothesizing that weight gains resulted from an interaction of phenothiazine intake with the hospital milieu rather than from either factor alone.

Tardive Dyskinesia

Tardive dyskinesia in adults has been extensively reviewed and Crane's (Crane, 1971; Crane & Naranjo, 1971) clear delineation of subtypes has facilitated more sophisticated studies in this area. Unfortunately, these long-lasting neurological effects are frequently undetected until neuroleptics have been discontinued or reduced in dosage. Interestingly, acute dystonic reactions tend to occur early in phenothiazine therapy and males appear to be twice as susceptible as females. Yet, in persistent tardive dyskinesia, such reactions take place late or after discontinuation of treatment and occur much more frequently in females (Ayd, 1967; Duvoisin, 1968). Some authors (Edwards, 1970; Faurbye, Rasch, Petersen, Brandborg, & Pakkenberg, 1964; Kline, 1968) believe that organic brain damage predisposes to development of tardive dyskinesia. Other investigators point out the lack of apparent correlation between dosage, duration of intake, time of onset or intensity of tardive dyskinesias. In two cases involving children, long-lasting neurological effects were attributed to inappropriately toxic doses of phenothiazines (Angle & McIntire, 1968; Dabbous & Bergman, 1966). It appears that the youngest reported patient with tardive dyskinesia emanating from phenothiazine treatment was 27 years of age (Rodova & Nahunek, 1964).

Impaired Learning

Many reported studies of the effects of phenothiazines on learning appear to be in some disagreement. LeVann (1959) noted increased attention span and increased accessibility to training in mentally retarded patients treated with Trifluoperazine. Freed and Peifer (1970) suggested that the learning process was facilitated in hyperactive children receiving Chlorpromazine. A study by Lehmann and Knight (1959) indicated that Trifluoperazine dampened sensory input and decreased psychomotor speed, while increasing attention, concentration and general vigilance in a group of normal volunteers. A detrimental effect of Chlorpromazine on attention, as judged by decreased performance on a paired associate measure and the Proteus mental age score, was reported by Helper, Wilcott, and Garfield (1963).

Werry, Weiss, Douglas, and Martin (1966) noted that Chlorpromazine had a slight depressant effect on intellectual functioning in the one-to-one test situation. Fish and her colleagues have repeatedly emphasized that the sedative effect of phenothiazines may be associated with decreased functioning including decreased learning if dosage is not properly adjusted (Campbell, Fish, Shapiro, & Floyd, 1970; Fish, 1960).

Ocular Changes

In 1964, Greiner and Berry first reported corneal and lens opacities associated with long-term, high-dose phenothiazine administration. Their observations have been confirmed by numerous investigators as well as by several recent studies based on large samples (Crane, Johnson, & Buffaloe, 1971; Greiner & Berry, 1964; Prien, DeLong, Cole, & Lavine, 1970). These reports have generally highlighted changes in adults. However, two cases of ocular changes in children exposed to long-term phenothiazine treatment have been reported by Geiger and Lesser (1967) and Goldman (1968). The case reported by Goldman is particularly interesting in that the 11-year-old patient received only 343 grams of Chlorpromazine, in contrast to larger total doses reported in other studies.

No special observations or guidelines have been established for children, but in adults both the total dosage and duration of phenothiazine treatment are significant in the development of ocular changes in susceptible patients (Crane, Johnson, & Buffaloe, 1971; Wilson, 1970). However, if the total cumulative Chlorpromazine intake is below 300 grams, or if the daily intake is less than 300 mgms, the possibility of developing such opacities in adults is considerably smaller than at higher doses (Wilson, 1970). Nevertheless, the smallest total dose of Chlorpromazine accompanied with ocular changes was found to be 213 grams (Crane, Johnson, Buffaloe, 1971) and Galbraith, Gibson, Crock and Pearce (1966) reported 13 patients who developed such changes after receiving a total of less than 500 grams of phenothiazines. The intense interest in the subject notwithstanding, most authors have not detected significant reductions in vision even with severe opacities (Buffaloe,

Table 1

Diagnostic Classification, Age and Sex of 52 Psychotic Children and Adolescents

Classification	Number			Age (years)	
	M	F	Total	Range	Median
Early infantile autism (Group A)	10	2	12	4-14	7
Psychosis with features of autism (Group B)	7	1	8	12-15	13
Psychosis complicated by organicity (Group C)	7	2	9	7-16	9
Acute schizophrenic episode	8	7	15	13-16	15
Chronic undifferentiated schizophrenia	1	3	4	14-16	15
Schizo-affective psychosis	2	–	2	14-16	15
Latent schizophrenia	–	1	1		14
Paranoid schizophrenia	1	–	1		14

Note.—Group A = classic infantile autism which excludes organicity and is characterized by early onset, withdrawal and inability to relate, speech problems, suspected deafness, and need for sameness; Group B = a serious, psychotic disorder which while not classic infantile autism, includes some of the features of infantile autism but is characterized especially by an onset later in childhood; Group C = probable psychosis but complicated by demonstrable organicity, known deafness, aphasia, or other evidence of brain damage.

Johnson, & Sandiper, 1967; Crane, Johnson, & Buffaloe, 1971; Prien, DeLong, Cole, & Lavine, 1970).

It should be noted that the literature generally, as well as this report, considers epithelial keratopathy as a clinical entity separated from the changes usually subsumed under eye opacities (a side effect of phenothiazine intake) (Johnson & Buffaloe, 1966).

SUBJECTS AND GENERAL PROCEDURE

The subjects of this study, all hospitalized at Winnebago State Hospital's Child-Adolescent Service at some time during the course of a recent 5-year period, had been admitted for treatment of psychosis or other severe disorders of personality or behavior. Such children and adolescents failed to respond to out-patient approaches in local treatment centers.

Of the 388 patients admitted for treatment during the period, 181 had

Table 2

Diagnostic Classification of 73 Patients with Personality, Behavioral, and Other Psychiatric Disorders

Classification	Number			Age (years)	
	M	F	Total	Range	Median
Personality Disorders					
Schizoid personality	1	2	3	13-15	14.0
Hysterical personality	0	3	3	13-15	14.0
Anti-social personality	3	0	3	12-15	15.0
Passive-aggressive personality	3	0	3	14-15	14.0
Behavior Disorders					
Hyperkinetic reaction of childhood	6	0	6	8-12	10.0
Withdrawing reaction of adolescence	2	2	4	15-16	15.5
Withdrawing reaction of childhood	3	1	4	6-12	11.5
Unsocialized aggressive reaction of adolescence	3	3	6	14-16	14.3
Unsocialized reaction of childhood	5	1	6	11-13	12.5
Group delinquent reaction of adolescence	0	3	3	15	15.0
Transient Situational Disturbances					
Adjustment reactions of childhood	6	0	6	6-13	11.2
Adjustment reaction of adolescence	3	4	7	13-15	14.0
Other Disorders					
Mild mental retardation	4	1	5	11-15	13.0
Nonpsychotic organic brain syndrome	9	1	10	7-15	11.0
Anorexia nervosa	0	1	1	13	13.0
Homosexuality	1	0	1	15	15.0
Depressive neurosis	1	1	2	14-15	14.5

received one or more phenothiazines as part of the treatment program. Twenty-three cases were excluded from the sample because the records were incomplete. Twenty-five additional cases involving concomitant use of several phenothiazines or phenothiazine intake concomitantly with anti-depressants or anorexics were also unsuitable for our analysis. Finally, 6 excluded patients on a low-calorie or other special diet reduced our sample to 125.

Tables 1 and 2 present the diagnoses of 86 boys and 39 girls ranging in age from 4 to 16 years (median = 13.58 years) comprising the sample of 125 selected from the total population on record.

Of the 52 psychotic patients, 29 had a diagnosis of infantile autism or childhood schizophrenia with onset prior to puberty. As shown in Table 1, this category comprising three groups initially delineated by Treffert (1970) included 12 autistic children (Group A), 8 children with a serious psychotic disorder encompassing some of the features of autism (Group B), and 9 psychotic children whose diagnosis was complicated by demonstrable organicity (Group C). Table 2 shows the variety of diagnoses, mostly personality and behavioral disorders, in the nonpsychotic group of children and adolescents.

The four related studies were carried out retrospectively. Anamnestic analysis was supplemented, whenever necessary, by clinical observation and in some instances by serial video tapes.

The records of patients with any of the four selected side effects of phenothiazine intake were analyzed for variables with which such complications might have been clearly associated. The variety of phenothiazines received by each patient during the course of the retrospectively examined period was taken into account. We have determined that 86 of the 125 patients were only on one drug while 39 received more than one phenothiazine prescribed at different times during the same period of hospitalization. Thioridazine and Chlorpromazine were used most frequently.*

Whenever possible, an attempt was made to isolate the effect of phenothiazines from other factors in the hospital milieu. In the analysis of data, the Sign Test was utilized to measure significance of weight changes and the Mann Whitney U Test to test significant differences between group medians.

STUDY 1

In this study, complete weight records prior to and during treatment were available for 30 children on Thioridazine, 16 on Chlorpromazine, and 14 on Trifluoperazine. These groups were studied over a 3-month period and compared with a random sample of 33 non-medicated children.

---

* Each phenothiazine was used singly or sequentially as follows: Thioridazine, 78 times; Chlorpromazine, 41 times; Trifluoperazine, 36 times; Chlorprothixene and Fluphenazine, 6 times; Carphenazine, 4 times; Perphenazine and Triflupromazine, 3 times; and Prochlorperazine, once.

Table 3

Weight Changes in 60 Medicated and 33 Non-medicated Children Over a 3-month Period

Group	Number				Median weight change (in lbs.)	p
	With weight increase	With weight decrease	With no weight change	Total		
On Chlorpromazine	10	6	–	16	+ 4.00	NS
On Trifluoperazine	6	6	2	14	0.00	NS
On Thioridazine	29	1	--	30	+10.50	<.001
Non-medicated	17	13	3	33	+ 0.83	NS

Table 3 shows the median weight changes as well as the number of children with increased or decreased weights in each group. Thioridazine was significantly associated with increases in 20 out of 30 children.* Weight percentile score increases ranged from 4 to 53 with a median positive change of 18 points. These changes had an occurrence median of 7 months with a range of 1 to 18 months and a daily dose range of 25 to 400 mgms.

Nine patients whose weights were tabulated before, during, and after Thioridazine intake were in a position to serve as their own controls. All gained on the drug and lost weight after its discontinuation. In this smaller group, the median weight percentile score increase of 18 points (over a median of 9 months) closely paralleled the median decrease of 17 points (over 6 months) following discontinuation. This weight gain on Thioridazine followed by loss after discontinuation was significant ($p < .002$).

STUDY 2

Ten children in the present study, 9 boys and 1 girl (8 to 15 years of age), had developed tardive dyskinesia. Seven had a diagnosis of childhood schizophrenia, and the remaining three hyperkinetic reaction of childhood and unsocialized aggressive reaction. In all, onset occurred after discontinuation of phenothiazines. The first symptoms were noted from 3 to 10 days after the end of drug intake and the syndrome sub-

---

* In this group, no significant changes in height percentile scores were noted on the University of Iowa Height and Weight Scales before and during treatment.

sided in 3 to 12 months. Facial tic, noted during the first month, was evident in 6 of these 10 children.

All afflicted children exhibited extraneous movements of upper extremities. Such movements were rhythmical and myoclonic-like, more evident distally than proximally, and could be voluntarily inhibited for brief periods. Also present in all patients was akathisia of an unique variety not accompanied by anxiety or other forms of subjective distress. Impairment was hardly in evidence in such activities as drinking from a glass or writing. The children failed to demonstrate cogwheel rigidity, tremor, or other Parkinsonian changes excepting akathisia. No motor reflex or sensory changes were elicited. The possibility of Sydenham's Chorea, raised in three cases, was excluded after complete laboratory workups. It was difficult to diagnose two children because of psychotic mannerisms and bizarre posturing present prior to medication. However, longitudinal observations showing gradual improvement over several weeks allowed greater precision.

Part A

In an attempt to isolate factors related to the development of tardive dyskinesia, we compared the 10 afflicted children with 64 (40 boys and 24 girls, 5 to 16 years of age) who had remained asymptomatic over a 1-month period after having been abruptly withdrawn from phenothiazines. In order to compare total drug intake as well as termination dosage of multiple drugs, Chlorpromazine was used as the standard. Thus, all phenothiazines were calculated in terms of Chlorpromazine equivalents in accordance with the standard dose conversion table utilized by Hollister (1970) as given in Table 4.

Table 4 reveals significant differences between the symptomatic and asymptomatic groups in terms of total gram intake, duration of treatment, and daily termination dosage. The median gram intake in the asymptomatic group (87) is in marked contrast with the 403 grams in the symptomatic. An equally dramatic difference is reflected in the comparison of duration of intake (c.4 vs. 32 months). The median daily termination dose was also significantly dissimilar ($p < .001$ for all variables).

Part B

Three patients were followed with serial video-taping from onset to the conclusion of their dyskenesias. Olaf, a 12-year-old boy whose symptoms had developed 3 days after abrupt discontinuation of his 400 mgm.

Table 4

Duration of Intake and Dosage of Phenothiazines in the Development of Tardive Dyskinesia

Variable	Symptomatic group (N = 10)*	Asymptomatic group (N = 64)†	U	z	p
Median duration of drug intake	32.50 months	3.92 months	22.5	4.71	<.001
Median total drug intake	403.00 grams	8.70 grams	18	4.78	<.001
Median daily termination dose	399.83 mgms.	99.57 mgms.	60.5	4.13	<.001

Note.—The total and daily termination doses are expressed in terms of Chlorpromazine equivalents whereby 100 mgms. was equated with 5 mgms. of Trifluoperazine, 100 of Chlorprothixene, 50 of Triflupromazine, 100 of Thioridazine, 2 of Fluphenazine, 10 of Perphenazine. *Median age = 12 years; in this group, 3 received Thioridazine, 1 Perphenazine, 1 Fluphenazine, and the remaining 5 various sequentially administered doses of Thioradizine, Chlorpromazine, Perphenazine, Trifluoperazine and Fluphenazine. †Median age = 13.5 years; all received singly and in various sequentially administered doses of Thioridazine, Chlorpromazine, Trifluoperazine, Fluphenazine, and Chlorprothixene.

daily dose of Thioridazine, exhibited a marked decrease in facial tic as well as alleviation of extraneous movements of upper extremities when the drug was reinstated for 24 hours, 7 days after the onset of symptoms. The other two, a 13-year-old boy named Jacob withdrawn from Thioridazine and a boy named Larry (15 years of age) from a combination of Trifluoperazine and Chlorpromazine, showed only a slight amelioration of their dyskinesias with brief reinstitution of the offending drugs. All three manifested mild symptoms 6 months after onset, but were asymptomatic 4 months later.*

A comparison was made between a group comprising Olaf, Jacob and one additional boy (Mac, 14 years old) on Thioridazine and 20 boys and 8 girls, 4 to 15 years of age) who did not develop tardive dyskenesia after sudden withdrawal from Thioridazine.

Table 5 once again demonstrates significant differences ($p < .01$) between the symptomatic and asymptomatic patients. Duration of intake

---

* Not unlike the adults with tardive dyskenesia receiving major neuroleptics (Crane, 1968), these 3 cases proved refractory to treatment with the usual anti-Parkinsonian drugs.

Table 5

Duration of Intake and Dosage of Thioridazine in the Development of Tardive Dyskinesia

Variable	Symptomatic group (N = 3)*	Asymptomatic group (N = 28)†	U	z	p
Median duration of drug intake	24 months	4 months	3	2.61	<.01
Median total drug intake	198 grams	7.13 grams	2	2.68	<.01
Median daily termination dosage	200 mgms	75.22 mgms	2	2.72	<.01

*Median age = 13 years; †Median age = 12.5 years.

had differed by 20 months and the total and daily termination dosages, by 190.87 grams and 124.7 milligrams.

Quite evidently, the incidence of tardive dyskenesia was high in most children who received large doses of phenothiazines over extended periods. The syndrome was in evidence in 10 out of 16 young patients whose total phenothiazine intake over a period of 15 months or longer had exceeded 130 grams,* and in 6 out of 10 whose daily termination doses were higher than 200 milligrams.

Such incidence was even higher among patients on Thioridazine, with 3 cases out of 4 whose total intake, lasting 22 months or longer, was higher than 145 grams; the syndrome had developed in as many as 3 out of 5 whose daily termination doses were 150 milligrams or higher.

Part C

To assess whether organic brain impairment might have enhanced the vulnerability of the 10 patients with tardive dyskinesia to that syndrome, we proceeded to compare this symptomatic group with the asymptomatic group of 64 mentioned in Part A. The comparison was based on a rating scale, devised for the purpose, which encompassed clinical, neurological, historical, laboratory, and psychological test findings. Impairment scores on the scale could range from 0 to 15. Independent ratings of each patient by each author yielded rather minor disagreements of no more than one point on the scale.

---

* As calculated in terms of Chlorpromazine equivalents on the basis of standard dose conversion parameters utilized by Hollister (1970).

The median rating for the asymptomatic group was 0.96 with a range of 0 to 9, closely approximating a median impairment score of 1.25 in the symptomatic group with a range of 0 to 7. Assuming that only impairment scores of 3 or higher were of clinical significance, we also compared the numbers with such scores in each group. The 2 out of 10 in the symptomatic group closely approximated the 10 out of 64 in the asymptomatic. With due reservations, these results may tend to lead to conclusions that organic brain damage in these young patients did not predispose them to the development of the tardive dyskinesia.

STUDY 3

A review of the academic records of patients investigated in this study disclosed an interesting finding. Three nonpsychotic children with normal intelligence quotients who had received Thioridazine to alleviate hyperactivity and aggressiveness, showed marked increases in achievement when tested on the Stanford Achievement battery after discontinuation of the drug. The changes in median achievement scores, on and off medication, for these three patients are presented in Figure 1.

In the first patient, a 12-year-old boy named Arthur, there was an increase in the battery median score of 0.4 years over an 18-month period on Thioridazine but an increase in achievement level of 2.8 years during the one-year period off Thioridazine. A second patient, a 13-year-old boy named David, made a total gain of only 2.2 years during 4 years on Thioridazine. During one year off medication, his achievement level increased 2 years. The third 13-year-old patient (Stanley) decreased his achievement level 0.7 years during the year he was receiving Thioridazine, and increased his battery median score by 1.6 years over his previous highest level during one year off medication. Arthur's daily dosage of Thioridazine had varied from 50 to 400 mgms., David's from 50 to 400, and Stanley's from 50 to 125 mgms.

These achievement scores were compared with those of 9 other children tested at similar times and intervals to rule out the possibility of relating some results to differences in the way the tests were administered or scored. None of these 9 children showed a battery median score increase of more than one year. The difference between the group of 3 and the second group of 9 was significant ($p < 0.01$). The 3 boys were thoroughly investigated to determine whether the dramatic increases in academic performance might have been related to changes in teachers, increased motivation, or a variety of other factors and none could be immediately correlated. While the achievements of Arthur, David, and

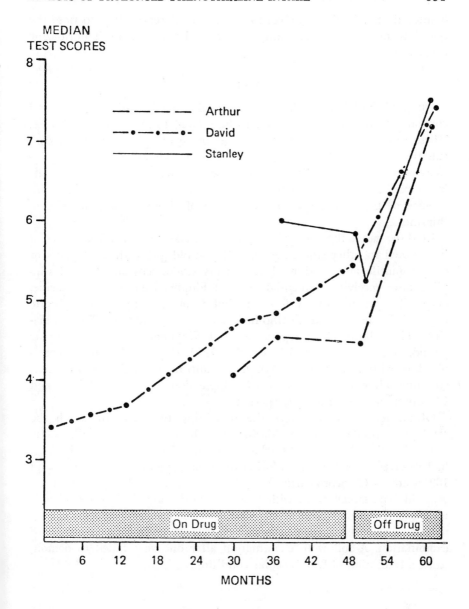

FIG. 1. Stanford Achievement Test scores of 3 patients during and after Thioridazine treatment:

Stanley do not lend themselves to statistical inference, they do raise the question of impaired learning that may be traced to Thioridazine intake.

Our review of 125 case histories revealed 5 manifestations of lens and corneal stippling which were felt to be related to phenothiazine intake. These cases were identified during the course of ophthalmological consultations which had been requested for refractive errors or other symptoms unrelated to the stippling. Since we did not routinely employ slit lamp examinations, no statement could be made regarding the true incidence of this side effect in our sample of children receiving phenothiazines.

In three cases, the total phenothiazine intake exceeded 750 grams, a level noted in other studies. Ann, a 15-year-old girl with a diagnosis of early infantile autism, showed moderately severe lens and corneal stippling after receiving sequential doses of Fluphenazine, Chlorpromazine, and Trifluoperazine over a 5-year period. George, a 14-year-old psychotic boy with features of autism who had received high doses of Chlorpromazine, Thioridazine, Trifluoperazine, and Fluphenazine over an 8-year period, also showed marked lens and corneal stippling. Ralph, a 15-year-old boy with a qualified diagnosis of autism, showed moderate lens stippling after receiving sequential high doses of Thioridazine and Chlorpromazine over a 5-year period.

Of particular interest were the remaining two cases in which the total gram intake of phenothiazines had been relatively small. A 12-year-old autistic boy named Carlos, who showed moderate lens stippling, had received 45 grams of Thioridazine over a period of 5 months and 169 grams of Chlorpromazine over 20 months. The other patient, a 14-year-old boy named Leon with a nonpsychotic organic brain syndrome who had received a total of 187 grams of Chlorpromazine over an 18-month period, also showed typical moderate lens stippling on slit lamp examination. A follow-up examination after one year failed to demonstrate a resolution of Leon's ocular condition.

The incidence of serious side effects in our sample of 125 should lend a note of caution in the prolonged use of high doses of phenothiazines in children. In major child mental illness, such drug intervention may sometimes be necessary. At times high doses may be required since, once a drug is deemed necessary and started, dosage must be gradually increased until either a satisfactory clinical response or toxic side effects are in evidence. However, the risks of such side effects will continually need to be weighed against the possible therapeutic benefit.

The author's experience with phenothiazines in the treatment of major mental illness in children has led to increasing discrimination in their use. In fact, in order to separate drug effects from those of the milieu in assessing therapeutic gain, a routine double blind placebo procedure has been introduced for each patient on psychotropic drugs. This procedure serves the double purpose of facilitating evaluation of the initial therapeutic effect of phenothiazines as well as that of periodically assessing their effectiveness when administered over prolonged periods of time. Drug and placebo are periodically interchanged so that neither the physician, nursing personnel, or patient are aware of the nature of intake at any given time. Because of the relatively slow excretion rates associated with phenothiazines, the changes from drug to placebo and in reverse are made at intervals of not less than one-month duration. Later, the observations of staff members and subjective impressions of the patient are combined. By comparing the drug-placebo period with changes in behavior, a clear differentiation of drug effects from those of the milieu can be accomplished. When continuous need for medication is prompted by beneficial changes in the clinical picture, drug holidays are used, whenever possible, to decrease the total drug intake.

CONCLUSION

Our retrospective investigation disclosed significant weight gains in 29 out of 30 patients that were related to Thioridazine intake. Tardive dyskinesia, found in 10 patients, was traced to total drug intake, duration of treatment and termination dosage; no relationship could be demonstrated to support assumptions that organic brain impairment predisposes to the development of that syndrome.

In 3 patients, achievement appeared to be accelerated after discontinuation of Thioridazine, suggesting a relationship to impaired learning. Less stippling occurred in 2 patients whose cumulative Chlorpromazine intake was relatively moderate.

We are inclined to suggest that therapeutic advantage must be continually weighed against the risks of using phenothiazines in the treatment of major mental illness in children. When such drug treatment is required over an extended period of time, a double blind individual procedure using the patient as his own control may facilitate judicious administration.

REFERENCES

AMDISEN, A.: Drug-produced obesity. *Danish Medical Bulletin*, 1964, 11, 182-189.

ANGLE, C. R. & McINTIRE, M. S.: Persistent dystonia in a brain-damaged child after ingestion of phenothiazine. *Journal of Pediatrics*, 1968, 73, 124-126.

AYD, F. J.: Persistent dyskinesia: A neurologic complication of major tranquilizers. *Medical Science*, 1967, 18, 32-40.

BUFFALOE, W. J., JOHNSON, A. W., & SANDIPER, M. G.: Total dosage of chlorpromazine and ocular opacities. *American Journal of Psychiatry*, 1967, 124, 154-155.

CAFFEY, E. M.: Experience with large scale interhospital cooperative research in chemotherapy. *American Journal of Psychiatry*, 1961, 117, 713-719.

CAFFEY, E. M. & KLETT, C. J.: Side effects and laboratory findings during combined drug therapy of chronic schizophrenics. *Diseases of the Nervous System*, 1961, 22, 370-375.

CAMPBELL, M., FISH, B., SHAPIRO, T., & FLOYD, A.: Thiothixene in young disturbed children. *Archives of General Psychiatry*, 1970, 23, 70-72.

CASTELNUOVO-TEDESCO, P., TANGUAY, P. E., KRAUT, B. M., & BURGESS, E. C.: Galactorrhea, headache and weight gain during treatment with Thioridazine. *American Journal of Psychiatry*, 1963, 119, 1178-1179.

CRANE, G. E.: Tardive dyskinesia in patients treated with major neuroleptics: Review of the literature. *American Journal of Psychiatry*, 1968, 124, 40-48.

CRANE, G. E.: Persistence of neurological symptoms due to neuroleptic drugs. *American Journal of Psychiatry*, 1971, 127, 1407-1410.

CRANE, G. E., JOHNSON, A. W., & BUFFALOE, W. J.: Long-term treatment with neuroleptic drugs and eye opacities. *American Journal of Psychiatry*, 1971, 127, 1045-1049.

CRANE, G. E. & NARANJO, E. R.: Motor disorders induced by neuroleptics. *Archives of General Psychiatry*, 1971, 24, 179-184.

DABBOUS, I. A. & BERGMAN, A. B.: Neurologic damage associated with phenothiazine. *American Journal of Diseases of Children*, 1966, 111, 291-296.

DiMASCIO, A.: Psychopharmacology in children. In S. Chess and A. Thomas (Eds.), *Annual Progress in Child Psychiatry and Child Development*. New York: Brunner-Mazel, 1971.

DUVOISIN, R. C.: Neurological reaction to psychotropic drugs. In D. H. Efron (Ed.), *Psychopharmacology: A Review of Progress*. Washington, D. C.: United States Government Printing Office, 1968.

EDWARDS, H.: The significance of brain damage in persistent oral dyskinesia. *British Journal of Psychiatry*, 1970, 116, 271-275.

EVELOFF, H. H.: Psychopharmacologic agents in child psychiatry. *Archives of General Psychiatry*, 1966, 14, 472-479.

FAURBYE, A., RASCH, P. J., PETERSEN, P. B., BRANDBORG, G., & PAKKENBERG, H.: Neurological symptoms in pharmacotherapy of psychoses. *Acta Physiologica Scandinavica*, 1964, 40, 10-27.

FISH, B.: Drug therapy in child psychiatry: Pharmacological aspects. *Comprehensive Psychiatry*, 1960, 1, 212-227.

FISH, B.: Drug use in psychiatric disorders of children. *American Journal of Psychiatry*, 1968, 124, 31-36. (Supp.)

FREED, H. & PEIFER, C. A.: Treatment of hyperkinetic emotionally disturbed children with prolonged administration of chlorpromazine. *Archives of Neurology*, 1970, 22, 176-180.

GALBRAITH, J. K., GIBSON, B. L., CROCK, G. W., & PEARCE, T. A.: Chlorpromazine therapy. *Medical Journal of Australia*, 1966, 1, 481-483.

GEIGER, L. A., & LESSER, L. I.: Ocular side effects of chlorpromazine in a child. *Journal of the American Medical Association*, 1967, 202, 916.

GOLDMAN, D.: Prolonged treatment of psychotic states. *Diseases of the Nervous System*, 1968, 29, 51-57. (Supp.)

GORDON, H. L. & GROTH, C.: Weight change during and after hospital treatment. *Archives of General Psychiatry*, 1964, 10, 187-191.

GREINER, A. C. & BERRY, K.: Skin pigmentation and corneal and lens opacities with prolonged chlorpromazine therapy. *Canadian Medical Association Journal*, 1964, 90, 663-665.

HELPER, M. M., WILCOTT, R. C., & GARFIELD, S. L.: Effects of chlorpromazine on learning and related processes in emotionally disturbed children. *Journal of Consulting Psychology*, 1963, 27, 1-9.

HOLLISTER, L. E.: Choice of antipsychotic drugs. *American Journal of Psychiatry*, 1970, 127, 186-190.

JOHNSON, A. W. & BUFFALOE, W. J.: Chlorpromazine epithelial keratopathy. *Archives of Ophthalmology*, 1966, 76, 664-667.

KLETT, C. J. & CAFFEY, E. M.: Weight changes during treatment with phenothiazine derivatives. *Journal of Neuropsychiatry*, 1960, 2, 102-108.

KLINE, N. S.: On the rarity of "irreversible" oral dyskinesias following phenothiazines. *American Journal of Psychiatry*, 1968, 124, 48-54. (Supp.)

LEHMANN, H. E. & KNIGHT, D. A.: Psychophysiologic testing with a new phenotropic drug. In Henry Brill (Ed.), *Trifluoperazine: Clinical and Pharmacological Aspects*. Philadelphia: Lea & Febiger, 1958.

LEVANN, L. J.: The use of trifluoperazine as a tranquilizing agent in mentally defective children. In John H. Moyer (Ed.), *Further Clinical and Laboratory Studies*. Philadelphia: Lea & Febiger, 1959.

PRIEN, R. F., DELONG, S. C., COLE, J. O., & LAVINE, J.: Ocular changes occurring with prolonged high dose chlorpromazine therapy. *Archives of General Psychiatry*, 1970, 23, 464-468.

RODOVA, A., & NAHUNEK, K.: Persistent dyskinesias after phenothiazines. *Ceskoslovenska Psychiatrie*, 1964, 60, 250-254.

SINGH, M. M., DEDIOS, L. V., & KLINE, N. S.: Weight as a correlate of clinical response to psychotropic drugs. *Psychosomatics*, 1970, 11, 562-570.

SLETTEN, I., MOU, B., CAZENAVE, M., & GERSHON, S.: Effects of caloric restriction on behavior and body weight during chlorpromazine therapy. *Diseases of the Nervous System*, 1967, 28, 519-522.

TREFFERT, D. A.: Child-adolescent unit in a psychiatric hospital: Five years later. *Archives of General Psychiatry*, 1969, 21, 745-752.

TREFFERT, D. A.: Epidemiology of infantile autism. *Archives of General Psychiatry*, 1970, 22, 431-438.

WERRY, J. S., WEISS, G., DOUGLAS, V., & MARTIN, J.: Studies on the hyperactive child. *Journal of Child Psychiatry*, 1966, 5, 292-312.

WILSON, D. J.: Ocular changes due to phenothiazine derivatives—a survey. *Transactions of the Ophthalmological Societies of the United Kingdom*, 1970, 89, 963-964.

Part X

PEDIATRICS AND MENTAL HEALTH

The psychological aspect of pediatric functioning is discussed in the two brief but pertinent papers in this section. Both reports deal with the pediatrician's obligation to be sensitive to the psychological status of his patients, but each approaches this subject from a different point of view.

Carey and Sibinga survey the type of mistakes a physician can make in his handling of acute minor illnesses that lead to unfavorable psychological consequences for the child. Stocking and his colleagues examine the incidence of psychopathology in a random sample of children admitted to a pediatric hospital and consider the role of the pediatric hospital as a mental health resource.

38

AVOIDING PEDIATRIC PATHOGENESIS IN THE MANAGEMENT OF ACUTE MINOR ILLNESS

William B. Carey, M.D., and

Maarten S. Sibinga, M.D.

From the Departments of Pediatrics, University of Pennsylvania Medical School at the Children's Hospital of Philadelphia and Temple University Medical School at St. Christopher's Hospital for Children, Philadelphia

ABSTRACT. The management of acute minor illnesses constitutes a major portion of a physician's work. The impact of such illness on the child's development and the physician's positive or negative influence on the child's and the parents' emotional adjustment are considered here. Very few data are available in the literature. Suggestions for management and research are presented.

Diagnosis and therapy of acute minor illness are far from uniform or agreed upon. Accurate diagnosis and reasonable treatment are the pediatrician's first responsibility. Over-, under-, and misdiagnosing and treating are to be avoided. Secondly, he should nurture the sick child by reducing stress and by promoting his adjustment to the illness situation. The child's emotional health suffers from the pediatrician's neglect, over-involvement with or mismanagement of his feelings during illness. Thirdly, the pediatrician should sup-

Reprinted with permission from Pediatrics, Vol. 49, No. 4, April, 1972, pp. 553-562. Copyright © The C. V. Mosby Co., St. Louis, Mo.

Presented in abbreviated form at the XIII International Congress of Pediatrics, Vienna, Austria, September 1971.

port the parents by helping them to deal with the specific illness and by promoting their capacity to cope with illness in general. If, instead, the pediatrician is overly dominant or submissive, neglectful or punitive in handling the parents' needs, they may become frightened, dependent, demanding, confused, or angry. Their feelings of incompetence in handling illnesses affect their general child-rearing abilities.

In recent years many pediatricians have shown an increased interest in the psychosocial aspects of their patients, such as intellectual function and personality development. Relatively less attention has been given to psychological factors in illness, and of that more emphasis has been placed on chronic disease (1) than on acute minor illness.

This is a curious omission when one realizes that, apart from well child examinations, acute minor illnesses are the pediatrician's principal area of activity and a major opportunity for a constructive role. These illnesses are a source of considerable stress for parent and child and occur more often in the formative period of early childhood than in later life (2).

The result of this inattention is that much ignorance, folklore, and pediatric pathogenesis pervade the area of management of minor illness, especially as the diagnosis and therapy of acute minor illness are far from uniform or agreed upon. Also no basic set of principles of behavior has evolved for the pediatrician.

Yet, teachers and practitioners need explicit guidelines and researchers need hypotheses for study. Psychologists and child psychiatrists may have areas of competence that overlap with ours in the handling of problems of intellectual function and personality development, but we pediatricians are usually the only professional persons involved in the care of acute minor illnesses. Nobody else has our continuing contact with the family or our particular professional expertise. We must use them more effectively.

This paper considers the illness, the child, the family, and the pediatrician as separate, but interacting, participants in the acute illness situation. We wish to examine (a) the needs of each, (b) how these needs may at times be improperly met by the pediatrician, (c) why this happens, and (d) what the consequences may be. Finally, we shall make suggestions as to how management might be improved to avoid iatrogenic complications. Material is drawn from the sparse, fragmentary literature, from our combined experience in clinical practice and teaching pediatric residents and from numerous discussions with colleagues.

By acute minor illness we mean to refer to such problems as the common infections, particularly of the respiratory and gastrointestinal tracts, and the common physical traumata, which are experienced by all children. Chronic illnesses and those requiring hospitalization are deliberately excluded. While most minor illnesses are stressful for parents and children, they vary from such trivial complaints as coryza up to the possibly stiff neck which brings the patient to the brink of hospitalization.

THE ILLNESS

The various acute minor illnesses that beset the child require diagnostic and therapeutic measures too numerous to mention here. Current management of jaundice in the newborn due to breast milk provides an example of how the diagnosis and therapy of acute minor illness can be far from uniform. The treatment varies all the way from denial of the significance of the phenomenon to permanent cessation of nursing and placement of the baby under phototherapy in the intensive care unit. Certain general problems in management deserve mention:

1. Overmanagement: Probably the most common error pediatricians make in management of the illness itself is overdiagnosing and overtreating (3). Problems which are generally minor may be made to seem major by the pediatrician who, for example, hospitalizes all cases of croup. In other instances, insignificant findings such as a functional heart murmur or a slight injection of the eardrums during fever may be overinterpreted, made into a "pseudo-disease" or "nondisease" (4) and managed with greater attention than is deserved.

Physicians apparently err in this direction for reasons which lie in two broad categories. On the one hand, the problem may be within the physician. For example, he may have poor professional training or judgment leading to overdiagnosis of heart disease (5). He may have neurotic anxiety that makes him afraid he will miss some important, but unlikely, condition. He may be influenced by the imbalancing effect of a recent frightening experience. He may consciously or unconsciously exaggerate illness for his own profit, or rarely even take unconscious sadistic pleasure in inflicting pain on someone. He may need the diagnostic exhibitionism of dramatization of trivia or of displaying expert knowledge of serious disorders not present. He might even overstate the seriousness of a situation as an expedient to justify referral of a tedious problem to a consultant. He may be prey to the rigidity of judgment which fails to appreciate the variations of normal.

On the other hand, the doctor may overmanage illness as the result of pressure from the family. This overmanagement ranges from the common irrational measures to decrease the frequency or duration of upper respiratory infections (6) to the extreme of the physician's allowing himself to be manipulated into making serious diagnoses where they are not justified (7).

There may be several results of this overmanagement: (a) Unnecessary fear may be generated in the family and child, who think of the child as being sicker or more vulnerable than he really is. Inappropriately extensive or repeated diagnostic measures may reinforce the importance of the symptom in the mind of parent and child, making the physician a "pathogenic agent" (8). (b) Unnecessary harm may be done to the child with excessive use of modern diagnostic and therapeutic agents, exposing the child without justification to iatrogenic physical disease, such as the "diseases of medical progress" (9) like acute diarrhea from antibiotic treatment, speech problems after early physical restraint (10), or jaundice from chlorpromazine. (c) Dependence on drugs may be encouraged.

2. Undermanagement: The opposite error in the management of illness is underdiagnosing and undertreatment. This may consist of overlooking disease that is present or of underestimating its extent or significance.

While this may arise from denial or from withholding of information by the family, it also occurs from superficiality or specific blind spots of the doctor. For example, the relative inattention of pediatricians to behavioral, as opposed to somatic, complaints has been well documented (11). The doctor's emotional reactions to dealing with the poor can make him less sensitive to their needs (12).

The consequences of underdiagnosis or treatment are, obviously, that some problems do not get sufficient attention and the patient is neglected, while his problems may persist or worsen.

3. Mismanagement: Improper diagnosing or treatment of the illness owing to poor judgment or inadequate knowledge can be disastrous and need not be elaborated upon here.

Pediatrician's Role—Treat the Illness

The primary responsibilities of the pediatrician are: 1) the appropriate treatment of illness in the child, which means that over-, under-, and misdiagnosing and treating are to be avoided, and the treatment administered competently, faithfully, and with compassion; 2) the avoidance of the pitfalls of diagnosis or treatment of "pseudo-diseases" or "nondiseases"; and 3) the taking of any reasonable steps to help the parent and child to prevent recurrences or spread of the illness. These things cannot be done well without consideration both for the child and for the family.

THE CHILD

It is the child who is the host of the acute illness and the focus of the parents' and physician's concern.

Several authors have described the stresses and needs experienced by the acutely ill child (13-19). Most commonly mentioned are: 1) the discomfort of the illness itself and its treatment; 2) the emotional reactions to the illness, such as feelings of guilt or of being bad, fears, anger, depression, and apathy; 3) the loss of normal social contacts at school and elsewhere outside the home; 4) the restrictions, such as bed rest and diet, within the home and the decreased or altered sensory input, and 5) the changed relationship with his parents, who may display indulgence or hostility.

While these stresses of acute minor illness have been described from the clinical experience of pediatricians and psychiatrists, very few studies have actually examined longitudinally the behavioral changes induced in children who are sick, but treated at home. Shrand (20) pointed out the transient changes in behavior attributable to the illness itself without hospitalization. Mattsson and Weisberg (21) demonstrated a shift in the predominant reaction from dependence in 2-year-olds to withdrawal in 3- to 4-year-old children.

One may suspect that there are other changes in reactions with age. Other variables may affect the individual child's reaction to his illness: sex difference (22, 23); the family's definition of illness and pattern of illness behavior (24); cultural, racial, and class differences (25, 26); variations in response to the disease-producing agent and its treatment; past experience with illness and pre-morbid personality.

The common problems in the physician's management of the sick child are:

1. Overattention to illness, neglect of the child: Probably the most common failure of the physcian managing the sick child is his treating the illness but neglecting the child himself, that is, being inadequately sensitive and attentive to the emotional needs of the sick child. The cause is usually a narrowness of interest or a lack of empathy or sensitivity on the part of the physician. Such a preoccupation with the technicalities of the illness and its management without adequate consideration

of the child results commonly in unnecessary injections and other painful procedures, overuse of hospitalization, unnecessary restrictions of activity, and failure to give the child reasonable reassurance. There is generally a greater chance that the minor illness will become a frightening, destructive experience for the child.

> Dr. Blinkers is known for his thoroughness and accuracy of diagnosis. He is held in high repute by his colleagues but his patients are terrified by him. They are reluctant to report that they are sick lest they have to see him.

2. Overattention to feelings: Just as he may ignore or be unaware of them, the pediatrician may be overly sensitive and attentive to the feelings of the child. By overidentification with the child the pediatrician becomes excessively involved emotionally, as with his own children, those of his friends (27), or of his colleagues (28). Such overconcern about discomfort and psychic trauma to the child may mean that proper diagnosis and management are in jeopardy.

> Dr. Mixer believes that he can provide better medical care for his own children than anyone else. In his concern for minimizing the discomfort and inconvenience of their respiratory infections, however, he employs far more antibiotics that he knows is proper.

3. Inappropriate handling of the child: Unsuitable reactions to a sick child, such as inappropriate facetiousness, dishonesty or punitive, rejecting attitudes, come from a variety of sources and usually stem from problems in the personality of the pediatrician. They must invariably make the illness experience more psychologically hazardous for the child.

> Before giving injections Dr. Blarney informs his patients that they will not hurt. As they dry their tears, he hands them lollipops and reminds them that they did not have any pain.

No reports can be found of the long-range results of the improper management of minor illnesses by physicians *per se*. Methodological problems in such a longitudinal study would be formidable. Any experienced pediatrician, however, can think of illustrative examples, such as the child who is treated for years as a semi-invalid because a physician had felt compelled to reveal the existence of a functional heart murmur without considering the impact of this information on the child and his parents.

Several psychiatric works comment on enduring abnormal reactions of children resulting from the total acute illness experience. Kanner (29) found excessive fear of physical hurt, hypochondriasis, enjoyment of attention in illness by rejected children, and disruption of scholastic progress. Other observers have described feelings of inferiority and isolation (13) and persistent dependency reactions and rebellion (14). Gordon, et al. (30) discovered significantly more severe childhood physical illness in the histories of adult psychiatric patients than in the histories of controls. It appears that no single stress or specific combination of stresses is nearly so great a statistical risk for adult mental health as an accumulation of various stressful factors in childhood, illness among them, the risk being proportional to the sum total of such factors (31).

Pediatrician's Role—Nurture the Sick Child

The pediatrician must not only treat the illness; he must also nurture the sick child. There are several ways he can do this:

1. The physician should reduce the stress of the illness as much as he can. The diagnosis and treatment must be as supportive and nonthreatening as possible (32). Physical discomfort and psychic trauma should be minimized. Unnecessary restrictions such as bedrest should be eliminated unless clearly indicated. Hospitalization, which frightens most young children (33), should be avoided unless clearly necessary and should be preceded by adequate preparation when possible. A prompt restoration of the child's equilibrium and normal relationship with his parents and surroundings should be encouraged.

2. The physician should promote the child's adjustment to the illness. Only by listening to the child and his parents can the doctor be aware of the needs of the child in the particular situation. Like the parent the child can be relieved of much anxiety if he can ventilate his rational and irrational fears. It is helpful if the pediatrician can acknowledge with honesty to the child that the illness or treatment produce discomfort. Having built the doctor-child relationship in this way, the pediatrician is in a better position to impart useful information to the child about what has happened and what he can expect to come. The child's cooperation in the program of treatment is then more likely.

3. Ideally, the pediatrician should make the illness an opportunity for the child's psychosocial growth. By learning about the illness and his ability to tolerate discomfort and to overcome a problem with the help of his family and physician, the child can grow in self-confidence and avoid developing a sense of physical inferiority or personal inadequacy. We should not overlook the child's ability to gain strength by identifying with the pediatrician (34).

THE FAMILY

Finally, we consider the family of the sick child, especially the parents, who are his primary caretakers. The family can interact with the sick child in several ways: 1) it may be the source or cause of the illness; 2) it is surely a factor affecting the illness' outcome; 3) it generally determines whether and when the child is taken to the doctor, and 4) it reacts to the illness (35).

The stresses for the parents of a sick child have been outlined by several authors (15-19, 24, 25, 36), and are of two principal sorts. They are: 1) the stresses that arise from the illness experience itself, for the parent, like the child, suffers fears and anxieties, anger, guilt, fatigue, depression, and distortions and misconceptions; and 2) the extraneous factors that complicate the parents' reaction to the situation. The latter include: (a) problems in the parents themselves, such as memories of previously disturbing experiences with illness, chronic emotional disorders like sado-masochism, or a transient imbalance of feelings, as in premenstrual tension (37); (b) problems in the child, such as preexisting illness or a difficult temperament; or (c) situational stresses, such as unemployment or marital discord. Such stresses may also have played a part in producing the illness (35, 38).

It appears that in many instances an "early infancy health crisis" (39), defined as an actual illness or the mere threat of it in the early months of life, presents an unusual challenge to the parents' capacity to adapt and act appropriately, the "vulnerable child syndrome" being a possible unfavorable outcome of the experience (40).

It is important that the parents be able, in spite of these various stresses, to cope effectively with the management of the illness and sick child. A basic requirement for their best functioning is that they be emotionally mature, united, and warmly attached to the child (41). Ineffective coping consists of (a) inappropriate feelings or understanding, such as too much or too little anxiety, persistent misconceptions about the illness or its treatment, an excessive sense of narcissistic injury (42); or (b) inability to muster appropriate behavior to meet the illness, such as difficulty in carrying out a reasonable share of the treatment process in conjunction with the doctor, as evidenced by noncompliance with the treatment plan (43, 44), or distortion of the handling of the sick child by overcontrol, oversubmissiveness, infantilization, or rejection.

The reactions of other members of the family, especially siblings, must be remembered as a part of the total family interaction.

Problems in the management of the family are of three principal kinds:

1. Overdomination and submission in the pediatrician-parent relationship. Some pediatricians make a practice of overwhelming parents with more information than they can successfully utilize, or of assuming so great a role in planning the program of treatment of the child that the parents are given little opportunity to assume responsibility themselves. The unskilled or distrusting pediatrician thereby keeps the family frightened and overly dependent on him. This exercise of his "apostolic function" (45) stifles self-reliance in parents.

> Dr. Snow complains that his patients' parents frequently bother him at all hours of the night with questions and appeals for help. After reporting to them all the physical findings, the differential diagnosis, and details of management, he cannot understand why they need to tax his wisdom any further.

On the other hand, oversubmissiveness to the wishes of the parents, usually due to insecurity in the pediatrician or an undue wish to please the parents, as when they are friends (27), wealthy or socially prominent, results in overuse of antibiotics and similar deviations from good medical practice. Once he has communicated to the family the message that he can be manipulated in this way, the physician has a hard time restoring himself as the impartial professional advisor. Pleasing parents (36) is a reasonable objective but it cannot be the pediatrician's organizing principle. It would mean that he is failing to utilize his expertise and long-term relationship with the family for the overall benefit of parent and child.

> Dr. Putty used to believe that the parents of the sick child should always leave his office with some kind of medicine, preferably something suggested by them. After several years of ingratiating himself with parents he realized that neither he nor the parents were acting responsibly. He sought refuge in the seemingly simpler world of academic medicine.

2. Neglect of the parents entails not giving sufficient attention to their feelings, their need for information or help in the management of the illness. Instead of appropriate discussions addressed to the parents' real concerns, the pediatrician may monopolize the discussion with his own interests or concerns. Overly hurried medical care ("volume business") also breeds neglect of parents. Handled in this way, parents can only become confused and helpless.

Dr. Blitz seldom sees less than 40 patients in a day. The parents of his patients marvel that he is so busy and important, but for guidance on all matters outside of medicine doses they have to turn elsewhere: to the druggist, the bridge club, and the lady next door.

3. Wrong handling of parents occurs when doctors give them misinformation about their child's illness or its management or do anything that needlessly upsets them. One wonders what the doctor had in mind when he told the parents of the child that he had "almost pneumonia." What is the physician up to when he says that he has caught the baby's sore throat or allergic rhinitis "just in time"? We must speculate that a variety of antisocial or ego-defective impulses may be at work: avarice, pride, hostility or a need to inflate one's own role or importance, for example. The various unfortunate consequences of such physician behavior include an increase in parental feelings of incompetence and an attachment of the parents to the doctor through fear or misguided gratitude.

Dr. Salvatore believes in preventive medicine and particularly warns parents about accidents. Whenever an accident does occur, he reminds them that they are responsible, whether consciously or unconsciously, for what has happened.

Pediatrician's Role: Support the Parents

Most pediatricians would agree that part of our proper role is to provide emotional support for parents. Few, however, would probably be able to conceptualize the exact nature and details of this important function.

Emotional support is not present at all in the "activity-passivity model" of the doctor-patient relationship in which the doctor does everything and the patient does nothing, as when the patient is comatose (46). In the "guidance-cooperation model" the patient or parent seeks and follows the doctor's advice. This is the usual situation in those acute illnesses. The "mutual-participation model" refers to the setting where the physician helps the patient or parents to help themselves. This kind of help, appropriate for many of the acute minor illnesses of children, is a great opportunity for emotional support.

The precise nature of emotional support, at least in the psychiatric situation, has been well described by Burnand as "the expectation of help if needed" while the supported person works toward gaining the confidence and competence to get along on his own (47).

In the pediatric setting support of parents seem to consist specifically of the following elements: 1) determining their needs and expectations, 2) helping them deal with the illness and sick child, and 3) promoting their general self-confidence in handling illness.

1) First of all, the pediatrician must determine the parents' needs. Success in the management of the illness situation depends on a knowledge of the parents and the reason for their call for help. Is it simply for information about the illness? Is the chief complaint unrelated to the real concern about the child (48)? Is it a "ticket of admission" (35) for some family problem? The parents' expectations of the pediatrician must also be understood, since they are varied and not always rational.

2) Helping the parents deal with the illness and the sick child consists of: (a) giving them information about diagnosis and treatment; (b) helping them to adapt to the realities of the illness situation; and (c) being available in case of further need.

Giving parents the information they need combats their confusion and helps them to shift from a position of relative helplessness to active participation in the recovery process. Thus, the pediatrician is doing for the family what they cannot do for themselves. Great care must be exerted by the physician not to give needlessly disturbing information, such as the fact that otitis media can develop into meningitis. A misguided sense of duty or a desire to protect himself or his reputation should not make the pediatrician say things that will not be helpful for the parents but only arouse their anxiety. The elder Oliver Wendell Holmes said this well in the last century, "The patient has no more right to all the truth than he has to all the medicine in your saddlebag. He should get only so much as is good for him" (46).

Assisting parents to adapt to the physical and emotional realities of the illness situation requires considerable skill from the physician. In this function he is helping them to help themselves, rather than providing precise directions. This means, for example, general suggestions on symptom relief, diet and activity, as opposed to exact antibiotic doses. If he can empathize with the parents' distress, he is likely to be in a better position to build an acceptable plan of management. If he can help them to get rid of inappropriate feelings and ideas about the illness and unsuitable plans, his own plan of therapy stands a better chance of being carried out. Irate parents (49) and those who are unreasonable or uncooperative (25) require the highest skills the pediatrician possesses. Parental pressures to alter therapy are best understood in terms of their anxiety and are best managed confidently without anger (50).

If extraneous but contributory physical or psychosocial problems become evident in the course of the acute illness, plans for their resolution can be scheduled for another time.

The physician is supporting the competence of the parents if he allows them to use their own understanding of the illness and their own plans for management whenever these are appropriate. Nothing builds confidence in a mother quite so much as being told she has done well on her own.

The advice provided by the pediatrician must be understandable and acceptable. Indefiniteness, lack of assurance, uncertainty, undue gravity, or silence may be very upsetting (46).

Finally, the pediatrician or a close associate should be available in case of further need. Parents appear to appreciate the physician's availability as much as his competence and attentiveness. Continuity of care is the best guarantee that the pediatrician will be available.

3) In his role of supporting parents the pediatrician should strive not only to determine their needs and help them cope with the present illness, but ideally also to promote their general self-confidence and capacity to handle illness. Even minor illnesses can be viewed as developmental crises (51) for the parents, from which they may emerge frightened and confused or with a feeling of mastery or accomplishment, although perhaps fatigue as well. This favorable outcome is most likely to happen when the pediatrician serves as a teacher and treatment partner as well as a healer (25). Parents too can gain strength through identification with the pediatrician (34). Inexperienced parents need more support but some continue to require extensive assistance because of their personality or because of the view that only the doctor knows what is right.

Advantages of a well-balanced parental self-reliance are considerable. There is a greater likelihood that the total management of the illness will be done right. The physician is enabled to spend less time attending to details, such as giving the same instructions repeatedly for the same problem. The parents' increased sense of competence in this area will probably spread into other important spheres, such as child-rearing practices.

SPECULATIONS AND QUESTIONS FOR THE READER

1) First of all, why is it that we have given so little attention previously to this major practical area? Are we embarrassed or unable to take a good look at what we are doing with minor illnesses? 2) How prevalent are the various types of management listed above? 3) How much physical and psychological disability results from these errors? 4) To what extent

can the above suggestions actually reduce iatrogenic complications? 5) If these suggestions are mistaken, what is a better approach? 6) What factors in the pediatrician makes him most helpful and least pathogenic: personality, training, or experience? 7) How can a doctor find out if he is making these errors and learn to change his ways? Will he profit, for example, by going over recorded interviews with respected colleagues as Balint described (45)? Finally, can nurse practitioners be trained to handle these problems instead of or in addition to pediatricians? If pediatricians have thought so little about it, what are they teaching them?

SUMMARY

The management of acute minor illnesses constitutes a major portion of a physician's work. The impact of such illness on the child's development and the physician's positive or negative influence on the child's and the parents' emotional adjustment are considered here. Very few data are available in the literature. Suggestions for management and research are presented.

Diagnosis and therapy of acute minor illnesses are far from uniform or agreed upon. Accurate diagnosis and reasonable treatment are the pediatrician's first responsibility. Over-, under-, and misdiagnosing and treating are to be avoided. Secondly, he should nurture the sick child by reducing stress and by promoting his adjustment to the illness situation. The child's emotional health suffers from the pediatrician's neglect, over-involvement with, or mismanagement of his feelings during illness. Thirdly, the pediatrician should support the parents by helping them to deal with the specific illness and by promoting their capacity to cope with illness in general. If, instead, the pediatrician is overly dominant or submissive, neglectful, or punitive in handling the parents' needs, they may become frightened, dependent, demanding, confused, or angry. Their feelings of incompetence in handling illnesses affect their general child-rearing abilities.

REFERENCES

1. GREEN, M.: Care of the child with a long-term life-threatening illness: Some principles of management. *Pediatrics*, 39:441, 1967.
2. VALADIAN, I., STUART, H. C., & REED, R. B.: Studies of illness in children followed from birth to eighteen years. *Monogr. Soc. Res. Child Develop.*, 26: No. 3, 1961.
3. KEITEL, H. G.: Summary of pitfalls in clinical practice. *Pediat. Clin. N. Amer.*, 12:377, 1965.
4. MEADOR, C. K.: The art and science of nondisease. *New Eng. J. Med.*, 272:92, 1965.

5. BERGMAN, A. B. & STAMM, S. J.: The morbidity of cardiac nondisease in school children. *New Eng. J. Med.*, 276:1008, 1967.

6. MORTIMER, E. A., JR.: Frequent colds. In M. Green and R. J. Haggerty (Eds.), *Ambulatory Pediatrics*. Philadelphia: W. B. Saunders Company, p. 211, 1968.

7. WINKELMEYER, R., JUDD, A. B., & STEARNS, R. P.: Two mistaken diagnoses of fatal illness in brothers. *Pediatrics*, 40:390, 1967.

8. APLEY, J.: *The Child with Abdominal Pains*. Oxford: Blackwell Scientific Publications, p. 78, 1959.

9. MOSER, R. H.: Diseases of medical progress. *New Eng. J. Med.*, 255:606, 1956.

10. SIBINGA, M. S. & FRIEDMAN, C. J.: Restraint and speech. *Pediatrics*, 48:116, 1971.

11. STARFIELD, B. & BORKOWF, S.: Physicians' recognition of complaints made by parents about their children's health. *Pediatrics*, 43:168, 1969.

12. McMAHON, A. W. & SHORE, M. F.: Some psychological reactions to working with the poor. *Arch. Gen. Psychiat.*, 18:562, 1968.

13. BEVERLY, B. I.: The effect of illness upon emotional development. *J. Pediat.*, 8: ECC, 1936.

14. LANGFORD, W. S.: Physical illness and convalescence: Their meaning to the child. *J. Pediat.*, 33:242, 1948.

15. FREUD, A.: The role of bodily illness in the mental life of children. *Psychoanal. Stud. Child*, VII:69, 1952.

16. KORSCH, B.: Psychological principles of pediatric practice: The pediatrician and the sick child. *Advances Pediat.*, 10:11, 1958.

17. APLEY, J. & MACKEITH, R.: *The Child and His Symptoms*. Philadelphia: F. A. Davis Company, Chapter 17, 1962.

18. PRUGH, D. G.: Toward an understanding of psychosomatic concepts in relation to illness in children. In A. J. Solnit and S. A. Provence (Eds.), *Modern Perspectives in Child Development*. New York: International Universities Press, Inc., pp. 324-330, 1963.

19. RAIMBAULT, G. & ROYER, P.: How do mother and child react to a child's illness? *Clin. Pediat.*, 8:255, 1969.

20. SHRAND, H.: Behavior changes in sick children nursed at home. *Pediatrics*, 36: 604, 1970.

21. MATTSSON, A. & WEISBERG, I.: Behavioral reactions to minor illness in preschool children. *Pediatrics*, 46:604, 1970.

22. MECHANIC, D.: The influence of mothers on their children's health attitudes and behavior. *Pediatrics*, 33:44, 1964.

23. WEINBERG, S.: Suicidal intent in adolescents: A hypothesis about the role of physical illness.

24. BLOOM, S. W.: *The Doctor and His Patient. A Sociological Interpretation*. New York: Russell Sage Foundation, 1963.

25. BLUM, R. H.: *The Management of the Doctor-Patient Relationship*. New York: McGraw-Hill, 1960.

26. MARSHALL, C. L., HASSANEIN, K. M., HASSANEIN, R. S., & PAUL, C. L.: Attitudes toward health among children of different races and socioeconomic groups. *Pediatrics*, 46:422, 1970.

27. CAREY, W. B. & SIBINGA, M. S.: Should pediatricians provide medical care for their friends' children? *Pediatrics*, 42:106, 1968.

28. KENNELL, J. H. & BOAZ, W. D.: The physicians' children as patients. *Pediatrics*, 30:100, 1962.

29. KANNER, L.: *Child Psychiatry*, ed. 3. Springfield, Illinois: C. C Thomas, p. 49, 1957.

30. GORDON, R. E., SINGER, M. B., & GORDON, K. K.: Social psychological stress. *Arch. Gen. Psychiat.*, 4:459, 1961.

31. LANGNER, T. S. & MICHAEL, S. T.: *The Midtown Manhattan Study. Life Stress*

and *Mental Health*. Free Press of Glencoe, Chapters 9 and 13. London: Collier-Macmillan Limited, 1963.

32. KORSCH, B.: Pediatrician-patient relations. In M. Green and R. J. Haggerty (Eds.), *Ambulatory Pediatrics*. Philadelphia: W. B. Saunders, p. 118, 1968.

33. VERNON, D. T. A., FOLEY, J. M., SIPOWICZ, R. R., & SCHULMAN, J. L.: *The Psychological Responses of Children to Hospitalization and Illness. A Review of the Literature*. Springfield, Illinois: C. C Thomas, 1965.

34. SOLNIT, A. J.: Psychotherapeutic role of the pediatrician. In M. Green and R. J. Haggerty (Eds.), *Ambulatory Pediatrics*. Philadelphia. W. B. Saunders, p. 159, 1968.

35. HAGGERTY, R. J.: Family crises: The role of the family in health and illness. In M. Green and R. J. Haggerty (Eds.), *Ambulatory Pediatrics*. Philadelphia: W. B. Saunders, p. 774, 1968.

36. THOMPSON, H. C. & SEAGLE, J. B.: Management of office practice—A philosophy. *Pediatrics*, 26:141, 1960.

37. DALTON, K.: Children's hospital admissions and mother's menstruation. *Brit. Med. J.*, 2:27, 1970.

38. MUTTER, A. Z. & SCHLEIFER, M. J.: The role of psychological and social factors in the onset of somatic illness in children. *Psychosom. Med.* 28:333, 1966.

39. CAREY, W. B.: Psychologic sequelae of early infancy health crises. *Clin. Pediat.*, 8:459, 1969.

40. GREEN, M. & SOLNIT, A. J.: Reactions to the threatened loss of a child: A vulnerable child syndrome. *Pediatrics*, 34:58, 1964.

41. MOORE, T.: Stress in normal childhood. *Human Relations*, 22:235, 1969.

42. STEIN, E. H., MURDAUGH, J., & MACLEOD, J. A.: Brief psychotherapy of psychiatric reactions to physical illness. *Amer. J. Psychiat.*, 125:1040, 1969.

43. FRANCIS, V., KORSCH, B. M., & MORRIS, M. J.: Gaps in doctor-patient communication. *New Eng. J. Med.*, 280:535, 1969.

44. GORDIS, L., MARKOWITZ, M., & LILIENFELD, A. M.: Why patients don't follow medical advice: A study of children on long term anti-streptococcal prophylaxis. *J. Pediat.*, 75:957, 1969.

45. BALINT, M.: *The Doctor, His Patient and the Illness*. New York: International Universities Press, Inc., 1957.

46. HOLLENDER, M. H.: *The Psychology of Medical Practice*. Philadelphia: W. B. Saunders Company, Chapters 1, 2, and 9, 1958.

47. BURNAND, G.: The nature of emotional support. *Brit. J. Psychiat.*, 115:139, 1969.

48. YUDKIN, S.: Six children with coughs. The second diagnosis. *Lancet*, 2:7202, 1961.

49. SCHULMAN, J. L.: The management of the irate parent. *J. Pediat.*, 77:338, 1970.

50. RICHMOND, J.: The pediatric patient in illness. In M. H. Hollender (Ed.), *The Psychology of Medical Practice*. Philadelphia: W. B. Saunders Company, Chapter 8, 1958.

51. CAPLAN, G.: *Prevention of Mental Disorders in Children*. New York: Basic Books, Inc., Chapter 1, 1961.

39

PSYCHOPATHOLOGY IN THE PEDI-ATRIC HOSPITAL—IMPLICATIONS FOR COMMUNITY HEALTH

Myron Stocking, M.D., William Rothney, M.D., George Grosser, Ph.D., and Rhoda Goodwin, M.A.

Departments of Psychiatry and Pediatrics
Tufts-New England Medical Center

PURPOSE

With the hope of contributing knowledge to a neglected area the authors undertook a study designed: 1) to find the incidence of psychopathology in children admitted to a pediatric hospital; 2) to delineate how often such psychopathology is not recognized by the pediatric staff; and 3) to find the frequency with which children are hospitalized unnecessarily.

The medical literature includes a number of studies which have revealed a high incidence of psychopathology in adults admitted for medical care within the general hospital. Zwerling et al. (1) studied 200 surgical admissions to a general hospital and found diagnosable mental disorders in 86% of the patients studied. Kaufman et al. (2), studying a sample of the medical admissions to a general hospital, found 66.8% to have some form of psychiatric disorder. Shapiro et al. (3) have reported

Reprinted from AMERICAN JOURNAL OF PUBLIC HEALTH, April, 1972, pp. 551-556.

This study was supported in part by PHS grant MH15037 and MH10731 from the National Institute of Mental Health and by a research grant #27516 from the New England Medical Center Hospitals.

.that in a random sample of 102 patients on the medical service of a general hospital 64% had severe psychopathology.

There are no comparable studies of children admitted to the pediatric hospital reported in the medical literature.

METHODS

A random sample of every twentieth child admitted to a pediatric hospital over a ten-month period was selected for study.* The parent (with one exception, the mother) of each child was interviewed by a child psychiatrist within the first 48 hours of the child's admission to the hospital. This screening interview was designed to reveal those children who were experiencing significant difficulties in personality development or emotional adaptation of severity sufficient to warrant psychiatric consultation.

An interview outline was evolved which was designed to be implemented flexibly by an experienced interviewer. Our goal was that the semi-structured interview could be implemented in one hour. The interview was to include consideration of these issues:

Present illness—The interviewer reviewed briefly the medical history of the illness leading to the current hospitalization.

Psychological functioning of the child at onset of present illness— Questioning was in detail and organized around the following points:

- School performance
- Areas of independence, interest and activity
- Quality of friendships and number
- Relationship to key family figures
- Relationship to adults outside family
- Overt neurotic symptomatology (including evidence of persistent or unresolved anxiety)
- Evidence of conscience formation
- Impulse and how handled
- Self-Image

Past history—Attention was devoted to obtaining data concerning: Mother's attitude and experiences during pregnancy with the hospitalized child; description of mother's experiences and attitudes at birth and neonatal period; description of the climate and quality of early

---

* The pediatric hospital in which the study was conducted is the principal clinical facility of a medical school department of pediatrics. Within the hospital there is a high standard of pediatric care. There has been a tradition of awareness and sensitivity to the overall needs of the child which has been reflected in the introduction of major modification in pediatric care pioneered within the hospital (4-6).

adaptation between mother and infant including a review of early feeding, motor development, and the approach to toilet training.

The interview was to be guided on the basis of the clinical intuition of the interviewer. If evidence of significant difficulty within a particular area existed, attention was devoted to delineating the difficulty rather than attempting to cover each interview topic in a uniformly comprehensive manner.

On a basis of this initial interview the child psychiatrist recorded his impression as to whether the child had been experiencing significant emotional difficulty in adapting to his illness or its treatment, and whether the child was experiencing significant problems in emotional development independent of the illness leading to hospitalization. He designated those instances in which psychiatric consultation was needed for an adequate formulation of comprehensive medical care. These ratings were not shared with the pediatric ward staff who were not informed of the nature or purpose of the screening interviews.

Specific psychiatric diagnoses were not established on each child, because thus far the field of child psychiatry has not established a single system of nosologic classification which can be applied with a high degree of reliability. The need for, as well as some of the major difficulties in establishing such a scheme, have been well discussed by M. Rutter (7).

To minimize the influence of subjective factors in the child psychiatrist's assessment of the presence of significant psychopathology and the need of psychiatric consultation, two different child psychiatrists took part in conducting the screening interviews. Each reviewed a subsample of the protocols of the screening interviews he had not personally conducted, in order to establish an independent rating of the presence of significant psychopathology and the indication for psychiatric consultation. Agreement between raters on the subsample was 95%.

Six months following discharge from the hospital, a home visit was conducted by a clinical psychologist from the research team. In this home visit mother and child were observed directly. The mother was interviewed to obtain follow-up data on the child's emotional adjustment following hospitalization and to gain a picture of the child's overall adjustment to his medical treatment.

As a further control of the validity of the child psychiatrist's assessment of the presence of significant psychopathology in the children studied, a third interviewer conducted the subsequent home visits. Protocols of the interviews at the time of the home visits were studied in order to assess whether there were any instances in which it appeared that our assessments of the presence of significant psychopathology on the basis of the screening interview might have been unwarranted. In no instance did this additional data leave us with the impression that we had described psychopathology initially when it did not exist.

In each instance when a child was judged to have either preexisting psychopathology or to have evidenced significant emotional difficulties in adapting to his illness or his treatment, a review was conducted to find out if psychiatric consultation had been requested. In instances where no psychiatric consultation was requested the medical record was scrutinized to find if the evidence of psychopathology or of difficulty in adapting to illness had been recognized and assessed by the pediatric staff and whether the regime of medical care was modified appropriately to deal with the existing problems.

Following completion of the screening interviews and the home visits a child psychiatrist reviewed the cases studied. He reviewed the admission interview data, the records of home visits, and the hospital medical records in order to rate the necessity of hospitalization for each child. A pediatrician made an independent rating of the necessity of hospitalization for each child based on his review of the hospital medical record.*

FINDINGS†

1. Incidence of Psychopathology in Hospitalized Children

The child psychiatrist found that 51 of the 80 children (63.7%) had significant psychopathology or difficulties in emotional adaptation which in his opinion warranted psychiatric consultation. Of these children eight (10%) had need of consultation because of emotional difficulties which were primarily related to adapting to the illness which caused their admission to the hospital. Forty-three children (53.7%) had emotional difficulties which were not a reflection of the emotional stress of adapting to preexisting medical illness or its treatment.

2. Incidence of Psychopathology Not Recognized by the Pediatric Staff

The pediatric ward staff requested psychiatric consultation on nine children (11.3% of the random sample). For 42 children regarded by

* The authors wish to express their appreciation to Dr. Aubrey Milunsky for his participation in these ratings.

† The authors wish to express their appreciation to Phyllis Schmitt for her assistance in data collection and data analysis.

the child psychiatrist as having significant psychopathology or difficulties in emotional adaptation warranting consultation, no consultation was requested. Scrutiny of the medical records gave no evidence that the emotional difficulties were recognized, or played a role in the formulation of case management by the pediatrician.

3. Frequency of Unnecessary Hospitalization

The need of hospitalization of the children in the study sample was assessed independently by a child psychiatrist and a pediatrician.

In the opinion of the child psychiatrist, 52 children (65%) clearly required hospitalization for optimal diagnosis and treatment. Four children (5%) were judged to have problems for which adequate diagnosis and treatment were possible without hospitalization, but for whom the advantages of hospitalization were regarded as outweighing its damaging effects. In the opinion of the child psychiatrist 24 of the children studied (30%) clearly did not require hospitalization for adequate diagnosis and treatment.

In the judgment of the pediatrician, hospitalization was clearly required for 56 children (70%). He regarded hospitalization as not required but nonetheless advantageous for 14 children (17.5%). He regarded hospitalization as clearly not necessary for ten children in the sample (12.5%).

4. The Nature of the Case Material

We would like to provide the reader a more detailed picture of some of the instances of psychopathology in particular children studied so he may have a basis for forming an impression of the range and quality of clinical data we encountered.

A. Children where psychopathology was recognized by pediatrician and psychiatric assessment was requested.

Nine psychiatric consultations were requested from the group of 80 children studied.

Three children had medical pathology which was either caused or aggravated by psychological factors: one child was asthmatic; one had ulcerative colitis; and the third was a ruminating infant who had failed to gain weight properly in the absence of any demonstrable underlying organic defects and in the presence of a disturbance in the early emotional climate between mother and child.

Three children had marked psychopathology manifested by grossly disturbed behavior. These children had been specifically admitted to the hospital for psychiatric assessment. There was no issue of physical illness. Each child lived in either a difficult or disorganized home environment and there were positive indications for undertaking psychiatric assessment on an inpatient basis.

Two children were admitted for assessment of atypical seizures. In each the possibility of psychological disturbances in the absence of underlying organic neurological disorder was to be assessed.

One child was a dwarf who was referred for psychiatric assessment of his overall emotional development.

B. Children rated by child psychiatrist as likely to benefit from psychiatric assessment for whom no psychiatric consultation was requested.

Review of the 42 mother-child pairs in this group revealed four subgroups. (In two instances a mother-child pair fell into two different subgroups.)

1) Psychiatric consultation was regarded as advisable for twelve infants of less than two years of age, in which the mother and child demonstrated difficulties in their early adaptation to one another.

Example

A ten-and-a-half-month-old child was admitted for treatment of meningitis. The child had had an upper respiratory infection for the previous two weeks.

The child's mother described herself as a nervous mother who "bugs her pediatrician" and "is always calling him." She had always been fearful that her child would develop a serious illness. Her apprehensiveness led her to take the infant's temperature almost hourly during the first two weeks of what appeared to be an uncomplicated respiratory infection.

This mother's apparent over-anxiousness served her well. On the fifteenth day of illness, the infant had a sudden elevation of temperature and began to look more ill. The mother called her pediatrician insisting on an immediate examination. The diagnosis of meningitis was made, apparently only shortly after the onset of meningeal involvement. Adequate treatment of the infectious process was implemented quickly and effectively. The child's hospital course was uncomplicated.

There was no comment on the mother-child relationship in the work-up of the ward pediatrician.

The psychiatric screening interview revealed that the mother had felt apprehensive, "mean and miserable" throughout her pregnancy.

She had been disappointed at the birth of a girl. To the mother's relief, the infant was quite easy to care for. The mother had worried about how her older daughter (15 months of age) would respond to the birth. She expected and feared feelings of rivalry, jealousy and hurt in the older child. To deal with this anticipated reaction the mother was careful to concentrate her attention on the older child, tending to leave the small infant unattended upstairs in a crib during the daytime hours, where she was "out of the main stream of things." When she fed or changed the infant she tried to do so out of sight of the older child, "so she wouldn't be jealous."

A home visit following hospitalization confirmed the impression of disturbance in the early mother-child relationship. The mother told the interviewer that by sixteen and one-half months the patient had become "a ravenous eater." "She eats more than her older sister who is two years and four months." The child by this time was a consistent thumb sucker. When asked about the child's use of toys or objects the mother replied, "She plays with everything, but the only thing she really likes is her thumb. She'd be a blanket baby if I let her—she sits and holds her dress and sucks her thumb."

The interviewer noted that although the child was up during the home visit, the mother did not pick her up, play with her, or talk to her. The only contact between the two was when the child fell out of her walker. The mother picked her up from the floor and placed her somewhere else.

2) Sixteen children over two years of age showed patterns of emotional disturbance. While in the opinion of the child psychiatrist the symptomatology sounded serious enough to warrant assessment for possible intervention, difficulties appeared to be either independent of the medical illness for which the child was hospitalized, or did not complicate its medical treatment.

Fifteen of the children in this group appeared to have either developmental difficulties of a general kind, or specific neurotic conflicts. In one instance the possibility of more serious psychopathology (either psychosis or an emerging borderline character structure) seemed likely.

3) Children whose maladaptation to either their illness or treatment regime seemed unlikely to interfere with effective implementation of their medical treatment. Eight children fell into this group.

4) Instances of significant psychiatric disorder in parents unrecognized by pediatric staff.

In eight instances in which children were evidencing difficulty in emotional adaptation, a decisive contributing factor was the presence of psychopathology in the parents for which psychiatric intervention appeared warranted. In general, the pediatric house staff focus their attention on the child directly—in no instance was a psychiatric consultation requested because of parental pathology in its own right, which might prevent the mother from caring adequately for her child. The pediatric house staff appeared to have only limited skill in differentiating evidence of significant parental psychopathology from the ranges of normal parental anxiety.

Example

A nine-year-old boy was admitted to the hospital on the basis of his mother's concern about "bloody" stools during an acute episode of gastroenteritis. The mother alleged that the child had lost at least a quart of blood with his stools. The boy himself minimized the bleeding, and following admission he did not appear seriously ill. His diarrhea quickly subsided with conservative medical management and there was no evidence of blood in his bowel movements thereafter.

Psychiatric screening interview revealed a mother who had been suffering a significant depression accompanied by moderate anxiety symptoms for several weeks prior to the boy's illness. Precipitating causes seemed to be a deteriorating relationship with her husband, and approaching middle age.

The mother expressed concern that she was babying her youngest son, the patient. She stated that as her family grew up it was hard for her to see the youngest one mature, and she found herself trying to keep him as a small boy.

Thus far, the boy himself appeared to be doing well in most spheres of his development. His mother complained during a follow-up home visit that her boy was spending so much time on his own, and "growing so independent." "He is so busy with projects he is giving me the brush-off and won't come on errands with me. He is too busy to play the piano with me in the evenings. I was much happier when the boys were small. I am miserable now that they are older and they know their own minds. If he and his father go off during the day, when they call I'll say did you miss me and he says 'no,' "

During the home visit the interviewer noted that the mother babied her son. She asked him if he would go for a drive with her later and he replied no. He said he was going out to play baseball. The mother said she would drive him to the game. As the boy talked his way out of the ride she was stroking his hair. When she asked him how he felt he replied "Fine." She asked "Were you dizzy today?" "Maybe a little." The mother turned to the interviewer and said, "You see, I told you he gets dizzy ever since he was in the hospital."

1. *Incidence of Psychopathology*

To assess the incidence of psychopathology in a special population such as that of the hospitalized child, one must compare it to the incidence of psychopathology in the population of children at large. Over the years a number of epidemiological studies have been undertaken to determine the incidence of psychopathology in childhood (8-10). These studies, conducted on populations of school-age children, have revealed an incidence of emotional difficulties ranging from 6% to 12% of the children studied. Comparatively an incidence of difficulty in emotional adaptation experienced by 63.7% of a population of hospitalized children seems high.

What factors may explain this high incidence? Our study does not provide definitive answers to this question. Two factors appear to us to be decisive. First, medical illness of a degree serious enough to warrant hospitalization constitutes a psychological stress of significant proportion, which many children do not master without symptom formation. In the children we studied, eight of those who had significant psychopathology (10% of the random sample) were experiencing emotional difficulties which were primarily related to difficulty in adapting to the illness for which they were hospitalized.

Of the remaining children with psychopathology in the random sample we studied, 53.7% had difficulties unrelated to adapting to medical illness that led to hospitalization. This incidence is approximately 40% greater than for the population at large. We believe this high frequency of emotional disorder may reflect a pattern of adaptation employed by many parents when they perceive signs that their child is in emotional distress. Often parents find it hard to integrate the awareness that their child is having psychological difficulties. A natural means of avoiding such an awareness is to focus on the child's physical problems whether they be real or imagined, whether primary or only peripheral to his overall adjustment.

If this assumption is correct, we would expect an unusually high incidence of emotional difficulties in any children hospitalized without clear-cut need. Of the twenty-four children judged by the child psychiatrist to have been hospitalized without need, twenty-one had been independently rated as having significant psychopathology and in need of psychiatric consultation. In short, one-third of the children studied in the hospital may not have needed to be there, and of those children, nine out of ten had significant emotional difficulties.

IMPLICATIONS FOR ORGANIZATION OF PSYCHIATRIC SERVICE IN THE PEDIATRIC SETTING

1. The Need for Psychiatric Screening

Our study suggests that often the pediatrician does not recognize significant psychopathology in the hospitalized child. In 42 of 51 children with significant psychopathology or difficulties in emotional adaptation, the ward pediatrician did not recognize evidence of failure in emotional adaptation. If this finding is representative, pediatrician and child psychiatrist need case-finding methods which will successfully spot the instances in which a child has emotional problems which would not otherwise be recognized. While many child psychiatrists rely increasingly on psychiatric ward rounds or comprehensive care rounds on the pediatric ward to provide the opportunity to observe directly the broader population of hospitalized children, it is our impression that only screening each pediatric admission, or screening a random sample of pediatric admissions would reveal accurately the range and incidence of emotional difficulties in the hospitalized children.

Even in hospitals where the limited availability of psychiatrists makes it impossible to expand consultation services, it is important that a representative group of the children with emotional difficulties be identified. Apart from his intervention in direct service to the child, the child psychiatrist on the pediatric wards serves by teaching the pediatrician to recognize the child who is failing in psychological adaptation and by helping the pediatrician to develop his ability to take care of such children. Those instances in which the pediatrician has not observed a child's emotional difficulty often provide particularly rich clinical material for child psychiatric teaching.

2. Implications for Programs in Community Mental Health

The possible usefulness of hospital pediatric services to programs of of Community Psychiatry has until the present received little emphasis. In a community of 75,000 people, 4,200 children under fifteen are likely to be hospitalized in each year.* On a basis of our study findings it

---

* In the United States in the year 1965-66, of children under fifteen, 56 per 1000 of the population were admitted for care in hospital pediatric services (11).

appears likely that approximately 2,500 of these children will have emotional difficulties warranting psychiatric intervention. It is our impression that this reservoir of children constitutes a problem in public mental health that has been previously unrecognized. Few of these children currently come to the attention of mental health professionals. Their needs remain largely unrecognized or unacknowledged. Our experience leads us to believe that child psychiatric programs implemented within the pediatric ward setting provide the best means for reaching the group of children we have described. These children are more accessible to therapeutic intervention while they are in the hospital than at any other time. Although most of the parents of the children we studied were not psychologically minded, as a group they were actively concerned for their children's welfare, and actively responsive to intervention at the time of their child's hospitalization. We found in the 81 families selected for the study only one parent refused to participate in the initial interview and subsequent home visit.

We found a high degree of parental cooperation despite the fact that many of the parents we interviewed initially were anxious, defensive, and sometimes distrustful. Nonetheless the interviewers in their role as hospital staff were able to establish a friendly alliance in almost every instance. By the time a mother had had a home visit usually the relationship with the interviewer was strong enough that it could have been used to help parents who otherwise might have become too defensive or hostile at the idea of psychiatric referral to seek psychiatric assessment of their child's development.

Programs of service relevant to the population encountered would include:

a) For mothers of infants under two years, regular home visits by trained child care workers who themselves have been effective mothers. These workers would be chosen on a basis of their personal capacity to empathize with young mothers as well as with their babies.

b) Individual psychotherapy for children with emerging internalized emotional conflicts.

c) Family group therapy for those families in which the parents' inner needs lead them to see a child with difficulty in emotional adaptation as physically ill.

d) Activity group therapy for those pre-adolescent children whose action orientation might make them unlikely candidates for individual psychotherapy.

We believe programs of psychiatric intervention designed to use to maximum advantage the context of the pediatric ward setting could constitute a crucial resource for any comprehensive program of community mental health designed to meet the needs of children.

SUMMARY AND CONCLUSION

1. We found a high incidence of psychopathology in a random sample of children admitted to the pediatric hospital. Of the children in the sample 63.7% were in need of psychiatric consultation.

2. The pediatric ward staff requested psychiatric consultation on only 11.3% of the sample.

3. Child psychiatrist and pediatrician agreed that approximately 70% of the children clearly needed hospitalization. The child psychiatrist felt that for 30% it was not necessary and was disadvantageous. The pediatrician regarded admission as not essential, but advantageous, for approximately 17% of the sample, and as clearly neither needed nor advantageous for 12.5% of the children studied.

4. In the group of children for whom hospitalization was judged unnecessary, the incidence of psychopathology was particularly great. Twenty-four of the twenty-seven children were independently judged to show signs of emotional disturbance.

Our study suggests to us that the pediatric hospital is already serving as a mental health resource to a large number of children, without any well-planned program to meet their needs. The hospital's usefulness as a resource is currently limited by the fact that too often hospitalization is used by the parent, and the doctor as well, to deny the child's emotional difficulty, rather than to delineate the child's emotional needs to help the child and his parents to achieve a realistic psychological adaptation.

REFERENCES

1. ZWERLING, I., TITCHENER, J., & GOTTSCHALK, L. ET AL.: Personality disorders and the relationship of emotion to surgical illness in 200 surgical patients. *Am. J. Psych.,* 112:270, 1955.
2. KAUFMAN, M. R., LEHMAN, S., FRANZBLAU, A. N. ET AL.: Psychiatric findings in admission to a medical service in a general hospital. *Journal of the Mt. Sinai Hospital,* 26, 2:160-170, 1959.
3. SHAPIRO, L. N., GROSSER, G. H., & VAILLANT, G. E.: The treatment gap in the general hospital: A study of the medical care needs of patients. Presented at the Annual Meeting of the American Psychiatric Association, Boston, Mass., May, 1968.

4. TISZA, V. B. & RICHARDSON, M. S.: The integration of a Mental Health program and a child psychiatry unit into a pediatric hospital. *Pediatrics*, 17, 1 (Jan. 1956).

5. TISZA, V. B. & ANGOFF, K.: A play program and its function in a pediatric hospital. *Pediatrics*, 19, 2 (Feb., 1957).

6. SHORE, M. F., GEISER, R. L., & WOLMAN, H. M.: Constructive uses of a hospital experience. *Children*, 12, 1 (Jan-Feb., 1965).

7. RUTTER, M.: Classification and Categorization in Child Psychiatry. *Journal of Child Pathology and Psychology* (Nov., 1965), pp. 71-83.

8. ULLMAN, C. A.: Identification of maladjusted school children. U.S. Public Health Service Monograph #7, Washington, 1952.

9. ROGERS, CARL: Mental Health findings in three elementary schools. *Educ. Research Bulletin* #21, 1942.

10. RUTTER, M. D. & GRAHAM, P. J.: Psychiatric Disorder in 10- and 11-year-old children. *Proc. Roy. Soc., Med.*, 59:382-387, 1966.

11. HEW, National Center for Health Statistics, Series 10, #50, Persons Hospitalized. February 1969, p. 4.

Part XI

ADULT OUTCOME OF CHILDHOOD DISORDER

Child psychiatrists frequently determine intervention strategies on the basis of their estimate of the long-term consequences of the deviant behavior displayed by a child. Actual data on the adult outcome of childhood disorders are, therefore, crucial information for the child psychiatrist.

Rutter's review article covers reports from several different countries and deals with the continuities and discontinuities of some well-defined child and adult disorders. Mellsop's paper describes a follow-up study of several thousand Australian children referred for behavior disorders to assess their rate of psychiatric impairment in adulthood, 20 years later. Although he found that the risk of being an adult patient was four times higher in these children than in the general population, he indicates the difficulty of identifying predictive indices of adult illness in childhood.

40

RELATIONSHIPS BETWEEN CHILD AND ADULT PSYCHIATRIC DISORDERS

Some Research Considerations

M. L. Rutter

The Institute of Psychiatry (London)

It is frequently assumed that psychiatric disorders have their roots in childhood and child psychiatrists have sometimes claimed that psychiatric treatment at an early age "goes a long way toward guaranteeing emotional health in the adult" (Howells, 1965). Would that it did, but unfortunately there is not a scrap of evidence that this is the case. Nevertheless, information on continuities and discontinuities from child psychiatric disorder to adult mental illness is of importance to both child and adult psychiatrists. The present paper considers the topic in terms of recent research findings—mostly from epidemiological investigations (Rutter et al., 1971) and long-term follow-up studies (Robins, 1971). A development approach will be followed in an attempt to delineate possible mechanisms underlying the relationships between child and adult psychiatric disorders. Possible links with childhood will be examined, taking each of the main adult psychiatric syndromes in turn—starting with the schizophrenic psychoses.

Reprinted from ACTA PSYCHIATRICA SCANDINAVICA 48, pp. 3-21, 1972. Read before the Nordic Psychiatric Society Conference, Bergen, Norway, May 26-28, 1971.

SCHIZOPHRENIC PSYCHOSES

Autism

Until recent years it has been generally assumed that infantile autism, the "psychosis" most characteristic of the infancy period, was the earliest manifestation of schizophrenia. In fact, autism was often considered under the heading of "schizophrenic syndrome in childhood" (Creak, 1961). There is now good evidence that this view was mistaken and that whatever the nature of infantile autism, it has nothing to do with schizophrenia.

A consideration of the clinical features of infantile autism and of schizophrenia emphasize the marked differences between the two disorders (Rutter, 1968). The sex ratio differs: autism is much commoner in boys whereas schizophrenia occurs with about equal frequency in the two sexes. Social class background differs: autistic children tend to come from professional and middle-class families but schizophrenics do not. The two disorders differ in terms of a family history of schizophrenia: this is common with schizophrenics and rare with autistics. Mental subnormality is a common feature of autism but it is not a characteristic of schizophrenia. The pattern of cognitive abilities also differentiates the two disorders. Delusions and hallucinations are very common symptoms in schizophrenia but they are quite rare in autistic children even after they reach maturity. Marked remissions and relapses are well recognized in schizophrenia but are decidedly uncommon in autism.

Kolvin and his colleagues (1971) in their systematic comparison between infantile psychoses and psychoses beginning in later childhood have found similar differences. Early and late childhood psychoses differ in symptomatology, family and social background, maternal characteristics, and cognitive factors. The psychoses beginning in later childhood appeared generally similar to adult-type schizophrenia. It may be concluded that schizophrenia may begin with psychotic symptoms in later childhood but only rarely are these psychotic symptoms overt before age 7 or 8 years.

Several independent studies of the children of schizophrenic mothers have shown that they do *not* develop infantile autism whereas they do have a much increased rate of schizophrenia and schizophreniform psychoses (Reisby, 1967; Heston, 1966; Rosenthal et al., 1968). There is also probably some increase in the rate of mental subnormality and antisocial behavior.

Finally, studies following autistic children from early childhood into adult life have shown that even when adult they are quite unlike schizophrenics (Rutter, 1970a; Kanner 1971). In particular, they do not develop delusions and hallucinations. Language abnormalities usually persist, interpersonal relationships improve but remain deficient, and obsessive-like oddities of behavior diminish but do not disappear. Perhaps the most striking finding to emerge from the follow-up studies of autistic children is the major difference in outcome between those of normal intelligence and those with associated mental retardation. The autistic child of low IQ has a poor prognosis in all respects and is likely to develop epileptic fits. Nearly all of those with an IQ below 50 will end up in long-term institutional care. In sharp contrast, the autistic child of normal IQ has a much better prognosis. Although very few will recover, some two-fifths will improve sufficiently to hold a steady job.

Much has yet to be learned about the causation of infantile autism but it seems reasonably certain that the disorder is quite distinct from adult schizophrenia. Whereas the exact nature of the basic defect in autism has still to be defined, the evidence points to some kind of cognitive, perceptual, or language deficit (Rutter, 1971a).

Schizophrenia

If schizophrenia does not begin as autism, what are its origins in childhood? Evidence is gradually accumulating on this question and it is clear that individuals who develop overt schizophrenia in adult life have frequently shown abnormalities of a non-psychotic type in childhood (Lane & Albee, 1965, 1966; Frazee 1953; Bower et al., 1960; Robins, 1966; Michael et al., 1957; Morris et al., 1954, 1956; Gardner, 1967; Stabenau & Pollin, 1967; Barthell & Holmes 1968). They are likely to have had a slightly lower birthweight than their sibs, a somewhat lower IQ (although possibly not a falling IQ as once thought (Lane & Albee, 1968)), poorer achievement at school, greater social isolation, oddity, and impaired relationships. In personality traits they most commonly have shown a mixture of introverted and extroverted characteristics. When they have shown overt psychiatric disorder in childhood, it has not followed any distinctive pattern; there may have been neurotic or antisocial problems but perhaps most commonly the disorders showed features of both.

While these studies undoubtedly indicate that schizophrenia often begins with prepsychotic abnormalities in childhood, the abnormalities do not constitute a sufficiently distinctive pattern to be used for predictive purposes. However, the findings do suggest that there may be a dichotomy between schizophrenics who have difficulties in childhood before the onset of psychosis and those who do not (Offord & Cross, 1969).

Anthony (1968) in the U.S.A. and Mednick & Schulsinger (1968) in Scandinavia have both undertaken prospective studies of the offspring of schizophrenic parents in an attempt to provide more specific indicators of a liability to schizophrenia. Anthony has not yet published definitive findings but the Scandinavia study showed that the children of schizophrenic mothers who eventually break down have had more obstetric complications in their birth history and have exhibited deviant autonomic nervous function. These findings are still too general to be used for the detection of children who will become schizophrenic in adult life but they take us one step in that direction.

NEUROSIS

Emotional disorders in childhood involving anxiety, phobias, obsessions, hypochondriasis, and the like are usually termed neurotic disorders. Although, perhaps, these disorders tend to be less clearly differentiated and less fixed in childhood than in adult life, they have much the same phenomenology as adult neurosis and it is usually assumed that there is a continuity between child neurosis and adult neurosis. This is implicit in case history-taking schemes for adult patients which generally include a section for "neurotic symptoms in childhood" (Slater & Roth, 1969). However, rather surprisingly, recent research suggests that, at least in part, this view may be mistaken.

This unexpected finding is most clearly shown in an exceptionally thorough and well-planned 30-year follow-up study of some 500 child psychiatric patients and a suitably chosen control group of 100, undertaken by Lee Robins (1966). She found that neurosis in adult life was more common in her child clinic patients than in her control subjects. Most of the children referred for neurotic type problems were *not* neurotic as adults, although fewer were psychiatrically normal compared with controls.

Taken in isolation this finding would carry little weight, in spite of the high quality of the study. The number of neurotic children was quite small and there is doubt on how far children referred to clinics for neurotic disorder in the 1920's, when the clinic emphasis was largely on delinquency and antisocial behavior, are similar to neurotic children attending today's clinics. But there is confirmatory evidence. The Dallas follow-up study of "shy, withdrawn" children (Michael et al., 1957) found most to be functioning well as adults—how well cannot be determined as no control group was used. A variety of medium-term follow-up studies of neurotic children and adolescents have shown that most have a good prognosis (Robins, 1971). Short-term investigations of response to treatment also show that neurotic children have the best outcome of all groups. On the other hand, Pritchard & Graham (1966) showed that of those neurotic children who *were* under psychiatric care as adults, most exhibited some form of neurotic or depressive condition. It must be concluded that there is some continuity between child neurosis and adult neurosis but that possibly this continuity applies to only a *minority* of each. Most neurotic children become normal adults and most neurotic adults develop their neurosis only in adult life.

This poses the question: What is the difference between the emotional disorders of childhood which clear up without trace and those which persist or recur to become adult neurosis? So far there are only very preliminary and partial answers to this question. Perhaps the clearest difference concerns phobic disorders (Marks & Gelder, 1966; Rutter et al., 1970) where there are important clinical distinctions according to age of onset. Agaraphobia begins at any time from late childhood to middle life, social anxieties usually start after puberty, specific situational phobias have no characteristic age of onset, and specific animal phobias *always* begin in childhood. The fears that specifically begin in childhood—such as fear of the dark or fear of animals—are ones which show a regular and pronounced fall with increasing age (Shepherd et al., 1971). Possibly, they are also ones which frequently occur in isolation without other evidence of general emotional disturbance. Thus, animal phobias in adults frequently occur as an isolated symptom.

The other difference between child and adult neurotic disorders concerns the sex ratio. In childhood, neurotic disorders have an almost equal sex ratio although they are slightly commoner in girls (Rutter et al., 1970). In adults, however, neurotic disorders are *much* commoner in women (Shepherd et al., 1966). This change in sex distribution of neurosis takes place during adolescence. Up to age 15 years males outnumber females among psychiatric referrals. From then onwards the predominance of female patients increased (Baldwin, 1968) with neurosis as the single commonest diagnostic category (Henderson et al., 1967; Kidd & Dixon, 1968).

That this sex difference by age may have some meaning is suggested by findings from studies examining associations between parental neurosis and child neurosis in members of the same family. Shepherd et al. (1966) studying general practice found that whereas *daughters* of neurotic mothers had higher rates of neurosis than did the control girls, the difference was less marked for sons. We found exactly the same when studying the children of patients attending psychiatric clinics. The daughters showed more disorder than controls but the difference for sons was smaller and not statistically significant (Rutter, 1970b). More recently, the finding has been replicated once more in an investigation of the families of 10-year-old children on the Isle of Wight. Neurosis in the mother was associated with emotional and behavioral problems in *daughters* but not in sons.

Possible explanations for these findings have been considered previously (Rutter, 1970a) with the tentative conclusion that the effect of parental neurosis on girls is largely genetic. Where there is continuity between child neurosis and adult neurosis, hereditary factors may be largely responsible. As adult neurosis is so much commoner in women than in men, this continuity would be more evident in girls than in boys.

If this continuity is genetically based, and this remains a hypothesis still to be tested, are the genetic factors concerned with personality variables such as "neuroticism" or are they concerned with "illness?" The former seems more likely. There are quite strong associations between the personality characteristic of "neuroticism" and the presence of neurotic illness (Eysenck, 1960). Although temperamental stability is much less marked in the preschool years (Rutter, 1970b), there is evidence of continuity from middle childhood to adult life for the neuroticism personality dimension (Bronson, 1969). However, the continuity of neuroticism as measured by the scales used in adults (Eysenck & Eysenck, 1969) has still to be empirically demonstrated.

What then is the explanation for those varieties of child neurosis which are entirely transitory and unrelated to adult neurosis? It will be clear that no satisfactory answer is yet possible. Nevertheless the scanty data available do suggest some tentative conclusions. Many "neurotic" manifestations in childhood are no more than exaggerations of normal developmental trends. Separation anxiety is entirely normal in the toddler but in some children it is more marked and more persistent than average. A fear of dogs is exceedingly common in preschool children and forms part of a normal maturational sequence. In some children, it is more severe and prolonged than in others. The same may be said of numerous other emotional "symptoms." Indeed, perhaps, it is inappropriate to regard them as "symptoms" at all—they are not manifestations of illness when mild and possibly also they are not when severe.

Extending this argument, it could be said that those emotional disorders which are not precursors of adult neurosis are more likely to be an exaggeration of normal developmental features. Thus, on this hypothesis, separation anxiety in the young child should be less likely to lead adult neurosis than separation anxiety in an older child. There is not much evidence on this point but in keeping with this view is the finding from one study that school phobia in the child just starting school has a better prognosis than school phobia in the eleven-year-old (Rodriguez et al., 1959). If this is a general finding the conclusion would be that where a neurotic manifestation is age-appropriate in type (although abnormal in severity or persistence) it is more benign than where it is age-inappropriate.

On the same grounds, the prognosis should be better where the neurotic feature occurs in isolation rather than as part of a more general emotional disturbance. This seems highly likely but evidence on the point is lacking.

If neuroses continuing into adulthood are strongly related to the personality feature of neuroticism, one might expect the transitory disorders of childhood to be less strongly tied to personality characteristics and perhaps more influenced by environmental circumstances. If this is so, neuroses in children of a non-neurotic personality or where there are environmental features which have played a crucial role in pathogenesis should have a better prognosis. This could be tested but it has not yet been done.

However, indirect support is provided by Sundby & Kreyberg's finding (1969) that the quality of a child's emotional relationships and his ability to form friendships were important prognostic factors in child neurosis. A similar association was found by Roff (1961) with respect to later antisocial conduct.

If transitory "neurotic" disorders are more often directly due to environmental stresses, why should they occur more often in boys (as would seem to be the case as the more persistent familial neuroses are mainly in girls)? Again, there is no well-established answer, but there is evidence that at least in some circumstances boys are more susceptible to environmental stresses than are girls (Rutter, 1970b). Certainly, boys are more prone to suffer ill effects from physical hazards and some findings suggest they are also more vulnerable to psychological and social influences.

Finally, in so far as continuity of neurosis is a function of continuity of personality one might expect neuroses in the preschool child to be more often transitory because temperamental features are less well established and show less constancy at that age. Wolff's follow-up study of preschool children attending a psychiatric clinic (1961) does not really support this view, but once more evidence is lacking.

This discussion has moved a long way into the realms of speculation and relevant facts are rather sparse. My reason for straying so far from established findings is simply that if we are to understand the nature of childhood neurosis, it is essential that we think of ways of examining how child neurosis differs from adult neurosis and of testing hypotheses about the psychological mechanisms underlying these differences. What is clear is that only some neuroses in childhood persist into adult life. Those that do not persist seem to differ in some important respects from neurotic disorders as they occur in adults. It is suggested that the continuity from childhood to adult life in this instance may be related to the presence of personality attributes which have an important genetic component. Those emotional disorders in childhood which are purely transitory, in contrast, may be due more often to developmental changes or to transient environmental stresses. Whether or not this hypothesis is correct, the nature of associations and lack of associations between child neurosis and adult neurosis warrants careful study.

"NEUROTIC TRAITS OF CHILDHOOD"

Before passing on to other disorders, a word is necessary on so-called neurotic traits of childhood. In the Slater & Roth (1969) history-taking scheme these included thumb-sucking, nail-biting, faddiness about food, stammering, and bed-wetting. Other schemes include similar features.

Epidemiological studies have clearly demonstrated that whatever these items represent, they do not represent neurosis of the child or adult variety (Rutter et al., 1970). Nail-biting is extremely common, being present in about a third of school age children, and it has little association with any general measure of neurosis, maladjustment, or psychiatric disorder. It may reflect some degree of tension but there is good evidence that it should not be equated with psychopathology. Thumb-sucking, similarly, is a very common feature in preschool children and of no particular significance. In older children it may indicate some emotional immaturity but it is only weakly related to neurosis. Food fads, too, are very frequent, and in only a minority of cases do they form part of a neurotic disorder. The cause of stammering is ill-understood but there is no reason for regarding it as a neurotic trait (Andrews & Harris, 1964). Bed-wetting in young children is mainly a developmental disorder which occurs in isolation and has little to do with neurosis. However, enuresis has multiple origins and in some children bed-wetting does form part of a general psychiatric disorder. But even in these cases the association is not particularly with neurosis; enuresis is just as likely to be linked with delinquency and antisocial behavior.

All in all, it is evident that there has been considerable conceptual confusion in choosing items to measure "neurotic traits in childhood." This part of the history-taking procedure needs radical revision.

DEPRESSION

Affective disorder is one of the most common psychiatric conditions in adult life but it is only rarely diagnosed in prepubertal children. Depression does not even appear in the index of Kanner's textbook on child psychiatry (1957). Indeed, Slater & Roth (1969) have claimed that "children . . . are almost immune to lasting changes of mood. The capacity for prolonged mood changes appears at puberty." Almost certainly this goes too far. Depression can and does occur in childhood. Nevertheless, it does appear to be the case that mood changes tend to be less persistent before puberty and numerous studies support the claim that depressive disorder is diagnosed much more frequently in adults than in children.

General practice studies in Britain have shown affective disorder to occur in about 10 per 1000 adults over a one-year period (Rawnsley, 1968), whereas a British total population study of 10- to 11-year-old children found a one year period of prevalence of only 1.4 per 1000 (Rutter et al., 1970). Hospital statistics show even bigger differences. In the Maudsley Hospital, for example, manic-depressive disorder and neurotic depression between them account for over two-fifths of all new outpatient referrals (Hare, 1968). In contrast, in childhood, depression does not even warrant a category of its own. Manic-depressive psychosis is almost unknown (Anthony & Scott, 1962) and neurotic depression is rarely diagnosed before puberty. Figures for suicide and attempted suicide follow the same pattern. Suicide is exceedingly rare before puberty and then shows a rising incidence during adolescence (Schaffer, 1971). Suicidal attempts are more frequent but again are uncommon before puberty and show a rising incidence during the teenage years (Connell, 1965). The meagre evidence on reactions to bereavement also suggests that grief is usually milder and of shorter duration in children than in adults (Marris, 1958; Burlingham & Freud, 1942, 1944).

All these findings would seem to support the notion that depressive disorder is essentially confined to adults. However, this view has recently come under sharp attack—particularly from Frommer (1968) working at St. Thomas' Hospital, London. She has claimed that about a quarter of her child psychiatric patients suffer from depression. Annell (1969) in Sweden, reporting on the use of lithium carbonate with manic-depressive illness in children, has also suggested that this is a more common condition in childhood than previously thought.

Several issues are involved in this controversy. The first is whether depression—as a symptom—occurs in childhood. The findings in this connection are reasonably clear-cut. Children rarely complain of depression as such, but misery and unhappiness are common symptoms as shown by studies of children in the general population (Rutter et al., 1970) as well as in those attending psychiatric clinics (Rutter, 1966). However, unhappiness as a symptom and depressive illness are not the same thing.

The second issue is whether the clinical syndrome of manic-depressive psychosis as seen in adults occurs in childhood. Again there is little disagreement. The syndrome is a rare occurrence before puberty. However, even in adults, neurotic depression is a much commoner disorder than a cyclic psychosis. There is more doubt on the question of how frequently a straightforward neurotic depression occurs in children. Frommer's figures (1968) suggest that this may be more common than previously supposed, but the matter requires further study.

The most important issue is the third: that is, whether depression occurs in childhood but does so in a form which differs from that in adult life. Various writers other than Frommer have suggested that depression in children may manifest itself in a masked form as somatic symptoms, antisocial behavior, enuresis, and accident proneness (Toolan, 1962; Faux & Rowley, 1967; Glaser, 1967). This is certainly possible. There are several disorders in which symptoms change with age. For example, severe *over*activity in early childhood changes to *under*activity in later childhood and early adolescence (Rutter et al., 1967). The issue is an important one. If depressive illness really does begin in childhood in a disguised form, this would be a matter of great theoretical and practical concern to both child and adult psychiatrists.

Unfortunately, the evidence to date is rather unsatisfactory. Frommer (1968) and Annell (1969) have both followed the strategy of examining the efficacy of anti-depressant medication in children they have regarded as depressive. Their clinical observations suggest that mono-amide oxidase inhibitors, tricyclic antidepressants and lithium carbonate may all be beneficial. Regrettably, this strategy is of very limited usefulness for several quite different reasons. First, the efficacy of these drugs in children has not yet been systematically evaluated through controlled trials. Until such trials have been undertaken, the uncontrolled clinical findings must be treated with considerable reserve and caution. Second, the value of some of these drugs in adult depressive disorders is not entirely certain and may well vary with the type of depression (Pare, 1968; Blackwell & Shepherd, 1968; Melia, 1970). Third, anti-depressants have other therapeutic effects, such as relieving enuresis (Shaffer et al, 1968). Accordingly, in order to use drugs to test the validity of a diagnosis of depression in childhood, it is necessary not only to show that anti-depressants are more effective than a placebo (even this is still a task for the future) but also to demonstrate that the effect is specific to children with symptoms thought to indicate depression.

This might be carried out as part of a study of symptom patterns in childhood. If a group of symptoms suggesting depression could be found by some kind of cluster or principle components analysis, then the validity of using these to diagnose depressive *disorder* (as distinct from depressive symptoms) might be assessed by determining whether children with these symptoms differed from other clinic children in any systematic way. In other words, do depressive thieves differ from other thieves? One comparison would be on the efficacy of anti-depressive medication. In each case the comparison would have to be made with children who share the same symptoms apart from depression. As well as on the response to drugs, the groups might be compared on a wide range of other variables including family history, precipitating factors, duration, nature of onset, sex, intellectual and scholastic attainment. If the presence of depressive symptoms proved to be linked with other features differentiating the groups, this would go some way towards showing the validity of depression as a diagnosis in prepubertal children.

Short-term follow-up studies would also be useful. If depression is thought to *underlie* the development of other symptoms such as abdominal pain, aggression, and truancy, the question is what happens to these other symptoms when the child ceases to be depressed, either as a result of medication or as a consequence of the natural course of the disorder. If the other symptoms persisted in spite of the loss of depression, then some doubt would be cast on the concept of depressive illness unless some additional reason were found to explain their non-disappearance. Yet another study waiting to be undertaken.

Family history studies might be of more value if the genetic basis of depressive illness in adults was more clear-cut and better understood. As it is, the findings are complex and difficult to interpret (Price, 1968), so that comparisons with childhood are likely to be of only very limited use. Even so, some light might be thrown on the concept of depressive illness in childhood if either (A) the *children* of depressed adults could be shown to have particular features, or (B) if the *parents* of children thought to be depressed had specific characteristics. Neither has been demonstrated up to now. In a clinic study of associations between parental mental illness and psychiatric disorder in the child, no relationship could be found between the parental diagnosis and the child's diagnosis or the parental symptoms and the child's symptoms (Rutter, 1966). Disorders in the children of depressed parents did not differ from those in the children of parents with other types of psychiatric disorder. Conversely, when the child had symptoms of depression, sleep disorder, abdominal pain, and the like, there is nothing characteristic about the parental disorder. The same conclusions apply to preliminary findings from a recent investigation (Rutter, 1970b) examining the effects of parental illness on the children. Disorders in the children of depressed parents do not seem to differ significantly from those in the children of schizophrenic, anxious, and alcoholic parents. Frommer (1968) found, as we did, that mental illness was common in the parents of children with all sorts of psychiatric disorder and that the rate of parental illness was not significantly higher in children thought to be depressed. She implied that depression may be commoner in the parents of depressed children than in the parents of "neurotic" children but gave no figures to support this. Further studies are needed but the evidence to date provides no support for the concept of adult-type depressive illness in prepubertal children.

Another approach would be to examine disorders in childhood which appear to have a depressive component in order to determine what features they have in common with adult depressive illness. Frommer (1968) has provided some data of this kind. Looking at symptoms it is immediately apparent that only a *minority* of children diagnosed as depressive complain of depression or early waking, but this might be just an age difference in the expression of symptoms, as moodiness and weepiness were common complaints in children. Perhaps the most striking feature of her findings is that in two out of her three depressive groups, boys predominate. This stands in sharp contrast to the findings in adult depressives when women outnumber men by 2 to 1 (Rawnsley, 1968).

The most direct way of determining whether depressive illness starts in childhood, as suggested, is to find out whether child psychiatric disorder of any type leads on to depressive illness in adult life. The available studies seem to indicate that this does *not* usually happen. I have already referred to Robins' long-term follow-up study of children who had attended a child guidance clinic (Robins, 1966). She found that clinic children when adult did *not* have a higher rate of either manic-depressive disease or of anxiety neurosis compared with control children. Similarly, Huffman & Wenig (1954) found no relationship between psychoneurosis or manic-depressive disease in adult life and any form of childhood problem behavior. Or again, similar findings stemmed from Pritchard & Graham's study (1966) of a group of patients who had attended both the child and adult departments of the Maudsley Hospital. They showed that parental illness in this group was *less* likely to be depressive than in the group of Maudsley patients as a whole, suggesting that depression usually began in adult life and was not preceded by any childhood disorder. The matter requires further investigation but so far the findings all indicate that it is quite *un*common for child psychiatric disorder of any type to develop into depressive illness in adult life.

Obviously, many ends remain untied and the controversies regarding depression in prepubertal children are far from resolved. The evidence seems to suggest that depressive symptomatology is rather commoner in prepubertal children than sometimes supposed and investigations into the use of anti-depressive medication would be very worthwhile. On the other hand, it appears that adult-type depressive illness only rarely begins in childhood and, for the most part, childhood depression is not the same as manic-depressive psychosis. These conclusions are necessarily very tentative. Their confirmation or refutation is an important task for further research. Answers to the problems posed on childhood depression would shed important light both on the origins of adult depressive illness and on the nature of psychiatric disorders in childhood.

ADOLESCENT "TURMOIL"

Adolescence has long been held to be a period of turmoil and upheaval and psychiatric disorders appearing at this time are frequently attributed to the difficulties consequent upon puberty and its psychological sequelae (Masterson, 1968). As a result of this view the diagnosis of "situational adjustment reaction" has been widely used for adolescents admitted to American mental hospitals (Rosen et al., 1968). Implicit in this diagnosis is the assumption that the conditions are reactive to temporary stresses and should prove to be transient.

Several follow-up studies have shown that this concept is mistaken—at least with regard to the adolescents who get referred to psychiatrists.

Masterson (1967) found that the outcome varied according to clinical picture in much the same way as in other age groups. Sociopaths did poorly, neurotics did very well, and the outcome for schizophrenics varied according to previous personality and the presence of depression or confusion. The same pattern at follow-up was found for adolescents seen at psychiatric outpatient clinics (Capes, 1971) and those admitted to inpatient psychiatric units (Annesley, 1961; Warren, 1965). Neurotics do well, those with antisocial disorders less well, and schizophrenics worst of all.

It must be concluded that psychiatric disorder in adolescence is not appreciably different from that in other age groups. If there is a clinical syndrome approximating that seen in adults, the prognosis is similar to that in adults and there is no good reason to consider the condition a reflection of "adolescent turmoil." Milder emotional problems not amounting to overt psychiatric disorder may well be a function of the developmental changes associated with adolescence but, even so, epidemiological studies suggest that the frequency of psychological disturbance in adolescence has been much exaggerated in the past (Weiner, 1970). While there are important developmental issues to be resolved at this age period, most youngsters emerge unscathed. In this connection it should be noted that as judged both by general practice studies and by clinic referral rates (Innes & Sharp, 1962; Kessel & Shepherd, 1962), psychiatric disorder is not at a peak in adolescence. The rates are still rising in late adolescence to reach a peak later in middle life.

PSYCHOPATHY

In the conditions considered so far, the links between child and adult psychiatric disorder have been rather uncertain or rather nonspecific. The one adult condition with reasonably reliable and specific antecedents is psychopathy (Robins, 1966). In Robins' long-term followup of child guidance clinic attenders, psychopaths were most likely to have shown a wide range of repeated antisocial behavior in childhood, the delinquent acts occurring in the community at large as well as at home and at school, and leading to at least one juvenile court appearance. Only about half such children will become psychopaths but very few psychopaths will not have shown this behavior in childhood. Antisocial behavior was most likely to persist into adult life if the child's parents and grandparents were also antisocial (Robins & Lewis, 1966). As shown also in other studies (e.g., Otterstrom, 1946), when antisocial behavior persists, it is frequently accompanied by a wide range of other social and psychological handicaps including marital disruption, poor work record, alcoholism, alienation from relatives, poor health, and financial dependency. Whereas many essentially normal individuals commit isolated delinquent acts (Belson, 1968), the prognosis for the child with repeated delinquency in several different settings is quite poor.

Moreover continuity of behavior does not begin with the delinquency. Several studies (Mulligan et al., 1963; Conger & Miller, 1966; Havighurst et al., 1962) have shown that delinquents are differentiable from other children even before delinquency begins. Delinquents-to-be are retarded in their educational attainments, unpopular, resentful of authority, impulsive, and aggressive. Wolff (1971) has shown that aggressive disobedient behavior and frank delinquency constitute different clusters of symptoms but the two clusters have similar correlates with external variables (Rutter et al., 1970) and longitudinal studies show that children aggressive at one age are often delinquent when older.

The reasons for this continuity between childhood antisocial disorder and adult psychopathy need to be explored. It might be thought that such persistence of abnormal behavior in conjunction with the fact that antisocial disorders frequently "run in families" must mean a genetically determined disorder of some kind, but this is probably *not* the case. Twin studies of antisocial and delinquent children show a high level of concordance in *both* monozygotic and dizygotic pairs, implying an environmental rather than a genetic basis to the disorder (Slater, 1953). Furthermore, the association between criminal behavior in the parents and antisocial disorder in the children is also probably environmentally determined. Bohman (1970) showed that criminality in the biological parents was *not* associated with disorder in their children when the children had been adopted in infancy, in sharp contrast to the situation when children are reared by their criminal parents.

These findings are only explicable in environmental terms. Our own studies have shown that the association between parental disorder and antisocial disorder in the sons is determined by the presence of marital discord and disharmony (Rutter, 1971). West's prospective study (1969) has also shown that once the effect of family variables has been partialled out, the presence of a criminal father does not add to the risk of the child's becoming delinquent.

Taken together, these findings all point to the importance of environmental factors in the genesis of delinquency. It is also known that temperamental characteristics (Rutter, 1971b; West, 1967), which may well have a large genetic component, affect the likelihood of a child's becoming delinquent. Also, it is uncertain how far the findings on environmental influences apply to the hard core of persistent psychopaths as distinct from the wider field of antisocial behavior. It could be that genetic factors may be more important in this smaller group of severe and persistent disorders. But on the evidence to date, it seems that the link between antisocial parents and delinquency in their children is mediated in large part by environmental influences. In so far as this is so, it should theoretically be possible to prevent the development of antisocial problems in some children. Unfortunately, attempts to do so in the past by counselling methods or group discussions with parents have proved singularly unsuccessful (Powers & Witmer, 1951; Tait & Hodges, 1962; Gildea et al., 1967) and psychiatrists up to now have not been able to produce any satisfactory answer to the question of how delinquency should be prevented. However, no problem is more worthy of study and no solution is likely to be more rewarding, for there should be no mistake about the dimensions of the public health challenge we face. Robins (1966) showed that antisocial children frequently had antisocial parents and grandparents, these children often became sociopathic adults, and the final chapter to the story concerns their children who are now showing evidence of problem behavior-continuity over four generations!

One other syndrome of childhood which needs mentioning with respect to the development of psychopathy is the hyperkinetic syndrome, characterized by poorly organized overactivity, distractibility, short attention span, and impulsiveness. Marked mood fluctuations, aggressive and destructive behavior also commonly occur, and the syndrome is often accompanied by minor neurologic abnormalities and learning difficulties (Werry, 1968). Not much is known about the eventual outcome of these children except that the prognosis for overall social adjustment is poor. A few develop psychosis and many have persisting abnormalities of personality often associated with criminal behavior (Menkes et al., 1967).

CONCLUSION

Although we have learned a lot about relationships between child and adult psychiatric disorders, this survey has shown that some of the most important questions remain unanswered. Now that it appears very likely that infantile autism has no connection with schizophrenia, it is all the more necessary to delineate precisely which childhood behaviors are portents of schizophrenia. In spite of the surface similarities between child neurosis and adult neurosis, research findings suggest that there are also important differences between the two conditions which require further exploration. Also many of the so-called neurotic traits of child-hood are now known not to be anything of the kind. Depression can occur in childhood but how often it does so remains a matter of controversy and the continuities and discontinuities between depression in young children and depressive illness in adults have still to be established. Adolescent turmoil has been found to be less important as a cause of psychiatric disorder than once thought and disorders in adolescence have few distinctive features. Psychopathy is the one disorder which has its roots most firmly set in childhood with repeated and widespread antisocial behavior in early life often leading to later persisting disorders of personality. In spite of the persistence of this behavior from childhood to adult life, it appears that environmental factors are most important in its genesis. This finding illustrates the fact that whether or not a disorder is transient is not a good guide to its pathogenesis.

REFERENCES

ANDREWS, G. & HARRIS, M. (1964): The syndrome of stuttering. (Clinics in Developmental Medicine No. 17.) Spastics Medical Education and Information Unit in association with Heinemann Medical Books, London.

ANNELL, A. L. (1969): Manic-depressive illness in children and effect of treatment with lithium carbonate. Acta Paedopsychiat., 36, 292-301.

ANNESLEY, P. T. (1961): Psychiatric illness in adolescence: presentation and prognosis. J. Ment. Sci., 107, 268-278.

ANTHONY, E. J. (1968): The developmental precursors of adult schizophrenia. J. Psychiat. Res., 6, Suppl. 1, 293-316.

ANTHONY, F. & SCOTT, P. (1962): Manic-depressive psychosis in childhood. J. Child Psychol., 1, 53-72.

BALDWIN, J. A. (1968): Psychiatric illness from birth to maturity: An epidemiological study. Acta Psychiat. Scand., 44, 313-333.

BARTHELL, C. N. & HOLMES, D. S. (1968): High school yearbooks: A non-reactive measure of social isolation in graduates who later became schizophrenic. J. Abnorm. Soc. Psychol., 73, 313-316.

BELSON, W. A. (1968): The extent of stealing by London boys and some of its origins. Advanc. Sci., December, 171-184.

BLACKWELL, B. & SHEPHERD, M. (1968): Prophylactic lithium: Another therapeutic myth? Lancet, 1, 968-971.

BOWER, E. M., SHELLHAMER, T. A., & DAILY, J. M. (1960): School characteristics of male adolescents who later become schizophrenic. Amer. J. Orthopsychiat., 30, 712-729.

BRONSON, W. C. (1969): Stable patterns of behavior; the significance of enduring orientations for personality development. In: J. P. Hill (Ed.): Minnesota Symposia on Child Psychology, Vol. 2. Minneapolis: University of Minnesota Press.

BURLINGHAM, D. & FREUD, A. (1942): Young Children in Wartime London.

BURLINGHAM, D. & FREUD, A. (1944): Infants Without Families. London: Allen & Unwin,

CAPES, M. (1970): Stress in Youth—A Study of the Psychiatric Treatment, Schooling and Care of 150 Adolescents. London: Oxford University Press.

CONGER, J. J. & MILLER, W. C. (1966): *Personality, Social Class, and Delinquency.* New York: J. Wiley.

CONNELL, P. H. (1965): Suicidal attempts in childhood and adolescence. In J. G. Howells (Ed.): *Modern Perspectives in Child Psychiatry.* New York: Brunner/Mazel.

CREAK, M. (Chairman) (1961): Schizophrenic syndrome in childhood: Progress report of a working party. *Cerebr. Palsy Bull.,* 3, 501-504.

EYSENCK, H. J. & EYSENCK, S. B. G. (1969): *Personality Structure and Measurement.* (Ed.): *Handbook of Abnormal Psychology.* London: Pitman.

EYSENCK, H. J. & EYSENCK, S. B. G. (1969): *Personality Structure and Measurement.* London: Routledge & Kegan Paul.

FAUX, E. J. & ROWLEY, G. M. (1967): Detecting depressions in childhood. *Hosp. Community Psychiat.,* 18, 51-58.

FRAZEE, H. E. (1953): Children who later became schizophrenic. *Smith College Studies in Social Work,* 23, 125-149.

FROMMER, E. (1968): Depressive illness in childhood. In A. Coppen & A. Walk (Eds.): *Recent Developments in Affective Disorders. Brit. J. Psychiat.* Spec. Publ. No. 2. London: R.M.P.A.

GARDNER, G. C. (1967): The relationship between childhood neurotic symptomatology and later schizophrenia in males and females. *J. Nerv. Ment. Dis.,* 144, 97-100.

GILDEA, M. C. L., GLIDEWELL, J. C., & KANTOR, M. B. (1967): The St. Louis School Mental Health Project: History and evaluation. In E. L. Cowen, E. A. Gardner & M. Zax (Eds.): *Emergent Approaches to Mental Health Problems.* New York: Meredith Publishing Co.

GLASER, K. (1967): Masked depression in children and adolescents. *Amer. J. Psychother.,* 21, 565-574.

HARE, E. H. (1968): *Triennial Statistical Report, Years 1964-1966.* London: Bethlem Royal Hospital and the Maudsley Hospital.

HAVINGHURST, R. J., BOWMAN, P. H., LIDDLE, G. P., MATTHEWS, C. V., & PIERCE, J. V. (1962): *Growing up in River City.* New York: J. Wiley.

HENDERSON, A. S., McCULLOCH, J. W., & PHILIP, A. E. (1967): Survey of mental illness in adolescence. *Brit. Med. J.,* 1, 83.

HESTON, L. L. (1966): Psychiatric disorders in foster home reared children of schizophrenic mothers. *Brit. J. Psychiat.,* 112, 819-825.

HOWELLS, J. G. (Ed.) (1965): *Modern Perspectives in Child Psychiatry.* New York: Brunner/Mazel.

HUFFMAN, P. W. & WENIG, P. W. (1954): Prodromal behavior patterns in mental illness. (Department of Public Welfare, State of Illinois, mimeo), cited by Robins (1971).

INNES, G. & SHARP, G. A. (1962): A study of psychiatric patients in North-East Scotland. *J. Ment. Sci.,* 108, 447.

KANNER, L. (1957): *Child Psychiatry.* 3rd ed. Springfield, Ill.: Thomas.

KANNER, L. (1971): Follow-up study of eleven autistic children originally reported in 1943. *J. Autism Childh. Schizophrenia,* in press.

KESSEL, N. & SHEPARD, M. (1962): Neurosis in hospital and general practice. *J. Ment. Sci.,* 108, 159-166.

KIDD, C. B. & DIXON, G. A. (1968): The incidence of psychiatric illness in Aberdeen teenagers. *Hlth Bull.* (Edinb.) 26, No. 2.

KOLVIN, I. (1971): Psychoses in childhood—a comparative study. In M. Rutter (Ed.): *Infantile Autism: Concepts, Characteristics and Treatment.* London: Churchill.

LANE, E. A. & ALBEE, G. W. (1966): Childhood intellectual differences between schizophrenic adults and their siblings. *Amer. J. Orthopsychiat.,* 35, 747-753.

LANE, E. A. & ALBEE, G. W. (1966): Comparative birth weights of schizophrenics and their siblings. *J. Psychol.,* 64, 227-231.

LANE, E. A. & ALBEE, G. W. (1968): On childhood intellectual decline of adult schizophrenics: A reassessment of an earlier study. *J. Abnorm. Soc. Psychol.*, 73, 174-177.

MARKS, I. M. & GELDER, M. G. (1966): Different ages of onset in varieties of phobia. *Amer. J. Psychiat.*, 123. 218-221.

MARRIS, P. (1958): *Widows and Their Families.* London: Routledge & Kegan Paul.

MASTERSON, J. F. (1967): *Psychiatric Dilemma of Adolescence.* Boston: Little, Brown & Co.

MASTERSON, J. F. (1968): The psychiatric significance of adolescent turmoil. *Amer. J. Psychiat.*, 124, 107-112.

MEDNICK, S. A. & F. SCHULSINGER (1968): Some premorbid characteristics related to breakdown in children with schizophrenic mothers. In D. Rosenthal & S. S. Kety (Eds.): *The Transmission of Schizophrenia.* Oxford: Pergamon.

MELIA, P. I. (1970): Prophylactic lithium: A double blind trial in recurrent affective disorders. *Brit. J. Psychiat.*, 116, 621-624.

MENKES, M. M., ROWE, J. S., & MENKES, J. H. (1967): A 25-year follow-up study on the hyperkinetic child with minimal brain dysfunction. *Pediatrics*, 39, 393-399.

MICHAEL, C. M., MORRIS, D. P., & SOROKER, E. (1957): Follow-up studies of shy withdrawn children. II. Relative incidence of schizophrenia. *Amer. J. Orthopsychiat.*, 27, 331-337.

MORRIS, D. P., SOROKER, E., & BARRUSS, C. (1954): Follow-up studies of shy, withdrawn children. I. Evaluation of later adjustment. *Amer. J. Orthopsychiat.*, 24: 743.

MORRIS, H. H., ESCOLL, P. J., & WEXLER, R. (1956): Aggressive behavior disorders of childhood: A follow-up study. *Amer. J. Psychiat.*, 112, 991-997.

MULLIGAN, G. J., DOUGLAS, J. W. B., HAMMOND, W. A., & TIZARD, J. (1963): Delinquency and symptoms of maladjustment: The findings of a longitudinal study. *Proc. Roy. Soc. Med.*, 56, 1083-1088.

OFFORD, D. R. & CROSS, L. A. (1969): Behavioral antecedents of adult schizophrenia. *Arch. Gen. Psychiat.*, 21, 267-283.

OTTERSTROM, E. (1946): Delinquency and children from bad homes. *Acta Paediat.* (Uppsala) 33, Suppl. 5.

PARE, C. M. B. (1968): Recent advances in the treatment of depression. In A. Coppen & A. Walk (Eds.): *Recent Developments in Affective Disorders. Brit. J. Psychiat.* Spec. Publ. No. 2. London: R.M.P.A.

POWERS, E. & WITMER, H. (1951): *An Experiment in the Prevention of Delinquency.* New York: Columbia University Press.

PRICE, J. (1958): The genetics of depressive behavior. In A. Coppen & A. Walk (Eds.): *Recent Developments in Affective Disorders. Brit. J. Psychiat.* Spec. Publ. No. 2. London: R.M.P.A.

PRITCHARD, M. & GRAHAM, P. (1966): An investigation of a group of patients who have attended both the child and adult department of the same psychiatric hospital. *Brit. J. Psychiat.*, 112, 603-612.

RAWNSLEY, K. (1968): Epidemiology of affective disorders. In: A. Coppen & A. Walk (Eds.): *Recent Developments in Affective Disorders. Brit. J. Psychiat.* Spec. Publ. No. 2. London: R.M.P.A.

REISBY, N. (1967): Psychoses in children of schizophrenic mothers. *Acta Psychiat. Scand.*, 42, 8-20.

ROBINS, L. N. (1966): *Deviant Children Grown Up.* Baltimore: Williams & Wilkins.

ROBINS, L. N. (1971): Follow-up studies investigating childhood disorders. In E. H. Hare & J. K. Wing (Eds.): *Psychiatric Epidemiology.* London: Oxford University Press.

ROBINS L. N. & LEWIS, R. G. (1966): The role of the antisocial family in school completion and delinquency: A three generation study. *Sociol. Quart.*, 7, 500-514.

RODRIGUEZ, A., RODRIGUEZ, M., & EISENBERG, L. (1959): The outcome of school phobia: A follow-up study based on 41 cases. *Amer. J. Psychiat.*, 116, 540.

Roff, M. (1961): Childhood social interactions and young adult bad conduct. *J. Abnorm. Soc. Psychol.*, 63, 333-337.

Rosen, B. M., Kramer, M., Redick, R. W., & Willner, S. G. (1968):Utilization of Psychiatric facilities by Children: Current Status, Trends, Implications. (Public Health Service Publication No. 1868.) Washington, D. C.: U.S. Dept. of Health, Education and Welfare.

Rosenthal, D., Wander, P. H., Kety, S. S., Schulsinger, F., Welner, J., & Øster-gaard, L. (1968): Schizophrenics' offspring reared in adoptive homes. In D. Rosenthal & S. S. Kety (Eds.): *Transmission of Schizophrenia*. Oxford: Pergamon.

Rutter, M. (1966): *Children of Sick Parents: An Environmental and Psychiatric Study*. (Maudsley Monograph No. 16.) London: Oxford University Press.

Rutter, M.: (1968): Concepts of autism: A review of research. *J. Child Psychol.*, 9, 1-25.

Rutter, M. (1970a): Autistic children: Infancy to adulthood. *Sem. Psychiat.*, 2, 435-450.

Rutter, M. (1970b): Sex differences in children's responses to family stress. In E. J. Anthony & C. Koupernik (Eds.): *The Child in His Family*. New York: Wiley Interscience.

Rutter, M. (Ed.) (1971a): *Infantile Autism: Concepts, Characteristics and Treatment*. London: Churchill.

Rutter, M. (1971b): Parent-child separation: Psychological effects on the children. *J. Child. Psychol.*, in press.

Rutter, M., Greenfeld, D., & Lockyer, L. (1967): A five to fifteen year follow-up study of infantile psychosis. II. Social and behavioral outcome. *Brit. J. Psychiat.*, 113, 1183-1199.

Rutter, M., Tizard, J., & Whitmore, K. (Eds.) (1970): *Education, Health and Behavior*. London: Longmans.

Shaffer, D. (1971): Unpublished paper.

Shaffer, D., Costello, A. J. C., & Hill, I. D. (1968): Control of enuresis with imipramine. *Arch. Dis. Childh.*, 43, 665-671.

Shepherd, M., Cooper, B., Brown, A. C., & Kalton, G. W. (1966): *Psychiatric Illness in General Practice*. London: Oxford University Press,

Shepherd, M., Oppenheim, B., & Mitchell, S. (1971): *Childhood Behaviour and Mental Health*. London: University of London Press,

Slater, E. T. O. (1953): *Psychotic and Neurotic Illnesses in Twins*. London: H.M.S.O.

Slater, E. & Roth, M. (1969): *Clinical Psychiatry*. 3rd ed. London: Cassell.

Stabenau, J. R. & Pollin, W. (1967): Early characteristics of monozygotic twins discordant for schizophrenia. *Arch. Gen. Psychiat.*, 12, 723-734.

Sundby, H. S. & Kreyberg, P. C. (1968): *Progress in Child Psychiatry*. Oslo: Universitetsforlaget; and Baltimore: Williams & Wilkins.

Tait, C. D. & Hodges, E. F. (1962): *Delinquents, Their Families and The Community*. Springfield: Charles C Thomas.

Toolan, J. M. (1962): Depression in children and adolescents. *Amer. J. Orthopsychiat.*, 32, 404-415.

Warren, W. (1965): A study of adolescent psychiatric in-patients and the outcome six or more years later: II. The follow-up study. *J. Child Psychol.*, 6, 141-160.

Weiner, I. B. (1970): *Psychological Disturbances in Adolescence*. New York: Wiley.

Werry, J. S. (1968): Developmental hyperactivity. *Pediat. Clin. N. Amer.*, 15, 581-599.

West, D. J. (1967): *The Young Offender*. London: Penguin Books.

West, D. J. (1969): *Present Conduct and Future Delinquency*. London: Heinemann.

Wolff, S. (1961): Symptomatology and outcome of pre-school children with behavior disorders attending a child guidance clinic. *J. Child Psychol.*, 2, 269-276.

Wolff, S. (1971): Dimensions and clusters of symptoms in disturbed children. *Brit. J. Psychiat.*, 118, 421-427.

41

PSYCHIATRIC PATIENTS SEEN AS CHILDREN AND ADULTS: CHILD-HOOD PREDICTORS OF ADULT ILLNESS

Graham W. Mellsop

Consultant Psychiatrist, Auckland Hospital, New Zealand

INTRODUCTION

The natural history of psychiatric illness is a subject in which most express interest, many believe they understand, but on which relatively few systematic studies have been published. Despite the widespread conviction that adult behavior patterns are largely laid down in childhood, few attempts have been made to reassess persons seen in childhood, when they become adults.

Longitudinal studies on children have generally been concerned only with a short follow-up not extending into adulthood (Levitt et al., 1959; Shepherd et al., 1966; Perez-Reyes and Lansing, 1967), with small numbers of patients (Morris et al., 1954; Michael et al., 1957), without adequate controls (Witmer and Keller, 1942; Bronner, 1944; Morris et al., 1956), or with a highly selected childhood diagnostic group (Otterstrom, 1946; Warren, 1960; Robins, 1966; Rutter et al., 1967). Studies were either totally retrospective (Olcinick et al., 1966), concerned with nonpsychiatric childhood populations (Birren, 1944; Skodak and Skeels, 1949;

Reproduced from the JOURNAL OF CHILD PSYCHOLOGY AND PSYCHIATRY, Vol. 13, 1972, pp. 91-101 with the permission of Microforms International Marketing Corp., licensee. © Pergamon Press Journal back files.

689

Tuddenham, 1959; Stewart, 1962), or with only one category of outcome, for example schizophrenia (Frazee, 1953; Gardner, 1967). Most of the quoted studies differ from the present one on more than one of the above variables.

The biases and disadvantages of retrospective studies of the natural history of personality development and psychiatric illness are well known as are the difficulties of prospective studies. The present work has used medical records as a basis for a study of the natural history of psychiatric illness, in which the child presentation data has been used retrospectively but was obtained at the time of the childhood attendance and therefore not reconstructed in the light of the child's adult status.

The overall aims have been: to determine whether and to what extent children referred to the Department of Psychiatry of the Royal Children's Hospital, Melbourne, subsequently become patients of the Victorian Mental Health Department; what features of the childhood presentation and patient are associated with adult illness; what connection there is between the child and the adult clinical picture; and to determine, by interviewing adults, the reliability and validity of their perception of their own childhood referral.

This paper is a report on the first phase of this study.

AIMS

(1) To determine whether psychiatric disorders in childhood lead to a higher incidence of psychiatric morbidity in adulthood.

(2) To determine what childhood clinical, social, or demographic factors are most likely to be associated with subsequent adult illness.

METHOD

The names and dates of birth of all children (3370) referred to the Department of Psychiatry, Royal Children's Hospital, during the decade 1 January 1945 to 31 December 1954 who were born prior to 1946, were obtained from the records of that Department. The names of all the females were submitted to the Commonwealth Bureau of Census and Statistics who provided the relevant married names. The Central Patients' Register (Krupinski and Stoller, 1962) of the Victorian Mental Health Department was then searched to determine which names from the above two lists were recorded as having been patients of the Mental Health Authority during the period June 1961-June 1969, this being the period during which the present register had been in operation.

Of the patients common to the Department of Psychiatry, Royal

Children's Hospital, and the Victorian Mental Health Department, all those of both sexes born prior to 1943 and 50 per cent of those born during 1943-1945 inclusive were selected as the cohort. (The 50 per cent excluded were randomly selected, the purpose being simply to reduce the amount of data to be handled and inspection showed the greater number of the children to have been born in the period 1943-1945). A similar sized group, matched for sex and year of birth, was selected from the Department of Psychiatry, Royal Children's Hospital list, to act as controls in that they were similar to the cohort in all respects except that they did not, as adults, become patients of the Victorian Mental Health Department (they could of course have become patients elsewhere).

The names of all the patients in both cohort and control were presented to the author, who was not aware of which patients belonged to which group, and he extracted in a uniform manner data concerned with social class, family constellation, psychiatric symptomatology, temporal relations, intelligence and diagnosis from the Royal Children's Hospital case histories. Diagnoses were made by the author on each of the three axes of the proposed "Tri-axial Classification" (Rutter et al., 1969). An additional method of classification used was by "reason for referral" (Buckle, 1970). This provides for eight mutually exclusive referral categories which are largely self-explanatory. Social class was assigned according to the method suggested by Krupinski and Stoller (1968).

The childhood presentations of cohort and control were then compared in detail and the results analyzed statistically.

RESULTS

Twelve per cent (406) of the (3370) children who presented to the Department of Psychiatry at the Royal Children's Hospital during the decade 1 January 1945 to 31 December 1954 had already been adult patients of the Victorian Mental Health Department by early 1969, when their ages would have been within the range 25-40 years. The male to female ratio was about two to one in both childhood and adult referrals.

To assess whether these children had a greater than expected rate of admission, as adults, to the Victorian Mental Health Departments facilities, the first admission rates of all persons, born between 1931 and 1945 inclusive, for the period 1961-1969 were added (*Statistical Bulletins* 1-8). This cumulative admission rate was 3 per cent and so it is apparent that the child psychiatric referrals have a four fold increase, over the general population, in their risk of being adult patients of the Victorian Mental Health Department by the ages reached at the time of this study. There was a non-significant tendency for the females from the child referrals, and from the total population, to have a higher referral rate as adults.

When those suffering from mental subnormality were excluded then of the 2982 original child referrals 298, or 10 per cent, were on the Victorian Mental Health Authority's register. This represents a referral rate, as adults, of three- and one-third times the expected.

From the 406 adult patients the names of 104 females and 188 males were taken to form the cohort as described under Method. The control group of 118 females and 220 males was selected (see Method) from the children who did not become adult patients.* Six of the cohort and eight of the controls were subsequently discarded as they had never arrived for their childhood consultations and two of the cohort and eight of the control group were discarded as the history sheets of their childhood presentation had vital information (for example history of illness) missing. This left 101 females and 183 males as the cohort for comparison with 112 female and 210 male controls, in terms of the childhood presentation.

In both males and females the onset of symptoms was more often during the first year of life ($p < 0.001$) in the total cohort group than in the controls though this difference disappeared *when the mentally retarded were excluded.*

The mean age at presentation was 7.7 years (range 1-14 years) for both males and females with a nonsignificant tendency for cohort to be younger than controls.

Reasons for referral (Table 1) did not distinguish at a significant level between the sexes or between those who became adult patients and those who did not.

When each referral category was taken separately there were no significant differences between those who did well and those who did badly for age at onset except in the case of males referred because of their behavior in society. Of the 34 males in this category, in 11 of the cohort and 3 of the controls, the onset of the behavior was at a preschool age compared with a later onset in 8 cohort and 12 controls. This tendency for the symptoms to appear earlier in the future adult patients is significant ($p < 0.05$).

---

* A technical oversight in the selection of the control group resulted in an excess of subjects with no matching in 27 male and 11 female subjects.

TABLE 1. NUMBERS IN EACH REFERRAL CATEGORY

| Referral category | Male | | Female | | Total | |
	Cohort	Control	Cohort	Control	Number	%
Handicaps (mental or physical)	59	66	39	38	202	33
Behaviour at home	40	39	12	20	111	18
Medical symptoms (e.g. enuresis, anxiety, nightmares)	24	39	18	22	103	17
Educational difficulties	24	34	21	17	96	16
Behaviour in society	18	16	4	9	47	8
School refusal	10	8	2	2	22	4
Behaviour at school	5	6	5	3	19	3
Withdrawal or other serious generalized psychiatric symptoms	3	2	0	1	6	1
Totals	183	210	101	112	606	100

Though the overall ratio of males to females was 2:1 this did not apply to the first axis diagnosis (Table 2) of mental subnormality where the numbers were nearly equal. In both sexes mental subnormality was significantly more common in those with the worse prognosis.

Personality disorder was more common in males in the cohort and in females in the control group. The diagnoses adaptation reaction and normal variation were less common in the future adult patients than in the controls, though, in males the former and in females the latter differences were not significant. Normal variation, adaptation reaction, developmental disorder and neuroses, combined, were less common among the cohort than among the controls (p < 0.05). Conversely, the remainder, combined, were more common among those destined to be adult patients.

On the second axis of intellectual level (Table 3) the findings of the first axis with respect to subnormality were confirmed and the cohort were more often subnormal than the controls ($p < 0.01$ for males and $p < 0.001$ for females) and females more often subnormal than males (p < 0.05).

On the third axis of "associated or etiological factors" where each child could receive more than one coding, in about 28 per cent of each group "no known factor" was recorded. The only variable which predicted prognosis was "disease or disorder of the central nervous system" which occurred in about 28 per cent of the cohort and 14 per cent of the controls ($p < 0.001$). When the subnormals were excluded from anal-

TABLE 2. DISTRIBUTION OF FIRST AXIS DIAGNOSES

| | Males | | | | | | Females | | | | | | Total | |
| | Cohort | | Control | | Total | | Cohort | | Control | | Total | | | |
	No.	%	No.	%	No.	%	No.	%	No.	%	No.	%	No.	%
Mental subnormality only	39**	21	21**	10	60*	15	37***	36	16***	14	53	25	113	18
Personality and conduct disorders	27***	15	11***	5	38	10	3*	3	11*	10	14	7	52	9
Other clinical syndromes	17	9	12	6	29	7	7	7	10	9	17	8	46	8
Neurotic disorders	32	17	48	23	80	20	21	21	18	16	39	18	119	20
Specific developmental disorder	21	12	36	17	57	15	9	9	14	13	23	11	80	13
Adaptation reaction	45	25	72	34	117	30	21*	21	35*	31	56	26	173	28
Normal variation	2*	1	10*	5	12	3	3	3	8	7	11	5	23	4
Total	183	100	210	100	393	100	101	100	112	100	213	100	606	100

The differences between cohort and controls in each sex or between the totals of males and females are significant when indicated by asterisks.
*$p < 0.05$, **$p < 0.01$, ***$p < 0.001$.

TABLE 3. SECOND AXIS DIAGNOSES

		Normal		Mild		Subnormal Moderate		Severe	
		No.	%	No.	%	No.	%	No.	%
Male	Cohort	125	68·3	38	20·8	19	10·5	1	0·5
	Control	172	81·8	29	13·5	7	3·5	2	1·0
Female	Cohort	56	54·4	27	26·7	15	14·9	3	3·0
	Control	86	76·8	19	17·0	4	3·5	3	2·7

TABLE 4. OCCURRENCE OF SYMPTOMS IN CERTAIN AREAS PER 100 PERSONS

	Male		Female		Total
	Cohort	Control	Cohort	Control	population
Neurotic	44	42	35	31	39
School	36	40	25	29	34
Speech	32	35	36	34	34
Conduct	42	32	24	29	33
Slow learning	37**	22**	48*	29*	32
Toilet	15	15	15	18	15
Sleep	13	17	7	13	13
Psychosomatic	10*	18*	9	11	13
Habits	11	9	7	5	9
Eating	8	6	9	4	7
Sexual	2	2	2	4	2

Differences between cohort and control non-significant except when marked by asterisks. *p · 0·025, **p · 0·005.

ysis "disease or disorder of the central nervous system" remained more common in cohort (15 per cent) than in controls (9 per cent) and this difference also reached significance ($p < 0.05$). Amongst the factors which did not aid prediction were "congenital malformations," "social and material," or "emotional and attitudinal" environmental factors.

The areas in which the children had symptoms are presented in Table 4. The average number of areas in which children had symptoms clustered about a mean of 2.3 per child. Slow learning ability was more common in females than in males and in both sexes, was more common in those who did worse on follow-up. No other variable distinguished cohort from control at a significant level except that psychosomatic symptoms were associated with a good outcome in males. There was a non-significant trend for symptoms of disturbed conduct to be associated with a good outcome in females and a bad outcome in males.

When the area of complaint was considered within different ages at presentation, the female cohort were soon to have more symptoms dur-

TABLE 5. TOTAL NUMBER OF ATTENDANCES

	Male		Female		Total
	Cohort	Control	Cohort	Control	
1	65	49	28	32	173
2-5	69	99	51	44	263
6 or more	49	62	22	36	170

TABLE 6. SOCIAL CLASS DISTRIBUTION AT CHILDHOOD REFERRAL, BASED ON FATHER'S OCCUPATION

		I	II	III	IV	V
Male	Cohort	2	13	8	75	60
	Control	5	11	9	62	84
Female	Cohort	2	10	6	30	32
	Control	0	8	10	41	33
Total		9 (2%)	42 (8%)	33 (7%)	208 (41%)	209 (42%)

ing infancy than the controls ($p < 0.001$) and the male cohort to have more during their pre-school years than the controls ($p < 0.01$). When the separate areas were compared on age at presentation the only feature of significance in either sex was a tendency for the females with conduct problems to have their symptoms at a pre-school age whereas in the controls they only became apparent later ($p < 0.05$).

Within diagnostic groups on the first axis there were no significant differences in age at onset or presentation between sexes or between cohort and control, except that male personality disorders presented prior to adolescence more often than female ($p < 0.05$) and in females, subnormal cohorts presented prior to adolescence more often than controls ($p < 0.05$).

Duration of symptoms prior to presentation did not distinguish future Mental Health Department patients from the others or male from female, either within separate diagnostic categories or in total.

When the number of attendances were compared (Table 5), the subnormal attended less often than the normal ($p < 0.001$) in both sexes and persons referred because of educational difficulties and handicaps attended less often than those in other referral categories ($p < 0.05$ and $p < 0.01$ respectively) for males only and those females referred because of medical symptoms attended less often than those in other referral categories ($p < 0.05$). In terms of first axis diagnoses, male subnormals attended less often than the rest and male adaptation reactions, developmental disorders and neurotics attended more often (each $p <$ 0.01) than the rest. Amongst the total female group subnormals attended less frequently and adaptation reactions and neurotics more frequently (both $p < 0.001$) than the rest. In comparing cohort with control there were no significant differences in females on any of the first axis diagnoses. In males, however, controls attended more often than cohort ($p < 0.01$) and within separate diagnostic categories the only significant difference was that those of the future adult patients suffering from "subnormality only," attended less often ($p < 0.05$) than the subnormals who did not become patients of the Victorian Mental Health Department.

It was only possible to assign social class to 84 per cent of the males and 81 per cent of the females, due to the parents' occupations not being recorded in the remainder.

Social class at referral (Table 6) did not distinguish males from females or adult patients from non-patients. The social class of the total population at risk was not available for comparison.

Within females there were no significant differences between cohort and control but in males social class IV was more common ($p < 0.05$). With social class comparison between referral categories no significant differences emerged.

When the children were compared in terms of family unity (Table 7), assessed simply by comparing those living with both parents, those living with one parent and those not living with any parent, no significant differences between the sexes or between cohort and control emerged. When prognosis was considered within separate diagnostic and referral categories the only significant difference was in those males referred for medical symptoms where the cohort were less likely ($p < 0.05$) than the controls to be living with both parents.

DISCUSSION

The results indicate that 20 years after their referral to the Department of Psychiatry, Royal Children's Hospital, the adults have a four-fold increase over the comparable general population in their risk of being patients of the Victorian Mental Health Department. This under-estimates the total adult morbidity of this group as it does not take into account those who have attended general hospitals or private practitioners for their psychiatric morbidity. It is probable that those forming the cohort will include most of the children destined to develop serious

TABLE 7.   PARENTAL CONSTELLATION AT TIME OF CHILDHOOD REFERRAL

| | Male | | | | Female | | | | Total | |
| | Cohort | | Control | | Cohort | | Control | | | |
	No.	%	No.	%	No.	%	No.	%	No.	%
Living with both parents	140	76	172	81	77	76	85	76	474	78
Living with one parent	29	16	24	11	12	12	13	12	78	13
Not living with any parent	14	8	14	7	12	12	14	14	54	9

or chronic adult morbidity as other work (Krupinski, et al., 1967; Mellsop, 1969) has shown that even where factors mitigate against admission to the Victorian Mental Health Department's facilities, these are operative to a much smaller degree in schizophrenia than in neuroses.

When analyzing the figures (from Tables 1-4) it must be remembered that as the total child psychiatric population had a fourfold increase (three- and one-third if subnormals excluded) in their chance of becoming adult patients, for any individual diagnosis or category to be associated with no increased adult morbidity, the ratio in that category of cohort to control would have to be less than 1:4. This was not the case with any diagnosis, referral category or symptom type.

As expected, those children diagnosed as intellectually subnormal were overrepresented in the cohort and this was particularly evident in the females. Of the other diagnoses, most did not distinguish but "adaptation reaction" and "normal variation," as the glossary implies (Rutter et al., 1969), were under-represented in the cohort. Personality and conduct disorders in males were associated with a very bad prognosis and this is perhaps consistent with the findings of Robins (1966) on delinquents, and Morris, et al. (1956) on children with behavior disorders. However in females the opposite situation pertained and this may be contrasted with other reports (Morris, et al., 1956; Annotation, 1969) indicating that delinquent girls and girls with behavior problems have a markedly increased incidence of psychiatric illness as adults. The most likely explanation for this discrepancy is that the mean age of presentation of the delinquents referred to in the other studies was about 13-14 years whereas the girls in this study presented at a mean age of 7.7 years. The two populations are therefore not directly comparable and are in fact probably rather different. In addition the term "personality and conduct disorders" is much broader than delinquency.

The findings with respect to area of complaint support the above, as when the child's unwanted behavior was concerned with symptoms of disturbed conduct (e.g., aggressiveness, lying, disobedience, cruelty), independent of diagnosis; then a poor adult prognosis was found for males and relatively good prognosis for females. Complaints related to slow learning ability in the child were associated with a bad prognosis in both sexes, consistent with the poor prognosis of the subnormals.

The relatively benign nature, at least in terms of being associated with serious psychiatric illness in adulthood, of the neurotic disorders and developmental disorders is indicated by their inability to distinguish cohort from control. This does not contradict the findings of other workers who have found childhood neurosis associated with adult neuroses (Warren, 1960) and psychosis (Gardner, 1967) as the ratio of cohort to control, being markedly greater than one to three- and one-third, indicates these children have an increased expectancy of adult morbidity. As mentioned above, however, the present follow-up is also likely to have underestimated subsequent adult neuroses.

The significant excess of subnormals in the cohort is not the total explanation of the finding that "disease or disorder of the central nervous system" was the only one of the "associated or etiological factors" considered to distinguish cohort from controls as this difference, though reduced, remained when the subnormal were excluded. That is, evidence of organic damage to the central nervous system exerts an adverse effect upon prognosis independent of intellectual subnormality. The findings that various types of environmental factors, as recorded in the histories, did not differ in prevalence between cohort and control was more of a surprise. Of some relevance to this was the finding that the percentages of "broken homes" (not living with both parents) was similar in cohort and controls. Other workers (Robins, 1966; Rutter, et al., 1967b) have also found that the presence or absence of a "broken home" does not influence the prognosis of childhood psychiatric illness.

It is probable that in most of those not assigned to a social class, the reason the occupation of the "head of the house" was not recorded was related to unavailable parents due, for example, to a "broken home." This would mean that many of those would probably be in social classes four and five, but the distribution between cohort and control would still remain comparable. Robins (1966) and Morris, et al. (1956) also found social class no use as a predictor. Though comparison of social class with that of the population at risk was not possible, inspection of the figures in Table 6 strongly suggests that social classes four and five are over-represented in all childhood referrals to the Royal Children's

Hospital. If this is so then it is probable that to be referred from the first three social classes, a child would need to be more severely disturbed. This suggests that though social class did not appear to have any influence on adult prognosis it may be that it exerted its influences in determining the original child referral. Therefore it is not possible to claim that measures to improve the maternal situation or social class standing of patients are unlikely to directly influence their risk of later psychiatric illness, from the findings of the present study alone.

The childhood condition associated with the worst prognosis, mental subnormality, was also that for which the least attendances were prescribed. The three conditions associated with the greatest number of attendances, adaptation reaction, developmental and neurotic disorders, were those with the best prognoses. It may be that children with the best prognosis anyway receive the most treatment, as suggested by Eisenberg (1969) or alternatively, it could be claimed that the treatment was more effective in these groups of children than in the remainder. Either way it suggests that serious consideration should be given to the idea that long term follow-up studies of childhood psychiatric patients throw more light on the natural history of the disease than on the efficacy of therapy. This is supported by the work of Witmer and Keller (1942) which led them to conclude that child guidance led to better current functioning, but not any difference in long term prognosis.

There are no completely comparable published studies of a follow-up on a children's general hospital department of psychiatry with which to compare the overall distribution of childhood diagnoses, age at presentation, duration of symptoms, social class or reason for referral. The next step in the utilization of the present data must be to compare the childhood and adulthood clinical pictures of the same patients.

SUMMARY

Of the 3370 children referred to the Department of Psychiatry, Royal Children's Hospital, Melbourne, during the decade 1 January 1945 to 31 December 1954 and who were born prior to 1946, 12 per cent were, as adults, patients of the Victorian Mental Health Department between June 1961 and June 1969. This represents a fourfold increase in expected rate. When the mentally subnormal were excluded from consideration the rate was $3\frac{1}{3}$ times greater than expected. Of the non-subnormal diagnostic groups, male personality disorders had the worst prognosis. Comparing the children on such variables as reason for referral, behavior complained of, age at onset of symptoms, age at presentation, duration of symptoms, social class and amount of treatment, little of predictive value emerged.

Acknowledgments—I wish to thank the Department of Psychiatry, Royal Children's Hospital, Melbourne, for access to their records, Dr. J. Krupinski and Dr. D. Buckle for advice and assistance, Dr. R. Ball for encouragement and advice, Miss L. Pidriz and my wife for clerical assistance, the Victorian State Actuary, for providing the names of those who had married, and the Victorian Mental Health Authority for funds and permission to publish this paper.

REFERENCES

ANNOTATION (1969): Delinquent girls. Lancet, 1, 713.

BIRREN, J. E. (1944): Psychological examinations of children who later became psychotic. *J. Abnorm. Soc. Psychol.*, 39, 84-96.

BRONNER, A. F. (1944): Treatment and what happened afterward? *Am. J. Orthopsychiat.*, 14, 28-35.

BUCKLE, D. (1970): Personal communication.

EISENBERG, L. (1969): Child psychiatry: The past quarter century. In Heseltine (Ed.), *Psychiatric Research in Our Changing World*. Amsterdam: G.F.D. Pub. Excerpta Medica Foundation.

FRAZEE, H. E. (1953): Children who later became schizophrenic? *Smith College Studies in Social Work*, XXIII, 125-149.

GARDNER, G. G. (1967): The relationship between childhood neurotic symptomatology and later schizophrenia in males and females. *J. Nerv. Ment. Dis.*, 144, 97-100.

KRUPINSKI, J. & STOLLER, A. (1962): A statistical system introduced for the evaluation of the epidemiology of psychiatric disorders in Victoria, Australia. *Health Bull. Melb.*, 3 ,127-128.

KRUPINSKI, J., BAIKIE, A. G., STOLLER, A., GRAVES, J., O'DAY, D. M., & POLKE, P. (1967): A community health survey of Meyfield, Victoria. *M.J.A.*, 1, 1204-1211.

KRUPINSKI, J. & STOLLER, A. (1968): Occupational hierarchy of first admissions to the Victorian Mental Health Department, 1962-1965. *Aust. & N.Z.J. Sociol.*, 4, 55-63.

LEVITT, E. E., BEISER, H. R., & ROBERTSON, R. E. (1959): A follow-up evaluation of cases treated at a community child guidance clinic. *Am. J. Orthopsychiat.*, 29, 337-349.

MELLSOP, G. W. (1969): The effect of distance in determining hospital admission rates. *M.J.A.*, 2, 814.

MICHAEL, C. M., MORRIS, D. P., & SOROKER, E. (1957): Follow-up studies of shy withdrawn children—I. Evaluation of later adjustment. *Am. J. Orthopsychiat.*, 24, 743-754.

MORRIS, H. H., ESCOLL, P. J., & WEXLER, R. (1956): Aggressive behavior disorders in childhood: A follow-up study. *Am. J. Psychiat.*, 112, 991-997.

OLEINICK, M. S., BAHN, A. K., EISENBERG, L., & LILIENFIELD, A. M. (1966): Early socialization experiences and intrafamilial environment. *Arch. Gen. Psychiat.*, 15, 344-353.

OTTERSTROM, EDITH D. (1946): Delinquency and children from bad homes. A study of their prognosis from the social point of view. *Acta. Paediat. Stockholm*, 33, Suppl. 5.

PEREZ-REYES, M. & LANSING, C. (1967): The diagnostic evaluation process. A follow-up of 49 children studied in an out-patient clinic. *Arch. Gen. Psychiat.*, 16, 609-620.

ROBINS, L. N. (1966): *Deviant Children Grown Up*. Baltimore: Williams & Wilkins.

RUTTER, M. & LOCKYER, L. (1967a): A five to fifteen year follow-up study of infantile psychosis—I. Description of sample. *Br. J. Psychiat.*, 113, 1169-1182.

RUTTER, M., GREENFIELD, D., & LOCKYER, L. (1967b): A five to fifteen year follow-up study of infantile psychosis—II. Social and behavioral outcome. *Br. J. Psychiat.,* 113, 1183-1199.

RUTTER, M., LEBOVICH, S., EISENBERG, L., SNEZNESVSKIJ, A. V., SADOUN, R., BROOKE, E., & LIN, T. (1969): A tri-axial classification of mental disorders in childhood. *J. Child Psychol. Psychiat.* 10, 41-61.

SHEPHERD, M., OPPENHEIM, A. N., & MITCHELL, S. (1966): Childhood behavior disorders and the child-guidance clinic: An epidemiological study. *J. Child Psychol. Psychiat.,* 7, 39-52.

SKODAK, M. & SKEELS, H. M. (1949): A final follow-up study of 100 adopted children. *J. Genet. Psychol.,* 75, 85-125.

Statistical Bulletins: Victorian Mental Health Department. Numbers 1-8 (1963-1970).

STEWART, L. H. (1962): Social and emotional adjustment during adolescence as related to the development of psychosomatic illness in adulthood. *Genetic Psychol. Monographs,* 65, 175-215.

TUDDENHAM, R. D. (1969): The constancy of personality ratings over two decades. *Genetic Psychol. Monographs,* 60, 3-29.

WARREN, W. (1960): Some relationships between the psychiatry of children and of adults. *J. Ment. Sci.,* 106, 815-826.

WITMER, H. L. & KELLER, J. (1942): Outgrowing childhood problems: A study of the value of child guidance treatment. *Smith College Studies in Social Work,* XIII, 74-89.

Part XII

EFFECTS OF INSTITUTIONALIZATION

The trend toward concrete studies of the specific effects of institution-alization, rather than global generalizations, noted in the Annual Progress Volume two years ago, continues. The study of language development in institutionalized children by Tizard and her colleagues reaffirms other recent reports which do not find any "institutional retardation" as such. They found that the children's level of language development correlated significantly with specific characteristics of the organization and func-tioning of the residential nursery. Zigler and Yando in their study of imitative behavior also found no generalized institutional effect. As with the other authors, their concern is with identifying specific correlations which might illuminate the dynamic mechanisms involved in imitative learning.

42

ENVIRONMENTAL EFFECTS ON LANGUAGE DEVELOPMENT: A STUDY OF YOUNG CHILDREN IN LONG-STAY RESIDENTIAL NURSERIES

Barbara Tizard, Oliver Cooperman,

Anne Joseph, and Jack Tizard

Institute of Education, University of London

Observational studies of 85 children aged 2-5 years were made in 13 residential nursery groups. The aim was to relate the language development of the children to the amount and quality of adult talk directed at them, and both these factors to the way in which the nursery was organized. No "institutional retardation" was found, and the mean test scores on both verbal and nonverbal tests were average. Significant correlations were obtained between the language comprehension scores of the children and both the quality of the talk directed to them and the way in which the nursery was organized.

In discussions of the effect of the environment on language development, it is customary to refer to the detrimental effect of institutional care, which is presumed to be mediated by inadequate verbal stimula-

Reprinted from CHILD DEVELOPMENT, 1972, 43, pp. 337-358. © 1972 by the Society for Research in Child Development, Inc. All rights reserved.

The study was made possible by a grant from Dr. Bernardo's Society and by the cooperation of the staff in nurseries under the auspices of Dr. Bernardo's Society, the Church of England Children's Society, and the National Children's Home.

tion. Most of the evidence for such an effect is now very out of date (e.g., Burlingham & Freud, 1944; Goldfarb, 1945; Kellmer Pringle & Bossio, 1958). In the intervening years residential institutions for young children in England, at any rate, have enormously improved, and it would seem appropriate to ask whether their verbal environment is not, in fact, superior to that of many private families. More specifically, one might ask how different institutions differ in their verbal environment, and whether the language development of children growing up in them can be related to the observed differences in verbal stimulation.

Earlier discussions have usually assumed that "institutional retardation" is caused by a lack of verbal or other stimulation. However, preliminary observations suggested to us that the important difference among present-day residential nurseries was in the quality rather than the quantity of the adult talk. In some nurseries a large proportion of adult talk appeared to be concerned with giving instructions to the children, without explanation, or with meaningless comments of the "That's pretty, aren't you a lucky boy" kind. Both categories of talk tended to involve a restricted vocabulary and short sentence length and were unlikely to provoke a verbal response from the child. In such nurseries extended conversations were rarely heard, and the staff's time was mainly occupied with the physical care of the children, moving the children from place to place, getting out and putting away equipment, and sitting watching the children. In other nurseries the staff's talk appeared to be much less restricted; they were heard offering the children opinions, information, and explanations, and they seemed to spend more time playing with the children, rather than supervising them.

If such differences in staff behavior among nurseries can be established, and relationships found with the level of the children's language development, it would seem important to discover the reason for them. Our basic viewpoint is that the way in which staff behave and talk within an institution is much influenced by its organizational structure. An earlier series of studies showed that in institutions for the mentally retarded both the child-care practices of the staff and the attainments of the children were significantly related to aspects of the formal organizational structure of the institution, that is, to "sociological" factors rather than to the psychological characteristics of the staff (King, Raynes, & Tizard, 1971; Tizard, 1970).

The residential nurseries in the present study did not present gross organizational differences of the kind found among institutions for the retarded, and it was known that the staff in the different nurseries had received a similar training and education and came from the same social class. Nevertheless, we believed that there were important differences in the way in which the nurseries were organized, which would affect the quality of staff talk and behavior, and hence the children's level of language development. It was therefore decided to seek relationships among three independent sets of data. The first set, obtained from records and by interview, was concerned with the organizational structure of the nurseries; the second, obtained through direct observation using time-sampling techniques, measured the "verbal environment" of the children; the third, obtained through formal psychological testing, comprised measures of both verbal and nonverbal development.

METHOD

An initial period of 3 months was spent making preliminary observations; developing time-sampling techniques, codes, and predictions; and making estimates of observer reliability. The main inquiry was undertaken in 11 residential nurseries, run by three major British voluntary societies which provide care for dependent children. In all, 13 nursery groups (see below) were studied. Systematic time-sampling observations were made over a period of 5 days in each nursery group; nursery staff were interviewed on another occasion, by a different examiner; and the children were tested by an experienced clinical psychologist within a few weeks of the observational study.*

The nursery setting.—The long-stay residential nurseries which we studied were very different from the grim foundling homes described by Spitz and earlier workers. Most of our nurseries were characterized not only by a high standard of physical care but by a concern for the psychological well-being of the children. The majority contained 15-25 children, organized into a baby unit and two or three mixed age groups of six children, ranging in age from about 12 months to the upper age limit of the nursery, which varied from 4½ to 7 years. Each group had its own suite of bedroom, bathroom, and living room, with its own nurse and assistant nurse. The nurse in charge of the group was usually a qualified nursery nurse, and the assistant was a student trainee. Two or more staff were on duty with the group each day, and since most of the cleaning and cooking was done by domestic staff, they could devote themselves to child care. The living room was furnished in a homelike style, with adult rather than kindergarten furnishings,

---

* The observations were carried out by O. B. C. and A. J., and the interviewing of nursery staff, by B. T. Psychological testing was done by Mrs. Liz Tregenza. Frances Cherry gave statistical advice and was responsible for computer analyses.

and plentifully supplied with toys and books; outside was a large garden containing further play equipment. In all the nurseries children over 3 attended a play group, where sand, paint, water, etc., were available, and the children were always read to at least once a day. Most of the nurseries made considerable efforts to broaden the children's experiences by organizing shopping expeditions, excursions, car and bus rides, and occasional weekend visits to the homes of staff members. The nurseries were rarely short of staff and indeed had a long waiting list of applicants. This is probably because the job of nursery nurse, which involves obtaining a certificate at the end of 2 years' practical and college training, has a relatively high status in England. Moreover, since each student on entering had to agree to remain for 3 years, staff turnover in all the nurseries was relatively low.

Differences in nursery organization: predictions and measurement of variables.—Despite these similarities, there were certain differences among the nurseries in social organization. Of these the most important was considered to be the autonomy of the group. Some nurseries were run very like hospitals, most decisions being made on an entirely routine basis or else referred to the matron. Each day was strictly timetabled, the matron made frequent inspections, and the freedom of both nurse and child was very limited. Thus, the children were not allowed to leave the group room unattended, and the nurse had to ask permission to take the children for a walk or to turn on the television set. In this situation the nurse had very little responsibility, and her tasks were so well defined that someone else could easily take her place. Such an arrangement is administratively convenient because staff become interchangeable and inexperienced staff can be put in charge of a group, but it results in very restricted role playing by the staff, whose function is reduced to maintaining order and "minding" the children on behalf of matron. Very often the intellectual and emotional energy of the nurse appeared to be invested elsewhere, and her responses to the children appeared mechanical and superficial. Because the staff were given little autonomy, they could not offer it to the children. More important, perhaps, the ethos of an institution where decisions are made at the top and each grade knows its position in the hierarchy favors the development of obedience rather than child autonomy. Such a social structure has implications in terms of verbal interchange; with a rigid framework of rules and routine there was little occasion for discussion either among staff or between staff and children; the expectation of group conformity was so pervasive that it was rare to hear a child offered a choice of any kind or given an explanation for any request. Even during play the children were often assigned a passive role; for example, they might be pushed on a swing or expected to sit quietly while a book was read. Since the staff generated little interesting stimulation, the children appeared uninterested in them; the children addressed rather few remarks to the staff and often did not answer their remarks.

In somewhat less centralized institutions the nurse in charge of the group might be given responsibility for allocating domestic work, or allowed to organize expeditions outside the nursery. In the most decentralized institutions, each group was separately housed in a cottage or flat, and the staff prepared their own meals and arranged their own day. The children could move freely about the house and garden, and the staff only rarely referred a decision to the matron. Their role, in fact, approximated more closely to that of a foster mother. Since they could plan their own day and were not under constant surveillance, they could treat the children more flexibly, and discussion became possible on such topics as the day's menu, how to spend the afternoon, or which television program to watch. Staff talk was therefore more varied and interesting, and children appeared to both address and answer the staff more often.

The first prediction, therefore, was that the more autonomous the group, the higher the quality of staff-child interactions—that is, the more often the staff would converse and play with the children, rather than passively "mind" them, the more often they would give the children explanations for orders, the more often both staff and children would answer each other's remarks, and the more often children would address remarks to the staff. When the staff were playing with the children or reading to them, it was predicted that the more autonomous the group, the more the child would be assigned an active role in the play or reading situation. Further, it was predicted that these differences in staff-child interaction would result in superior language development in the children in the more autonomous groups. The autonomy of the nursery group was measured by a score based on the number of day-to-day decisions staff and children could make for themselves.

Unfortunately, groups of nurseries could not be found which differed only in autonomy, and it was considered necessary to measure differences in associated organizational variables which might affect staff behavior and/or language development. Thus there was a tendency for low autonomy to be associated with low staff stability. By staff stability is meant not staff turnover, which, as explained above, was everywhere relatively low, but the length of time staff worked with a particular group of children. Since all the nurseries were training centers, the junior staff on any one group were constantly changing; as students they attended college 2 days a week and were switched from group to group for "experience." In addition, in some nurseries both students and trained staff did night duty for 1 or 2 weeks every 2 months and at these times and when free were replaced by "floating" staff. In other nurseries greater stability was achieved by employing special night staff, and by appointing two permanent trained nurses to each group, so that when one was off duty the other was on. The measure of staff stability used was the number of trained nurses who had worked on the group for at least a week in the past 2 years. It seemed likely that low stability would affect staff behavior in much the same way as low autonomy, since staff who only stayed for a short time with the children would tend to "mind" them, and the children would tend to talk to them and answer them less often.

Second, in some nurseries the children were moved on to all-age homes at the age of 4+, so that half or more of each group were under the age of 3. In others, children could remain until they were 7, and each group had one or two children aged 5 or older. Because of the burden of physical care and the more restricted vocabulary and syntax likely to be used with a young group, it seemed likely that the lower the mean age of the children in the group, the lower the level of language development of the children.

Finally, although all the nurseries were generously staffed by most standards, some were much better staffed than others; for example, in the best-staffed nurseries there were always at least two staff present with each group of six children, some of whom were away for part of the day at school, while in the worst-staffed nurseries only one staff member was on duty with the group during most of the morning and afternoon.

A measure of staff-child ratio was obtained for each nursery group by dividing the number of staff hours worked per week by the number of children present for all or part of each day. It seemed likely that the better the staff-child ratio, the more often would the staff be able to converse and play with the children, and the better would be the language development of the children.

Selection of nurseries.—A large number of nurseries were visited and the staff in them interviewed, to obtain scores on these four variables. It was hoped to select groups of nurseries so that the effect of at least some variables could be seen in isolation, for example, groups with high autonomy and good stability but with differing staff ratios or mean ages. In fact, scores on all the variables proved to be rather highly correlated; thus only one nursery could be found with relatively high autonomy and low mean age, and only one with a relatively high autonomy and low staff ratio. Eleven nurseries were finally chosen which included the extremes of social organization found, and in nine of these nurseries one group of children was chosen for observation, on the basis that (1) during the week of observation the customary staff would be on duty, and (2) when possible the group should include at least one child aged 2, 3, and 4 years old. In two nurseries, which were large "village" communities, two groups differing in social organization were chosen, so that in all 13 nursery groups were observed.

THE CHILDREN

Data were collected on two sets of children, those actually observed ($N = 46$) and those tested ($N = 85$). The first set comprised all children aged between 24 and 59 months in the 13 nursery groups observed. The second set comprised all children, whether observed or not, in the 11 nurseries who were between the ages of 24 and 59 months and who had been at least 6 months in the nursery, whose medical record showed them to be healthy, full-term babies, and who were not considered by their doctors to be handicapped in any way. Thirty-four of these children were aged 2.0-3.0 years, 26 were 3.05-4.0 years, and 25 were 4.05-4.95 years. Two-thirds of the children were boys. Slightly less than half of the children were white, 24 children were of mixed race, with white mothers, and 22 were of West Indian parentage. The majority of the children had been admitted as infants: 70% of those tested had been admitted before the age of 12 months, and only 14% after the age of 24 months. The chief reason for admission was illegitimacy: about a quarter of the children were visited regularly by their mothers, who would probably take them home eventually, but nearly two-thirds were without family contacts. In most cases these were children whom their mothers had placed in the nursery for adoption but who had not been adopted because of their color or family background, for example, a family history of epilepsy, psychopathy, or depression. In fact, since our study quite a number of these children have been adopted. There was no information available about the IQs of the parents or the occupation of nearly one-half of the fathers. The occupations of all the mothers were known: significantly more were from Social Class 5 (unskilled workers) and significantly fewer from Social Class 3 (skilled workers) than would be expected from the London and South East England Census (1961).

Measurement of staff behavior: observational techniques.—Five days were spent by one of the two observers in each of the 13 nursery groups. The observer lived in the nursery and spent the evenings in friendly informal contacts with the staff. Considerable efforts were made to explain the project to the staff and to allay their anxieties. They were told that the study was concerned with the effect that such factors as staff ratio and mean age had on the way that staff and children spent the day, but they were not told that staff talk was being recorded. The first day was used as a "warm-up": observations were made but not used. On the next four days observations were made from the time the staff came to dress the children until midday, or from midday until the children were in bed. Time-sampling techniques were used to record the ways in which staff used their time (staff activity: the first 10 seconds in every 30 seconds; staff talk and child talk: the first 5 seconds in every 30 seconds). An attempt was made to record exactly what was done or said during this time.

The three schedules were alternated throughout each half day, in the approximate proportions of staff activity, 1; staff talk, 0.66; child talk, 0.33; so that, in all, 2 complete working days were observed. One staff member or child was observed for 3 minutes. At the end of this period the observations were coded, and another staff member or child was observed. At the time of each observation, the location, time of day, and number of staff and children present were noted, as well as whether the staff member being observed was at that moment the most senior one present.

The staff activity schedule aimed to measure the amount of time staff spent in "social" activities, which were considered likely to further the children's language development, that is, playing or reading with children, teaching them, conversing with them, or responding affectionately to them. Play and reading were further subclassified into "active" and "passive" according to whether the child actively participated in the given activity or was the passive recipient. For example a child might be "read to," or the reading might involve a discussion with the child about the pictures or the story; the nurse might build a tower of bricks for the child, or nurse and child might both take part in a construction.

The major codes of staff activity used were housework (cleaning, cooking, etc.), physical child care (toileting, dressing, washing children, etc.) and supervisory activities (taking equipment out and putting it away, watchng the chldren, moving them from place to place, disciplining children). In each observation period it was also noted whether the staff spoke to another nurse or a child, and if so, to whom.

The staff talk schedule aimed to measure the frequency with which the staff made "informative" remarks, that is, remarks considered likely to further the children's language development, for example, reading to the child, telling or asking the child something about present, past, or future activities, naming objects, asking for or giving an opinion, an explanation, or a piece of information. The other major codes for staff talk were negative control (instructions to terminate an activity), positive control (instructions to initiate an activity), expressions of pleasure and affection, expressions of displeasure and anger, offering the child a choice, and "supervisory" talk, a category of talk used by adults when they wish to respond to children but have no real communication to make.

The flavor of the staff talk is best conveyed by examples. The following remarks were coded as *informative*: "Do you know where your coat is?" "That's not a sweet, it's a piece of a puzzle." "John doesn't need a haircut." "Your Mummy is coming soon." By contrast, *supervisory* remarks repeated, confirmed, or disconfirmed what the child had said— for example, "Did you?" "Mark pulled his tail, did you say?" "Yes, it is yours" (the child having said it was his); were ritual accompaniments to certain actions—for example, "Here you are," "Off we go," "Thank you," "Hello," "Goodbye"; or were ritualistic responses to a child's demand or comment—for example, "That's nice," "Aren't you clever," "Lucky boy." All remarks made with the intention of initiating or terminating a child's activity were coded as *negative* or *positive* control. Some of these remarks did contain information—for example, "Do that again and you'll be put out of the room"—but were coded as *control* remarks. However, in most cases control remarks were terse: "Stop it," "Come on," and "Hurry up" were the most frequently occurring. In the case of commands, a note was made of whether a verbal explanation of any kind was given with the command. A note was also made of what child was addressed and whether he replied. A large number of minor codes were used in both the Staff Activity and Staff Talk Schedules; for instance, 18 types of housework were coded and 10 types of informative talk. However, only the major codes described above were used in the analysis.

In the Child Talk Schedule the speech of the child was not recorded, but only whether he spoke during the observation period, to whom he spoke, and whether the staff answered him, as well as whether the staff spoke to him during the observation period and whether he replied. Only children aged 2.0-4.1 years were observed.

As far as possible visits were made alternately to nurseries with low and high autonomy, and each of the two observers visited approximately equal numbers of nurseries with high, low, and medium autonomy. Although the observers were not responsible for the selection of the nurseries or for the interviewing of the staff, the characteristics of the nursery organization were of course apparent to them.

Psychological testing.—After the observations had been made a clinical psychologist, who was not part of the research team and not informed about our expectations, tested all the healthy 2- to 5-year-old children in the nurseries visited (as further specified earlier) with the Reynell Developmental Language Scales and the nonverbal scale of the Minnesota Pre-School Scale. The Reynell Developmental Language Scales have been developed and standardized on an English preschool population (Reynell, 1969). They consist of two independent scales, which assess language comprehension and expression separately.

The Verbal Comprehension Scale assesses the child's ability to understand language, without requiring him to use it, since all responses may be made by demonstration. At each point in the scale the child is presented with a number of pictures or objects. Success at the early stages involves showing an understanding of simple verbal labels—for example, by pointing to the correct picture or toy when asked, "Where is the spoon?" At later stages success depends on understanding attributes such as color, size, and position—for example, the child is told, "Turn the little table upside down"—or correctly carrying out a sequence of instructions—for example, "Put all the pigs in the box and give me a brown horse." According to the author (Reynell, 1969, p. 11) the scale is intended "to follow the developmental process of verbal comprehension without too much dependence on increasing the difficulty of the vocabulary used." However, it is not possible to know how far success or failure on any item depends upon the child's vocabulary.

The Expressive Language Scale, which is composed of three sections, is intended to assess the child's ability to use spoken language. The child's syntax is assessed by noting whether at any point during the examination he is heard to use various constructions, such as questions or complex sentences. The second section requires him to give the names of a variety of objects and pictures, and at a higher stage to define words. The third section tests his ability to describe pictures: his responses to the instruction, "Tell me about the picture," are scored according to the number of ideas expressed, regardless of perceptual or grammatical inaccuracies. Separate standard scores are not available for these three sections.

The Reynell scores take the form of standard scores for each age and sex. In order to facilitate computation, each score was multiplied by 10 and 100 was added to it, giving the test a mean of 100, with a standard deviation of 10. As recommended in the instructions, the Minnesota nonverbal scale was only administered to children 3 and over. Whenever it seemed best, the child's nurse was present, and on three occasions an unresponsive child was retested a few days or weeks later. Apart from this, no particular difficulty was encountered in testing the children; in no case was the child considered untestable, or so unresponsive or distractable that the psychologist had serious doubts about the validity of the test results.

It was predicted that there would be no significant difference between the mean scores of the children in different nurseries on the Minnesota nonverbal scale, but that there would be significant positive correlations between the mean Reynell Comprehension and Expression scores of children in each nursery and (a) the scores for nursery organization and (b) the observed frequency of "social" activity, "informative" talk, explanations given with commands, staff answering children, children answering staff, and children talking to staff. No significant correlation was expected between the frequency of staff talk and the children's test scores.

RESULTS

Reliability of observational data.—During the pilot study the reliability of each of the schedules used was tested by assessing the agreement between the two observers over each of approximately 200 observation periods. For the categories of *staff activity* the concordance was 88% or better, except for agreement on the subcode active/passive, when it was 77%. The agreement on *staff talk*, ignoring periods when nothing was said, was 74% and on the coding of what was said, and whether the child replied, 80%. The reliability of *child talk* was lower: concordance was between 50% and 60% except for the category "child answers staff" where it was only 25%. Probably the number of different events to be observed was too high on this schedule. In the analysis of results the score for each institution on "percentage of children answer staff" was taken from the Staff Talk Schedule, where reliability was acceptable. The correlation between the frequency with which the codes were used by the two observers was very high on all three schedules, $r = .99$, .94, and .95.

In the main study it was possible to check on interschedule agreement because some categories of behavior were recorded in two different

TABLE 1

INTERCORRELATION OF ORGANIZATIONAL VARIABLES

	Stability	Age	Autonomy	Ratio	Loadings on First Component
Staff stability	1	...	...	...	0.852
Mean age of group ...	0.58*	1	...	...	0.858
Group autonomy	0.71**	0.84***	1	...	0.928
Staff ratio	0.62*	0.48	0.59*	1	0.775

$*\ p = <.05.$
$**\ p = <.01.$
$***\ p = <.001.$

schedules. The correlation between the percentage of observation periods in which staff in each group were observed to speak in the Staff Activity and Staff Talk Schedules was $r = .80$, $p < .001$, $N = 13$. The correlation between the percentage of observations in which each child was spoken to by staff, calculated from these two schedules, was $r = .66$, $p < .001$, $N = 79$. The correlation between the frequency with which children were observed to answer staff on the Staff Talk and Child Talk Schedules was $r = .66$, $p < .01$, $N = 13$. The reliabilities calculated from the pilot study data were obtained by comparing individual observations made by different observers at the same time but using different watches; the coefficients of agreement reported from the main study are based on comparisons between observations made by the same observer on two separate occasions.

Measures of social organization.—Table 1 shows that all but one of the intercorrelations between the scores on the four nursery organization questionnaires were significant. With only 13 sets of scores, significant differences between the correlations of each variable and the observational data could not be obtained, nor could significant partial correlations; hence the effect of each variable could not be examined separately. Each nursery group was therefore given a single composite score, derived by a principal-component anlysis from the correlation matrix. Since the first component accounted for 73% of the variance, and the highest loading on the second component, staff ratio, was not significant, each group was given a score on the first component. They were thus finally ranked from "best" to "worst" according to their combined scores on the four questionnaires.

The groups whose composite scores were more than one standard deviation above the mean all had high autonomy, stable staffing, and a high staff ratio, and in all of them more than half of the children were

TABLE 2

STAFF ACTIVITIES AND NURSERY ORGANIZATION

	OBSERVATIONS IN WHICH DIFFERENT ACTIVITIES OCCURRED, ALL GROUPS COMBINED (%)		CORRELATION OF STAFF ACTIVITY (MEAN %) PER GROUP WITH GROUP COMPOSITE ORGANIZATION SCORE	
	Mean	SD	r ($N = 13$)	p
Administrative and personal	2.1	1.18	.09	...
Work (household chores)	11.7	5.28	.05	...
Physical child care	23.8	3.76	—.10	...
Supervisory activities	46.3	7.51	—.52	...
Social activities	15.8	5.91	.72	$<.01$
Play with child in which child active	3.0	2.20	.60	$<.05$

NOTE.—Mean number of observations per group = 625, SD 80.4.

aged 3 or over, while in the three groups whose composite scores were one standard deviation or more below the mean the reverse was the case. In the intermediate seven groups there was a variety of combinations of score.

Social organization and staff activity.—Table 2 shows that for the nurseries as a whole most staff time was spent in physical and supervisory child care. As predicted, a correlation was found between the manner in which the nursery was organized (the nursery composite score) and the amount of staff "social" activity (reading, playing, chatting to the children) and also between the amount of social activity in which the child was active rather than passive and the composite score.

Social organization and staff talk.—Table 3 shows the overall frequency of various kinds of staff talk. There was no shortage of verbal stimulation; in half of the observation periods the staff observed were speaking to a child. However, the largest category of talk was commands: the frequency of high-quality talk—that is, talk likely to enrich the child's language and to stimulate a reply—was relatively low.

Table 3 also gives the correlation between the various categories of staff talk and the composite social organization score of each nursery group. In nurseries which scored high on the measure of social organization there was more informative talk than in other nurseries, and explanations were more often given with commands. These nurseries also gave fewer negative commands. It should be noted, however, that there

TABLE 3

STAFF TALK AND NURSERY ORGANIZATION

	OBSERVATIONS IN WHICH DIFFERENT KINDS OF TALK OCCURRED, ALL GROUPS COMBINED (%)		CORRELATION OF CATEGORY OF STAFF TALK (MEAN %) PER GROUP WITH THE GROUP COMPOSITE ORGANIZATION SCORE	
	Mean	SD	r ($N = 13$)	p
Talk to other staff	8.1	3.11	.20	...
Talk to children	51.4	7.48	.31	...
Informative talk	13.8	4.72	.75	<.01
Explanation with commands	2.4	1.33	.57	<.05
Negative commands	9.4	3.02	—.61	<.05
Positive commands	11.9	2.7	.45	...
Displeasure and anger	1.3	0.90	—.07	...
Affection and pleasure	1.2	0.63	—.33	...
Supervisory	10.7	3.17	—.13	...
Choice offered to child ...	1.0	0.55	.20	...
Humor	1.6	1.07	.04	...
Staff remarks which child answers	21.78	10.88	.55	<.05

NOTE.—Mean number of observations per group = 383, SD 47.9.

TABLE 4

CHILD TALK AND NURSERY ORGANIZATION

	OBSERVATIONS IN WHICH DIFFERENT KINDS OF CHILD TALK OCCURRED, ALL GROUPS COMBINED (%)		CORRELATION OF CATEGORY OF CHILD TALK (MEAN %) PER GROUP WITH THE GROUP COMPOSITE ORGANIZATION SCORE	
	Mean	SD	r ($N = 13$)	p
Observations in which child spoke	36.0	5.83	.22	...
Child's remarks which staff answered	61.9	8.45	.62	<.05
Observations in which child talks to staff	18.0	4.59	.44	...
Observations in which child talks to self	7.0	3.94	.06	...
Observations in which child talks to other children	11.0	5.05	.47	...

NOTE.—Mean number of observations per group = 258, SD 60.6.

was no significant correlation between the proportion of occasions during which staff were observed to talk to the children and the composite organizational score of the nursery group.

Social organization and child talk.—Tables 3 and 4 show that the children were observed to talk much less frequently than the staff and to answer them much less often. Contrary to our prediction, no significant correlations were found between the amount the children talked to the staff and the composite score for the nursery group, but significant correlations were obtained between both the frequency with which children replied to staff and the frequency with which staff answered children, on the one hand, and the organizational score, on the other.

Frequency of response to different types of staff talk.—Children answered "informative" remarks by the staff significantly more often than "supervisory" remarks—35% informative remarks answered, 20% supervisory remarks, $\chi^2(1) = 33.84$, $p < .001$. Negative control remarks were only answered on 11.8% of occasions, and positive control, on 15% of occasions.

Staff sentence structure related to other variables.—During the 5-second observations of staff talk, the first remark made, which may have extended beyond this period, was recorded verbatim. Significant product-moment correlations were found between the mean sentence length of the staff and the composite score of the nursery, $r = .64$, $p < .02$, $N = 13$; the mean sentence length and the Reynell comprehension score of the children in the nursery, $r = .57$, $p < .05$, $N = 13$; the percentage of complex sentences with subordinate clauses, and the composite score of the nursery, $r = .72$, $p < .01$, $N = 13$; and the percentage of complex sentences and the Reynell comprehension score of the nursery, $r = .62$, $p < .02$, $N = 13$. Since the most frequent category of talk was commands, and explanations were rarely offered (Table 3), most staff talk had a very simple structure. Overall mean sentence length was 4.75 (SD 0.57, range 3.72-5.50); the overall mean percentage of complex sentences used was 5.95 (SD 3.16, range 0.96-12.9).

Staff and child talk related to age of children.—Since the mean age of children in nursery groups differed, it was considered important to determine how far the quality and quantity of talk was affected by the age of the child addressed. There was no overall relationship between the age of the child and the amount of talk addressed to him, but the youngest children were addressed less often; there was a significant increase in percentage of talk to children up to, but not beyond, the age of 3, slope $= 0.49$, SE 0.14, $t(30) = 3.62$, $p < .01$. Significant regressions of staff talk on age were found for percentage of informative talk, which increased significantly with the age of the child addressed, slope $= 0.03$, SE 0.01, $t\,(48) = 3.31$, $p < .01$, and percentage of talk by the child to other children, which increased significantly with the age of the child speaking, slope $= 0.37$, SE 0.10, $t\,(40) = 3.55$, $p < .01$.

Psychological test results.—Table 5 shows that these residential nursery children were not retarded. As described above, the Reynell standard scores were converted to give a mean of 100, and a standard deviation of 10. Thus Reynell standard scores of 1.0 and —1.0 became 110 and 90, respectively. There was a tendency for the older children to obtain higher scores on the Reynell Verbal Comprehension Scale, although not on the other tests (product-moment correlation age of child and Reynell comprehension score, $r = .26$, $p < .05$, $N = 85$), and this correlation remained, $r = .24$, after the composite score of the nursery had been partialed out. This tendency was caused by the significantly lower scores of the youngest children—mean Reynell comprehension score of children aged 2.0-2.5 years $= 98.07$, SD 8.6, $N = 14$; 2.55-4.95 years $= 106.68$, SD 8.7, $N = 71$, $t\,(84) = 2.86$, $p < .01$. Differences in test scores between the sexes were very small and not significant. There was no significant difference between the language scores of white children and those of children of mixed or West Indian parentage, but the mean Minnesota nonverbal score of the latter group was significantly higher.

Social organization and test results.—As predicted, there was a significant correlation between the mean Reynell comprehension score of the nursery group and its composite score, $r = .71$, $p < .01$, $N = 13$, but not between the mean Minnesota nonverbal score of the nursery group and its composite score, $r = .36$, $N = 13$. Table 5 shows that the difference between the mean Reynell comprehension score of the nurseries is not only significant but large. If the nurseries are divided into three, according to whether their composite score is within 1 SD below the mean, then the difference between the mean score of the children in the "best" nurseries and the "worst" nurseries is 1.5 SD. There was no significant correlation between the mean Reynell expression score and the composite score, $r = .35$, $N = 13$, but an F test, with more degrees of freedom, showed significantly lower expression scores for the children in the "worst" nurseries, $F\,(2,78) = 4.27$, $p < .05$ (table 5).

Test scores and observational data.—Table 6 shows that, as predicted, there were significant correlations between the mean Reynell comprehension score of the nursery group and the frequency of "informative" staff talk, staff "social" activity, the frequency with which staff answered the children's remarks, and the amount of play in which the child was actively rather than passively involved.

TABLE 5

TEST SCORES OF 85 RESIDENTIAL NURSERY CHILDREN

	REYNELL COMPREHENSION			REYNELL EXPRESSION			MINNESOTA NONVERBAL		
	N	Mean	SD	N	Mean	SD	N	Mean	SD
All nursery children	85	104.6	9.7	85	98.5	9.7	54	104.9	9.6
Girls	30	104.1	8.1	30	98.3	7.4	17	104.5	9.7
Boys	55	104.8	10.6	55	98.7	10.9	37	105.1	9.8
White children	39	102.6	10.0	39	98.5	11.2	24	101.3	11.1
Children of mixed or West Indian parentage	46	106.3	9.4	46	98.6	8.5	30	107.7	7.4
	$t = 1.70$, N.S.			$t = 0.02$, N.S.			$t = 2.51$, $p < .02$		
Children in groups with composite score more than 1 SD above mean	9	114.9	6.2	9	100.0	10.6	7	106.7	8.4
Children in groups with composite score within 1 SD of mean	43	104.7	8.7	43	100.7	9.1	29	105.2	10.6
Children in groups with composite score more than 1 SD below mean	27	99.4	9.2	27	94.1	9.6	15	100.6	5.9
	$F(2,78) = 11.08$, $p < .001$			$F(2,78) = 4.27$, $p < .05$			$F(2,50) = 1.58$, N.S.		

NOTE.—In this comparison six children in "village" nurseries where the composite score of the cottage was unknown were excluded.

TABLE 6

CORRELATIONS BETWEEN OBSERVED AMOUNTS OF STAFF BEHAVIOR PER GROUP
AND MEAN REYNELL SCORES OF EACH GROUP

CATEGORY OF STAFF BEHAVIOR	CORRELATION WITH COMPREHENSION SCORE		CORRELATION WITH EXPRESSION SCORE
	r	p	r
Informative staff talk	.81	<.001	.07
Staff answer children	.77	<.01	.35
"Social" activity by staff	.62	<.05	.39
Play with staff in which child is active	.68	<.02	.01
Explanation with commands	.13	...	—.18
Talk by staff to children	.42	...	—.08

NOTE.—$N = 13$.

There was, however, no significant correlation between the frequency with which explanations were given with commands and the Reynell comprehension score. As predicted, there were no significant correlations between the frequency of staff talk to the children and any of the test scores. It was considered possible that such a relationship existed but was masked by differences in staff-child ratio, since in some nurseries the same output of talk by the staff had to be shared among more children. A cumulative observed staff-child ratio for each nursery was calculated from the information recorded with each observation of the number of staff and children in the room. The percentage of staff talk to the children for each nursery was then weighted by this staff-child ratio, but the correlation with the mean Reynell comprehension score of the group remained nonsignificant, $r = 0.30$, $N = 13$. There was also a significant correlation between the individual Reynell comprehension scores of the children and the frequency with which informative talk was directed at them, $r = .51$, $p < .001$, $N = 46$, but not between these individual test scores and the frequency with which the child was spoken to, $r = .19$, $N = 46$. Against prediction there were no significant correlations between the mean Reynell expression scores of the nursery group and any of the observation data, except for a correlation between the mean expression score of the nursery groups and the frequency with which the children in the group were observed to talk, $r = .69$, $p < .01$, $N = 13$. As predicted, there were no significant correlations between the mean Minnesota non-verbal scores of the nursery groups and any of the observation data.

Effects of variation in numbers of staff and children present on staff be-

havior.—Although, as explained above, the effect on staff behavior of differences between nurseries in staff ratio could not be examined separately, since a high staff ratio tended to be associated with high autonomy, our data allowed us to look at the behavior of staff when different numbers of children were present. It was expected that on occasions when the staff-child ratio was high—for instance, because extra staff were on duty or some children had been taken out—the staff would talk to and play with the children more, while on occasions when it was low —for instance, because of staff illness—the reverse process would occur. In order to standardize the comparison, only play periods were considered, and one nursery where there were never fewer than three children present was excluded. Comparisons were made between staff talk and behavior when one staff was present with one to two children, three to six children, and seven or more children. There were no significant differences in the amount of staff "informative" talk, "social" activity, or percentage of talk to the children as the number of children present increased, and this was equally true of the behavior of two staff present with one to two, three to six, and seven or more children. The nurses appeared to have a style of responding to the children, influenced perhaps by their conception of their role, which was not much affected by the number of children present. However, an interesting finding emerges if one compares the behavior of staff when the number of children is constant but when either one or two staff are present.

Table 7 shows that the presence of two staff by no means doubles the amount of stimulation; situations A and D represent the same staff-child ratio, but in Situation A, when only one nurse is on duty, the children get much more staff attention. There are two reasons for this: first, when two staff were together they often talked to each other rather than to the children; second, because in all the nurseries there was a marked staff hierarchy, one of the two staff was always understood to be in charge, and the staff member not in charge tended to interact with the children much less (see next section).

Effect of differing roles on staff behavior.—Besides each observation a note was made of whether the staff member observed was in charge of the children at the time. There was a marked staff hierarchy in all the nurseries, including those with high autonomy, often expressed by differences in uniform and privileges; and it was always clearly understood who was in command. First-year students had a higher status than assistants but were subordinate to second-year students; trained nurses with two years experience were senior to newly certificated trained nurses. It was therefore possible to make two sets of staff comparisons, between

TABLE 7

STAFF BEHAVIOR, AS PERCENTAGE OF OBSERVATIONS, WITH VARYING NUMBERS
OF STAFF AND CHILDREN PRESENT

	Mean	SD
A. One staff, one or two children present:		
"Social" activity	28.2	19.4
Talk to children	64.9	9.3
Informative talk	18.2	3.5
B. One staff, three to six children present:		
"Social" activity	26.8	20.0
Talk to children	60.1	12.5
Informative talk	19.1	5.1
C. Two staff, one or two children present:		
"Social" activity	12.8	11.8
Talk to children	39.7	9.2
Informative talk	13.0	11.8
D. Two staff, three to six children present:		
"Social" activity	16.6	11.5
Talk to children	41.0	9.4
Informative talk	9.7	6.4

trained and untrained staff and between staff in charge and not in charge
(students or assistants, usually not in charge, would take charge of the
children when trained staff were off duty or merely out of the room).

Overall, trained staff talked to the children significantly more often
than untrained, $\chi^2(1) = 58.04$; $p < .001$; but there was no significant
difference between the frequency of talk of trained staff in charge and
untrained staff in charge. Regardless of training, whoever was in charge
talked more (percentage of talk: staff in charge, 56%; not in charge,
29%; $\chi^2(1) = 2.314$, $p < .001$); used more informative talk (staff in
charge, 15%; not in charge, 6%; $\chi^2(1) = 52.34$, $p < .001$); and played
more with the children (social activity: staff in charge, 17%; not in
charge, 10%; $\chi^2(1) = 43.37$, $p < .001$). The only significant difference
between the behavior of trained and untrained staff in charge was a
slight tendency for the untrained staff to play more with the children
and allow them to be more active (percentage of social activity: trained
staff in charge, 16.3%; untrained, 18.6%; $\chi^2(1) = 4.93$; $p < .05$; percentage of "social active" trained staff in charge, 2.6%; untrained in
charge, 3.6%; $\chi^2(1) = 5.59$, $p < .025$).

Effect of social organization on behavior of staff playing different roles.
—The composite score of the nursery group was correlated with the
observed talk and behavior of staff in various roles. Only the trained
staff and the staff in charge were greatly affected by the organization of

the nursery; there were no significant correlations between the composite score and the behavior of staff not in charge, except that the lower the composite score, that is, the "worse" the nursery, the more negative commands were used by staff not in charge, $r = -.76$, $p < .01$, $N = 13$.

Social class background and other characteristics of staff and children in different nurseries.—There is no reason to believe that children were selectively placed in the nurseries, and there was no significant difference between the social class distribution of the mothers of the children in the three "best" and the three "worst" nurseries. The staff in all the nurseries were studying for, or had achiveed, the same diploma (N.N.E.B.). All were the daughters of skilled workers or small shopkeepers, and all had left school at the age of 15 or 16 with from zero to four "O" levels. There was no significant correlation between the number of "O" levels obtained by the staff and the composite score of the nursery, $r = -.34$, $N = 13$. However, there was a significant tendency for the "better" nurseries to be staffed by more experienced nurses —composite score of group and years of experience of nurse in charge, $r = .70$, $p < .01$, $N = 13$. This tendency appeared to be related to the autonomy of the group; only inexperienced staff would accept a very low level of autonomy, while only experienced staff would be given the responsibility of an autonomous group.

DISCUSSION

Our evidence strongly suggests that intellectual retardation is not a necessary consequence of institutional placement; even in our "worst" nurseries the mean test scores were all near average, while in the "best" nurseries the children's language comprehension scores were considerably above average. Since many of the children were of lower-working-class parentage, it seems likely that intellectually they had in fact benefited from their institutional upbringing.

There are probably two reasons why the retardation reported elsewhere was not found. First, the children in this study were all healthy and without a history of premature or difficult delivery; most had been admitted as infants and had not suffered from the early neglect or frequent environmental shifts of many children who come into residential care.

Second, not only were the physical care and the provision of books and play equipment excellent in these nurseries, but the organization of the children into smaller mixed age groups with a relatively high staff ratio and few household duties for the staff resulted in a high frequency of adult talk. The percentage of observation periods in which the observed staff spoke to a child ranged in different nurseries from 36.8% to 61.5%. No comparable study has been made in private families, but pilot observations suggest that the frequency of maternal talk is usually of a much lower order. One reason for this difference is probably that in private families children are not always with their mothers—they may play in another room or out of doors. In the residential nurseries, however, children are not allowed to be out of sight of the staff. Further, while the mother at home tends to divide her attention among a variety of duties—as cook, cleaner, wife, hostess, friend, as well as mother—the nurse is expected to confine her attention mainly to child care.

Whatever the quality of staff talk, then, the large quantity observed in all the nurseries together with daily reading sessions appears sufficient to promote an average level of language development. If the quantity of staff talk falls significantly below this level, the children's language development may suffer: we found a lower mean language comprehension score in the youngest group tested, who were talked to significantly less than the older children. Children under 2 were spoken to even less, and an earlier study showed slight language retardation in these children at 24 months (Tizard & Joseph 1970).

Although the frequency of staff talk was sufficient in all the nurseries to promote average language development, the level of development was related to the quality of staff talk. Very significant correlations were found between both the frequency of "informative" staff talk and the frequency with which the staff answered the children, and the language comprehension scores of the children. Since there was no evidence that children were selectively placed, and since there were no significant differences between the mean nonverbal scores of the nurseries, this finding would seem to be strong evidence of the effect of differing verbal environments on language development, uncontaminated by genetic influences. It should be noted that the range of verbal quality we observed was relatively narrow: no nurse talked like a graduate mother, the longest staff mean sentence length per nursery was 5.50 words, and explanations were rare even in the "best" nurseries. This fact may account for the failure to find a significant correlation between language comprehension scores and the frequency of explanations.

In this study we were able to show not only that the children's language scores were related to differences in their verbal environment but also that both these factors were related to differences in the way in which the nurseries were organized. Unfortunately it was not possible to isolate the effect of any one organizational variable. Thus, in the nurseries where the children's comprehension scores were highest, and the most "informative" staff talk was heard, not only were the nursery groups more autonomous, but the staff tended to be more experienced; and staff stability, staff-child ratio, and the mean age of the children all tended to be higher.

However, a variety of evidence suggests that the crucial variable in determining the quality of staff behavior was the social relationship obtaining at any given time among the staff and between staff and children. Thus, within any given setting when the staff-ratio improved, perhaps because some children were away, the staff did not change their style of response to the children or begin to play with them or talk to them more often. But their style of response did dramatically change according to whether at the time of observation they were in charge of the children. When in charge, the behavior of trained and untrained staff could not be distinguished, except for a slight advantage to the untrained staff. When not in charge, both the quality and quantity of their behavior fell significantly.

Moreover, the differences between the way in which the nurseries were organized affected all the staff in charge, whether trained or not, in the same way. Thus, in the high-autonomy groups all staff in charge tended to play and converse with the children more than did the staff in charge of low-autonomy groups. However, staff not in charge behaved very similarly in every nursery. All these data suggest that staff autonomy, whether momentary or long-range, has a decisive effect on staff behavior; if assigned a limited role, staff tend to behave in a limited way.

Contrary to prediction, we did not find any relationship between the children's ability to use language (Reynell expression scores) and the quality of the verbal environment; moreover, the correlation with the composite organizational score of the nursery was not large. This negative finding may have been due to the greater unreliability of the expression scores, which depend on the amount of talk which the child is willing to produce in the test situation, or to the fact that in some respects the staff-child relationship was similar in all the nurseries. It will have been noted (Tables 3, 4) that the pattern of talk in the nurseries studied appears unlike that of a middle-class family. The adults talked more and the children less than would have been expected, while the frequency of affect-laden speech and choices offered to the child appear very low. Initiation of both speech and action tended to come from the staff, and even in the "best" nurseries the children seemed uncommunicative. We can only speculate about the reasons for this. Although the frequency with which the staff answered children's talk was fairly high (Table 4), the type of response—for example, "that's nice"—probably provided little reinforcement. In all the nurseries close relationships between staff and child were actively discouraged (Tizard & Tizard 1971); in institutions where this is not the case a different pattern of communications might be expected.

In conclusion, we would argue that in view of the wide variety of institutional settings, and the evidence from this and earlier studies (e.g., King, Raynes, & Tizard 1971) of their varying effects on development, it is perhaps time to abandon the concept of the "institution" as a factor in development, and to replace it with a consideration of the effects of different institutional regimens on different aspects of development.

REFERENCES

BURLINGHAM, D. T. & FREUD, A.: *Infants Without Families.* New York: International Universities Press, 1944.

GOLDFARB, W.: Effects of psychological deprivation in infancy and subsequent stimulation. *American Journal of Psychiatry,* 1945, 102, 18-33.

KELLMER PRINGLE, M. L., & BOSSIO, V. A study of deprived children. *Vita Humana,* 1958, 1, 142-170.

KING, R., RAYNES, N., & TIZARD, J.: *Patterns of Residential Care: Sociological Studies in Institutions for Handicapped Children.* London: Routledge & Kegan Paul, 1971.

REYNELL, J.: *Reynell Developmental Language Scales.* Slough, Buckinghamshire: National Foundation for Educational Research, 1969.

TIZARD, B. & JOSEPH, A.: Cognitive development of young children in residential care. *Journal of Child Psychology and Psychiatry,* 1970, 11, 177-186.

TIZARD, J.: The role of social institutions in the causation, prevention and alleviation of mental retardation. In H. C. Haywood (Ed.): *Social-Cultural Aspects of Mental Retardation.* New York: Appleton-Century-Crofts, 1970.

TIZARD, J. & TIZARD, B.: The social development of two-year-old children in residential nurseries. In H. R. Schaffer (Ed.): *The Origins of Human Social Relations.* New York: Academic, 1971.

43

OUTERDIRECTEDNESS AND IMITATIVE BEHAVIOR OF INSTITUTIONALIZED AND NONINSTITUTIONALIZED YOUNGER AND OLDER CHILDREN

Edward Zigler

Yale University

and

Regina Yando

Harvard University and Fernald State School

Four groups of 48 children, institutionalized and noninstitutionalized younger and older children of normal intelligence, were administered a measure of outerdirectedness. The task, which was designed to elicit imitative behavior, allowed for comparison of performance under conditions where (a) the task was presented as a problem or no problem, and (b) cues were provided by an adult or by a machine. Younger children were found to be more imitative than older children. More imitation was found in the machine-cue than in the adult-cue condition. Younger noninstitutionalized children were found to be more imitative than younger institutionalized children, but only if the task

Reprinted from CHILD DEVELOPMENT, 1972, 43, pp. 413-425. © 1972 by the Society for Research and Child Development, Inc. All rights reserved.

did not require the solution of a problem. The relationship of these findings to reinforcement and contiguity-mediational theories of imitation was discussed.

Outerdirectedness has been defined by Zigler and his colleagues (Achenbach & Zigler 1968; Balla, Styfco, & Zigler 1971; Sanders, Zigler, & Butterfield 1968; Turnure & Zigler 1964; Yando & Zigler 1971) as a style of problem solving characterized by reliance on concrete situational cues rather than by active attempts to deduce abstract relationships. The extent to which a person manifests outerdirectedness is believed to depend both on his level of cognitive development and on his experience of success or failure in the employment of his cognitive resources. Since outerdirectedness is generally more conducive to successful problem solving than is reliance on poorly developed cognitive abilities, the lower the cognitive level of a person the more outerdirected he should be. However, the degree of outerdirectedness evidenced by a person is also influenced by his willingness to employ his cognitive abilities, and such willingness should depend in part on that person's history of success and failure in the use of his abilities.

It is the success-failure dimension of the outerdirectedness formulation that has been most actively tested. Studies (Achenbach & Zigler 1968; Balla et al. 1971; Sanders et al. 1968; Turnure & Zigler 1964; Yando & Zigler 1971) have repeatedly confirmed the prediction that a child with a history of intellectual failure is more outerdirected than a child at the same level of cognitive development who has not experienced such failure. Investigatory efforts concerning the general developmental aspect of outerdirectedness, however, have been limited, and findings (Achenbach & Zigler 1968; Balla et al. 1971; Yando & Zigler 1971) have been inconsistent in regard to the prediction that children who have attained higher levels of cognitive development are less dependent on concrete external cues than are children at lower cognitive levels.

A recent study (Yando & Zigler 1971) has indicated that life experiences other than a child's history of intellectual success or failure influence his willingness to employ cues dispensed by adults. In this study, non-institutionalized children of average intellect were found to utilize cues provided by an adult significantly more than did institutionalized children of average intellect. On the basis of previous findings from the literature concerned with the motivational dynamics of social deprivation (Harter & Zigler 1968; Irons & Zigler 1969; Shallenberger & Zigler 1961; Zigler 1963; Zigler, Balla, & Butterfield 1968; Zigler & Williams 1963), Yando and Zigler (1971) argued that socially deprived children of average intellect have experienced such negative treatment by adults that they become suspicious of adults and the cues they provide.

A major goal of the present study was to compare the performance of socially deprived (i.e., institutionalized) and nondeprived children of average intellect on a measure *presented* as: (a) a task in which any of the child's responses were acceptable, or (b) a task having only a single correct solution (but which was in fact insoluble). The expectation was that on the "nonproblem" task, where the child could choose whether he would or would not use the cues provided by the adult, deprived children, due to their wariness of adults, would be less imitative than nondeprived children. However, given the formulation that outerdirectedness essentially reflects a child's effort to solve problems, one would expect nondeprived children to manifest a similar degree of outerdirectedness on an insoluble task presented as a problem having numerous alternatives but only a single solution. In such a situation, even the child reluctant to use cues provided by an adult has little choice but to do so.

In order to provide additional data relevant to the hypothesis that outerdirectedness decreases with cognitive development, children of two MA levels were employed. In addition, the salience for children of cues provided by an adult was compared with that of machine-dispensed cues. Although Turnure and Zigler (1964) suggested that cues provided by human models may be more salient to an outerdirected child than are nonhuman cues, studies (Balla et al. 1971; Sanders et al. 1968; Yando & Zigler 1971) which have investigated this prediction have failed to verify it.

METHOD

Subjects

A total of 192 predominately white children,* 96 boys and 96 girls, served as Ss. The population consisted of four equal groups ($N = 48$) of children: lower MA, younger CA, institutionalized; lower MA, younger CA, noninstitutionalized; higher MA, older CA, institutionalized; and higher MA, older CA, noninstitutionalized. No child in the sample was retarded (i.e., IQ below 85) or showed evidence of gross motor, sensory, or psychotic disturbances.

The noninstitutionalized population was obtained from an elementary

---

* The sample included five black children, four of whom were institutionalized.

TABLE 1

MEAN MA, CA, AND IQ FOR EACH GROUP OF SUBJECTS

GROUP	N	MA (IN YEARS) $\overline{X}$	SD	CA (IN YEARS) $\overline{X}$	SD	IQ $\overline{X}$	SD
Younger subjects:							
Noninstitutionalized:							
Human–problem	12	7.08	1.05	5.82	0.14	113	12.57
Human–no-problem ...	12	7.01	1.01	5.90	0.28	112	11.70
Nonhuman–problem ...	12	7.19	1.03	6.03	0.24	114	12.53
Nonhuman–no-problem	12	7.16	1.11	5.94	0.22	114	12.61
Institutionalized:							
Human–problem	12	7.18	1.01	7.11	0.94	100	9.17
Human–no-problem ...	12	6.99	0.97	7.52	1.20	95	5.92
Nonhuman–problem ...	12	7.28	1.04	7.58	1.26	97	9.38
Nonhuman–no-problem	12	7.07	1.18	7.63	1.64	94	7.00
Older subjects:							
Noninstitutionalized:							
Human–problem	12	11.61	1.29	9.63	0.51	121	14.32
Human–no-problem ...	12	11.71	1.50	9.59	0.44	120	12.37
Nonhuman–problem ...	12	11.79	1.32	9.86	0.52	120	13.23
Nonhuman–no-problem	12	11.60	1.11	9.81	0.44	118	11.45
Institutionalized:							
Human–problem	12	11.53	1.34	11.39	0.89	99	8.43
Human–no-problem ...	12	11.48	1.45	10.94	1.51	104	12.00
Nonhuman–problem ...	12	11.83	1.43	11.46	1.95	104	12.00
Nonhuman–no-problem .:..........	12	11.55	1.16	12.08	0.81	96	8.77

school in a suburb of Boston, Massachusetts. The institutionalized (socially deprived) population was selected from 11 state and private residential child-care facilities in Massachusetts, Rhode Island, and New Hampshire. All institutionalized children had been removed from their homes for such reasons as neglect, abandonment, divorce, or emotional problems of the parents. Nonuniformity of record keeping and such factors as frequent placement and removal from foster homes made it impossible to control for length of institutionalization.

Subjects were matched by MA and sex for the four experimental conditions at each of the two MA levels. The mean CA, MA, and IQ of each group are presented in Table 1. Children in the various institutions were randomly assigned to each condition. Group IQ scores (Kuhlmann-Anderson) were acquired from the school records for the noninstitutionalized older children. For the younger noninstitutionalized and some institutionalized children, IQ scores were obtained from the Peabody Picture Vocabulary Test Form B, administered by a trained E prior to experimental testing. For the remainder of the institutionalized children, Stanford-Binet Form L-M or WISC IQ scores were obtained from the institutional records.

Apparatus

Materials for the imitation task consisted of marbles of four colors and two identical "marble holders," one used by S and one used either by the adult (human condition) or in conjunction with a mechanical marble dispenser (nonhuman condition). The marble holders were inverted wooden bowls with wide rims approximately 30 cm in diameter, divided into quadrants, with each quadrant painted a different color (purple, gold, brown, and orange). A battery-operated doorbell, used only in the problem condition, was placed inside the S's marble holder. A Gerbrand's Model A automatic candy dispenser was modified to release marbles. The dispenser was mounted on a 30 × 30 × 30-cm plywood box in such a manner as to ensure that the marbles dropped from the dispenser onto the center of the marble holder. Two switches, hidden from S's view, enabled E to control the dispenser and the doorbell. The red, blue, green, and yellow marbles were kept in separate compartments in two identical partitioned plastic boxes.

Procedure

Each S was tested individually by a trained E, a young female with teaching experience, who was unaware of the hypotheses being tested.

The imitation task consisted of 60 trials and was administered in four conditions: human-problem; human-no problem, nonhuman-problem; nonhuman-no problem. Subject's task was to show which color marble he liked to put with which color quadrant of his marble holder (no-problem conditions), or to solve the "problem" of which color marble belonged to a specific quadrant (problem conditions). Employing the other marble holder, E (human conditions) or the marble dispenser (nonhuman conditions) provided the cues which S could imitate.

Children were taken into the experimental room by E, who seated them on the floor in front of the apparatus. After introducing the task as a "color-go-together" game, E proceeded to ascertain whether or not each S knew the colors of the materials employed.

Human and nonhuman conditions.—In the human conditions, S was told that he could place any color marble he liked onto any of the four quadrants of his marble holder. Before S made his choice, however, E placed a marble onto her marble holder so that S might see "how some colors look together." Each trial of S was thus preceded by E placing a marble onto a quadrant of her marble holder. The marble remained on E's marble holder until S completed his trial. After S made his choice of both marble and quadrant, both E and S returned their marbles to their respective plastic marble boxes. The E followed a predetermined pattern of marble/marbleholder color placement. The pattern consisted of all possible color combinations randomized in four blocks of 16 trials (with four trials dropped from the last block).

In the nonhuman conditions, the procedure was the same with the exception that the marble dispenser dropped a marble onto the marble holder before S made his selection of marble and quadrant. The machine dropped marbles in such a way as to guarantee randomness in respect both to the color of the marble and to the quadrant onto which the marble fell. Prior to the first trial, E demonstrated how the machine worked. As S watched, E filled the dispenser with marbles and showed S that it cycled automatically, but did not explicitly reveal that she controlled the machine.

No-problem and problem conditions.—In the no-problem conditions, S was informed that he was being asked to play the game for no other reason than that E was interested in seeing what colors boys and girls liked to see "go together." The E, carefully refraining from either positive or negative comments, remained neutral throughout the trials and accepted whatever choices S made.

In the problem conditions, S was informed that his task was to discover which color marble went on which color quadrant. He was told that when he was right the bell in his marble holder would ring, and the bell was then demonstrated for him. Regardless of the S's selections, he was reinforced on the basis of a 33% randomized reinforcement schedule. In addition, each time the bell rang, E commented upon his performance with such statements as "good" or "that's right." Therefore, although S was led to believe there was a correct solution, there in fact was not. After the last trial, children in this condition were praised for their performance, being told among other things that they had done much better than other children who had played the game.

RESULTS

CA and IQ Analyses

It can be seen in Table 1 that, while all groups were matched on the MA variable, the institutionalized Ss were slightly older chronologically and had lower IQs than the noninstitutionalized Ss. Earlier findings (Yando & Zigler 1971), however, have revealed that CA effects, independent of MA, do not influence the degree of outerdirectedness. On the other hand, several studies (Achenbach & Zigler 1968; Turnure & Zigler 1964) have indicated that IQ is related to outerdirectedness, though it should be noted that these IQ-outerdirectedness relationships were obtained with groups differing much more widely on IQ than did the institutionalized and noninstitutionalized groups presented in Table 1.

In order to assess CA and IQ effects in the present study, Pearson product-moment correlations were obtained between these subject variables and the dependent variable. Since one would expect all of the younger Ss to be more outerdirected than all of the older Ss, separate correlational analyses were performed for each of these two MA groups (both of which included institutionalized and noninstitutionalized Ss). The older MA subject analysis revealed CA and IQ to be unrelated to the dependent variable. For younger MA subjects, IQ was also found to be unrelated to the dependent variable; however, CA was found to be significantly related to the measure of imitation ($r = -.21$, $p < .05$). Although this finding barely reached the .05 level of significance and was not supported by the remaining correlational data, an analysis of covariance was performed. A test of nonadditivity indicated that the regression coefficient between CA and the dependent variable was not significant ($b = .11$, $F < 1$).

Dependent-Variable Analyses

Imitation was measured by assigning one point for each trial on which the child both (a) chose the same color as that used by the E or dispensed by the machine, and (b) placed that marble on the same quadrant of the holder as did E or the machine (a maximum score of 60 possible). In order to assess the usefulness of the task as a measure of imitation, the mean imitation scores for all groups were compared with that level which could be anticipated by chance. The expectation was that at least one homogeneous group would show above chance-level imitation.* the performance of younger children across all conditions was in keeping with this expectation.

Since the means and variances of the imitation scores were correlated, the problem was corrected by performing all analyses on logarithmically

---

* According to a binomial model with $p = .0625$ and $N = 60$, raw score values of 6.50 and over are greater than would be likely by chance alone at the $p < .5$ level, whereas values of 8.00 or more reach the $p < .01$ level of significance.

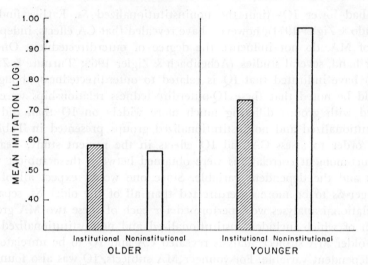

FIG. 1.—Mean log imitation scores for younger and older children

transformed scores. The log imitation scores were subjected to a $2 \times 2 \times 2 \times 2 \times 2$ (Institutionalization $\times$ MA $\times$ Type of Cue $\times$ Problem Condition $\times$ Sex) analysis of variance. Significant main effects were revealed for MA, $F(1,160) = 21.36$, $p < .001$, and type of cue, $F(1,160) = 6.95$, $p < .01$, indicating that younger children ($\bar{x} = .85$ log, 12.47 raw) imitated more than older children ($\bar{x} = .57$ log, 5.79 raw) and that all children imitated more in the presence of nonhuman cues ($X = .79$ log, 11.16 raw) than human cues ($\bar{x} = .63$ log, 7.10 raw).

Of the two-way interactions, only MA $\times$ Institutionalization, $F(1, 160) = 4.87$, $p < .05$, proved significant. As can be seen in Figure 1, whereas the performance of the older noninstitutionalized ($\bar{x} = .56$ log, 6.06 raw) and institutionalized ($\bar{x} = .58$ log, 5.52 raw) children was approximately the same, the noninstitutionalized younger children ($\bar{x} = .97$ log, 16.02 raw) imitated more than the institutionalized younger children ($\bar{x} = .73$ log, 8.92 raw). A Newman-Keuls comparison of the means revealed that noninstitutionalized younger children differed significantly ($p < .01$) from all other groups; no other differences proved significant. The only other significant finding was an MA $\times$ Institutionalization $\times$ Problem Condition interaction, $F(1,160) = 6.91$, $p < .01$, which is represented in Figure 2.

In order to assess further this interaction, separate 2×2 (MA $\times$ Institutionalization) analyses of variance were conducted for the problem

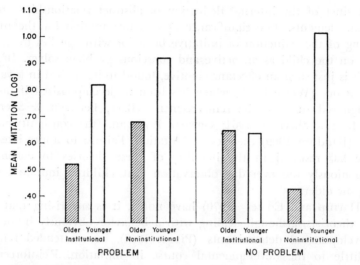

FIG. 2.—Mean log imitation scores for problem and no-problem groups

and no-problem data. The problem-condition analysis revealed only a main effect for MA, $F(1,92) = 8.97$, $p < .005$, indicating that younger children (institutionalized $\bar{x} = .82$ log, 11.42 raw; noninstitutionalized $\bar{x} = .92$ log, 15.13 raw) imitated more than older children (institutionalized $\bar{x} = .52$ log, 5.17 raw; noninstitutionalized $\bar{x} = .68$ log, 8.13 raw). The analysis of the no-problem groups revealed a main effect for MA, $F(1,92) = 12.42$, $p < .001$, and an MA × Institutionalization interaction, $F(1,92) = 12.96$, $p < .001$. A Newman-Keuls comparison of the means of the four no-problem groups indicated that younger noninstitutionalized children ($\bar{x} = 1.01$ log, 16.92 raw) imitated more than older noninstitutionalized ($\bar{x} = .43$ log, 4.00 raw), younger institutionalized ($\bar{x} = .64$ log, 6.42 raw), and older institutionalized ($\bar{x} = .65$ log, 5.88 raw) children at the .05 level of significance. None of the latter three groups differed significantly from each other.

DISCUSSION

Younger children proved to be more imitative than older children. This finding is consistent with the outerdirectedness formulation within which the child is viewed as intrinsically motivated to solve problems. As the chld develops and becomes more cognitively proficient, successful problem solving becomes less dependent upon cues from others and more the product of the internal deduction of abstract relationships among problem elements. The significance of this formulation for the understanding of the reduction of imitative behavior with age lies in its emphasis on the child as an active and conscious problem solver. In contrast, it is just such an effectance motive, found to be critical in a variety of behaviors (White 1959), which has been underemphasized if not totally ignored in both the reinforcement (Baer, Peterson, & Sherman 1967; Baer & Sherman 1964; Gewirtz 1971) and the contiguity-mediational (Bandura 1969) theories of imitation. Failure to appreciate this motive has resulted in the inability of these theories to encompass parsimoniously the everyday observation that children imitate less as they grow older.

As Hartup and Coates (1970) have noted, it is surprising that imitation theorists, although dealing with a behavior obviously influenced by developmental determinants (Piaget 1952), have attended remarkably little to the developmental course in imitation. Reinforcement theorists (Gewirtz 1971), while admitting that developmental factors could affect the "contents and limits" of imitation, nonetheless assert that developmental changes do not influence the basic modes of acquisition and maintenance of imitative responses. Imitative behavior, as viewed by these theorists, is simply a derivative case of instrumental conditioning.

Contiguity-mediational theorists (Bandura 1969), while constructing a highly differentiated theory of imitation supported by a number of empirical efforts, have been even less explicit about the effects of age, either chronological or mental, on imitation. Imitative learning, according to their view, depends on the "acquisition" by the observer of behaviors emitted by a model. "Acquisition," in turn, depends on a variety of attentional, symbolic, and other cognitive-mediational processes which improve with development. Contiguity-mediational theory therefore implicitly generates the prediction that, *with the incentive* for imitative responding held constant, imitation increases wth age. Such a prediction, however, is completely at variance with a major finding of the present study, namely, that with increasing age children imitate less.

The cause of this disparity between prediction and observation may lie in having neglected the child's motive for imitating. Contiguity-mediational theory has emphasized the unquestioned fact that developing attention, memory, and other cognitive processes progressively augment the growing child's ability to imitate. But while the ability to assimilate and reproduce behaviors emitted by a model is an important factor in the imitative process, the child's desire and need to imitate are much more important determinants of the extent to which he will display imitative behavior. Thus, by emphasizing motivational factors, the outer-directedness formulation is able to predict not only that younger children will in general be more imitative than older children, but also that individuals of any age will become more imitative when encountering ambiguous situations or problems beyond their cognitive ability (Britt 1971).

The outerdirectedness formulation offers additional explanatory advantage over other imitation theories in that it makes comprehensible the variability in imitation found among groups of children with varying social histories but of the same age. In the present study, as in an earlier study (Yando & Zigler 1971), younger noninstitutionalized children were found to be significantly more imitative than younger institutionalized children. It should be noted that the institutionalized children had all been removed from their families for such reasons as physical abuse and abandonment. It is therefore plausible to assume that the past experiences of the institutionalized children led them to view the E as a non-nurturant adult, whereas the past experiences of the noninstitutionalized children led them to view the E as a nurturant adult. If this assumption is correct, the finding of more imitation in noninstitutionalized than in institutionalized children is consistent with the finding of greater imitation by children of models with whom they had had previous nurturant interactions (Bandura & Huston 1961).

What remains at issue is *why* a model viewed as nurturant generates a higher frequency of imitation than does a model viewed as nonnurturant. An explanation advanced by Bandura (1969) holds that nurturant models enhance "observational learning by eliciting and maintaining strong attending behavior" (pp. 136-137). Such an explanation, however, appears inadequate in view of the finding (Yando & Zigler 1971) that institutionalized children of normal intellect actively avoided utilizing the cues provided by an adult. Such avoidance would necessitate that the child attend closely both to the model and to the cue being offered. The decision not to imitate would, therefore, appear to have little to do with the child's attentional processes but would, rather, turn upon the child's attitude toward the adult and the cues he provided. Considerable evidence now exists to show that institutionalized children are highly suspicious of adults (Zigler, in press) as a result of the negative treatment they have received from them. It is hypothesized that this suspiciousness (actually verbalized by children in the earlier study with such statements as "You're trying to fool me") results in a reduction in reliance on cues provided by adults. It should be noted that in both the present and in the earlier study (Yando & Zigler 1971) a difference in imitation across conditions was found only between the younger institutionalized and noninstitutionalized children. The failure to find such a difference between the two older groups is probably due to the general tendency of all older children not to imitate.

Further evidence that the child's motivation to solve problems is an important determinant of imitation was contained in the findings related to the problem—no-problem condition. Consistent with the expectation generated by the outerdirectedness formulation, the behavior of institutionalized and noninstitutionalized children was more similar in the problem than in the no-problem condition. If the task was not presented to the child as a problem, the younger noninstitutionalized child imitated significantly more than the younger institutionalized and the older institutionalized and noninstitutionalized groups. However, when children were presented with an insoluble problem-solving task, no institutional effect was found; the only significant effect was that all younger children imitated more than all older children. It thus appeared that younger institutionalized children overcome their reluctance to utilize adult cues when confronted with a problem that cannot be solved by employing their own intellectual resources. As has been found with retarded children in such situations (Yando & Zigler 1971), whatever the institutionalized child's attitude toward adults might be, in a difficult problem situation he has little choice but to utilize whatever cues are available.

The present study, then, generates the conclusion that the amount of imitation in which a child engages is complexly determined by (a) the cognitive level of the child, (b) his attitude toward the adult who is providing cues which may be imitated, and (c) the nature of the task that confronts him.

Finally, the study lends no support to the prediction that the human cue situation produces more imitation than the nonhuman situation. As in an earlier study (Yando & Zigler 1971), precisely the opposite was found. It is to be noted that there may be a considerable difference between the experimental designation of conditions as "human" and "nonhuman" and the phenomenological experience of a child in these conditions. In the nonhuman condition, the adult was continuously present, sat next to the apparatus which emitted the "nonhuman" cues, and possibly led the child to perceive these cues as under the control of the E and therefore "human." If this analysis is correct, then the generally higher imitation in the nonhuman condition could be ascribed to the novelty and attention-drawing power of the apparatus employed in that condition. However, one other hypothesis must be entertained. Given the technological emphasis of our current era, children may believe that cues emitted by machines are less fallible and therefore more trustworthy guides to action than those emitted by adults.

REFERENCES

ACHENBACH, T. & ZIGLER, E.: Cue learning and problem learning strategies in normal and retarded children. *Child Development*, 1968, 39, 827-848.

BAER, D. M., PETERSON, R. F., & SHERMAN, J. A.: The development of imitation by reinforcing behavioral similarity to a model. *Journal of the Experimental Analysis of Behavior*, 1967, 10, 405-416.

BAER, D. M. & SHERMAN, J. A.: Reinforcement control of generalized imitation in young children. *Journal of Experimental Child Psychology*, 1964, 1, 37-49.

BALLA, D., STYFCO, S. J., & ZIGLER, E.: Use of the opposition concept and outer-directedness in normal, familial retarded, and organic retarded children. *American Journal of Mental Deficiency*, 1971, 75, 663-680.

BANDURA, A.: *Principles of Behavior Modification*. New York: Holt, Rinehart, & Winston, 1969.

BANDURA, A. & HUSTON, A. C.: Identification as a process of incidental learning. *Journal of Abnormal and Social Psychology*, 1961, 63, 311-318.

BRITT, D. W.: Effects of probability of reinforcement and social stimulus consistency on imitation. *Journal of Personality and Social Psychology*, 1971, 18, 189-200.

GEWIRTZ, J. L.: Conditional responding as a paradigm for observation, imitative learning and vicarious-reinforcement. In H. W. Reese (Ed.): *Advances in Child Development and Behavior*. Vol. 6. New York: Academic, 1971, in press.

HARTER, S. & ZIGLER, E.: The effectiveness of adult and peer reinforcement on the performance of institutionalized and noninstitutionalized retardates. *Journal of Abnormal Psychology*, 1968, 73, 144-149.

HARTUP, W. W. & COATES, B.: The role of imitation in childhood socialization. In R. A. Hoppe, G. A. Milton, & E. C. Simmel (Eds.): *Early Experiences and the Processes of Socialization*. New York: Academic, 1970. Pp. 109-142.

IRONS, N. & ZIGLER, E.: Children's responsiveness to social reinforcement as a function of short-term preliminary social interactions and long-term social deprivation. *Developmental Psychology*, 1969, 1, 402-409.

PIAGET, J.: *Play, Dreams, and Imitation in Childhood*. New York: Norton, 1952.

SANDERS, B., ZIGLER, E., & BUTTERFIELD, E. C.: Outerdirectedness in the discrimination learning of normal and mentally retarded children. *Journal of Abnormal Psychology*, 1968, 73, 368-375.

SHALLENBERGER, P. & ZIGLER, E.: Rigidity, negative reaction tendencies, and cosatiation effects in normal and feebleminded children. *Journal of Abnormal and Social Psychology*, 1961, 63, 20-26.

TURNURE, J. E. & ZIGLER, E.: Outerdirectedness in the problem-solving of normal and retarded children. *Journal of Abnormal and Social Psychology*, 1964, 69, 427-436.

WHITE, R. W.: Motivation reconsidered: The concept of competence. *Psychological Review*, 1959, 66, 297-333.

YANDO, R., & ZIGLER, E. Outerdirectedness in the problem-solving of institutionalized and noninstitutionalized normal and retarded children. *Developmental Psychology*, 1971, 4, 277-288.

ZIGLER, E.: Rigidity and social reinforcement effects in the performance of institutionalized and noninstitutionalized normal and retarded children. *Journal of Personality*, 1963, 31, 258-269.

ZIGLER, E.: The retarded child as a whole person. In H. Adams & W. K. Boardman III (Eds.): *Advances in Experimental Clinical Psychology.* Vol. 1. New York: Pergamon, in press.

ZIGLER, E., BALLA, D., & BUTTERFIELD, E.: A longitudinal investigation of the relationship between preinstitutional social deprivation and social motivation in institutionalized retardates. *Journal of Personality and Social Psychology,* 1968, 10, 437-445.

ZIGLER, E. & WILLIAMS, J.: Institutionalization and effectiveness of social reinforcement: a three year follow-up study. *Journal of Abnormal and Social Psychology,* 1963, 66, 197-205.

This work was supported by research grant HD-MH-03008, the Gunnar Dybwad Award of the National Association for Retarded Children, and by grant 12-HSP-096. The authors wish to express their appreciation to the administration and staff of the following schools for their cooperation: Brook Farm, West Roxbury, Massachusetts; the Children's Center, Providence, Rhode Island; Children's Study Home, Springfield, Massachusetts; Lt. Joseph P. Kennedy Memorial School, Hyde Park, Massachusetts; New England Home for Little Wanderers, Jamaica Plain, Massachusetts; Saint Aloysius Home, Greenville, Rhode Island; Saint Charles Children's Home, Rochester, New Hampshire; Saint Vincent's Home, Fall River, Massachusetts; Manchester Children's Home, Manchester, New Hampshire; Chase Home for Children, Portsmouth, New Hampshire; Home for Italian Children, Jamaica Plain, Massachusetts; Williams School, Newton, Massachusetts. The authors especially wish to thank Susan Litzinger for running the subjects and David Blocker, Martin Grosse, Abby Sheldon, and Sylvia Goldstein for assistance with various aspects of this study. The authors are also indebted to David Balla and Susan Harter for their critical reading of an earlier version of this article. Requests for reprints should be sent to Edward Zigler, Department of Psychology, 333 Cedar Street, Yale University, New Haven, Connecticut 06510.

ANNUAL PROGRESS IN CHILD PSYCHIATRY
AND CHILD DEVELOPMENT

CONTENTS—Volume 1: 1968

743

744

ANNUAL PROGRESS IN CHILD PSYCHIATRY AND CHILD DEVELOPMENT

CONTENTS—Volume 2: 1969

745

746

ANNUAL PROGRESS IN CHILD PSYCHIATRY
AND CHILD DEVELOPMENT

CONTENTS—Volume 3: 1970

747

748

749

CONTENTS—Volume 4: 1971

751

ANNUAL PROGRESS IN CHILD PSYCHIATRY
AND CHILD DEVELOPMENT

CONTENTS—Volume 5 : 1972

XI. TREATMENT

XII. DELIVERY OF SERVICES